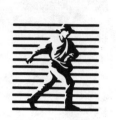

Staying Healthy in a Risky Environment: The New York University Medical Center Family Guide

Arthur C. Upton, M.D.
Medical Editor

Eden Graber, M.S.
Editor

Lewis Goldfrank, M.D.   Robert Nadig, M.D.
Anthony Grieco, M.D.   Philip Tierno, Jr., Ph.D.
Editorial Board

SIMON & SCHUSTER
New York   London   Toronto   Sydney   Tokyo   Singapore

SIMON & SCHUSTER
Simon & Schuster Building
Rockefeller Center
1230 Avenue of the Americas
New York, New York 10020

Copyright © 1993 by Graber Productions, Inc.

Designed by Irving Perkins Associates
Manufactured in the United States of America

10 9 8 7 6 5 4 3 2 1

Library of Congress Cataloging-in-Publication Data

Staying healthy in a risky environment: The New York University
Medical Center family guide / Arthur C. Upton, medical editor,
Eden Graber, editor.
     p.   cm.
     Includes bibliographical references and index.
     1. Environmental health—Popular works.   2. Environmentally
induced diseases—Popular works.   I. Upton, Arthur C., 1923–
II. Graber, Eden.   III. New York University Medical Center.
RA565.S73   1993
613'.1—dc20   93-2634
                                                       CIP

ISBN: 0-671-76815-8

The ideas, procedures and suggestions in this book are intended to
supplement, not replace, the medical and legal advice of trained
professionals. Laws vary from state to state, and if legal advice is
required, the services of a competent professional should be sought.
In addition, all matters regarding your health require medical supervision. Consult your physician before adopting the medical suggestions in this book, as well as about any condition that may
require diagnosis or medical attention.

The authors and publishers disclaim any liability arising directly or
indirectly from the use of this book.

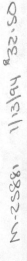

Contents

SECTION III. TWENTY COMMON SYMPTOMS OF EXPOSURE TO TOXIC ENVIRONMENTAL AGENTS

SECTION IV. THE SOURCES OF ENVIRONMENTAL HEALTH HAZARDS

SECTION V. **PREVENTION AND ENVIRONMENTAL ACTION**

SECTION VI. **APPENDICES**

Preface

Just as our landscape has been irrevocably altered by the inventions, constructions, and excavations of human civilization, so too has contemporary medicine. An appreciation of the importance of environmental factors has become an essential component in treating disease and in educating people to avoid illness.

New York University Medical Center was one of the first major health care institutions to recognize the importance of environmental factors in human health. In 1947, it established the Division of Industrial Medicine within the NYU School of Medicine to explore systematically the growing evidence that agents in the workplace and the environment may adversely affect health. By 1954, the division had grown into a full-scale institute; renamed the Norton Nelson Institute of Environmental Medicine (NIEM), it is now the largest and most productive university-based environmental health research institute in the world.

The Norton Nelson Institute reflects the philosophy and commitment of New York University Medical Center, a three-pronged mission of research, clinical care, and education, with each branch supporting and informing the others. Over the years, scientists and physicians at the Norton Nelson Institute have worked to identify the nature, extent, and mechanisms of actions of environmental health hazards and have developed and refined many of the scientific tools now used to investigate these matters.

Working in collaboration with specialists in other areas of medicine, Nelson Institute members have played a major role in isolating and defining the importance of numerous environmental health hazards and in helping to develop effective clinical treatments and preventive measures to foster public health.

The Norton Nelson Institute has become a significant scientific leader in shaping public policy, with members contributing their expertise to legislators and regulators and sitting on numerous advisory boards and councils, including the National Institute of Environmental Health Science, the National Cancer Institute, and the Environmental Protection Agency.

As we move through this last decade of the twentieth century and into the next millennium, environmental and occupational medicine will undoubtedly gain greater significance, particularly in the more developed regions of the world that have witnessed enormous strides in reducing deaths and disability caused by infectious diseases. Our well-being will depend on our understanding of the often subtle but significant interplay of genetics and environmental factors and our ability to modify risk factors that result from nature as well as from human behavior and design.

SAUL J. FARBER, M.D.
DEAN, NEW YORK UNIVERSITY
SCHOOL OF MEDICINE

Preface

Enormous environmental disasters have acquainted us with the importance of controlling the levels of chemicals that we put in our environment. The disasters examined in this book, such as the one at Minamata Bay in Japan, have killed thousands and potentially injured millions of people. The stories are both captivating and important and have taught us to be more careful about the chemicals in our environment.

The solutions to the problems of environmental contamination involve not only devising better ways to degrade chemicals but also devising new ways to control the emissions of certain toxic chemicals. For example, metals are persistent environmental chemicals since they cannot be biodegraded. If we continue taking the metals out of the earth's crust and putting them into our atmosphere and in our water, eventually toxic levels of such metals as lead, mercury, and cadmium will be reached, and developing ways to biodegrade these environmental toxicants will be very difficult.

One goal of the science of toxicology and environmental medicine is to identify the chemicals that are producing injury in humans. Another goal is to try and intervene in preventing human exposure before any diseases have occurred, since in most instances it is difficult to reverse a disease once it has appeared. In order for people to live longer, healthier lives they need to become aware of how to prevent the types of exposure to dangerous chemicals that are described in this book.

The investigators at the Norton Nelson Institute of Environmental Medicine are working to understand the mechanisms by which chemicals produce injury, and to develop strategies to intervene in disease prevention. Support comes primarily from the federal government in research dollars, which are used to study the science of dangerous chemicals in our environment, and of how they enter the human body to produce illnesses. This research effort has enabled us to become aware of many potentially dangerous chemicals before they can cause any diseases. We are only now starting to devise treatments and interventions for chemical-induced injuries. Most of our current efforts are in preventive medicine.

If you have any further interest in this area, please address all inquiries to the Norton Nelson Institute of Environmental Medicine, New York University Medical Center, 550 First Avenue, New York, New York 10016.

—MAX COSTA, PH.D.
Professor and Chairman
Norton Nelson Institute of
Environmental Medicine

Preface

During the last century, the average life expectancy of people in industrialized nations has virtually doubled, an encouraging statistic largely due to improvements in nutrition, sanitation, and public health. Although infectious diseases have been the major causes of disability and death, increasingly they are being supplanted by chronic ailments that are rooted in the interplay of genetic and environmental factors. Unhealthy life-styles and exposure to damaging chemical and physical agents—in air, water, soil, and food; in drugs, cosmetics, and consumer products; and in our houses, workplaces, and communities—are now being recognized as significant public health risks, deserving of careful attention and intelligent action.

We need to recognize the causal roles played by these environmental factors, not only to aid us in accurate diagnosis and management of the illnesses they cause but, more importantly, so we can assist in preventing those illnesses. For example, now that we have recognized that cigarette smoke is implicated in one of every five deaths in the United States, we've been able to launch major efforts to eliminate the smoking habit and thereby prevent the enormous burden of illness it causes.

Unfortunately, many environmental health issues are more complex and less completely understood than smoking. There are a large number of environmental risk factors that exert diverse effects on human health, and adequate information about them is not accessible when needed, particularly for the general public. We hope this book provides the necessary information in a clear, accessible format to help you both to understand the nature and extent of environmental health risks and to take intelligent action on your own behalf to prevent disease and maintain good health.

Although exhaustive treatment of the subject is beyond the scope of this book, its chapters have been designed to cover those topics of greatest general importance. We welcome questions or comments from you about any of the subjects discussed herein. Please address them to: The Norton Nelson Institute of Environmental Medicine, New York University Medical Center, 550 First Avenue, New York, NY, 10016.

—ARTHUR C. UPTON, M.D.
Former Director,
Norton Nelson Institute
of Environmental Medicine

Acknowledgments

To create a book as comprehensive in scope and unique in subject matter as this one required the knowledge, patience, and efforts of a great number of people. It is impossible to cite each of them individually, but some contributions must be acknowledged.

I am deeply indebted to each member of the editorial board. For three years, this very special group of physicians fit biweekly meetings into already packed professional schedules and gave up precious time on evenings and weekends to carefully scrutinize every word and every illustration in this book. They freely shared their expertise, stretched their imaginations to adapt medical literature for the general reader, and persevered through the Herculean task of reaching a consensus in order to present the many controversial issues discussed within these pages. I have never worked with a more dedicated and congenial group of professionals.

Special thanks go to John Deats, who as the gifted director of public affairs for NYU Medical Center, instituted a forward-thinking approach to communications with the public that was the catalyst for developing this project. I relied upon both his concrete and moral support at every step along this way.

Each of our chapters was reviewed by six or more specialists from diverse fields. I'd like to thank each of the more than one hundred physicians and scientists, nurses, and health care professionals from our faculty and other institutions who reviewed the chapters or advised us on specific sections. Special thanks go to the members of our external board of advisors, who participated in this project generously and with the selfless aim of ensuring that this first comprehensive presentation on environmental health for general readers be as accurate, balanced, and up-to-date as possible.

More than most health books, this one relied upon the special talents of medical journalists. Thanks go to Patricia Barnes-Svarney, Robert Barnett, Sue Berkman, Winifred Conkling, Ed Edelson, Oliver Fultz, Constance Grzelka, Dr. Jeanne Kassler, Larry Katzenstein, Lucy Kavaler, Carolyn Rice, Robin Rutsky, Dawn Stover, and Ellen Watson. Thanks also to those who assisted our efforts, namely John Barbour, William Check, Ann Eisenberg, Denise Grady, Carol Levine, Janet Raloff, and Rick Weiss.

We were also fortunate to have the talents of Nina Wallace and Michael Reingold, inventive medical illustrators, who created all of the art used in this book. Thanks as well to copy editors Barbara Ravage and Susan Male Smith.

Special thanks to our project's editor-in-chief at Simon & Schuster, Marilyn Abraham, whose enthusiasm and clarity both fueled and helped shape this project; to the diligent "hands-on" editor, Sheila Curry; and to the person responsible for bringing us together, agent Janet Manus.

A special note of appreciation goes to my editorial associates, James Poniewozik and Nancy Gagliardi, who were instrumental in helping to coordinate and execute the myriad administrative and research pieces of this project. Thanks also to David Sachs and Lynn Odell from the public affairs staff of the NYU Medical Center for their insights and professional efforts and to editorial assistants Susan Randel and Songhui Ma, who helped during the early stages of this project.

Many, many thanks to my family: my husband Richard Tilton, who supported and encouraged me and who withstood the pressurized periods before deadlines, and our children, Cassall and Alexander, for whose sake I first decided to explore this topic and who have accommodated having a part-time, somewhat preoccupied mother for three years of their young lives.

—EDEN GRABER

Affiliations

science communications and nonfiction books for children. For seven years she was the associate director of public affairs for New York University Medical Center and editor of its "New Dimensions Healthwire" news service produced in conjunction with the Associated Press. She is the coauthor of *The Fielding's Travelers Medical Companion* (Morrow, 1990) as well as numerous articles in trade and consumer publications. She holds a master of science degree in specialized journalism from Polytechnic Institute of New York.

EXTERNAL BOARD OF ADVISORS

Donald G. Barnes, Ph.D., Staff Director, Science Advisory Board, U.S. Environmental Protection Agency

Bernard Goldstein, M.D., Chairman, Department of Environmental Medicine, Robert Wood Johnson Medical Center, Piscataway, NJ

Richard J. Jackson, M.D., Chief of Hazard Identification and Risk Assessment Branch, Office of Environmental Health Hazard Assessment, Berkeley, CA

Nancy Kim, Ph.D., Director, Division of Environmental Health Assessment, New York Department of Health, Albany, NY

Donald Mattison, M.D., Dean, Graduate School of Public Health, University of Pittsburgh, Pittsburgh, PA

Gilbert Omenn, M.D., Ph.D., Dean, School of Public Health and Community Medicine, University of Washington, Seattle, WA

Maureen Paul, M.D., Director, Occupational Health and Reproductive Hazards Center, University of Massachusetts Medical Center, Worcester, MA

Herbert Rosenkranz, M.D., Chairman, Department of Environmental and Occupational Health, Graduate School of Public Health, University of Pittsburgh, Pittsburgh, PA

Kenneth Rosenman, M.D., Associate Professor, Department of Medicine, Michigan State University, East Lansing, MI

WRITERS AND ILLUSTRATORS

Writers

Patricia Barnes-Svarney
Robert Barnett
Sue Berkman
Winifred Conkling
Ed Edelson

Oliver Fultz
Constance Grzelka
Dr. Jeanne Kassler
Larry Katzenstein
Lucy Kavaler

Carolyn Rice
Robin Rutsky
Dawn Stover
Ellen Watson

Illustrators

Michael Reingold

Nina Wallace

PEER REVIEWERS

The editors are grateful to the expert reviewers who have helped to assure the accuracy and quality of the text.

Reviewers on the NYU Medical Center Faculty

Michael Albom, M.D., Clinical Associate Professor of Dermatology

Robert Asbell, M.D., Clinical Associate Professor of Ophthalmology

Arthur Bertolino, M.D., Ph.D., Clinical Assistant Professor of Dermatology

Ronald Blum, M.D., Professor of Medicine

Istvan Boksay, M.D., Ph.D., Research Assistant Professor of Psychiatry

William Borkowsky, M.D., Associate Professor of Pediatrics

Ronald Brancaccio, M.D., Clinical Associate Professor of Dermatology

Ronald Carr, M.D., Professor of Ophthalmology

Hosakere K. Chandra Sekhar, M.D., Associate Professor of Clinical Otolaryngology

Mitchell Charap, M.D., Associate Professor of Clinical Medicine

Jay Cooper, M.D., Professor of Radiology

Max Costa, Ph.D., Professor of Environmental Medicine and Pharmacology

Robert Cykiert, M.D., Clinical Assistant Professor of Ophthalmology

Vittorio Defendi, M.D., May Ellen and Gerald Jay Ritter Professor of Oncology; Chairman, Department of Pathology

Martin Doerfler, M.D., Assistant Professor of Medicine

Lance D. Dworkin, M.D., Associate Professor of Medicine

Kenneth Eng, M.D., Professor of Surgery

Hugh Evans, Ph.D., Professor of Environmental Medicine

Enrico Fazzini, D.O., Ph.D., Clinical Assistant Professor of Neurology

Joseph Fetto, M.D., Clinical Associate Professor of Orthopedic Surgery

Toni Field, M.D., Clinical Assistant Professor of Emergency Medicine

Alexander Fisher, M.D., Clinical Professor of Dermatology

George L. Foltin, M.D., Assistant Professor of Clinical Pediatrics; Director, Pediatric Emergency Services, Bellevue Hospital

Arthur Fox, M.D., Professor of Medicine, Chief of Cardiology

Irwin M. Freedberg, M.D., George Miller MacKee Professor and Chairman, Department of Dermatology

Michael L. Freedman, M.D., Professor of Medicine, Diane and Arthur Belfer Professor of Geriatric Medicine

George Friedman-Jimenez, M.D., Research Assistant Professor of Environmental Medicine; Director, Occupational and Environmental Health Clinic, Bellevue Hospital

Stuart Garay, M.D., Assistant Professor of Clinical Medicine

Shirley Garnett, R.N., M.S., Manager, Education Center

Seymour Garte, Ph.D., Associate Professor of Environmental Medicine

Aaron Gindea, M.D., Instructor of Medicine

Melvin C. Gluck, M.D., Associate Professor of Clinical Medicine

Albert Goodgold, M.D., Professor of Clinical Neurology

Govindan Gopinathan, M.D., Clinical Professor of Neurology

Paul Hammerschlag, M.D., Clinical Associate Professor of Otolaryngology

Naomi Harley, Ph.D., Research Professor of Environmental Medicine

Eugenia Hawrylko, M.D., Instructor in Clinical Medicine

Robert Hessler, M.D., Assistant Professor of Clinical Surgery and Emergency Medicine

Howard Hochster, M.D., Assistant Professor of Medicine

Ronald Hoffman, M.D., Clinical Associate Professor of Otolaryngology

Robert Holzman, M.D., Associate Professor of Medicine

Lawrence Horowitz, M.D., Associate Professor of Clinical Medicine

David Kamelhar, M.D., Clinical Assistant Professor of Medicine

Sandra Kammerman, M.D., Associate Professor of Medicine

Thomas Kantor, M.D., Professor of Clinical Medicine

Paul Kechijian, M.D., Clinical Associate Professor of Dermatology

Albert Keegan, M.D., Professor of Clinical Radiology

Martin Kohn, M.D., Ph.D., Assistant Professor of Clinical Surgery and Emergency Medicine; Director, Emergency Medicine Residency, Bellevue Hospital

Edwin Kolodny, M.D., Bernard A. and Charlotte Marden Professor and Chairman, Department of Neurology

Mathew Lee, M.D., M.P.H., Professor, Clinical Rehabilition Medicine, and Acting Chairman, Department of Rehabilitation Medicine

Richard I. Levin, M.D., Associate Professor of Medicine; Director, Laboratory of Cardiovascular Research

Neal Lewin, M.D., Clinical Assistant Professor of Medicine

Henry Wan-Peng Lim, M.D., Associate Professor of Dermatology

Arthur Lindner, M.D., Associate Professor of Medicine

Mack Lipkin, Jr., M.D., Associate Professor of Clinical Medicine

Morton Lippmann, Ph.D., Professor of Environmental Medicine

Eddie Louie, M.D., Clinical Instructor of Medicine

Joseph Lowy, M.D., Clinical Instructor of Medicine

Paula Marchetta, M.D., Instructor in Clinical Medicine

Janet Moy, M.D., Assistant Professor of Dermatology

Marion Nestle, Ph.D., M.P.H., Professor and Chair, Department of Nutrition, Food and Hotel Management, New York University

Kenneth Noble, M.D., Associate Professor of Clinical Ophthalmology

Margareta Nordin, B.S., Med. Dr., Research Associate Professor of Environmental Medicine

Catherine O'Boyle, R.N., M.S., Associate Executive Director, Bellevue Hospital

Wade Parks, Ph.D., M.D., Pat and John Rosenwald Professor and Chairman, Department of Pediatrics, Bellevue Hospital

Bernard S. Pasternack, Ph.D., Professor of Environmental Medicine

Arthur Penn, Ph.D., Research Professor of Environmental Medicine

Kent Peterson, M.D., Clinical Associate Professor of Environmental Medicine

Robert Pfeffer, M.D., Professor of Clinical Surgery

Donald Pizzarello, Ph.D., Professor of Radiology

Claudia S. Plottel, M.D., Instructor in Clinical Medicine

David Ramsay, M.D., M.Ed., Associate Professor of Clinical Dermatology

David M. Rapoport, M.D., Associate Professor of Clinical Medicine

Perry Robins, M.D., Associate Professor of Clinical Dermatology

William N. Rom, M.D., M.PH., Professor of Medicine and Environmental Medicine; Chief, Division of Pulmonary and Critical Care Medicine, Bellevue Hospital

Stanley Rosenthal, Ph.D., Associate Professor of Experimental Dermatology

Stephen Rothstein, M.D., Assistant Professor of Otolaryngology

Michael Ruoff, M.D., Clinical Associate Professor of Medicine

Miguel Sanchez, M.D., Assistant Professor of Dermatology

Ken Schneider, M.D., Associate Professor of Clinical Otolaryngology

Nancy Sculerati, M.D., Assistant Professor of Otolaryngology

Mindell Seidlin, M.D., Assistant Professor of Clinical Medicine

William Shapiro, M.D., Clinical Assistant Professor of Otolaryngology

Roy Shore, Ph.D., Professor of Environmental Medicine

Nicholas A. Soter, M.D., Professor of Dermatology

James Speyer, M.D., Associate Professor of Clinical Medicine

George Teebor, M.D., Professor of Pathology and Environmental Medicine

Walter Troll, Ph.D., Professor of Environmental Medicine

Paul Tunick, M.D., Clinical Associate Professor of Medicine

Susan B. Waltzman, Ph.D., Professor of Clinical Otolaryngology

Harold Weinberg, M.D., Ph.D., Clinical Associate Professor of Neurology

Roger Wetherbee, M.D., Clinical Assistant Professor of Medicine

Ron Wood, Ph.D., Research Associate Professor of Environmental Medicine

Sol Zimmerman, M.D., Associate Professor of Clinical Pediatrics

Arthur Zitrin, M.D., Professor of Psychiatry, Associate Dean for Student Affairs

Susan B. Zolla-Pazner, Ph.D., Professor of Pathology

External Peer Reviewers

Robert J. Barish, Ph.D., Chief Radiotherapy Physicist, Mary Immaculate Hospital, Catholic Medical Center of Brooklyn and Queens (New York, NY)

William Chang, M.D., Assistant Professor of Medicine, Brown University

Linda Cowan, Ph.D., Associate Professor of Statistics and Epidemiology, Oklahoma University

Thomas Hadley, M.D., Medical Director, Healthlink, div. Memorial Hospital (Freemont, OH)

Glendon Henry, M.D., Attending Physician, Emergency Services, Bellevue Hospital Center (New York, NY)

Mary Ann Howland, Pharm.D., ABAT, Clinical Professor of Pharmacy, St. John's University (Jamaica, NY), and Consultant, New York City Poison Control Center

Robert Mason, Ph.D. (C16), Division of Standards Development and Technology Transfer, Centers for Disease Control, National Institute for Occupational Safety and Health

J. Donald Millar, M.D., Director, National Institute for Occupational Safety and Health, Centers for Disease Control and Prevention

Gary Rosenthal, Ph.D., D.A.B.T., Group Leader, Pharmacology and Toxicology, Samatogen (Boulder, CO)

Russell Ross, Ph.D., Professor and Chairman, Department of Pathology, University of Washington School of Medicine

Steven Sheskier, M.D., Attending Orthopedic Surgeon, Hospital for Joint Diseases (New York, NY)

Richard Wang, M.D., Attending Physician, Emergency Services, Bellevue Hospital Center (New York, NY)

Richard Weisman, Pharm. D., Director, New York City Poison Control Center

Robert W. Wissler, Ph.D., M.D., Distinguished Service Professor of Pathology, University of Chicago Medical Center

Environmental Health Basics

Introduction

The notion that something in the environment can make people ill dates back to the Greek physician Hippocrates. In the fourth century B.C., "the father of medicine" suggested that illness can result from foul air, contaminated by the decay of dead plants and animals and other wastes. (This "miasma theory" of disease persisted for centuries and was used to explain outbreaks of diseases such as malaria and yellow fever.) Similarly, the ancient Greeks and Romans recognized the role played by certain environmental factors in the development of disease, in particular, the dangers of asbestos, lead, and mercury.

Today, many of us seem to have taken this awareness to an extreme. We live in an age of widespread anxiety about environmental hazards. We seem hemmed in on all sides by toxic threats, both synthetic and natural: Industrial chemicals and pesticides leaching into the soil and our drinking water, emissions from vehicles and smokestacks fouling the air, piles of trash looming as big as mountains, garbage barges wandering unwanted from country to country, torrents of sewage pouring into streams and rivers are some of the images that confront us daily as we open our newspapers over a cup of coffee or turn on the 6:00 news.

Judging by the reports, no area of the landscape, no aspect of our daily lives, escapes these perils. Newly installed carpets and floor tiles may release noxious, irritating vapors. Drinking water treated with chlorine to kill dangerous microorganisms may expose us to cancer-causing substances. We wonder if our dental fillings are releasing toxic mercury vapors, if our pots and pans are leaching aluminum into our food and causing senility, or if the electromagnetic fields around our electric blankets (and the alarm clocks at the bedside) are interfering with our fertility. The very products we once prized as modern conveniences now come under suspicion as high-tech menaces.

In this litany of environmental ills, each item is not equally threatening. There are ways to separate the serious hazards from the less serious, and timely concerns from those of marginal interest.

We now have access to more information than ever on possible environmental dangers. Unfortunately, instead of helping us to live our lives in a more healthy manner, this abundance of information causes many people to feel helpless and overwhelmed, to shrug their shoulders and give up. Their reponse: "*Everything* can kill you these days—what can I do about it?"

Staying Healthy in a Risky Environment: The New York University Medical Center Family Guide is a tool to help you "do something about it." There *are* steps you can take to safeguard your health and the health of those around you. We have collected, organized, and evaluated up-to-date information on environmental health, so that you can understand the issues of the day, distinguish serious threats from minor worries, and take control of your environment.

There are two important ideas to keep in mind while reading this book, as well as any other report on environmental issues. First, this is a subject area replete with controversies: there are many gaps in knowledge and many uncertainties in the information in this field. Second, the perspective of the source of information is an important part of the message that is communicated to you. The same environmental hazard—a toxic industrial chemical, for example—could be seen in quite different ways by a laboratory scientist studying its properties; by its manufacturer, defending itself against liability claims; by a worker who believes he or she became ill from on-the-job exposures to the chemical; by a consultant in charge of cleaning up sites where the chemical was dumped; by a family living by a river too polluted with the chemical to allow its use for swimming or for drinking water; or by a public health professional, attempting to counsel communities on the measures that could best protect them from the chemical.

This is a book written by scientists and physicians, working in tandem with professional journalists. It expresses a *public health viewpoint*, which means that we attempt to suggest the best steps, based on available information, that individuals and communities can take to protect their health and avoid exposures to toxic environmental agents.

We intend the book not only as a reference tool that provides specific information and facts, but also as an educational guide to make you aware of significant *concepts and principles* that you can apply in daily life and use to confront and comprehend new issues, to identify environmental health threats, to weigh the assessments of their importance, and to prioritize your concerns and your actions.

In the first section of the book, we introduce some basic concepts of environmental health: What is an environmental hazard? What is the difference between a hazard and a risk? What methods do scientists use to discover what the risks are and to assess which are of more or less concern?

In the section "The Environment's Effects on the Body," we examine closely the *internal* en-vironment—the various systems of the body—explaining how and why they are affected by agents in the external environment and what you can do to protect them from harm. In Section III, we examine twenty common symptoms of illness and explain which environmental agents can cause them. Though this section is not intended to be used for self-diagnosis, it provides information of which you should be aware when discussing your health with your physician.

In Section IV, "The Sources of Environmental Health Hazards," we break the external environment into several of its most significant component areas, including the air, the water supply, and the workplace, and examine these environments in terms of how they can pose hazards and how we can work to make them safer and cleaner. We also detail a number of methods by which you can safeguard your health. Finally, in Section V, "Prevention and Environmental Action," we examine ways in which to act on your knowledge of environmental health, we outline a preventive health plan and examine the political and social avenues for environmental change.

We hope that this book will provide a valuable source of information about environmental health, but we also hope that it will help you to feel confident, rather than terrified, about the prospects of living in today's world. It is worthwhile, after all, to ask ourselves why the world appears to be so risky when people actually live longer, better, and healthier than any of the preceding generations. It's worthwhile to become educated about the environment and to resist being overwhelmed by the crush of "Are You Toxic?" reports. Not all of the environmental hazards we hear about are equal in the dangers they pose; in fact, some of the ones that receive little attention actually cause the greatest damage. And not all of the things we consider "risky" belong in the list of our top priorities. There is much that we can do to clarify both the scope of environmental health threats and the actions that will help protect our health, the health of our communities, and the health of our planet.

CHAPTER 1

What Is an Environmental Health Hazard?

The small town of Dunsmuir is nestled amidst the forests and mountain streams of northern California. Until ten o'clock on the night of July 14, 1991, the area was a paradise for trout fishermen and nature lovers; many of its residents were self-styled refugees from the pollution of Los Angeles. On that summer night, however, a Southern Pacific freight train carrying a cargo of pesticide ran off its track while crossing the Sacramento River. Thirteen thousand gallons of the chemical spilled into the river and rapidly spread throughout the fast-flowing water. Within two days, the spill had reached Shasta Lake, 47 miles downstream.

The pesticide poisoned the water, killing fish by the thousands and depleting the flourishing populations of algae and other plankton on which they fed. A toxic cloud formed over the water and drifted to the riverbank habitats of otters, egrets, and herons. Of course, insects also died in great numbers, leaving birds and small animals at risk of starvation.

The residents of Dunsmuir were also affected by the poisonous vapor. Out of a population of but a few thousand, 400 people went to the nearest emergency room, suffering from asthma and other acute respiratory symptoms, gastrointestinal complaints, burning eyes and throat, skin rashes, and headaches. As a precautionary measure, public health officials recommended that pregnant women who had been close to the river when the spill occurred be tested for possible neurologic damage to the fetuses developing in their wombs.

The town of Dunsmuir is small, and at 13,000 gallons, the chemical spill could not be classified as major, but the incident stands as an example of the wide-ranging effects of such environmental hazards, how they can touch upon human health and the ecology in ways that linger and have the potential to harm future generations.

The creation of an environmental health hazard does not require a disaster such as Dunsmuir. The air we breathe, the water we drink, the noise we hear, the products we use, the way we live—all of these factors combine to make an environment that can preserve our health . . . or damage it.

THE MAJOR TYPES OF ENVIRONMENTAL HEALTH HAZARDS

The word *hazard* means a potential harm. An environmental health hazard is a substance or agent that has the ability to cause some type of adverse health effect, be it minor damage to a tissue, serious illness, or death.

Hazards are sometimes confused with risks,

though there is a distinction between the two: A risk is the *probability* that the potential danger of the hazard will actually be realized. If a person is not exposed to a hazard, however dangerous, there is no risk.

For example, a fire is a hazard (it causes burns), but the risk of being burned varies tremendously: A fire burning down the block from us may not incite us to evacuate our house (low risk of being burned), but if the flames are raging right next door and leaping to our roof, its time to get out quickly (high risk). What if the fire in progress is a quarter of a mile away but in a pesticide factory? Whether or not we decide to leave the area depends upon the likelihood of being exposed to something toxic. We need to know what substances are likely to be in that factory building, just how toxic they potentially are when ignited, and how far they are likely to travel from their source; in this case, the risks are a bit less certain and less familiar to us.

Box 1.1 HAZARDS VERSUS RISKS: ASBESTOS

When considering environmental health priorities, it is important to keep in mind the difference between a hazard and a risk. The case of environmental asbestos is a particularly illustrative example.

Asbestos is a group of naturally occurring fibrous minerals considered to be major environmental health hazards by the U.S. Environmental Protection Agency (EPA). When inhaled, certain types of asbestos fibers can cause both irreversible damage to the lung (asbestosis) and a rare form of cancer of the lining of the lung (mesothelioma). Asbestos was used as fireproofing and insulating material; asbestos shingles, tiles, steam pipes, and jackets and spray-on acoustic ceilings were common in houses, public buildings, and schools from the 1930s through most of the 1960s. The EPA ordered a phaseout of asbestos for many uses in 1974; even so, some 30 million tons have been used in this country since the turn of the century, and a great deal is still around.

There may be asbestos in the insulation around the pipes in the basement of a house. People who live in the house most likely have been in the *vicinity* of asbestos—which is enclosed in a protective casing—but they can only be *exposed* to it if the asbestos fibers are airborne. In other words, although encased asbestos constitutes a *hazard*, there is a *risk* of exposure only if the fibers enter the air. If the asbestos insulation around the basement pipes is intact, exposure to released fibers is highly unlikely. In fact, in the rush to remove the asbestos that they have heard is so hazardous, many people have actually created a greater health hazard for themselves: When not removed correctly, asbestos fibers are frequently released into the air where they can be inhaled, increasing exposure beyond what would have occurred had the asbestos been left in place (see Box 6.6, p. 127).

Despite their myriad forms, most environmental health hazards can be grouped into four categories. Most of us readily recognize the first three—chemical hazards, physical hazards, and biological hazards—many of us overlook or minimize the importance of the fourth—cultural hazards—although this is the area in which we have the greatest control regarding exposure.

Chemical Hazards

There are five principal types of chemical hazards. *Toxins* are chemicals that are harmful or fatal to humans in low doses. Most are neurotoxins, affecting the brain and nervous system. (Some scientists distinguish between toxins, which are naturally occurring substances, and synthetically produced toxicants. In this book, both are referred to as toxins.) Most of the chemical hazards are hazardous substances, but we use this term more narrowly to describe chemicals that cause harm because they are flammable or explosive, because they irritate or damage organs of the body (such as the skin or the lungs), or because they induce sensitivities and allergic reactions. *Carcinogens* are agents that cause or promote the growth of cancer. *Teratogens* cause birth defects. *Mutagens* are agents that cause changes in the genetic material found in chromosomes (mutagens can function as carcinogens or teratogens, depending on what cells they affect and what mutations they cause).

Chemical hazards come from the substances found in our air, water, and food; at our workplaces; in our homes and schools. Chemical toxins may be synthetic or natural. Aflatoxin, for example, is a potent chemical poison produced naturally by molds that grow on peanuts, almonds, and other nuts; animal feed corn; and cottonseed.

Box 1.2 CHEMICAL HAZARDS: MERCURY

The pages of medical history are filled with stories about toxic heavy metals, particularly lead and mercury. Hundreds of years ago madness among the mirror-makers of Venice and the hatters of London was linked to inhaling mercury vapors, which were a by-product of the manufacturing process (hence, the phrase "mad as a hatter"). Mercury is both a *hazardous substance* (as it can cause skin irritation) and a *toxin* (as it can have deadly effects on the nervous system); the latter is mercury's most well-known and serious threat.

The full extent of this hazard to human health was not appreciated until the 1950s, when more than one hundred people in Minamata, Japan, were stricken with brain and nervous system damage, including lesions and atrophy of the brain; forty-six people died of the symptoms. The ailment, now known as Minamata disease, was traced to mercury-laden wastes deposited in the bay waters by a chemical plant; since the 1950s, thousands of new cases were reported in the area. The people of Minamata were poisoned not by drinking the water, but by eating fish that had ingested and absorbed the mercury, which accumulated in levels high enough to harm humans (see Figure 17.1, pp. 600–601).

The outbreak at Minamata not only increased the understanding of mercury as a hazard to human health, but also demonstrated the far-reaching effects of damage to the ecology. When the fish that form an important part of our diet are contaminated, the poison will enter our systems, too.

Another even greater epidemic of Minamata disease occurred in December 1971, this time in Iraq. By the time it had run its course, 6,530 people in many parts of the country had become ill with disorders of the nervous system, and 459 died. After considerable medical detective work, the source of the epidemic was found in

(continued)

Box 1.2   CHEMICAL HAZARDS: MERCURY (*continued*)

what should have been the staff of life: homemade bread. A shipment of seed grain intended only for planting had been treated with a fungicide containing methylmercury before being shipped from Mexico to the southern Iraqi port of Basra. Instead of being planted, the seed was used for bread—with dire results.

Physical Hazards

Those aspects of the external environment that are sources of such bodily injuries as fractures, lacerations, abrasions, and burns are classified as physical hazards. The forces of the external world expose us to such devastating physical hazards as earthquakes, volcanoes, floods, cyclones, landslides, and fires.

Physical hazards in the workplace include noise, vibration, and ergonomic hazards (caused by the adverse effects of motions or body positions involved in performing a task) among other assorted circumstances that lead to bodily injury (see Chapter 21, "The Workplace").

Radiation is classified as a physical hazard, although its effects extend to damage to cells and the genetic material in them. As a culture, we still do not demonstrate much concern about exposure to nonionizing radiation in the form of the sun's ultraviolet rays, which we pursue to obtain a "healthy" tan, even though such radiation can cause significant damage. When absorbed by the skin and the eyes, however, these rays can cause sunburn, premature aging of the skin, cancer, and cataracts; looking directly at the sun in eclipse can result in blindness (see Chapter 4, "Skin Ailments"). We are usually more concerned about other forms of nonionizing radiation, such as microwaves, which can heat body tissues causing burns, and electromagnetic fields produced in the generation of electric power, which are currently being investigated for a variety of negative health effects.

Our greatest fears seem reserved for ionizing radiation, the type used in X rays and generated by nuclear power and weaponry. Large doses of this physical hazard can damage cells and tissues and may cause cancer in humans (see Chapter 16, "Radiant Energy").

Biological Hazards

Disease-causing biological agents include microorganisms, such as viruses and bacteria, parasites, molds, and fungi. Many of them cause transmissible illnesses that can be spread from person to person through air, water, food, bodily fluids, or, in certain instances, via insects.

Disease-causing pathogens are responsible for a wide range of ailments, from pneumonia, mumps, and toxic shock syndrome to gastrointestinal upsets and diarrhea, which characterize food poisoning, and to the deadly botulism toxin, which flourishes in improperly canned or bottled foods. Disease-causing microorganisms are considered the greatest safety threat to our food supply, and many of them, including *Salmonella* (which infects chickens and raw eggs), *Campylobacter jejuni*, and *Staphylococcus aureus*, thrive on foods that are not handled or stored properly (see Chapter 17, "Food Safety").

Ubiquitous in the world today are the sexually transmitted diseases, such as hepatitis B, acquired immune deficiency syndrome (AIDS), syphilis, gonorrhea, chlamydia, and herpes, caused by microorganisms.

People whose occupations, hobbies, or sports activities keep them out of doors (including farmers, loggers, gardeners, and hikers) can come into contact with insect-borne microorganisms. The bite of a tick can spread Lyme disease, Rocky Mountain spotted fever, and viral encephalitis. Abroad, the *Anopheles* mosquito may harbor and pass onto humans the parasites that cause malaria. Farmers and others who come in direct contact with soil or farm animals may be exposed to zoonotic disease (resulting from infectious agents that attack both humans and animals), such as rabies (see Chapter 21, "The Workplace").

The most widespread skin irritant is a biolog-ical hazard: the poison ivy plant (see Chapter 4, "Skin Ailments").

In indoor air, high concentrations of molds and fungi may be responsible for allergic reactions and ailments often attributed to "sick building syndrome" (see Box 14.7, p. 557). The droplets of water condensed and diffused by air conditioners have been linked to outbreaks of Legionnaires' disease (see Box 1.3).

Box 1.3   IDENTIFYING A BIOLOGICAL HAZARD: LEGIONNAIRES' DISEASE

When a mysterious outbreak of a particularly deadly form of pneumonia occurred among American Legion members during their annual convention in Philadelphia in 1976, epidemiologists were instrumental in identifying not only the cause of the disease—a previously unknown bacterium, which was promptly named *Legionella pneumophila*—but also the unexpected source of exposure: air circulating through the hotel's air-conditioning system in which colonies of *Legionella pneumophila* thrived.

In the early 1980s, there was a series of outbreaks of Legionnaires' disease in patients at a number of hospitals in the United States. As *Legionella pneumophila* was still considered a rare pathogen, health investigators were stumped: How was it that such a rare microorganism was suddenly infecting so many people in so many different geographic areas? Initially, doctors theorized that the patients affected must have had weakened immune systems due to other illnesses and were thus vulnerable to this rare bacterium. The theory fell apart, though, and it became apparent that many of those stricken were not among the sickest: All of those who came down with Legionnaires' disease had been well enough to take showers during their hospital stays. Inspecting the patients' hospital rooms, medical detectives uncovered another unexpected source of exposure. Lurking in the shower heads used by the people who had become infected were colonies of *Legionnella* bacteria.

Another outbreak of the disease occurred in 1989 in Bogalusa, Louisiana, where seventy citizens fell ill and two died of Legionnaires' disease. This time, the victims seemed to have nothing in common except grocery shopping. The trail began with this single clue and led health department investigators to supermarkets where they noticed that the fruit and vegetable bins are sprayed at frequent intervals to keep them cool and fresh. Probing further, the medical sleuths found that the sprays were fed from open troughs of water located in the back of the stores. As it turned out, the troughs were not cleaned regularly, providing a perfect breeding ground for the growth of algae, which in turn nourished colonies of the *Legionella* bacteria. The shoppers had all been exposed by the small misting of spray on their faces, which contained sufficient numbers of disease-causing *Legionella* bacteria to cause the infection.

Box 1.4 CULTURAL HAZARDS AND PREVENTIVE HEALTH

Many of the cultural hazards become acutely important when devising a preventive health plan. Some factors routinely considered are age, gender, and family history of disease and whether or not a person smokes tobacco or consumes alcohol. The importance of many of the other factors is only now being fully realized, including potential environmental exposures in the workplace; through recreational activities; or in general contact with air, soil, and water, as well as the role of diet and sexual practices. In Chapter 22, "The ABCs of Staying Healthy," we discuss these factors in the context of designing your own personal preventive health program.

Nonmodifiable Risk Factors

- Family history of disease
- Age
- Gender

Partially Modifiable Risk Factors

- Occupational environment
- Home and community

Modifiable Risk Factors

- Tobacco smoking
- Diet
- Stress
- Social support
- Alcohol or substance abuse
- Sexual practices

Cultural Hazards

Heart disease and cancer are the two main causes of death in this country, followed by stroke, chronic obstructive pulmonary disease, diabetes, and chronic liver disease. These disorders, once held to be inherited or primarily the results of aging, are now widely thought to be related to worksite conditions, diet, and smoking, as well as to exposure to toxic substances.

Scientists have long known that health is affected by complex, interrelated factors of heredity and environment. No two individuals respond to an environmental insult in exactly the same way. The wild card is heredity. We know, for example, that smoking tobacco and exposure to environmental tobacco smoke produce an assault that is damaging to the largest number of people; yet there are individuals who have smoked from puberty onward and die at the age of ninety from a cause totally unrelated to the tobacco habit. Arsenic is a well-recognized poison; but, as some would-be murderers have discovered, an amount of arsenic that sickens and kills one person may have little effect on another. Similarly, some people exposed to small quantities of arsenic in their drinking water become ill, whereas others are not affected by relatively large amounts.

Susceptibility versus resistance to disease stems from genes, the environment, or both. The two come together in the family setting. Familial predisposition to disease depends on both the genes inherited from parents and earlier forebears and the environment family members share. This includes diet, exercise, smoking, drinking habits, and even exposure to pollutants in a family business (see Chapter 22, "The ABCs of Staying Healthy").

RISKS TO THE ECOLOGY OF PLANET EARTH

A special group of hazards—changes in the ecosystem—is the most recent to gain recognition. In 1990, the Science Advisory Board to the EPA specifically recommended that the agency place as much emphasis on reducing ecological risk as on reducing human health risk. The two are related: If the ecosystem deteriorates, so will the quality of human life.

The health effect of an ecologic hazard can be immediate, as when the groundwater in an area becomes contaminated by runoff from toxic agricultural chemicals and pollutes well water used for drinking. More often, however, the damage does not appear until long after the environmental insult has taken place—often when the change in the ecosystem can no longer be reversed. Over the long term, protecting the environment is of major importance in protecting human health.

Depletion of the ozone layer is a classic example of an ecological hazard that will have an adverse effect on tomorrow's health. Ozone, the most active chemical form of oxygen, is a pollutant at ground level. High above the earth in the stratosphere, however, a layer of ozone serves a purpose important for all life on earth: It blocks a substantial amount of a recognized physical hazard—the sun's ultraviolet rays (see Box 14.5, p. 552).

Until well into the twentieth century, the ozone shield was unaffected by human activity. Then, in the 1930s, a new class of chemicals, chlorofluorocarbons (CFCs), was developed. CFCs became widely used as coolants in refrigerators, air conditioners, industrial solvents, and aerosol propellants and in the manufacture of styrofoam and a host of other products. After more than forty years of use, it was observed by chemists at the University of Michigan and the University of California, Irvine, that millions of pounds of CFCs escape into the atmosphere every year and that they destroy ozone when they reach the stratosphere.

This explains why the ozone layer has been thinning for some years, to such a degree that a "hole," or area of exceptionally low concentration, has appeared over the Antarctic, and the danger is spreading to other parts of the globe. A 1992 National Aeronautics and Space Administration study, making use of an upper-atmosphere research satellite, discovered an alarmingly high concentration of the ozone-depleting chemicals in the atmosphere over populated regions of North America, Europe, and Asia.

Ultraviolet radiation is the main cause of skin cancer, accounting for hundreds of thousands of cases and 8,500 deaths a year. Some scientists predict that this figure will at least double if ozone destruction continues unabated. Because ultraviolet light affects eyes as well as skin, a marked increase in cataracts can also be anticipated. Also, ozone destruction poses a threat to the world food supply because of ultraviolet radiation's damaging effects on crops and livestock.

In efforts to avert these dangers, the use of CFCs in aerosols was banned more than ten years ago, and an international agreement to bring production of the chemicals to a halt by the year 2000 has been signed by ninety-three countries. The U.S. phaseout is to be completed by 1996 (see Chapter 14, "Air").

Identifying hazards is the first step in the complex process of finding out where the risks in the environment actually exist. Making the link between an environmental agent and the harm it causes is part of this process and is the subject of the next chapter.

CHAPTER 2

Illness and the Environment: Finding the Links

When everyone who orders the lunch special at the local coffee shop comes down with diarrhea by the next morning, there is little doubt that something went wrong in the kitchen. Most environmental health threats, however, are not so easily identified.

A great many diseases, particularly chronic ones, originate from many factors. Although it is true that some cancers are clearly linked to a pollutant—for example, mesothelioma of the lung is considered a "sentinel event" pointing to asbestos exposure—such clear-cut incidents are rare. In general, scientists are hard-pressed to decide which and how many of the elements present in an individual's external and internal environment are working together to maintain health or create illness.

For the physician attempting to make a diagnosis, the situation is similarly complex. Faced with a patient with a variety of complaints, the physician may not be aware of exposure to an environmental hazard. Symptoms of environmentally caused diseases may be the same as those of diseases due to other causes.

If a child has difficulty in school, unless one has cause to suspect exposure to lead in the home, it is all too easy to attribute the problems to causes other than lead poisoning. Fatigue, shortness of breath, headache, gastrointestinal upset, a rash, are all symptoms that could be caused by influenza, pulmonary disease, mi-graine headaches, ulcers, an allergy, or they could be due to exposure to any of a wide variety of pollutants. Symptoms such as sleeplessness; lack of energy; and loss of interest in food, sex, and work can signal depression, but they may also result from low-level exposure to gases, metals, and dusts that damage the brain and nervous system.

People often do not remember that they have been exposed to a potentially harmful environmental agent, or they may remember but fail to see its relevance and, thus, do not mention the exposure when giving a medical history.

Symptoms can appear immediately after exposure (acute) or develop as the result of numerous or prolonged exposures to lower levels of an agent (chronic). A considerable period of time may elapse between exposure to a hazard and the onset of disease (latency period). Particularly with toxins that affect a developing fetus, a long latency period may mean that the adverse effects do not become evident until the offspring of the person exposed grows to adulthood. Such is the case with the prescription drug diethylstilbestrol, a hormone prescribed in the 1950s to prevent premature miscarriage but which later turned out to increase the likelihood of vaginal and cervical cancer *not* in the women who took the drug, but in their daughters.

Years of accumulated exposure may be required before the damage is expressed. Long periods of living in moderately polluted air may precede the onset of chronic respiratory illness, skin cancer may follow decades of exposure to the midday sun, and it takes years for high-cholesterol diets to result in fatty deposits in the arteries, and even more years for these deposits to induce heart disease.

Individual variation in the way people react is also a factor. People often vary widely in their responses to even known toxins. Several seemingly harmless quantities of toxins can also interact to produce markedly more serious reactions (see the case of the engineer on p. 756).

All of these factors conspire with human failure to remember an exposure to make it difficult for physicians to link cause and effect even for diseases known to have environmental origins.

EPIDEMIOLOGY: TEASING OUT THE LINKS

Despite its name, which reflects its historical roots in the study of epidemics, the modern science of epidemiology is the study of patterns of illness among human populations and among factors that might be responsible for influencing these patterns. Like Sherlock Holmes, epidemiologists make deductions based on clues—illness patterns and apparently associated factors—relying on mathematical computations and statistics to pin down the truth. Their observations are buttressed by information from other observations and from experiments on other animal species.

The approach has proved fruitful. Indeed, many, if not most, of the known links between illness and environmental factors have relied upon epidemiology. Following up observations that some diseases crop up much more frequently in a particular group of workers historically has been a major first step in identifying many environmental agents.

The observation that workers who manufactured batteries suffered from the same neurological symptoms led health investigators to identify on-the-job exposure to lead as the source. Similarly, in the 1930s, the observation that several hundred men who had worked on the same large tunneling project later suffered the same type of severe damage to the lungs cemented recognition of the damaging effects of occupational exposure to silica. Although silicosis had been known as an occupational risk be-fore then, this time the public demanded workers be protected from toxic substances. The result was the Walsh–Healy Act of 1936.

More recently, the appearance of a new and lethal form of pneumonia among a group of American Legion members attending the same conference led to the identification of a previously unknown organism that causes Legionnaires' disease, as well as clarifying an unexpected source of environmental exposures (see Box 1.3, p. 27).

Tracking Down a Mysterious Agent: The L-Tryptophan Case

Consider as a case study the fate of some 1,500 people who, beginning in the summer of 1989 and continuing into the early part of 1990, became seriously ill with severe muscle pain and weakness, coupled with eosinophilia, a rare blood disorder characterized by extraordinarily high counts of a type of white blood cell linked to inflammation. Confounded by the symptoms, doctors tested patients for an array of disorders, including parasite infestations and cancer. At least one patient underwent exploratory surgery for tumors; none were found.

Within a few months, the illness had a name: eosinophilia–myalgia syndrome, or EMS. Many of those who suffered (about 80 percent of those affected were women) also had fever, rash, swelling of limbs, hair loss, and trouble breathing; often, muscle and nerve damage developed. Hundreds were hospitalized; twenty-eight died.

Doctors discovered that their patients had one thing in common: Almost all had taken a dietary supplement called L-tryptophan. L-Tryptophan is an amino acid, one of the chemical building blocks that join in various combinations to form proteins. A "natural" substance, tryptophan is present in many foods. Because of studies suggesting that it may brighten mood and induce sleep, L-tryptophan became a big seller in health food stores in the 1980s; thousands, perhaps millions, of Americans took it in doses many times the level that would normally be consumed in food, seeking to alleviate depression or listlessness. Most of them believed that, as a natural product, L-tryptophan was "safer" than conventional drugs.

The Food and Drug Administration had never approved L-tryptophan for use as a drug—as it was being used—or tested the effects of the quantities in which people were taking it.

L-Tryptophan was marketed as a "food supplement"; as such, it was not subject to the stringent manufacturing standards or safety and efficacy requirements that apply to drugs.

Following up the observed association between symptoms of EMS and use of L-tryptophan, researchers in several states set up case–control studies, comparing EMS patients (the cases) with groups of healthy people matched for age, sex, and neighborhood (the controls) (see Box 2.2). There were no notable differences between the two groups in terms of their diets, use of vitamins or medications, or water supply; what was different was that all of the patients, but only a few of the controls, had taken L-tryptophan.

When the results were in, the researchers found that that difference—the use of L-tryptophan—was clearly related to the development of EMS; the association was statistically significant, making it highly unlikely that it resulted from coincidence.

Box 2.1 ASSESSING PROBABILITY: HOW GOOD WAS THE STUDY?

In analyzing the results of a study, scientists must measure the probability that the difference observed could have occurred by chance. Accompanying a scientific report is a P, or probability, value, which indicates the percentage chance that the results could be the result of chance. The lower the P value, the better; a P value of .05 or less—meaning that the odds of the result having been obtained by chance are no more than five out of one hundred—is considered good.

Few studies are more conclusive than that, but one must not overlook the fact that when $P = .05$, it does mean that five times out of one hundred, the findings could be wrong.

Based on this analysis, researchers suspected that a contaminant in the L-tryptophan pills had caused the sudden outbreak of illness.

The next step, described by one researcher as "gumshoe epidemiology," was to obtain bottles of L-tryptophan that had been used by people who had gotten sick and to trace them back to their source. If all the suspect product came from

a single manufacturer, that would support the theory of a contaminant.

All of the L-tryptophan sold in the United States had been manufactured by a half-dozen Japanese firms that exported bulk shipments of the powder to American companies, which in turn processed it into tablets and capsules and sold it under a variety of labels. Tracking the sources of the samples sometimes meant contacting four or five intermediaries, not all of whom kept accurate records. Complicating the task further, researchers could not even be sure that they were tracing the right samples since EMS might be one of those ailments with a delayed onset; some people had become ill with EMS months after stopping L-tryptophan, raising the possibility that the pills that the patients were taking when their symptoms arose might not have been the pills that caused the illness.

Despite these uncertainties, the trail did lead back to a single manufacturer of L-tryptophan and to batches of L-tryptophan that were produced after changes were made in the production process. (L-Tryptophan might not have seemed so pure and natural to its enthusiasts if they had known how it was made—fermented in vats of genetically engineered bacteria, from which it was chemically extracted and filtered.)

Another study was needed to compare EMS patients with other L-tryptophan users who did not become ill. Again, a statistically significant number of those who were ill had taken pills that could be traced back to the batches in question. A contaminant seemed more likely than ever.

Box 2.2   THE CASE–CONTROL STUDY

A major category of epidemiologic study involves comparing two (or more) different groups of people on the basis of some salient characteristics and then observing differing factors that may relate to the incidence of disease.

Case–control studies start with a group of people who have a health problem (the cases). They are then matched with another group of people who do not have the health problem but who are similar in age, occupation, activity, or other salient characteristics (the controls). The frequency with which the exposure and the problem occurs is compared in the two groups, and the comparison is evaluated for its statistical reliability.

For example, in the L-tryptophan incident, researchers initially set up case–control studies comparing EMS patients with control groups of healthy people matched for age, sex, and neighborhood to prove that the suspected association between L-tryptophan and the illness was real. Another case–control study was later needed to follow the trail of the suspected environmental contaminant, this time comparing people who used L-tryptophan who had become ill (and whose pills were from the suspect batch) with people who used L-tryptophan who did not develop EMS. This further validated suspicions that the cause of the disease was a contaminant in the pills.

Finding the contaminant, if indeed there was one, would prove difficult, however. Researchers had no idea what they were looking for. No chemical or microbe had ever been known to produce EMS before. Preliminary chemical analyses revealed that the L-tryptophan contained scores of other unidentified substances. Late in 1990, after months of testing, scientists at the Centers for Disease Control and Prevention in Atlanta identified a potentially toxic contaminant in the L-tryptophan produced by one Japanese company. Eventually, it became clear that this substance was far more common in L-tryptophan taken by EMS patients than in samples taken by people who had remained healthy.

Still, the job of identification was not complete. To implicate it conclusively, the contaminant had to produce EMS when given to test animals. Purified L-tryptophan also had to be tested and shown not to produce EMS in the same animals. Initially, it was not clear whether any species of animal was susceptible, until one type of rat did develop an EMS-like disorder after being fed contaminated L-tryptophan, and studies utilizing this species were able to proceed.

DESIGN OF EPIDEMIOLOGIC STUDIES

Epidemiologic studies provide a window on the human experience and can be designed to manipulate conditions so that the effects of a particular agent, microorganism, or chemical in the environment can be assessed with an acceptable degree of reliability.

When confronted with a disease, does what we suspect, based on what we see in the clinic, hold true in the population at large? Can we intervene to protect the health of the community? Are our actions really effective?

The design of an epidemiologic study depends on the particular research circumstances that must be dealt with—what questions need to be answered, what information is readily available, how quickly is an answer needed. Each type of study has its limitations and level of uncertainty.

Retrospective and Prospective Studies

Studies can look forward (prospective) or backward (retrospective) in time. In the EMS–L-tryptophan case, and in the Legionnaires' disease case discussed on p. 27, the matter was pressing and answers were needed right away; retrospective studies were used in these instances.

A *retrospective* study looks back over existing information and asks, in essence, What is the difference between people who already have a disease or symptoms and people who do not? Such studies are relatively inexpensive, can be undertaken quickly, and require relatively few subjects. However, they have their limits: In many cases, they are prone to error due to faulty human recall (recall bias) or the need to use existing data that has been collected for other purposes and must be fit to the new question of interest rather than data collected under circumstances specifically tailored to answer the question at hand.

Prospective studies look forward in time, starting with a group of people who do not have a disease and following them to see if or how the ailment develops. These studies tend to yield more reliable information than retrospective studies but are lengthy, relatively costly, and large in scale.

One of the most well-known and fruitful prospective studies is the Framingham study on cardiovascular disease. The study examined the relationship between heart disease and such factors as smoking, cholesterol, and high blood pressure among 5,287 adults in Framingham, Massachussetts. Beginning in 1950, researchers followed the health status, practices, and mortality rates of groups of Framingham citizens for over forty years, periodically comparing statistics between groups such as smokers and nonsmokers and people with low and high systolic blood pressure. Much of what we know about the role of diet and exercise, as well as high-risk practices such as smoking, in the development of heart disease depended upon long-term prospective studies such as this one.

When associations between a life-style and a disease recur consistently in such a large population, physicians and scientists are on sound ground in advising people to alter their diet and give up smoking and other unhealthy practices. Citizens also have the ammunition needed to demand environmental regulation of harmful substances, such as tobacco.

Box 2.3 THE CHINA STUDY

A currently ongoing prospective study is the China study, in which researchers are examining, over time, a number of parameters—diet, smoking habits, level of activity—and their effects on the incidence of certain diseases. The geographical area included in this study is vast and encompasses people with many different life-styles; the study began with 6,500 people living in sixty-nine counties in twenty-five provinces, and has subsequently been expanded.

Because most rural Chinese spend their entire lives in the province of their birth, there is consistency in findings on the incidence of cardiovascular disease: Cardiovascular disease is much lower in China than in the West, and the difference has been attributed to dietary differences. In the typical Chinese diet, fat provides no more than 10 to 15 percent of calories, compared with 40 percent in the West. As a result, among rural Chinese, the levels of cholesterol, the major risk factor for heart attacks, average below 140 milligrams per deciliter—well under the 200+ level frequently found in Americans.

As the international team of researchers has discovered, not all Chinese, even in the countryside, eat in so healthy a manner. In recent times, some of the counties studied have become more affluent, their inhabitants have increased their meat consumption, and the incidence rate for cardiovascular disease in these richer communities is fifty times higher than in poorer villages where the traditional low-fat Chinese diet is maintained.

Current observations of the changing Chinese life-style also point to an increased probability of disease over the next few years. Cigarette smoking has been increasing by leaps and bounds over the last twenty years to the point that about 80 percent of the men are now smokers. Although lung cancer is still less common than in the industrialized countries of the West, it is definitely on the rise. Since smoking contributes greatly to cardiovascular disease, predictions are for an increase in the latter as well. The China study should provide strong evidence linking various cultural hazards more precisely to the incidence of disease.

Intriguing Observations: Disease Clusters

When a collection of individuals develops the same disease in numbers that appear too large to be due to coincidence, public health officials stand up and take notice.

These so-called disease clusters can be most valuable in providing clues to a possible common source of exposure to an environmental agent. Sometimes, following up on the observation of an apparently high number of cases of disease in a particular area or at a particular time does prove to be fruitful. Certainly, recognition of the cluster of birth defects that appeared in Minamata, Japan, was important in tracking down the industrial contamination of the waters of Minamata Bay with the neurotoxin methylmercury (see p. 25).

A great many of what seem to be disease clusters, however, turn out to be false clues that lead nowhere. A disease cluster is only a clue, and it does not necessarily confirm the presence of a pollutant. It helps to maintain healthy skepticism, particularly when the reports are of a cluster of cancers that appear just after a pollutant has entered the environment: Cancer is a disease with a latency period of ten, twenty, or more years.

Clusters must be carefully followed up with well-designed studies and analyses. Often, it turns out that the number of cases actually falls within the expected range due to coincidence. When tracking a cluster over time, researchers may discover that the incidence of a cancer tapers off to average expected levels.

An example of this is a cluster of leukemia cases identified in a town in New Jersey where a chemical plant is located. Investigators studying a population in a second town in New Jersey, which had the same kind of chemical plant, found no more than the expected incidence of leukemia. After a few years, the number of cases of leukemia in the first town returned to normal levels.

On the other hand, an increased rate of leukemia in Plymouth, Massachusetts, persisted over so long a period of time that it appeared reasonable to link it to the presence of toxic chemicals in the area, and a number of local plants were therefore closed down.

As clues hinting at exposure to workplace toxins, disease clusters have been valuable, but they can be confusing if the work force is not particularly large. Suppose, for example, that in the general population the expected rate of deaths due to a particular cancer is 3 out of 1,000 people annually. If a factory with 1,000 workers has six cancer deaths over that period—twice the expected rate—the sample size is too small to disclose reliably whether exposure to a factor in the workplace is to blame.

Even clusters that do represent sufficient numbers of cases can fail to point to a cause. In west central Phoenix, Arizona, for example, forty-nine children developed leukemia between 1965 and 1986, twenty more than is consistent with the local rate. After two and a half years of detective work, however, the Arizona Department of Health Services was unable to link the cancers to proximity to any identifiable carcinogen.

TOXICOLOGIC STUDIES

Epidemiologic studies deal only with existing health conditions; they are not used to identify an etiologic or causative agent in advance. A different approach is needed when it is important to know beforehand whether a substance might cause a disease, harm a developing fetus, or affect the body's ability to regulate growth. In these cases—and when trying to determine what amount, or dose, of a substance causes harm—scientists rely heavily on toxicologic studies.

By law, a product containing a chemical must be subjected to toxicological testing before being released into the marketplace. Pesticides, ingredients in pesticide formulations, chemicals in drug formulations, and other potentially toxic substances are subjected to study. Tests are also designed to measure the efficacy of a product to be used prophylactically (to prevent disease) or therapeutically (to treat disease).

Although these tests are directed toward human applications, it is seldom ethical or feasible to use people as subjects. (It is one thing to ask people to agree to participate in a study requiring them to take low doses of aspirin [see Box 2.4] and quite another to have them ingest quantities of a potentially lethal drug.) Experiments measuring results in humans (clinical trials) are preceded by tests using computers, laboratory conditions, animals, and other experimental surrogates.

Box 2.4 THE CLINICAL TRIAL

Caution is essential in applying the conclusions of a study based on information about groups to individuals. So many risk factors are involved in the development of an illness that observational and descriptive studies can only suggest, not prove, connections. Clinical trials are used to track the development of disease in individuals with much greater specificity than the other experimental designs.

In a clinical trial, an individual is assigned to one of two groups—exposed or nonexposed—and then followed to see if the exposed group develops the disease or symptoms with statistically significantly different frequency than does the unexposed group.

A good example is the recently completed clinical trial, the physicians' health study, conducted by researchers at the Harvard Medical School, which asked the question, Will taking aspirin reduce a man's risk of a heart attack?

The hypothesis evolved out of the knowledge that clogged arteries induce heart attacks and that aspirin is a drug that inhibits blood clotting. More than 22,000 male physicians between the ages of forty and eighty-four were randomly divided into two groups of equal size. One group received an aspirin pill on alternate days; the other group took a placebo (a "dummy" pill) that resembled an aspirin tablet. The two groups were followed for an average of five years. By the end of that time, there had been a 44 percent reduction in the incidence of heart attack in the aspirin takers as compared with the group on placebo. This reduction occurred among men more than fifty years of age.

The aspirin study was terminated earlier than planned, because in view of the conclusion that small doses of aspirin taken regularly could indeed protect against heart attacks, the Harvard researchers felt it was no longer ethical to continue withholding the drug from the control group. (The study did not address the risks of bleeding from aspirin.)

Computational Approaches

Modern technology makes possible some type of research without using a living cell. Models relating chemical structure to toxicity can be created on a computer. If the goal is to predict the toxicity of a chemical or to find antidotes to a poisonous substance, numerous possibilities are drawn up, analyzing each alternative. The computer can be programmed for the scientist to call up and combine potential antidotes with a variety of doses given via different routes and times of administration. The configuration maps receptor sites, chemical and physiological interactions, adverse effects, desirable effects, and so on.

Animal Studies

In the EMS–L-tryptophan incident, part of the task of identifying the toxic agent required showing that the contaminant actually induced EMS. Because experiments on humans could not be used, tests were conducted on animal surrogates. Purified L-tryptophan also had to be tested and shown not to produce EMS in the same animals.

Animal experiments are used not only to identify a toxic agent but to determine how much of a particular suspect substance, such as a chemical found in contaminated soil or air, is needed to produce ill effects. The substance being studied is administered to test animals in gradually increasing doses until a limit is reached, which may be the onset of illness or death. Many experiments end at the maximum tolerated dose, the maximum dose that can be tolerated without causing death. The results are extrapolated to humans, taking into consideration such factors as body mass, to estimate the risk from a given level of exposure to the substance in humans.

Selecting the appropriate animal species is a crucial step of carrying out studies to determine toxic effects. The typical laboratory animals used for testing carcinogens are mice and rats, whereas guinea pigs, mice, and some primates are used for testing harmful microorganisms. (Research into leprosy lagged because no animal could be infected and used as a model. This investigative stalemate was broken about twenty years ago when leprosy was discovered in armadillos living in the wild in Louisiana and eastern Texas. Very large amounts of bacilli can be cultured from the armadillo, so this animal is now being used in research to develop a vaccine against leprosy.)

How accurately can results from animal studies be applied to humans? Caution is needed in interpreting the results. If an animal is injured by an environmental pollutant, does it follow, then, that a human being must be as well? The answer is: Often, but not always.

Although animals are like humans in many of the most basic physiologic ways, there are crucial differences between other animal species and humans that can affect the outcome.

Different species react in different ways when exposed to chemicals. In the case of dioxin, for example, rats, guinea pigs, and hamsters all developed abnormalities and lesions when exposed—but not in the same way. The liver in rats is most seriously affected, although guinea pigs appear to be 1,000 times more sensitive than rats to the toxic chemical. This leaves the tantalizing question of whether human reactions are more like those of the laboratory rat or the guinea pig.

Reactions to other chemicals also separate along species lines: Nitrobenzene, a chemical toxic to humans, affects cats and dogs but is far less potent for rats, rabbits, and even monkeys, the latter animal being physiologically closest to humans in most ways. The industrial chemical triorthocresyl phosphate damages nerve fibers in chickens as well as humans but not in dogs or rats.

A hazard toxic to one animal species is not necessarily toxic to humans. For example, when administered during pregnancy, cortisone can produce a cleft palate in infant mice but not in humans. In general, though, if toxicity is shown to occur in a number of species, the case for potential harm to humans is strengthened.

It also does not necessarily mean that substances safe for animals are not hazardous to humans. Perhaps the most tragic result of this type of inconsistency between species occurred with the drug thalidomide, which is effective in preventing nausea and inducing sleep. After being thoroughly tested for its general toxicity in tests with rats, it was prescribed to pregnant women (primarily in Europe) in the 1960s. The offspring of mother rats who had been given thalidomide had been perfectly normal; humans, however, metabolize thalidomide differently, and the drug proved to cause structural malformations to the fetuses developing in the wombs of women who had taken the drug (see Box 11.2, p. 232).

Box 2.5 POOLING RESULTS: METAANALYSIS

The need to increase the precision of the various scientific tools available led to the development of the technique of metaanalysis. The prefix *meta* means "sharing," and that is precisely how metaanalysis works. Researchers pool the results of a group of

(*continued*)

Box 2.5   POOLING RESULTS: METAANALYSIS (*continued*)

studies. The technique is particularly useful when individual studies are small and the results inconsistent; metaanalysis can help reconcile some of the questions of precision.

For example, let's say that eight toxicity studies of the effects of a pesticide give the following contradictory results: In three, a large number of cancers was induced; in another three, part of the control group did more poorly than the experimental animals, and in two, some animals died and others thrived. Comparable methods were used in all the studies, but the studies differed in size. Owing to this, the results may not be as contradictory as they seem. Metaanalysis of the eight studies would make an overall conclusion that is more precise than that of any of the eight singly.

---

*   *   *

The task of establishing links between elements in the environment and human health effects is obviously not a simple one. More often than not, it is an arduous process that can take many forms; can be complicated by myriad factors; and can require a great deal of time, resources, and deductive insight. However, it is also an area of science that has produced a number of proven methods for understanding the environment's role in disease and has yielded a number of valuable successes. Understanding the means by which scientists uncover these links can help us to explore the issues of environmental health with greater confidence and less fear of the unknown.

CHAPTER 3

How We Perceive Risks and How Scientists Measure Them

In a psychological study, participants were asked to rate the probability of a flood occurring in California and killing hundreds of people. The participants estimated the risk at virtually zero. They were then asked about the probability of an earthquake occurring in California and setting off a flood that would kill hundreds of people. They rated the probability of this occurrence as high.

Why would people come up with such wildly differing assessments? Neither judgment was based on more information about California than the other; the difference lay in the participants' *perception* of the facts. When the chance of flooding was linked with the chance of earthquakes which are well publicized in connection with the state of California, the perceived possibility of flooding suddenly became much greater.

This study highlights an important issue confronting those seeking to battle or avoid environmental health risks. We prioritize our public environmental policies and our private health habits based on what we perceive to be the greatest risks to our health, and often, these perceptions are at odds with what scientists have to say.

THE PERCEPTION GAP: THE EXPERTS AND THE PUBLIC

In 1987, the EPA assigned a task force of seventy-five environmental experts to rate in terms of their relative riskiness thirty-one environmental hazards that are regulated by the EPA. The task force based its evaluations both on four aspects of the hazard—did it cause cancer? cause other health effects? damage the ecology? damage welfare (materials and property)?—and upon the number of people potentially affected.

The group placed the hazards in general categories of high, medium, and low risk; they also attempted to rank the hazards within those categories where possible. Hazards that were judged high in three of the four categories and that also affected a great number of people were rated higher than hazards receiving high scores in just one or two categories, or those that affected fewer people.

(Note that the task force did not evaluate cigarette smoking, since it is not under EPA regulation. Had they included it, tobacco smoke, which covers both individual and environmental tobacco smoke, would likely have outstripped many of the other hazards in reaching the top positions, both in terms of damage that it causes and the number of people affected.)

One year later, the Roper Organization conducted a poll of Americans on their perceptions of environmental risks (see Table 3.1). Although subjects were not given the four criteria for judgment used by the EPA task force, their assignment was essentially the same: to rate a list of environmental hazards as high, medium, or low risk. It turned out that the public disagreed with the experts more often than they agreed: While both the public and the task force concur that worker exposure to chemicals in the workplace presents a major risk, their views or other issues diverged, sometimes dramatically.

What did the public rank as posing the greatest potential danger? Hazardous waste sites were selected by two-thirds of people questioned. The experts classify the risks associated with hazardous waste sites as medium to low on the basis that comparatively few people are potentially affected.

Industrial accidents releasing pollutants also received one of the highest risk ratings from the public. The experts felt it presented a moderate to low risk (for the same reasons cited above.)

Sixty percent of the public said accidental oil spills represent one of the greatest of all dangers. Once again, the experts did not agree; they rated

Table 3.1: PUBLIC VERSUS EXPERT RANKINGS OF ENVIRONMENTAL RISKS[a]

Roper Poll[b]	Experts
1. Hazardous waste sites	Medium to low
2. Workplace chemicals	High
3. Industrial waterway pollution	Low
6. Chemical leaks from underground storage tanks	Medium to low
7. Pesticides	High
8. Pollution from industrial accidents	Medium to low
9. Water pollution from farm runoff	Medium
10. Tap-water contamination	High
11. Industrial air pollution	High
12. Ozone-layer destruction	High
13. Coastal water contamination	Low
14. Sewage plant water pollution	Medium to low
15. Vehicle exhaust	High
16. Oil spills	Medium to low
17. Acid rain	High
18. Water pollution from urban runoff	Medium
19. Damaged wetlands	Low
20. Genetic alteration	Low
21. Nonhazardous waste sites	Medium to low
22. Greenhouse effect	Low
23. Indoor air pollution	High
25. Indoor radon	High

[a] Public rankings of twenty-two environmental risks, as measured by a 1988 Roper Organization poll, were compared with the assessments of the same risks by an EPA task force of seventy-five environmental experts.

[b] This listing omits four of the twenty-six hazards ranked in the Roper poll, because they were not rated by the EPA task force. These four hazards—nuclear accident radiation, radioactive waste, X-ray radiation, and microwave oven radiation—were ranked fourth, fifth, twenty-fourth, and twenty-sixth by the public, respectively. It also omits some categories assessed by the task force that did not correspond directly to any of the hazards on the Roper list.

it relatively low in relation to other environmental hazards.

The task force experts rated radon a top environmental health hazard, but an overwhelming majority of the survey's respondents—83 percent—overlooked it as a significant threat.

The public did agree with the EPA's evaluation that depletion of stratospheric ozone poses a great ecological risk, but they considered the effect on human health as negligible. (In fact, they did not rank it as a risk at all.) In contrast, the EPA experts put the effect on human health in the high-risk category.

Box 3.1 RISK PERCEPTION: A SELF-TEST

The following list contains a number of environmental issues that have received attention in recent years. While reading this list, ask yourself whether each hazard poses for you a relatively high risk, a medium risk, or a low risk:

- An industrial accident that releases toxic chemicals into the air.
- Radioactive radon gas, released from the soil, that seeps into homes through cracks in the basement.
- Deposits of buried hazardous waste.
- Oil spills resulting from accidents involving oil tankers and offshore drilling stations.
- Pollution of the waterways from industrial effluents.
- Pollution of the air in the home and office.
- Contamination of soil and groundwater from underground chemical and gasoline tanks.
- Acid rain resulting from industrial emissions.

A U.S. Environmental Protection Agency (EPA) task force of experts has ranked these hazards and others in terms of their relative riskiness. Hazards are ranked in descending order of perceived riskiness, with position number one considered to pose the greatest risk. You can compare your assessments with those of the task force as listed in Table 3.1. The difference may surprise you.

Such differences in perception are more than just a curiosity. If the public and the experts do not see eye to eye on precisely what are the greatest environmental risks, they are unlikely to agree on what measures should be taken to reduce health risks. Not surprisingly, elected officials and policymakers may be influenced by public opinion as much, if not more, than by scientific data. The existing governmental priorities toward environmental risks are more often in line with the public's opinions expressed in the Roper poll than the scientific experts' opinions.

Why Public Versus Expert Opinions Diverge

It is not surprising that the public does not see eye to eye with the experts on these matters considering that the two groups have significantly different vantage points on risk.

Experts define risk in terms of probability and populations—the odds of harm occurring to a certain percentage of the population and the overall severity of the damage. A major priority of the experts is to protect the greatest number of people the greatest amount of time (see Risk Assessment, p. 48).

On the other hand, the public views things from a personal vantage point, projecting themselves into the situation of the people affected by a given hazard. Their assessment of risk does not primarily depend upon the likelihood of a hazard being realized; rather, they will ask, "How seriously would this affect *me*—or my family or my community—if it were to happen here?" The individual counts most heavily in the public's equation of risk.

Viewed this way, it makes sense that hazardous waste sites—rated low by the experts because, *in general*, they do not pose a great threat for a significant portion of population—are viewed as high risks by the public: They might pose a high risk to *an individual* if he or she lived close to a hazardous waste site.

Human nature plays a role in the public's assessment of risk, and the cold facts of fatality and injury simply are not enough to convince us that something is dangerous or that it is safe. When judging their own health, for example, most individuals believe that their own fate will be better than that of their neighbors—a fallacy in reasoning that underlies the difficulty of convincing people to change even the most dangerous habits, such as engaging in unprotected sexual intercourse, driving while intoxicated, smoking cigarettes, not wearing seat belts, or eating meals that are low in fruits and vegetables and high in fats.

Our judgment of risks is also affected by psychological and cultural factors—deep-seated fears, moral and spiritual values, habitual patterns of thought—as well as by the manner in which information about risks is communicated to us.

The subject of how we perceive risk is of notable importance, therefore, in understanding how and why we act—or do not respond—in the face of environmental threats. Risk perception has been studied for the better part of two decades by a number of researchers. (In the section that follows, we have relied upon the extensive work of Dr. Peter Sandman and researchers at the Rutgers Environmental Communication Research Program, who have been among the leaders in this field.) What these researchers have pinpointed are a variety of factors—really, dichotomous qualities about an event—that will color how risky or safe we interpret circumstances to be (see Table 3.2).

Radon: An Ignored Threat

Radon is a classic example of how these dichotomies influence the perception of risk.

Radon is a naturally occurring, odorless gas that is generated by the natural breakdown (radioactive decay) of uranium present in certain rocks and soil; it can seep into the basements of houses built on such rocks and soil, accumulating to high levels. In the United States, between 5,000 and 30,000 lung cancer deaths *each year* are attributed to radon exposure.

The EPA and the New Jersey State Health Department estimate that almost one-third of the homes in northern New Jersey have enough radon seeping into their basements to pose a greater than one in one hundred lifetime risk of lung cancer. Initially, New Jersey public health officials prepared themselves to deal with the public panic they believed would ensue when this information was publicized. Instead, they have found themselves dealing with a quite different response: apathy.

Less than *5 percent* of North Jersey homeowners have availed themselves of the relatively simple, inexpensive tests available to monitor radon in the home (see Box 14.8, p. 559). The task that confronts New Jersey health officials is to educate a public that *underestimates* this risk.

How does the list of risk dichotomies account for the public's perception of radon as not risky? To begin with, radon is a natural hazard, not an artificial one. It is present in a familiar environment, the home, an environment over which we feel we exert great control. The hazard is diffuse

Table 3.2: COMPONENTS OF INTERPRETING RISK

Hazards having these characterics appear less risky	*Hazards having these characteristics appear* more risky
Voluntary (e.g., not wearing seatbelts)	Coerced (e.g., a garbage dump built without your permission)
Familiar (e.g., secondhand smoke)	Exotic (e.g., food irradiation)
Natural (e.g., radon)	Artificial (e.g., X rays)
Controllable (e.g., personal habits)	Uncontrollable (e.g., natural disasters)
Individual control (e.g., household pest spray)	Controlled by others (e.g., public insect spraying)
Fair (e.g., polluter gets hurt)	Unfair (e.g., one person pollutes, but another gets hurt)
Not memorable (a hazard that one has never seen or heard of)	Memorable (a hazard that one has experienced or seen in the media)
Not dreaded (e.g., one that causes emphysema)	Dreaded (e.g., one that causes cancer)
Not fatal (e.g., greenhouse effect)	Fatal (e.g., toxic gas release)
Chronic (happens consistently over time)	Acute (sporadic but intense, e.g., an oil spill)
High trust (e.g., pronounced safe by a physician)	Low trust (e.g., one pronounced safe by a chemical company)
Moral (e.g., equal risk to all)	Moral irrelevance (e.g., harms children)
Diffuse in time and space (e.g., kills 500 over the course of year)	Focused in time and space (e.g., kills 500 per decade, but all at once)
Immediate (effects of exposure certain and instant, e.g., gas explosions)	Delayed (effects of exposure take years to develop, e.g., asbestos)
Knowable (one knows if one is exposed, e.g., sunlight)	Unknowable (one does not necessarily know if one is exposed, e.g., invisible ionizing radiation)
Individual mitigation possible (e.g., poor diet)	No individual mitigation possible (e.g., toxic dumping into water)
Detectable (e.g., auto exhaust)	Undetectable (e.g., invisible radiation)

in time and space; if all 30,000 or even 5,000 deaths occurred on the same day, we would take more notice. Importantly, no one is coercing us into accepting the risks, since we choose to remain in our homes, and radon is a "natural" phenomenon.

A little twist to this story underscores these points: As reported in the EPA booklet by Peter Sandman, *Explaining Environmental Risk*, three New Jersey communities faced a radon problem due to an artificial source, a landfill that incorporated radioactive industrial wastes. Radon readings in these homes were *no higher* than those in many homes on natural hot spots, but fear and outrage in the community was so high and so successfully mobilized that the government was persuaded to spend hundreds of thousands of dollars per home to clean up the landfill.

When the state proposed to dilute the soil to near-background levels of radon and dispose of it in an abandoned quarry in the rural community of Vernon, it provoked the largest environmental protests in years.

Some Important Dichotomies of Risk Perception

As with radon, many cultural hazards—what people eat and drink; where and how they live and work; their sexual practices; and whether or not they smoke, consume alcohol, or sunbathe—are often underestimated because they are familiar, voluntary, and natural (particularly compared with chemical, physical, or biological hazards). Unfortunately, although cultural hazards *seem* less risky, they account for as much as 60 percent of the fatalities and illnesses associated with the environment (see Chapter 22, "The ABCs of Staying Healthy").

At the other extreme of this high-risk/low-risk schematic is the physical hazard of ionizing radiation (the type present in nuclear power plants and atomic explosions). Most people view radiation exposure in almost any form with fear and trepidation. Radiation has many of the hallmarks from the "more risky" column of Table 3.2: It is *artificial* rather than natural; it is *controlled by someone else* and involuntary; its technological complexity makes it seem *exotic* to most of us; it causes one of the more *dreaded* outcomes (cancer); it can be fatal; it affects both the innocent and the "guilty" (*unfair*); we associate it with horrific images of *memorable* events that crystallize its dangers (Hiroshima and Nagasaki, the explosion of the Chernobyl nuclear reactor); and we have had previous experiences that may cause us to question the *trustworthiness* of the authorities whose expertise we rely upon to protect us.

There is one classic exception to the public's fear of radiation: sunlight. Despite the fact that ultraviolet light from the sun is also a form of radiation (see Chapter 16, "Radiant Energy")—one that can cause sunburn, premature aging of the skin, skin cancers, and cataracts—millions of people expose themselves to this hazard voluntarily. The risks inherent in this behavior are increasingly well publicized, yet we respond to this *familiar, controllable, voluntary, unmemorable,* and *natural* hazard with the same type of apathy apparent in our regard for radon.

High Trust Versus Low Trust. A product comes on the market and is later suspected of possibly causing adverse health effects. In one case, it turns out that the company knew of the potential danger but concealed the data, and once the news was out, the corporate response was cold and unfeeling. The public's trust in this company and its product is shattered.

In another case, a company immediately admits its fault, compensates those who are wronged, and sets in motion the procedures for assuring that the safety of its products will be checked in the future. The public responds positively to such responsible behavior, and the product is not seen as quite so risky. For example, when benzene contamination was found in Perrier bottled water, the company's voluntary and immediate recall of 72 million bottles weighed heavily in its favor; although sales of Perrier obviously plummeted at first, public trust in this company and product allowed the bottled water to regain a large portion of its previous market share.

Familiar Versus Exotic. Residents who live near an abandoned hazardous waste site express their outrage most loudly when the cleanup of the site begins. Until that time, many are prepared to put up with the mess because they have become used to it—it is commonplace, part of their familiar background environment. The commonplace risk is transformed into an exotic, "riskier" risk as soon as high-technology equipment arrives on the scene and engineers dressed in protective "spacesuit" outfits begin working at the site.

Natural Versus Artificial. Artificial substances, such as food additives and pesticide residues, are seen as carrying more health risks than natural substances, such as disease-causing bacteria, lead, and aflatoxins contaminating food, even though the natural substances cause greater harm to a greater number of people.

Controlled by Individual Versus Controlled by Others.

Many of us are convinced that exposure to outdoor air pollution, over which we exercise little individual control, produces more cancers and respiratory disorders than smoking, a hazard within our individual control—even though the opposite is scientifically true.

Voluntary Versus Coerced.

A corporation purchases land in a community and announces that it is putting up a manufacturing plant that the community fears will release pollutants into the air or local waters. Despite the employment gains, the citizenry is outraged; they feel forced to assume health risks against their will and perceive the risks as high; community groups organize effectively enough to block—at least temporarily—the building of the plant.

In another scenario, representatives of the same company meet with the chamber of commerce and the citizens groups and offer to pay the community's costs of hiring independent experts to evaluate the site. The company promises that construction will begin only if an agreement is reached with the community and offers to compensate anyone who is affected adversely. The building of the plant proceeds unopposed (the risks are viewed as minimal), and the community appreciates the economic gains in terms of jobs.

It is not the compensation alone that overcomes the objections: The opportunity to say yes or no to the presence of the manufacturing plant makes it seem that the plant—effluents and all—is not as risky as initially perceived.

A Pitfall in Communicating Risk.

Most people bridle when presented with risk comparisons that juxtapose a voluntary risk and an involuntary risk. The association of sunbathing with exposure to radiation from a nuclear explosion, for example, strikes most people as belittling of their intelligence and the seriousness of their concerns.

Consider this hypothetical example: A committee of experts is convened to determine how to allocate a limited amount of funds for eliminating environmental health risks. Several community activists have urged the committee to concentrate the resources on reducing the dangers from a certain pesticide that has received much recent media attention. Instead, the committee recommends that the money be put toward efforts to reduce smoking, contending that the risks of heart disease and cancer from direct and passive smoke far outweigh the potential harm of the pesticide. Even though the committee would be on firm scientific ground—tobacco use is acknowledged to cause over 400,000 deaths annually in America—the public would likely be outraged at the recommendation. Many people would suspect that the committee (perhaps in collusion with the pesticide manufacturer) was dismissing their concerns and sending the message: Quit smoking, and stop demanding that companies make their products safer!

In reality, of course, such situations are rarely so clear-cut. Governments and groups allocate resources in varying amounts to a number of concerns, and whether one uses a certain pesticide is not inextricably linked with whether or not one smokes. Nonetheless, the principle of communication still applies in many real situations.

Moral Relevance Versus Moral Irrelevance.

Protecting children and other vulnerable groups is one of society's moral imperatives. Any risk that endangers children trespasses on this mandate and is consistently overestimated; even the most solid scientific evidence that challenges this perception will be resisted.

Moral relevance was at the heart of the public outcry in 1989 against the use of Alar, a chemical used primarily on apples to ripen them uniformly and enhance their red color. When Alar breaks down, one of the substances formed has been shown to cause cancers in animals. Exposure to carcinogens early in life is considered particularly dangerous. Since children are major consumers of apple juice, getting Alar off the market became the focus of a 10,000-member citizen's group called Mothers & Others for Pesticide Limits. The group was formed under the auspices of the National Resources Defense Council, whose studies of the cancer risk of Alar and other pesticides concluded that these risks are "intolerable" (see Chapter 17, "Food Safety"). Other risk assessment experts disagreed, stating that the danger posed was negligible (the quantities of the substance consumed by the test animals were enormous in comparison to the quantities consumed by human children). Since children were involved—and protecting them is a *moral imperative*—many parents (and many pediatricians in their advice to parents) decided to err on the side of caution and avoid apple juice, at least for one apple-growing season. Unable to withstand the outcry, the apple growers ceased using Alar, even though the EPA had not proposed a ban on it.

Beginning to Understand Our Choices

Appreciating human nature, the lens through which we perceive information about safety and danger, will help us to more effectively make the personal—and public—decisions that affect us and our communities. However, it is not just human nature and psychology alone that account for the difficulty of reconciling the assessments of experts with our own. We want the experts to give us solid information, and they give us the best that science has to offer. We suspect, though, that the "truth" cannot really be known. To some extent we are correct: The scientific enterprise involved in assessing the risks of environmental hazards does contain uncertainties.

Understanding, even generally, how scientists identify hazards and measure and evaluate the risks associated with them can help us to feel more confident in the face of conflicting reports. It is these scientific approaches that we will examine next.

RISK ASSESSMENT: CALCULATING THE ODDS OF HARM

When the EPA task force experts set out to prioritize the thirty-one hazards under the agency's purview (see p. 41), ranking them relative to each other using such criteria as the extent and seriousness of the potential damage, it was the first time that these EPA-regulated environmental hazards had been systematically evaluated. Their approach, however, was not novel; rather, it was a form of an established scientific practice termed *risk assessment*.

Risk assessment deals with probabilities (odds) and populations (large groups of people) rather than individuals to estimate how likely or unlikely is the chance that the group will suffer adverse effects of exposure to some factor. In this process, a scientist asks, "What is the agent that causes harm?" and then goes on to system-

atically compile information on a number of important aspects of the hazard. The ultimate goal is to come up with a number or rank order that, it is hoped, expresses the probability that a hazard will cause harm.

On the surface, the process that is used by the EPA as well as many other groups of scientists and policymakers seems straightforward and clear-cut. In reality, however, there are many uncertainties that are introduced or must be embraced at almost every step along the way. Some of the uncertainties stem from assumptions inherent in the scientific "tools" at our disposal (see Table 3.3, and Chapter 2, "Illness and the Environment: Finding the Links"), whereas others stem from a sheer lack of information.

EPA's Approach to Risk Assessment

The EPA uses a four-part model of risk assessment:

• *Identifying the hazard.* What is the agent that causes harm? What is its biological mechanism? How serious is the damage done?
• *Determining dose response.* What amount is toxic? Does the response follow a linear dose–response model or a threshold model?
• *Estimating exposure.* How much of the agent was present in the ambient environment? How much of it likely reached its target site in the body?
• *Characterizing the risks.* Just how risky is this hazard? What is the probability—in numbers—that it will harm us? How serious is the harm likely to be? Are any of us particularly susceptible to being harmed? How sure are we about our results?

Identifying the hazard. Singling out one hazard from all the others in the world is one of the greatest challenges in assessing environmental risks. Just as the background noise in a restaurant or busy city street can drown out the voices of two people trying to converse, there is a background level for disease. People are exposed to many different toxic agents, and it is almost impossible to consider and experimentally control for all variables that can potentially affect an observed association between a toxic agent and a particular substance. This problem often crops up when people react to substances in food, such as sulfites. The symptoms of such a reaction could also stem from causes as diverse as stress, household products, and substances handled at work. Even once the problem is diagnosed as stemming from food, the cause still must be sifted from a vast number of factors—where a person eats, how the food is prepared, all the foods and beverages that compose a diet.

Astute clinical observations and epidemiologic studies are often the basis for initially isolating a hazard. Finding out what kinds of harm it causes and its adverse biological effects are also part of the process of identification. Does this agent burn us (fire), starve our cells of life-giving oxygen (carbon monoxide), cause structural malformations to developing fetuses (thalidomide), induce cells to ignore the boundaries of their neighbors or interrupt the cell's mechanism to put a brake on growth (benzene), both of which could lead to tumor development? Does this hazard shorten life, cause a disabling illness or injury, cause a temporary and reversible ailment, or result in passing physical discomfort or psychological reactions?

Toxic agents exert their effects at particular points in the body, or *target sites.* Knowing their biological effects enables the researcher to identify a reasonable endpoint to study—damage to the lung's structures, growth of a particular kind of cancer, structural birth defects, as examples—in order to estimate the potential of the agent to harm.

Since not all harmful effects are equal—a skin rash may not be life-threatening, but damage to the nervous system may be—part of identifying the hazard is specifying how serious is the damage it causes.

Determining harmful amounts (dose–response curves). What quantity—or dose—of this agent is toxic? Most medical research, including what we know of the effects of environmental pollutants, poisons, and therapeutic drugs, relies on animal studies. (Such clinical research on humans is not considered ethical.) Results are then extrapolated from these studies to humans to predict how much of a chemical or agent is harmful.

Numerous uncertainties are introduced into this endeavor, only one reason being that animal subjects do not always respond as humans do (see Chapter 2, "Illness and the Environment: Finding the Links"). Taking the results observed using high doses and extrapolating to low doses—as is done in toxicology tests on an-

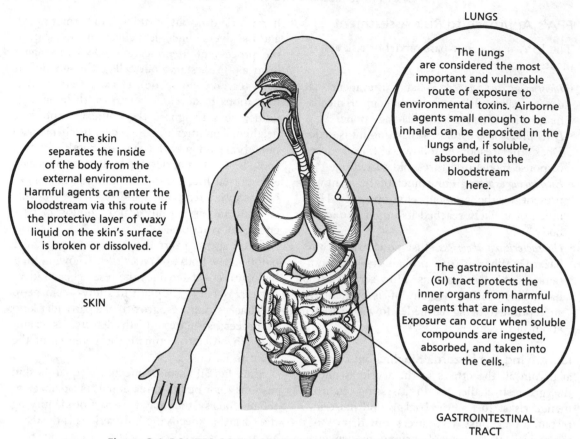

The skin separates the inside of the body from the external environment. Harmful agents can enter the bloodstream via this route if the protective layer of waxy liquid on the skin's surface is broken or dissolved.

SKIN

LUNGS

The lungs are considered the most important and vulnerable route of exposure to environmental toxins. Airborne agents small enough to be inhaled can be deposited in the lungs and, if soluble, absorbed into the bloodstream here.

The gastrointestinal (GI) tract protects the inner organs from harmful agents that are ingested. Exposure can occur when soluble compounds are ingested, absorbed, and taken into the cells.

GASTROINTESTINAL TRACT

Figure 3.1 ROUTES OF EXPOSURE TO ENVIRONMENTAL AGENTS.

Exposure to toxic substances in the environment occurs through three major pathways: the skin, the gastrointestinal tract, and the lungs.

imals—means making certain assumptions that are subject to debate.

If we start with a dose of a substance that causes most animals to sicken or die and then work down to a dose that can be assumed to be "virtually safe," we may assume that the harmful effects accrue in proportion to the dose, or in a linear manner. For example, this assumes that if 100 grams of a substance causes impairment, then 10 grams of the substance will cause one-tenth of the effect. This type of *linear dose response* is often assumed, particularly for potentially carcinogenic substances.

However, some substances are not observably harmful until an individual is exposed to a cer-

tain amount. Substantial harm is seen at 100 grams, for example, but no harm *at all* is seen until 30 grams is reached. This type of *threshold dose response* is exemplified by vitamin B_6; a valuable nutrient needed by the body, the vitamin becomes toxic when taken in high doses. Furthermore, it may be that harm does not accrue in a gradual manner but is relatively negligible at lower levels, then skyrockets as the dose is raised above a certain level.

The effects of these assumptions are not just academic. Depending on which assumption we choose about the *dose–response relationship*, we may come up with an entirely different standard for a safe dose. This is the source of a number of controversies surrounding policies for such substances as additives in food, in which no dose of a carcinogenic substance is considered safe (see Chapter 17, "Food Safety"), chemicals in the workplace, outdoor air pollutants, pesticide residues, and even the optimal percentage of fat in the diet.

Determining exposure. The type and extent of exposure to a hazard is key in determining its harmfulness. No matter how harmful an agent may be, we are not at risk if we are not exposed to it—and just being in the vicinity of a hazard does not mean we are exposed to it. (See the asbestos example, p. 24.)

Scientists have access to a number of tools and approaches for monitoring and analyzing substances at a site. The method chosen depends on the substance being measured and the goals of the study; for example, techniques or equipment that are adept at measuring the fluctuating concentrations of a substance at a given site over time may not be sensitive enough to measure minute amounts of substances at a specific time. Table 3.3 compares some methods that can be used to measure substances in the air.

To calculate exposure, researchers often collect data on a hazardous substance at the site where it is released, but by the time it has been diffused in air or water, changes may have occurred that transform it into a different substance altogether. Once a substance is inside the body, metabolic processes alter it further. Measurements *should* deal with the substance in all its forms, but such types of exposure data are difficult and expensive to collect.

The exposure that really counts is the amount that reaches the target site, where the agent can do damage.

Table 3.3: METHODS OF SAMPLING ENVIRONMENTAL POLLUTANTS

Method	Advantages	Disadvantages
Monitoring physical stresses (e.g., radiation) over time	Monitors placed in the field can measure long-term exposure levels	Monitor can disrupt area being monitored, jeopardizing integrity of measurement; equipment may be expensive
Sampling air for respirable-sized particulates	Data more directly predicts exposure within lungs	Overlooks particles too large to be respirated, which can affect mouth, nose, and throat
Sampling air for all particulates	Includes large particulates that can be absorbed through skin or ingested	Does not give specific data on lung exposure
Collecting settled particulate matter	Sample reflects a specific time period and region	Weather can disperse settled particles; only larger particles will settle
Collecting concentrated sample of gases	Can be analyzed in lab, so lower gas concentrations are detected more easily and accurately	Chemical reactions in lab or in sample may alter sample, so it may differ from air at collection site
Monitoring gases on-site	Data reflects conditions directly at site; study can be extended over time	Monitoring equipment and conditions may be less sensitive than those available in laboratory

Source: Dade W. Moeller, *Environmental Health* (Cambridge, MA: Harvard University Press, 1992), pp. 235–37.

It is obviously impractical, unethical, or infeasible to take such internal measurements. In some cases, scientists can gain valuable perspective on internal doses by searching for *biomarkers*—biochemical or cellular alterations that are produced in the metabolism of a toxin or created by the body's response to the presence of the toxin. Such biologic markers hold promise in opening up methods for determining individual susceptibility to environmental toxins, and as a more precise method for determining that exposure to a toxin in the environment has actually occurred at a meaningful site within the body. Biomarkers can also be used to detect signs of early effects of potentially toxic substances—signs that show up before the first stages of impairment or disease are evident.

The existence of so many uncertainties in estimating exposure explains, in part, why scientists often come up with markedly different estimates of risk—estimates that confound, confuse, and frustrate the public. Once again, these issues underlie debates on policies and standards that are intended to protect the public from exposure to harmful environmental agents.

Characterizing the risks. To put together all of this information, we also need to know if there are other factors that may be important, such as whether there are particular subgroups of people who are more susceptible to exposure or to the adverse effects (children, the elderly, people with certain diseases, women who are pregnant or their developing fetuses, or workers in certain occupations, for example). How do personal habits, diet, age, or genetic predisposition affect the risks?

Another very important factor is exposure to other hazards. For example, multiple hazards are often encountered together, and deleterious effects can arise when two or more harmful agents interact. The hazards can interact in a way that simply combines their potential destructive effects (additive) or in ways that increase them many times more (multiplicative or synergistic). Synergistic effects are not uncommon: The combined effects of tobacco smoke and radon encountered together are much greater than the sum of their individual effects, and the same holds true for tobacco smoke and asbestos (see Box 3.2).

Box 3.2   SYNERGISTIC EFFECTS OF TOBACCO SMOKE AND ASBESTOS

Both cigarette smokers and people who are exposed to asbestos increase their chances of developing lung cancer, but people exposed to *both* agents increase their vulnerability vastly. Compared to a person who neither smokes nor comes into contact with asbestos, a person who smokes two packs per day who is not exposed to asbestos is approximately ten times more likely to develop lung cancer. Someone exposed to asbestos and who does not smoke has a five times greater risk. A person who *both* smokes two packs per day and who is exposed to asbestos, however, has a *fifty* times greater risk of lung cancer—a risk much greater than the sum of the risks of asbestos and smoking separately.

There are thousands of toxic chemicals as well as nontoxic substances, such as medications, that can interact with them, and it is simply not feasible to test for all potential adverse interactions. Ultimately, the end result of the risk assessment is a *risk characterization*. Sometimes, it is a numerical expression of the risks (there's a 50–50 likelihood of harm occurring under such and such terms of exposure). Sometimes it is a ranking or rating relative to other risks, as in the case of the EPA task force rating of the thirty-one hazards discussed earlier (see Table 3.1).

Limitations of Risk Assessment

Risk assessment cannot adequately address a number of important hazards—such as electromagnetic fields, for which it is not possible to decide if there is a dose–response effect on the basis of animal experiments to date. Nonetheless, because it is crucial that we address the risks associated with such hazards, scientists at the National Academy of Sciences and the EPA currently are refining their approach and should release updated guidelines in the mid-1990s.

Risk assessments are also only as good as the data they are based upon, and much of the information about environmental health hazards is incomplete or relies on debatable (and hotly debated) assumptions. In many areas, we simply lack sufficient data.

The effects of many hazards depend on how long the exposure lasts and whether the dose is received at once or continuously over time. Many of these details of exposure are not yet quantified and cannot yet be adequately accounted for when making an assessment of risks.

Risk assessment, like all scientific endeavors, is imperfect, given the complexities of nature. However, like many other scientific activities, it still yields useful, relevant information. Judgments about risks are needed by legislators to set sensible national pollution standards, physicians to counsel their patients on which course of action to take to enhance health or treat a disease, and individuals to minimize their chances of being harmed by encounters with untoward agents and circumstances in the outside world.

The Environment's Effects on the Body

CHAPTER 4

Skin Ailments

As long as human beings have walked the earth, the environment has affected their skin. One of the earliest reports of an environmentally caused skin reaction came from ancient Egypt, where the sages of antiquity described the way contact with certain plants affect the skin in the presence of sunlight. Although the Egyptians did not specifically identify the chemicals in these plants, which are called *psoralens* and are activated by sunlight, their astute observation pointed to the complexity and the ubiquity of chemicals in our environment.

Three thousand years later, the list of environmental agents that can adversely affect the skin has greatly expanded to cover chemicals used at work or in the home, organisms that are found in plants and animals and their products, and, most important, chronic exposure to the sun. It is ironic that many people live in fear of exposure to chemicals in the environment, yet may regularly sunbathe despite the alarming rise in skin cancer related to sun exposure.

An estimated 30 percent of Americans each year develop a dermatological condition that requires treatment by a physician. On the work front (excluding injuries and accidents, which are responsible for most illness among workers), occupational skin diseases account for about one-half of all other work-related illnesses reported in the United States. It has been estimated that about 1 in every 1,000 workers develops an oc-cupational skin disease—primarily contact dermatitis (see p. 62). Skin problems that arise from the job environment may be simply annoying or may cause people to lose time from work or find a new occupation.

In rare cases, an outbreak of a dermatological "problem" can trigger public fear. A case in point was the mysterious "red sweat" that occurred in 1980 among flight attendants who worked on the New York to Miami route of a major airline. The symptoms were tiny red spots that appeared on the stewardesses' arms after takeoff; this phenomenon caused a great deal of alarm after several attendants developed it.

The airline called in a team of dermatologists from a major medical center in New York to solve the mystery. At first, the stewardesses were taken directly to the medical center for tests after landing, but by then the redness had disappeared. Next, a dermatologist flew to Miami with the crew to try to determine in flight what culprit was causing the red spots.

As the search for the offending agent continued, one medical investigator observed that on each flight, the stewardesses handled a demonstration life raft imprinted with a red stamp. The dermatologists took samples of the stamp and the red spots on the attendants' skin. A chemical analysis showed identical ingredients: tiny bits of red paint. The mystery was solved.

In this case, fear and anxiety were the main

symptoms. Fortunately, there was a solution to the problem and no lasting effect on the skin. More often, once a person develops a rash or skin irritation in response to some substance in the environment, it may become a chronic problem. Sometimes the cause is apparent, for instance, when the hands become itchy and red after using a corrosive oven cleaner. Other times, it takes persistence to deduce the cause of a long-time skin rash.

All kinds of substances in the environment can cause skin reactions, as can all sorts of activities. Work heads the list of activities that can put us into contact with irritants or toxins that may adversely affect the skin. However, doing household chores, using cosmetics, cooking, pursuing hobbies, and enjoying leisure-time activities also may lead to skin reactions.

While it is now possible to prevent some problems by avoiding exposure to toxic substances, numerous new chemicals are introduced in industry and consumer products each year, and the reaction to these chemicals usually is not known until people begin reporting skin problems. The bottom line is that it takes solid medical detective work to diagnose many skin disorders that occur in response to contact with environmental agents.

THE STRUCTURE OF OUR SKIN

The skin is our largest and most visible organ. It is not just a wrapper that holds muscles, tissues, and organs in place, but an external barrier and sensory organ that plays a crucial role in protecting us from environmental insult while helping us to adapt to the external world. On an average-size person, the skin accounts for about 10 pounds of body weight, and extends over a surface area of 2 square meters.

Absorption of chemicals through the skin is a major route of exposure to environmental toxins. When the skin's protective barrier has been damaged or is subject to prolonged contact with a toxic substance, harmful chemicals may gain access to other body systems by absorption through the skin (also called *percutaneous absorption*). Numerous chemicals can enter the body in this way and effect other organs, including aniline dyes, arsenic, benzene, cyanide salts, mercury, methyl-*n*-butyl ketone, halogenated hydrocarbons, and pesticides.

Layers of the Skin

The skin is a waterproof mantle that helps control body temperature and conserve heat and moisture. In cold weather, blood vessels near the skin's surface constrict, decreasing blood flow and thus preventing heat loss. Hot weather causes increased blood flow and signals millions of sweat glands in the skin to produce perspiration to cool the skin.

Sebaceous glands in the skin secrete a greasy substance that helps protect the skin's surface against invasion by infectious agents and keeps the skin from drying out. In addition, the skin serves as home to specialized cells that prevent infectious and toxic agents from entering the body. The skin is a sensory organ containing nerve endings sensitive to changes in temperature, pain, and pressure, thus allowing us to react quickly to possible danger. The skin also works at manufacturing vitamin D through a chemical reaction with ultraviolet rays in sunlight—a process that helps the body use calcium properly.

Like any other organ, the skin has specialized cells that perform a variety of tasks. Its three layers—the epidermis, dermis, and subcutaneous fat—each play important roles in the skin's defensive and adaptive functions.

Epidermis. The outer layer is a very thin surface that measures, on average, a mere twenty cells thick. The first part of this tough outer, or horny, layer of skin consists of the *stratum corneum*. It is formed of tightly packed cells that have worked their way up from the deepest level of the epidermis to the surface for shedding. (It takes about four weeks for a skin cell to reach the surface.)

As skin cells make their way toward the surface to renew the stratum corneum, their appearance slowly changes, as does their function (see Figure 4.1c). In moving from the basal—or bottom—layer of the epidermis, up through the spiny layer and into the granular layer, the living cells transform themselves into the flattened, lifeless cells of the surface.

The principal cells of the epidermis are called *keratinocytes* because of the major constituent protein, *keratin*, that they contain. Keratins are tough structural proteins from which hair and nails also are formed. Keratinocytes are responsible for providing the skin's barrier function and are now under study for their role in a variety of inflammatory and immune reactions.

Melanocytes, which produce *melanin*, the pigmented material that imparts color to the skin, are dispersed among the keratinocytes in the lower cell layers. Melanin also offers some degree of protection from the sun because it absorbs some of the sun's ultraviolet radiation. When little or no melanin is present in the skin, there is a higher risk of injury from the sun.

An important immune cell that also resides in the epidermis is the *Langerhans cell*. Its job is to be a watchdog that recognizes foreign substances and alerts other immune cells, which can then mobilize and destroy the invader. Langerhans cells play an important role in allergic contact dermatitis (see p. 62).

Dermis. Directly below the epidermis lies the dermis, a tough but flexible layer of skin. The resilient tissue of the dermis derives its strength and elasticity from a combination of components, such as water and connective tissue (elastic and collagen fibers). Blood vessels, nerves, and other cells abound in the dermis and offer nourishment to the epidermis. Sweat glands, sebaceous glands that produce oil, and hair follicles originate deep in the dermis and pass through the epidermis.

Subcutaneous tissue. The tissue underneath the dermis provides a fatty cushion of insulation and protection to the skin and to internal structures such as bones and organs. It also serves as a reserve supply of nutrients for the cells (see Figure 4.1a).

Hair and Nails

The hair and nails also are a part of the skin. Although hair helps to retain body heat and protect the scalp from sunburn, it tends to be more appreciated for its aesthetic function than for any other purpose. The nails shield the sensitive tissue on the tips of your fingers and toes from injury and foreign organisms in the environment (see p. 80).

CHEMICALS AND SKIN DAMAGE

Several skin disorders and diseases may originate in response to environmental factors on the job and are sometimes termed *occupational dermatitis* as a group. Among these are sensitivity to light as a result of handling certain chemicals, allergic and irritant contact dermatitis, absorption of toxic substances into the body through the skin, disfiguring acne from various chemical products, and loss of skin color or permanently stained skin.

Eczema and Dermatitis

An array of household and cosmetic products, as well as substances used on the work front constantly increases our chances of encountering an ever-expanding array of environmental chemicals that cause the skin to develop eczema or dermatitis. Eczema and dermatitis are terms that have long been used interchangeably. Eczema takes its name from a Greek word that means "to

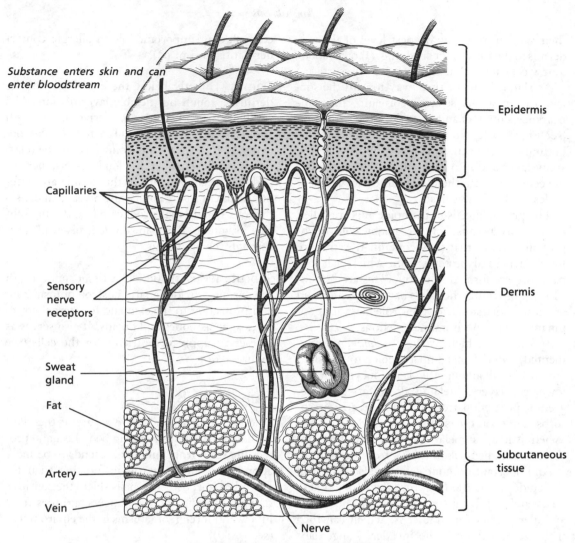

Substance enters skin and can enter bloodstream

Epidermis

Capillaries

Sensory nerve receptors

Dermis

Sweat gland

Fat

Artery

Subcutaneous tissue

Vein

Nerve

(a) THE MAJOR LAYERS OF THE SKIN

Figure 4.1 THE SKIN.

(a) The three major layers of the skin are shown: the epidermis, the dermis, and subcutaneous tissue. When potentially harmful environmental agents penetrate through breaks in the protective "horny" layer of the epidermis or gaps in the waxy coating secreted by the sebaceous glands, they can enter the dermis, attacking nerve receptors located there and/or entering the bloodstream.

bubble forth." Indeed, this description applies to the most acute phases of dermatitis, conditions characterized by a red and slightly scaly appearance, occasionally accompanied by blistering and itching.

Although the term *eczema* encompasses the many forms of dermatitis discussed in this chapter, including those that occur in response to the environment or a chemical agent that appears to have no clear cause, such as atopic dermatitis,

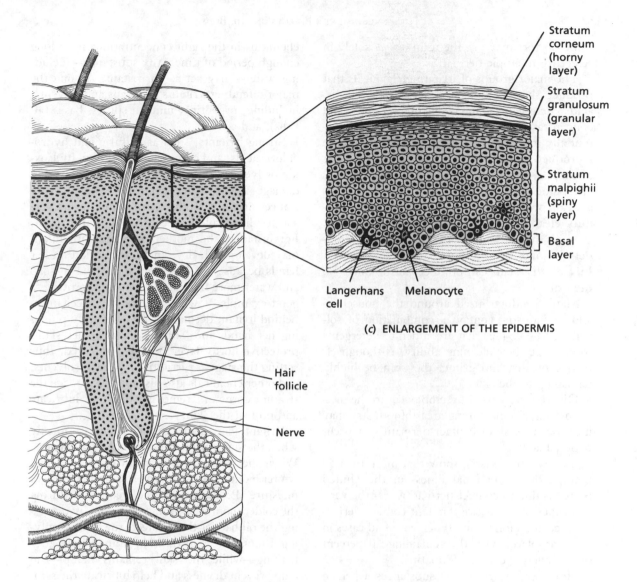

Stratum corneum (horny layer)

Stratum granulosum (granular layer)

Stratum malpighii (spiny layer)

Basal layer

Langerhans cell

Melanocyte

(c) ENLARGEMENT OF THE EPIDERMIS

Hair follicle

Nerve

(b) THE MAJOR LAYERS OF THE SKIN (CONTINUED)

Figure 4.1 THE SKIN.

(b) Hair follicles originate in the dermis and extend up through the epidermis.

(c) Close up of the epidermis. The appearance of skin cells changes slowly as they move from the bottom basal layer through the spiny layer (*stratum malpighii*) and the granular layer (*stratum granulosum*), becoming flattened, lifeless cells of the surface, or horny layer (*stratum corneum*).

some doctors may use the term *eczema* solely in reference to atopic dermatitis.

The major groups of irritating chemicals that produce skin reactions are classified as alkalis, acids, detergents, enzymes, solvents, oils, and concentrated salt solutions. Some of these potentially irritating substances may be present in a product in minimal amounts, such as in a bar of soap, which may be mildly alkaline. On the other side of the alkali spectrum are such items as drain openers, oven cleaners, and other heavy-duty cleaning products that can burn the skin.

Acids may be a major ingredient in such products as toilet bowl cleaners and drain openers. Like alkalis, acids can produce caustic burns on the skin.

Many products used around the household and in industry contain a combination of solvents and enzymes that are added to detergents to enhance their cleaning ability. Although effective on dirt and grime, they can be highly damaging to the skin.

Oils routinely used by employees in the metalworking and machining areas of industry may increase the risk of contact dermatitis or occupational acne.

Surveys of industry show that more than 50 percent of occupational illness in the United States is due to contact dermatitis: Of the various types of dermatitis, irritant contact dermatitis accounts for about 70 percent of all cases in the workplace, with the remaining 30 percent due to allergic contact dermatitis.

However numerous the substances a person may encounter on the job, an equally large number of potential irritants is encountered at home, including bleaches, dishwashing liquids, pesticides, abrasive cleaners, soaps, shampoos, floor cleaners and waxes, and bathroom and window cleaners. Gardeners and hobbyists can expect to encounter an equally wide array of irritants.

Irritant Dermatitis. This rash develops as a result of a direct physical insult by a chemical to the barrier of the skin. Anyone's skin can develop an irritant reaction if exposed to certain chemicals in the right concentrations for a long enough period of time. Any substance—including water—may act as an irritant. Among the major offending irritants are soaps and solvents, including turpentine, mineral spirits, bases (alkalis), and acids.

Strong irritants, such as sulfuric and hydrochloric acids, and bases, such as sodium hydroxide or lye, can produce blisters and severe skin damage shortly after exposure. Weaker substances may not produce a problem until a person has had prolonged contact with an irritant. For instance, the mother of a newborn infant may develop red, dry, and cracked skin on her hands because she has them immersed in soap and water more frequently. This case provides a good example of what may be the mechanism behind irritant dermatitis: By constantly plunging her hands into soap and water, her skin's protective horny layer becomes impaired, thus setting the stage for irritation. Alkalis, solvents, and other chemicals also disrupt and damage the stratum corneum, removing oils that lubricate and protect the skin.

Irritant dermatitis develops more quickly when the skin's barrier is weakened by dryness. When the humidity is low during the fall and winter months, the skin loses a greater amount of moisture. People who bathe frequently during the colder months encourage dry skin by removing the oil barrier that protects the skin. Applying a moisturizer to the skin immediately after bathing—while the skin remains damp—can help prevent dryness and help lubricate the skin.

Allergic Contact Dermatitis. This rash arises due to a different mechanism than that of irritant dermatitis. Unlike irritant dermatitis, in which the inflammation is due to direct injury from contact with a chemical, an allergic skin reaction occurs when the immune system recognizes and reacts to a particular substance.

Medical researchers believe that each of us is born with a repertoire of white blood cells, called *T cells*, that contain receptors for various environmental allergens. If we manage to live our lives without ever coming into contact with the allergens, we won't develop the allergies. However, if we encounter such a substance, the process of sensitization, or allergic response, begins. The first time a person who will become allergic to a substance comes into contact with it, he or she won't develop a rash. However, with each subsequent encounter, the population of T-cells continues to expand in size. The capability to react heightens with each exposure until it reaches the point when the person develops allergic symptoms such as redness, swelling, itching, and fluid-filled blisters after contact with the allergen (see Chapter 8, "Immunological Alterations," for a detailed description of the allergic response in contact dermatitis).

Box 4.1 PREVENTING CONTACT DERMATITIS

Contact dermatitis may develop more easily in people with sensitive skin, but those with normal skin are at risk, too. Here are some guidelines to follow that may help prevent an irritant or allergic skin reaction:

- Limit excessive contact with water because water dehydrates the skin.
- Wear rubber gloves when using cleaners, solvents, polishes, and even dish liquid at home and irritating chemicals at work. Perspiration can be a source of irritation for some wearers of plain or even cotton-lined rubber gloves. People whose hands are especially sensitive may need to wear cotton gloves *inside* rubber gloves to allow for more effective absorption of perspiration. If the liners become soaked with sweat, change them as necessary.
- Remove rings whenever coming into contact with soaps and detergents. If the residue from these products gets trapped under the ring, it can irritate the skin below.
- If you plan to have your ears pierced, find out in advance what kind of piercing needle will be used. Choose a vendor who uses a sterilized stainless-steel needle and request surgical steel studs as your starter pair of earrings. When the skin heals after a period of a few weeks, opt for 18-karat gold or stainless-steel earrings because they are less likely to cause a skin reaction.
- Shun irritating and drying cleansing soaps for hand washing and bathing. Instead, select a superfatted soap that contains moisturizers.
- After washing hands or bathing, seal in the moisture with an ointment or a cream applied to *damp* skin.
- Launder new clothing and bed linens before using them. If you've had an adverse reaction to the formaldehyde resins that are used in permanent press clothing, buy untreated fabrics instead.
- Read labels, especially if you know you're sensitive to certain ingredients.

THE LEADING ALLERGENS. There are thousands of allergens present in the environment. When you consider all of the chemicals that are present in food, manufactured goods, plants, and medications, it is impossible to predict which substance will trigger a reaction in any one person. Thousands of chemicals have been linked with allergic skin sensitization. Many people use a substance for a long period of time before becoming sensitized to it.

If the cause of a skin reaction isn't clear, your doctor may recommend a patch test to identify the offending agent that is causing the rash. In a patch test, the doctor places a small amount of different substances on the skin of the back and leaves them there for forty-eight hours or longer to see if there is an allergic reaction to the substance. If there is redness, swelling, or itching, there is a strong likelihood of a skin allergy to one of the substances.

Dermatologists generally agree that poison ivy, nickel, preservatives, hair dyes, formaldehyde, rubber, fragrances, flavors, and some ingredients in nail care products are the most common sensitizers that affect the skin.

Poison ivy: Plants of the *Rhus* family (poison ivy, poison oak, and poison sumac) are the leading skin sensitizers in the United States (see p. 163 for details of the reactions). As much as 70 percent of the population is allergic to poison ivy. The oil urushiol is responsible for producing the rash associated with these plants and can be found in the leaves, stems, and roots. Those at particular risk for coming in contact with this allergen are those with outdoor jobs (such as farmers, foresters, timber cutters, and landscapers), gardeners, hikers, and campers. One of the greatest dangers to people sensitive to poison ivy is breathing the smoke created from burning the plants; the allergen is released into the air and can create a similar reaction and swelling inside the lungs. People with this allergy should be extremely careful, for example, when burning weeds or lawn trimmings or when near a brush fire. Mangoes, which belong to the same family of plants as poison ivy and poison sumac, can also cause a reaction in people with this allergy.

Nickel: This metal is the second most common cause of allergic contact dermatitis.

People who are sensitized to nickel tend to be allergic to the metal for the rest of their lives. This is a problem because nickel is a component of so many objects that we use every day, from zippers, watches, and watchbands to costume jewelry, doorknobs, coins, bra hooks, paper clips, tools, cooking implements—even eyelash curlers, snaps, and metal eyeglass frames. In fact, anything that looks like metal is likely to contain nickel (see Box 4.2). (Nickel also is a component of stainless steel. However, the chemical bonding that takes place in the manufacture of stainless steel is so strong that the nickel it contains cannot be drawn into the skin.)

Women have a much higher incidence of nickel allergy than men, thought to result from their greater use of jewelry and ear piercing. Even gold jewelry contains varying amounts of nickel. While most people with nickel allergies can tolerate 18-karat gold jewelry, 14-karat gold, which may contain nickel, may precipitate a reaction in those who are allergic (such people are usually advised to avoid 10-karat gold, because it contains a relatively large amount of nickel).

Box 4.2 HOW TO TEST METALS FOR THE PRESENCE OF NICKEL

People who are sensitive to nickel usually handle such a variety of metal objects in the course of a day that it's often difficult to say with certainty which item is producing an allergic skin reaction. Until recently, there was no way to know whether an object or jewelry contained nickel until irritation occurred after contact. Now a test is available that can detect the presence of nickel in products easily.

The spot test employs the chemical dimethylglyoxime as the active ingredient that detects any nickel in a metal alloy. A few drops of dimethylglyoxime and an ammonium hydroxide solution are placed on a cotton-tipped applicator and rubbed

(continued)

Box 4.2   HOW TO TEST METALS FOR THE PRESENCE OF NICKEL (*continued*)

against the item to be tested: When nickel is present, the test yields a positive result: a red precipitate on the tip of the applicator.

Nickel-sensitive people who have unexplained bouts of dermatitis but haven't been able to pinpoint the source of their rash should find this test useful. It can be applied to jewelry, doorknobs, chair arms and legs, scissors, keys, knobs, furniture trim, wheelchair frames, and a multitude of other metal-containing objects.

Preservatives: Used to prevent the growth of bacteria and fungi, preservatives are the primary allergens in lotions, creams, and other cosmetics. Paraben preservatives, which were introduced in the 1970s, have emerged as much safer than they were once considered to be. The more frequently used preservatives that tend to cause problems with allergic dermatitis today include quaternium 15 (found in waterproof eyeshadow), imidazolidinyl urea (found in face powder), and dialozolidinyl urea (found in eyeliner and face powder), as well as thimerosal, a preservative used in eye care products, such as eye drops and contact lens solutions.

Hair dyes: Permanent hair dyes contain the chemical *para*-phenylenediamine, a known sensitizer. A typical reaction to this ingredient includes redness, scaling, oozing, and blistering. The scalp itself is relatively resistant to the sensitizing effects of hair dyes, but the forehead, ears, and the back of the neck are not and tend to be more severely affected.

(*Note of advice:* If you use permanent hair dyes, perform a patch test *each* time the product is used, even if you had no previous reaction to the dye.)

Formaldehyde: Although this chemical is most well known as a preservative used often in medical laboratories and mortuaries, it is also used as a preservative in many consumer products and as a finishing agent in permanent press clothing and paper products. Exposure to formaldehyde is widespread, commonly through contact with

clothing, cosmetics, insulation, cigarette smoke, automobile exhaust, or through exposure to free formaldehyde released from urea formaldehyde insulation, as well as carpets, particle board, and fabrics (see Chapter 14, "Air"). Many people have developed allergic contact dermatitis from exposure to formaldehyde in such items as paper, nail hardeners, carpet and fabric resins, air fresheners, and coolants. Exposure can affect the respiratory tract as well as the skin (see Chapter 6, "Respiratory Ailments").

Formaldehyde can be so irritating to the skin that Japan and Sweden have banned its use in cosmetic products. In the United States, formaldehyde is an ingredient in rinse-off cosmetic products, such as shampoos. When used this way, the formaldehyde is so rapidly diluted and rinsed away that the skin receives very limited exposure to it. Therefore, there are very few cases of allergic contact dermatitis of the scalp or face from contact with the chemical.

The problems that have occurred with formaldehyde in clothing are related not to the chemical itself but to resins that chemists have created from formaldehyde for use in industry. These resins, commonly used in permanent press garments, break down when they come into contact with the skin through normal body heat and perspiration. Following reports of allergic reactions to these resins in the 1970s and 1980s, the textile industry moved toward using resins that have been chemically modified to release much less formaldehyde. As a result, today's textile resins don't break down as easily as those used in the past. People who have had skin reactions to these chemicals have been allergic to these resins and *not* to the formaldehyde.

Rubber: Allergies to rubber may actually be to a protein in rubber and/or to chemicals, such as accelerators and antioxidants, added to rubber to make this gummy substance stretch and remain durable. These chemicals can cause symptoms such as itching, redness, and, occasionally, a watery, blistering rash. Manufacturers are not required to list any of these chemicals on product labels.

Latex rubber is the source of an increasing number of allergic reactions, and has now come under the scrutiny of the Food and Drug Administration (FDA). Latex rubber is the material used in condoms, gloves, and various medical devices. Many of these reactions have resulted from contact of latex rubber with the mucous membranes of the mouth, the vaginal and rectal areas, and the intestinal lining. The FDA has recommended that health care workers ask people who are scheduled for surgery or radiologic procedures whether they have ever had a sensitivity reaction to latex (for example, to ask whether the person ever developed itching or swelling around the mouth after blowing up a balloon).

Situations that involve contact with latex include oral exposure to latex gloves during dental procedures; vaginal contact with the use of condoms, diaphragms, and pessaries; and rectal contact during rectal examinations or from barium enema cuffs in a medical setting and through condoms used in anal sex. Anyone who must undergo surgery involving the intestines will encounter latex when glove-wearing surgeons touch the intestinal mucosa. In addition, when catheters are necessary during hospitalization or for medical reasons, the urinary tract is exposed to latex.

Increasing numbers of cases of latex sensitivity have been reported—among patients as well as medical personnel—as more health care workers routinely wear latex gloves as a part of universal infection control precautions (see Box 4.3). Some people develop the annoying and irritating skin rash from contact with the rubber accelerators or antioxidants, but those who become sensitized to latex are at risk of more severe reactions. They may develop anything from a mild response, to hives (urticaria), to a dramatic, life-threatening allergic reaction called *anaphylaxis*, which involves the lungs, blood vessels, and other blood systems as well (see Chapter 8, "Immunological Alterations").

(*Note:* Latex condoms are relatively effective as a means of protection against the human immunodeficiency virus [HIV], the acquired immunodeficiency syndrome [AIDS] virus, and other sexually transmitted diseases. As more sexually active Americans use these condoms, a certain number of them will develop a contact sensitivity to the rubber accelerators used in some of these products. Hypoallergenic condoms are now under development, but until these are ready for the marketplace, men with this sensitivity are advised to "double up": Wear a lambskin condom next to the skin, and place a latex condom over it. The natural skin condom will protect the skin of the penis but does not protect against HIV. If a man's sexual partner is latex-sensitive, the man should wear the lambskin condom over the latex condom.)

Rubber compounds can cause reactions wherever the rubber comes into contact with the skin. Problems with rashes have been reported by people using shower caps, waistbands, undergarments, swimsuits, athletic shoes, leather shoes held together by rubber cement, goggles for swimming, and full-body suits for scuba diving.

Box 4.3   COPING WITH RUBBER-GLOVE DERMATITIS

As hospitals and medical and dental offices have adopted the practice of requiring staff to wear rubber gloves as a safety precaution against contact with HIV, a growing number of doctors, dentists, and nurses are developing rubber-glove dermatitis.

The latex used in these gloves often contains the rubber chemicals mercaptobenzothiazole and tetraethylthiuram, which are the most common causes of allergic rubber glove dermatitis. In some cases, the cornstarch powder used inside the gloves also may produce contact dermatitis in some wearers.

Gloves that contain no latex protein have been developed for people who have experienced either skin irritation or hives in response to contact with natural latex. The substitute gloves contain an antioxidant known as zinc dithiocarbamate. Studies thus far have shown that reactions to this substance have been rare. These gloves, sold under the commercial name Elastyren, are available in sterile and nonsterile form.

Fragrances: These chemicals are placed in cosmetics, perfumes, soaps, room deodorizers, toilet tissue, and sanitary napkins and can cause a reaction in unsuspecting users.

Some fragrances can, by themselves, cause allergic dermatitis. A number of other fragrances induce a rash when they interact with sunlight. (Musk ambrette, for example, is a popular fragrance and a leading sensitizer in terms of these photoreactions.)

Fragrances are considered trade secrets and the list of ingredients on a cosmetic product label will simply read "fragrance," without specifying which one it contained.

There is a difference between a product that claims to be unscented and one that is fragrance-free: A product that claims to be fragrance-free is not supposed to contain any fragrance, while an unscented product has no scent but usually employs a fragrance to mask an odor. (Oils such as lanolin, for instance, tend to have a rancid odor and manufacturers add masking fragrances to neutralize the unpleasant smell.) For the most part, such unscented products contain a trace amount of fragrance. Although it is usually not enough to present a problem, people who are very sensitive to the fragrance have been known to develop allergic reactions.

Flavors: These chemicals impart either a flavor or an aroma to a substance and may be derived from natural sources or produced synthetically in the laboratory. Occasionally, a substance is a flavor as well as a fragrance. For example, balsam of Peru, a substance that is present in vanilla, can fall into either category, although it is not usually problematic. On the other hand, cinnamic aldehyde, a component of cinnamon, is a flavor and a fragrance that can produce an irritant reaction in some people, an allergic response in others, and *nonimmunologic contact urticaria*, commonly known as hives, in many more. (Commercial mouthwashes that include cinnamic aldehyde in the product produce a low-grade hiving reaction that makes the mouth "tingle.") Bakers who work with cinnamon often develop dermatitis. Sensitive individuals may develop an allergic reaction to toothpastes that contain cinnamic aldehyde. Other substances used both as flavors and fragrances include benzaldehyde, cassia (cinnamon oil), cinnamic acid, and menthol.

Nail cosmetics: As greater numbers of people use nail-care products, allergies to these substances are increasing. One ingredient, in particular, is responsible for these reactions: the *para*-toluene sulfonamide resin added to nail polishes to enhance their gloss, hardness, and adhesion.

Hardened and completely dry, the resin does not cause a problem, but when still wet, it can. Nail polish users who touch their skin, especially around the eye area, while the polish is drying are likely to develop allergic reactions around the eyelids and along the neck.

Other sensitizing substances include the acrylics in the instant glues used in nail sculpting. When the nail glue dries and the nail is filed down for sculpting, dust from the nail and the glue can settle on the eyelids, face, and neck, causing allergic reactions.

The acrylic glue methyl methacrylate was used in nail salons until it was banned by the FDA in 1976 because of the large number of allergic reactions that it caused. Orthopedic surgeons still use methyl methacrylate, an excellent adhesive, in joint replacement surgery. Typically, the surgical patient does not react to the substance, but the surgeons themselves do, becoming sensitized to this type of acrylic. (Methyl methacrylate may also be a peripheral neurotoxin.)

Medications: Medications that are applied externally to rashes can sometimes sensitize the area of skin that is affected by the rash. In some cases, inflamed skin can get worse when a sensitizing ingredient in a topical medication is applied.

Numerous topical medications have caused dermatitis in some people including: anesthetics, such as benzocaine, tetracaine, dibucaine, and butycaine; topical antibiotics, such as neomycin, streptomycin, penicillin, and sulfonamides; topical antihistamines, such as promethazine and diphenhydramine; and occasionally, topical antiseptics that contain mercury, such as merthiolate and mercurochrome.

Any drug that is taken in pills or by injection is capable of causing a drug allergy reaction, and such a response usually presents first on the skin. For example, reactions to penicillin, sulfa drugs, and barbiturates often begin with hives; and medications that contain iodides and bromides tend to produce an acnelike rash.

Delivering medications through skin patches (transdermally) may irritate or sensitize the users either to the medication itself, to the material from which the patch is made, or to the adhesive material that sticks the patch to the skin.

Box 4.4   COSMETICS SAFETY

While Americans spend an estimated $19 *billion* each year on cosmetics and toiletries, they may be unaware that there are few of the regulatory safeguards on these products that are in place for other consumer goods.

Federal regulations do require listing ingredients in cosmetics and toiletries in decreasing order of prominence, but manufacturers do not have to reveal trade secrets, specific fragrances or flavors, or ingredients that are present only in minute amounts. Unfortunately, some of these ingredients are sensitizing substances.

Consumers commonly assume that cosmetics, like drugs, must receive approval by the FDA before being marketed; in fact, this is not the case. There are very few federal standards that govern the cosmetics industry. The FDA relies upon the federal Food, Drug, and Cosmetics Act of 1938 to monitor this industry. Under this statute, adulterating or misbranding any cosmetic is prohibited. If the FDA determines that a cosmetic is not safe or that it contains false or misleading labeling, it can

(continued)

Box 4.4   COSMETICS SAFETY (*continued*)

take action, mainly to ask the manufacturer to voluntarily recall the product before the FDA bans its sale.

However, there is no formal system in place for collecting and reporting complaints and injuries associated with cosmetics use, which presents a problem since consumer complaints are the main source used by the FDA to monitor which products need evaluation; at this point, the agency evaluates just ten to twenty products each year.

Under current law, cosmetics manufacturers *voluntarily* register their products; about 40 percent of the almost 2,500 manufacturers and packagers of cosmetics had registered their products, according to a 1990 report issued by the U.S. General Accounting Office.

Since 1976, the cosmetic industry has relied upon its own watchdog system, called the Cosmetic Ingredient Review program (CIR), a self-review process sponsored by the trade group, the Cosmetic, Toiletry, and Fragrance Association. The CIR panel of experts evaluates the safety of cosmetic ingredients before they are placed on the market and also scrutinizes test results for signs of adverse effects.

The number of complaints related to cosmetic injuries is most likely vastly underreported. Rather than see their physician, a person who experiences an adverse reaction to a product on the market simply switches to another product, or treats him- or herself. Only when serious reactions occur in a number of people is it likely that a product will be recalled or banned for cosmetic purposes.

Atopic Dermatitis. Atopic dermatitis, a chronic form of skin inflammation, is marked by an extreme sensitivity to environmental influences and substances that don't produce a reaction in most people.

Researchers suspect that there is a familial tendency toward atopic dermatitis. About 70 percent of people with this disease have a family history of asthma, hay fever, and atopic skin inflammation. Many of those affected and their families tend to produce higher than normal amounts of a blood protein called immunoglobulin E; however, the significance of this finding is unclear.

Atopic dermatitis usually develops during infancy and then disappears, only to recur at intervals during childhood and young adult life. While it usually improves during the adult years, some people do not develop the condition until they reach adulthood.

Among the trigger factors that aggravate this condition are minor or sudden changes in temperature; contact with irritating fibers, such as wool; perspiration; and, possibly, stress. Dry and thickened areas of skin are the hallmark of atopic dermatitis, with the crease of the arm (about the elbow) and the leg (about the knee) most commonly affected.

Certain occupations may be best avoided by people with atopic dermatitis, especially jobs that involve constant contact with water; extreme changes in temperature; and heavy use of soaps, solvents, and detergents. However, this condition may flare up when neither occupation or environment is an issue.

Box 4.5 OTHER FORMS OF DERMATITIS

There are other forms of dermatitis whose cause is not linked to anything in the environment. They include the following:

Seborrheic dermatitis is an inflammation of the scalp and often the middle of the face, the eyebrows, chest, and upper back. Dermatologists have not determined the specific cause of this condition, with its characteristic red and scaling skin, but can easily treat it.

Stasis dermatitis occurs on the skin of the legs as the result of faulty blood circulation. Tiny red spots of discoloration appear on the skin around the ankles, and they eventually darken to produce brownish discoloration. These pinpoint spots indicate abnormal blood flow from the capillaries in the lower leg. Areas of redness, scaling, and itching may appear on the ankle. Advanced changes include leg ulcers.

Nummular dermatitis gets its name from the coin-shaped dry patches that develop on the skin of the legs, arms, and the trunk. Although the cause is unknown, a combination of factors including a dry environment, dry skin, and irritating substances such as wool and soap are thought to influence this condition.

Pigment Changes and Disorders

Contact with certain chemicals can bring about toxic vitiligo, an irreversible condition in which the skin's color-producing cells (melanocytes) stop working normally and the skin loses its pigmentation. Unlike cosmetic vitiligo, a disorder that causes melanocytes to stop producing pigment in the skin for no known reason, so-called toxic vitiligo is caused by exposure to chemicals that are derivatives of phenols or catechols. These substances, which are used as antioxidants and germicidal disinfectants, are typically encountered when working with photographic developing solutions, lubricating oils, plastic and adhesive resins, and institutional or industrial disinfectant cleaning solutions.

Staining of the Skin

Heavy metals, especially silver, mercury, and arsenic, may discolor the skin and stain the fingernails as well.

Mercury. Mercury is used widely in industry, used by tattoo artists to permanently stain the skin, and found in some cosmetics and drugs as an ingredient in various topical applications for the skin, such as moisturizers and ointments. (Until about 1970, several commercially available bleaching creams that were designed to get rid of "age spots" on the face and hands contained a form of mercury.)

Some people have developed slate gray pigmentation of the skin after lengthy use of a mercury-containing moisturizer. In other cases, short-term use of a skin preparation that included mercury has produced grayish-brown spots around the face.

Mercury can cause other skin problems apart from staining the skin. During World War II, for example, a number of people who worked in munitions factories developed contact dermatitis from working with mercury fulminate powder. Exposure to high levels of mercury also can produce respiratory irritation, disturbances of the digestive tract, neurologic impairment, and kidney damage.

Silver. Silver and its derivatives can cause the skin to become abnormally pigmented. Silver nitrate, a topical medication used to treat infections of the mucous membranes, appears to exit the body through the skin and may leave a silver or bluish-gray stain in its wake. This discoloration, known as *argyria*, also affects photographers and film developers who continuously work with silver salts in developing film. Constant contact with the silver causes their fingers and nails to develop a blue-gray discoloration.

Arsenic. Arsenic typically causes brown-colored areas of discoloration on the skin, typically described as "raindrops on a dusty road." When arsenic enters the body through the lungs or the gastrointestinal tract, it usually takes two to four weeks after exposure for it to appear in the skin, hair, and change the nail formation, causing Mee's lines (see p. 320). With chronic exposure to arsenic, some workers may develop multiple skin cancers from five to twenty-five years *after* exposure.

meta-Phenylenediamine. *meta*-phenylenediamine, used in color developing, may cause depigmentation and dermatitis.

Acne

Once believed to be an affliction solely confined to the population of growing adolescents, common acne, with its annoying flare-ups of inflamed, red pimples, affects a large percentage of the population at one time or another. One of the major causes is "overreactive" oil glands (sebaceous glands) in the skin. Stress and, in some people, contact with cosmetics can aggravate the condition. Two other forms of acne occur as a result of contact with certain chemicals.

Oil acne. Contact with certain oils causes an inflammation of the opening of the hair follicle, producing pimples, blackheads, and cysts on the backs of the hands and forearms. Areas of the skin that are exposed to oil-soaked clothing also may be affected. Mechanics, machinists, and workers who have direct contact with petroleum-based oils and greases may have a higher risk of oil acne.

Chloracne. One of the most severe forms of acne that is directly related to environmental exposure is chloracne. Characterized by the appearance of widespread cysts, especially on the face, chloracne is classically described as a reaction to 2, 3, 7, 8-tetrachlorodibenzo-*p*-dioxin (TCDD), commonly called dioxin. TCDD is produced as a by-product of chemical manufacture. Choracne has been associated with exposure to polyhalogenated aromatic hydrocarbons, including biphenyls (PCBs and PBBs), and dibenzofurans, although it may be that contamination of these chemicals with dioxin is the culprit.

Small amounts of these chemicals contaminate herbicides, some electrical insulating materials, and the fly ash and flue gases that are waste products of some industrial incineration processes.

Exposure to the dioxin-contaminated chemicals may also affect the liver and other organs besides the skin. Chloracne is a disease that does not always respond well to treatment. Industries that produce chemicals containing chlorinated aromatic hydrocarbons are required to completely enclose the manufacturing process so that workers cannot touch or inhale these substances.

VIBRATION SYNDROME

Work that involves the regular use of hand-held vibrating tools or equipment such as pneumatic hammers and chain saws may traumatize the affected fingers and hand, resulting in skin ailments. Raynaud's phenomenon, for example, may be the most well-known example of a condition that can result from repeatedly using vibrating instruments (see Chapter 18, "Noise").

Another vibration-related malady is vibratory angioedema, which is believed to be a hereditary condition that often leads to hives. This illness is characterized by local skin injuries, such as itching and redness, and swelling resulting from the ongoing vibratory stimulation.

Box 4.6   HOW THE OFFICE CAN GET "UNDER YOUR SKIN"

The risk of developing some type of skin ailment is inherent in almost every line of work, from auto mechanics to baking, floral arranging, printing, and health care. Numerous occupations, including barbers, cosmetologists, bartenders, restaurant workers, doctors, and nurses, involve some type of "wet work," in which the workers plunge their hands into water many times in the course of a day; this destroys some of their skin's protective oil surface and leaves them more vulnerable to skin problems.

Office workers, who previously thought themselves immune to such ailments, are increasingly reporting a variety of dermatologic symptoms, such as, itchy patches of redness and scaling, which have been attributed to *low-humidity occupational dermatoses* (lowering the room temperature, humidifying the air, and using a moisturizer regularly usually relieves this problem), or a burning, pricking sensation around the eyes, nose, and mouth, and, to a lesser extent, skin irritation, which may indicate allergic contact dermatitis reactions that occur from handling carbonless copy paper. Video display terminals have been implicated as the possible cause of *video display terminal dermatitis*, although experts disagree as to whether such a skin disorder really exists or whether working at a VDT simply aggravates an existing skin disorder.

SUN DAMAGE: SKIN AGING, SKIN CANCER, AND PHOTOSENSITIVITY

Armed with a mind-set that suntanned skin is "healthy" looking, millions of American sunbathers willingly subject themselves to dangerous ultraviolet radiation from the most deceptively dangerous source of environmental harm—the sun.

Anyone who has ever experienced a painful sunburn knows how powerful the sun's rays can be. Although all of the light emitted from the sun cannot be seen by the naked eye, scientists have measured solar radiation and have classified it as heat, visible light, and invisible ultraviolet light.

Ultraviolet radiation from the sun is further broken down into ultraviolet C (UVC), which largely does not reach the earth's surface; UVB, the shorter, high-energy rays that produce sunburn; and UVA, the longer, lower-energy rays that play an important role in tanning and in some allergic reactions to the sun. UVB has been found to damage cell membranes and the genetic material DNA and to contribute to skin cancer. UVA is a direct contributor to premature aging of the skin and skin cancer.

Sun Damage: A Cumulative Process

Much of what was thought to be biological aging is now known to be sun-induced skin damage. Although aging itself cannot be prevented, premature skin aging from sun exposure is something that can be controlled.

As much as 70 percent of the skin damage that

leads to premature aging comes from exposure to the sun. People tend to get their most intense exposure to sunlight during childhood, with an estimated 80 percent of sun exposure occurring before age eighteen. Unfortunately, skin damage due to exposure to the sun is cumulative; the clock begins running during childhood.

The sun can wreak havoc on the skin in a number of ways. Bronzing the skin year-round or every summer forces the production of more melanin, the dark pigment that your skin produces as a natural sun block to keep out damaging ultraviolet light rays. A suntan indicates that your skin's protective mechanism has been at work and that some damage has occurred.

The body's normal response to injury is to try to repair itself. However, when a person spends a large amount of time in the sun, the energy from sunlight is disruptive and destructive to the deoxyribonucleic acid (DNA) in the skin.

Ultraviolet B (UVB) rays cause the redness of a sunburn. At a cellular level, UVB rays damage the genetic material of cells in the outer layer of skin (increasing the risk of cancer). In the meantime, ultraviolet A (UVA) rays penetrate deep into the dermis, or second layer of skin, throwing the elastic and collagen fibers and other cells into disarray. What results is a breakdown of the skin's underlying structure and premature wrinkling and aging of the skin.

A single episode of sunburn with its blistering, peeling, and pain has the immediate disadvantage of discomfort, but once it heals you should be back to normal. The problems arise from repeated exposure to sunlight and constant tanning. The degenerative changes of long-term sun exposure take place slowly, beginning with dryness, wrinkling, uneven pigmentation, thickened and sagging skin, and benign or precancerous growths and often culminate in skin cancer.

Other than staying out of the sun and wearing clothes that completely cover the skin, sunscreens are considered the best protection from too much exposure to the sun.

Skin Cancer

By now we have all heard about the links between exposure to the sun's rays and the rise of skin cancer. What is less appreciated is the *degree* to which skin cancer rates now soar: In the United States, the annual incidence of new cases of skin cancer is now above 600,000, and over 32,000 of these new cases are of melanoma, the most serious, deadly form.

Skin cancer is largely a disease affected by environmental factors and, largely, by factors under our control—namely, exposure to the sun's rays, which is the primary cause for most forms of this cancer. Outdoor recreational activities, a penchant for sunbathing, and the global depletion of the protective upper layer of ozone that shields the earth from the sun's ultraviolet rays all contribute to the increasing incidence of this disease.

The risk of skin cancer is greater for people who labor for years in sunlight for several hours a day. Unintentional exposure to ionizing radiation, or X rays, by doctors, dentists, and other health care personnel also increases the risk of skin cancer. Workers who handle creosote, pitch, asphalt, and mineral oil are prone to developing growths called tar warts on areas of skin that were exposed to these substances, but only rarely do these develop into cancer.

There are three major types of skin cancer:

Basal cell carcinoma. Basal cell carcinoma is the most prevalent form of skin cancer, with about 500,000 cases reported annually in the United States. Fair-skinned people are more likely to develop this form of cancer, which initially arises at the junction of the epidermis and dermis and gradually penetrates deeper into the skin. Fortunately, it usually remains localized.

Squamous cell carcinoma. More than 100,000 cases of squamous cell carcinoma, the second most common skin cancer, are reported each year in this country. This type of cancer can develop from red and scaly precancerous spots called *actinic* or *solar keratoses* but often develops in otherwise healthy-looking skin. Squamous cell carcinomas grow in the epidermal layer and, in rare instances, can spread to other parts of the body. Long-term exposure to sunlight is a major cause of this type of skin cancer. Individuals who experience long-term exposure to chemicals, such as arsenic, can develop small indentations on the palms and soles called *arsenical keratoses*. Although these premalignant growths eventually can develop into squamous cell cancer, it is the areas of the skin that were *not* exposed to arsenic that tend to be the sites where this cancer develops. People employed in the ore smelting and refining industries and in the production of insecticides and weed killers may be exposed to arsenic in their work.

Malignant melanoma. Although it accounts for only 5 percent of all skin cancers, malignant melanoma is responsible for nearly 80 percent of all deaths due to skin cancer. Alarmingly, the rate of Americans developing melanoma has risen from 1 in every 1,500 people in 1931, to 1 in every 105 people in 1991. Moreover, its incidence is climbing at a faster rate than any other cancer in the United States; at the current rate, one in every seventy-five Americans will develop melanoma in the year 2000. Melanoma affects men and women equally. However, among young women—especially those between twenty-five and twenty-nine—malignant melanoma is the most frequently occurring cancer. In women thirty to thirty-four, the incidence of melanoma is second only to breast cancer. Studies have indicated that children and adolescents who had three or more episodes of severe blistering sunburns before age twenty have a five times higher risk of malignant melanoma than those who have never had any such episodes.

Experts have determined specific factors that may increase the risk of developing melanoma: having blonde or red hair; having large numbers of unusual "moles" called dysplastic nevi; having actinic, or solar, keratoses (rough red patches on the skin); having a family history of melanoma; working outdoors three or more years as a teenager; and experiencing five or more blistering sunburns as a child or adolescent.

All three types of skin cancer are curable if detected early. The earlier that skin cancer is detected, the better the chance of a cure. With early treatment, basal cell carcinoma and squamous cell carcinoma have better than a 95 percent cure rate. Malignant melanomas that are less than one thirty-second of an inch thick also can have up to a 95 percent cure rate.

Box 4.7   THE ABCDs OF SKIN CANCER

Certain skin changes call for immediate medical attention. If you notice any of the following signs or changes in your skin, see a personal physician or dermatologist:

Basal cell carcinoma

- A persistent spot or patch that may be itchy, have a scab, and may or may not be painful.
- A sore that doesn't heal or continues to bleed, ooze, and form a scab that keeps reopening.
- A bump on the skin that is indented in the center. The borders look rolled and blood vessels may later appear on the surface.
- A spot that looks waxy or pearly.

(continued)

> ### Box 4.7 THE ABCDs OF SKIN CANCER (*continued*)
>
> *Squamous cell carcinoma*
>
> - A red, rough, wartlike lump.
> - An ulcerated area of skin that has a raised border and crusted surface with a pebble-grained base.
>
> *Malignant melanoma*
>
> - Half of a mole or a sore that appears different from the other half.
> - The border of the sore or mole that is poorly defined, with irregular borders.
> - The mole's pigmentation is irregular: some parts are light in color, other parts appear dark.
> - The lesion begins to enlarge in diameter and becomes larger than a pencil eraser.

Photosensitivity

Photosensitive reactions are skin reactions caused by a combination of exposure to a substance and to sunlight. Photosensitivity, or light sensitivity, produces rashes, blistering, or redness (the rash that forms usually clears up when the offending substances and/or sunlight are avoided).

Photosensitivity reactions can be divided into two principal categories: phototoxic and photoallergic reactions. A phototoxic reaction is similar to an irritant reaction of the skin in the sense that anyone can develop an irritation if he or she uses a substance long enough. Photoallergic reactions, on the other hand, only affect certain individuals who have been previously sensitized to the substance.

Fragrances, such as oil of bergamot, lavender, and lime, are the most common cause of phototoxic reactions. Chemicals called psoralens, which naturally occur in limes and other vegetables, can react with ultraviolet light to produce a skin irritation characterized by a blistering burn (this commonly occurs when people squeeze lime juice into their beverages while they are out in sunlight).

Occupational exposure to certain chemicals and products can induce photosensitivity disorders. For example, people who handle creosote and tar and then encounter direct sunlight may suffer burning and stinging of the skin, followed by inflammation. Produce clerks and cashiers in supermarkets have been known to develop blistering rashes on their hands after handling fruits and vegetables and then being exposed to the sun. The phototoxic substances that prompt this reaction are called furocoumarins and are found in limes, lemons, figs, celery, carrots, parsley, parsnip, and dill.

The components of sunscreens may cause allergic skin reactions. *para*-Aminobenzoic acid, popularly known as PABA, is an effective sunscreen, but it may cause an irritant or allergic dermatitis in those who are sensitive to this chemical. People with PABA sensitivity can substitute sunscreens that are equally effective, including products containing benzophenones and cinnamates.

Photoallergic reactions can occur as the result of a combination of sunshine and an internally ingested medication or a topically applied one. Among the drugs that have caused phototoxic and allergic reactions in some people are the sulfonamide antibiotics; some of the oral medications for diabetes treatment; certain diuretics, including many of the thiazides (such as, benzthiazide, chlorothiazide, chlorthalidone, cyclothiazide, hydrochlorothiazide, chlorzide, metolazone, and polythiazide; and the phenothi-

Figure 4.2 HOW TO PERFORM A MONTHLY SKIN EXAMINATION.

Perform a self-examination of your skin at least once a month. Bring any changes you notice to your doctor's attention as soon as possible. The American Academy of Dermatology recommends that you follow these steps during your monthly self-exam.

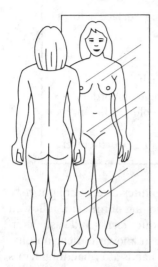

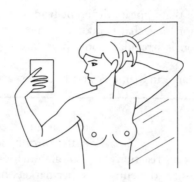

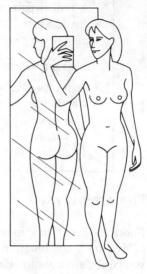

1. First examine the front and back of your body in the mirror, then, with your arms raised, examine the right and left sides.

2. Using a hand mirror, examine the back of your neck and scalp. Lift your hair so that you can look carefully at your scalp and hair-line.

3. Holding a hand mirror, check your back and buttocks.

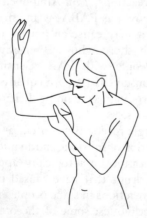

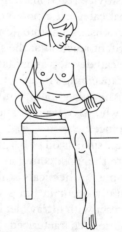

4. Bending your elbows, take a careful look at your forearms, upper underarm, and palms.

5. While sitting, look at the backs of your legs and feet. Be sure to examine the soles of your feet and the spaces in between the toes.

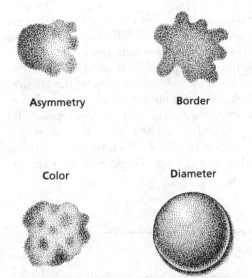

Figure 4.3 THE ABCDs OF SKIN CANCER.

ABCD is an acronym for the specific signs of skin cancer:
Asymmetry: When half of a mole doesn't resemble the other half.
Border: If the mole is irregular in shape or not clearly defined.
Color: A mottled mole.
Diameter: A mole larger than the size of a pencil eraser.

azines, a group of antipsychotic tranquilizer drugs, which may produce a sun sensitivity.

Some people develop a photosensitivity of unknown cause called *polymorphous light reaction*. This condition typically produces rashes that consist of raised red bumps. In some cases, the rash erupts upon the first significant exposure to sunlight in the spring or summer, only to lessen in severity or even disappear upon subsequent exposure to the sun as the skin tans.

Protecting Yourself from the Sun

Numerous over-the-counter sunscreens are available for blocking out the UVB rays that cause sunburn. These products are labeled in accordance with FDA guidelines that rate different categories of sunscreen products based upon their ability to block UVB rays.

The sun protection factor (SPF) number that is listed on each sunscreen label indicates how long you can stay in the sun before your skin will burn. A sunscreen bearing a label of an SPF 15 would allow you to get fifteen times more sun exposure without burning than you could normally tolerate without wearing a sunscreen.

The categories of sunscreens are as follows:

Sun Protection	SPF
Minimal	2–4
Moderate	4–6
Extra	6–8
Maximal	8–15
Ultra	15 +

(Many people have reasoned that the higher the SPF number of a sunscreen, the better the protection. As SPFs have shot as high as 50, confusion over numbers has increased as well. For the most part, an SPF of 15 is more than adequate protection for adults; higher numbers are often recommended for infants.)

There are no FDA standards for rating a sunscreen's ability to block out UVA radiation. Many sunscreens are formulated only to filter out UVB rays; others are called broad-spectrum sunscreens because they also offer some defense against UVA rays. This is important because UVA radiation, once thought to be the source of harmless tanning, has a significant role in both premature aging and skin cancer.

(UVA radiation emitted from the sun is one hundred times greater in quantity than the amount that comes from UVB rays [although much less strong]. Whereas UVB rays are strongest during the summer months, the intensity of UVA rays is pretty much the same year-round.)

Most experts advise using a broad-spectrum sunscreen as possibly the best approach to protecting yourself.

Broadspectrum sunscreens now on the market often contain benzophenones and cinnamates, chemicals that can absorb both UVA and UVB light waves. Sunscreen ingredients that are active in both spectra include oxybenzone, dioxybenzone, avobenzone, butyl methoxydibenzoylmethane, sulisobenzone, 2-ethylhexyl-2-cyano-3, diphenylacrylate, red petrolatum, and titanium dioxide. Many sunscreens employ PABA and its derivatives, such as padimate O, an ingredient that effectively absorbs UVB radiation.

Sunscreens are not visible once they are applied and rubbed into the skin, in contrast to sunblocks, which remain on the surface to provide a physical block. Sunblocks are typically creams or pastes that contain zinc oxide or titanium dioxide. Some sunscreens incorporate zinc oxide into their formulas, but these combination sunscreen/sunblock products are not as effective as the individual products used together. (Mixing sunscreen and sunblock reduces the amount of block, thus diminishing the total protection factor that is inherent in a sunblock product.) Finally, it is always wise to test a sunscreen on a small section of the skin before using it to be sure that you are not allergic to any of the ingredients.

Box 4.8 SUN PROTECTION FACTORS TO CONSIDER

While medical researchers have established that *any* repeated exposure to the sun can potentially have harmful effects, this doesn't mean that people shouldn't go outdoors, simply that they take certain precautions:

- Don't allow yourself to get a sunburn.
- Minimize sun exposure between 10 A.M. and 3 P.M. (when the sun's rays are strongest).
- Use a sunscreen when you're planning to spend any time outdoors during peak sun hours for longer than a few minutes. Incidental sun exposure can add up. Choose a broad-spectrum sunscreen with an SPF of at least 15.
- Apply the sunscreen forty-five to sixty minutes *before* venturing into the sun. The ingredients need some time to absorb into the skin to provide the most effective protection. If you have bald spots or areas of thinning hair, apply sunscreen to the vulnerable parts of your scalp and wear a cap with a visor.
- Reapply the sunscreen every two hours. Reapply it more frequently after perspiring heavily or swimming. Even sunscreens that are waterproof should be reapplied after swimming.
- Wear protective clothing. Wide-brimmed hats, pants, and long-sleeved shirts that are tightly woven help prevent ultraviolet radiation from penetrating the fabric.
- If you're a beachgoer, invest in a beach umbrella. Select an umbrella that has a tightly woven fabric as opposed to the see-through kind.
- Keep infants and toddlers out of the sun as much as possible. Apply sunscreen with an SPF of *at least* 15 to children over six months of age when you take them out in the sunshine. It's best to allow only moderate amounts of sun exposure to young children.
- Shun tanning parlors.
- Apply sunscreen even when staying in the shade. Ultraviolet rays can reflect from water, sand, and other surfaces and produce damage.

Box 4.9 TANNING PARLORS AND FAKE TANS

Each day, an estimated 1 million Americans visit a tanning salon or a sun room located in a beauty parlor, health club, or other business to bronze their skin. While tanning parlors claim that the UVA lights used in their establishments are safe and promote a healthy tan without burning the skin, scientific evidence suggests the contrary: Prolonged exposure to UVA light alone is now known to also contribute to skin cancer. (Moreover, the lights in these parlors emit some UVB rays as well.)

The UVA radiation penetrates both the outer and deeper layers of the skin and causes damage, promotes the breakdown of connective tissue that leads to premature aging, injures blood vessels, may even decrease the skin's immune function, and can cause skin cancer.

A survey of thirty-one salon operators in a midwestern city revealed that the managers of these parlors aren't always aware of the risks that are inherent in using a tanning booth. Researchers who conducted the study in Lansing, Michigan, found that the salon owners believed that tanning booths offered protection against sunburn and sun damage. Less than half of the salon operators had any age restrictions on access to the tanning booths. Some patrons were allowed to bring young children into the booths with them. Two-thirds of the tanning parlor operators said they always warned their customers that tanning increases the risk of skin cancer. All of those surveyed required that patrons wear protective eye goggles while tanning.

A growing number of states are enacting legislation that provides for the regulation of tanning salons. The laws place limits on access to minors, require the use of protective eyewear, call for signed statements by patrons who acknowledge that they are aware of the risks of tanning, and require operators to report any injuries that may occur.

Amid the onslaught of messages about the dangers of sunburn, tanning, and tanning parlors, cosmetics manufacturers have come to the consumer's rescue with what the industry calls the only safe tan: the tan in a bottle. Basically, there are two types of commercially available tanning products: bronzers and tanning agents that stain the skin.

A *skin bronzer* is like makeup in that it is applied to the skin and can be washed off. It contains a tint to mimic a tan and may even contain a sunscreen. If you use a bronzer, check to see if sunscreen is listed among its ingredients. If it contains no sunscreen and you're planning to be outdoors, apply a sunscreen before you use the bronzing product.

Self-tanning lotions or *creams* that stain the skin use dihydroxyacetone (DHA) to create a temporary color. The FDA has approved the use of DHA as a safe-to-use color additive. The compounds in DHA react with the dead cells in the outermost layer of the skin to produce a fake tan. As the skin sheds its old cells in the normal process of cell renewal, the artificially produced tan fades away. However, skin stains don't protect the skin from sun damage: Always apply sunscreen when you plan to spend time in the sun.

(continued)

Box 4.9   TANNING PARLORS AND FAKE TANS (*continued*)

Tanning pills—another way to obtain a fake tan—have been around since the early 1980s. Shortly after these pills were introduced, the FDA began issuing warnings not to use them. These pills contain synthetic β-carotene and a food coloring substance called canthaxanthin that can make the skin look orange. Besides tinting the skin, these colorants can accumulate in the blood, tissues, and organs and the side effects can be toxic or even fatal.

THE FORGOTTEN "SKIN"

Few of us realize that our hair and nails are also part of our skin. Like skin, they require a certain amount of care, attention, and protection from environmental assaults in order to stay healthy.

Hair Damage

Most hair damage is due to chemical injury, trauma from overgrooming the hair, and excessive environmental exposure to sunlight. The energy from the sun actually sets off a chemical reaction in the hair that can change the nature of the proteins of which hair is made. As a result, the hair may lighten, become more fragile, and develop more split ends. People who swim in chlorinated pools and then sit in the sun simply compound the amount of chemical damage.

By far, most hair damage is due to chemical products put on the hair to beautify it, such as dyes, permanent wave lotions, and hair relaxers. Mechanical damage created by the friction from combing or brushing the hair too frequently or from wearing tightly pulled back hairstyles also is a common problem.

Chemical treatments to relax hair and hairstyles in which the hair is pulled back tightly against the scalp place a great deal of mechanical stress on the hair follicle. This continued stress disrupts hair production and eventually damages the follicle's ability to make hair. Over time, the hairs coming from this follicle will be short, smaller in calibre, and possibly contain less pigment.

Hair dyes can be harsh and irritating to the skin and may cause allergic contact dermatitis. Permanent hair dyes can also cause chemical damage to the hair. (The chemical compounds in the dyes become imbedded in the hair fiber in order to produce the desired color change. Additional damage comes from stripping the hair to first remove the color and then applying the permanent dye.)

There's no set point at which it can be said that significant hair damage will occur after regular dyeing. Hair breakage and hair loss usually result after years of routine use of dye or too frequent use over a shorter period of time.

The agents used in permanent solutions are generally safe for healthy hair, although dryness and split ends may be a problem. Hair permanents can cause damage when done too often or too close in time to having the hair dyed. Hair should not be permed more frequently than at twelve-week intervals.

Hair Loss.

Alterations in the external environment, as well as in the internal systems of the body, can produce changes in the hair cycle. Among those that affect the telogen (resting) phase are illness, pregnancy, and crash diets. Exposure to heavy metals (such as arsenic and thallium), chemotherapy drugs, and low-level radiation therapy affect the growth phase, turning off the switch that keeps the hair follicle's production line in operation. Often, the hair cells resume their work, but sometimes regrowth never occurs.

In *telogen effluvium*, the hair loss is temporary. It results from a large number of hair follicles entering the resting phase of the growth cycle, leading to a rapid, synchronous shedding of hair. The condition usually clears up when any irritant is removed.

Alopecia areata is typically characterized by patches of hair loss on the scalp and other parts of the body.

The most common form of hair loss—*androgenetic alopecia* (common male-pattern baldness)—does not occur as a result of injury, illness, or environmental influences but is a genetically programmed process that affects numerous men and women (particularly after menopause).

Although there are plenty of ways to take better care of our hair, there's no single drug or treatment that can strengthen normal hair. As long as you're eating a normal, balanced diet and are in good health, rest assured that you're doing the best you can for the quality of your hair.

If you do have a hair loss problem, there are medical treatments that may be helpful.

Box 4.10 KEEPING THE HAIR HEALTHY

Moderation is the best approach to take in keeping your hair healthy. It is perfectly fine to dye, perm, or use an electric hot comb or dryer on your hair, *provided* that you aren't abusive to your hair.

Shampooing won't harm the hair. Contrary to popular belief, a daily shampoo doesn't encourage hair loss; it does keep the hair from looking matted, providing more apparent fullness.

Hair dryers, hot combs, and hair crimpers shouldn't cause a problem when used in moderation. Avoid high heat settings to prevent dryness and hair breakage. If possible, allow your hair to dry partially before finishing the job with a dryer.

If you want to color your hair, you may choose a rinse or a temporary dye instead of a permanent dye. If you do choose a permanent dye, carefully follow instructions on the label and be certain to test the product before each use to be certain that you are not allergic to any of its ingredients (typically, *para*-phenylenediamene). Some semipermanent dyes do not contain this ingredient and may be an alternative for people who are allergic.

Nail Damage

Nails can be affected by trauma, infections, overall health, or any variety of the chemicals and drugs that exist in the environment. Most damage to the nails, however, is the result of overexposure to one of the most common substances in the environment: water. Water is considered the primary cause of brittle nails.

Although tough looking, nails are highly absorbent. Placing the hands in water for prolonged periods causes the nails to swell. Upon removing the hands from water, the moisture evaporates, and the nails contract back to their normal size. This cycle of expansion and contraction repeats itself every time the nails are placed in water. Eventually, the nail becomes much more susceptible to breakage and splitting.

Cleaners, detergents, and solvents by themselves or added to water can also be damaging to the nails.

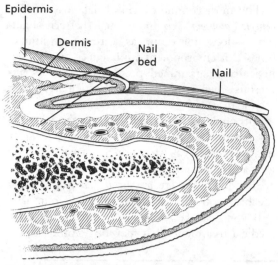

Figure 4.4 THE NAIL.

Nail Care Products.

Nail care products, such as enamels, polishes, and acrylic false nails, may produce allergies in certain users and may lead to situations that encourage infection in others.

Nail polish covers the nail and makes it waterproof. When the polished nails are placed in water and then removed, the water underneath the nail can't evaporate. The dampness may encourage colonies of bacteria and yeast to grow in the area and lead to infection. Similar problems also may occur when acrylic nails are placed over the natural nails.

While some people with brittle nails use nail polish to protect their nails, this may create more of a problem; when the polish is removed, solvents in the polish remover may dry the nails.

Manicures can create problems when the manicurist pushes the cuticle back too far or cuts this small piece of skin to remove it. By attaching to the nail, the cuticle protects the finger from infection. Cutting the cuticle provides an entry for

bacteria and solutions to enter the nail's growing area and sets the stage for infection. Cuticles should be treated gently.

Nail Injuries.

Trauma to the nail from an accident, for instance, slamming a door on a finger or bumping a toe, can produce a hemorrhage beneath the nail plate. This type of hemorrhage can be very painful because it occurs in a confined space, creating pressure on the surrounding tissue. The treatment for this kind of injury is surgical removal of the affected nail or the creation of a small opening in the nail to relieve the pressure.

In the case of a severe injury from an accident that crushes the nail, the nail plate may fall off and usually a new one will grow in its place. (Severe injuries should be evaluated by a physician.)

Brittle Nails.

Brittle and split nails are a common problem that usually results from overexposure to water. Occasionally, chronic illness is reflected in the nails and may produce painful and brittle nails or more serious nail symptoms (see the symptom chart, Nail Abnormalities, p. 320).

Any number of folk remedies have been employed to correct brittle nails. Although gelatin ranks at the top of the list of supposed cures for brittle nails, it does nothing to influence the strength of the nails or their rate of growth.

Swiss researchers have found that people with brittle fingernails who took small doses of the B vitamin biotin boosted the thickness of their nails by 25 percent. The group of people in the study received 2.5 milligrams of biotin a day for a six-month period. Biotin occurs naturally in such foods as cauliflower, lentils, milk, and peanut butter. Federal guidelines have not set an official recommended daily allowance for biotin.

Box 4.11 PROTECTING THE NAILS

As a rule, it's easier to protect the nails than to correct damage that has been done.

- Avoid prolonged exposure to water.
- When you must plunge hands into water for long periods of time, wear gloves for protection.
- Avoid biting nails or pulling at the cuticle because both of these activities can lead to infection.
- If you must use nail polishes and removers, use them with care. Keep nails *unpolished* for a few days between applications.
- Don't overgroom nails. Aggressively pushing back the cuticle can cause a space to develop in front of the nail's growing area that can lead to infection.

CHAPTER 5

The Brain and Nervous System

In "The Fumigation Chamber," medical mystery writer Berton Roueche describes the case of Dr. Betty Page, who, in the summer of 1984, began to experience intermittent bouts of fatigue, nausea, and abdominal cramping for no discernible reason. Over the course of the next year, she consulted numerous specialists—gastroenterologists, cardiologists, neurologists, orthopedists. Despite their best diagnostic efforts, Dr. Page's puzzling disease continued to progress, and her symptoms soon worsened to include muscle weakness, joint pain, and double vision. As a result, she was forced to leave her position as professor of medicine at a major medical school, work that she had found stimulating and enjoyable.

"I kept thinking, hoping, that tomorrow or the day after or the day after that I'd wake up feeling better," Dr. Page is quoted as recalling. "But nothing changed . . . I was getting worried, really worried."

Ultimately, the source of Dr. Page's symptoms proved to be an insecticide used at her summer cottage. Its potent formula combined an organophosphate compound with methyl carbamate, two chemical substances that can have a poisonous, or toxic, effect on the nervous system.

This chapter discusses the impact that poisons, or toxins, have on the body's master control center, the nervous system. There are literally thousands of neurotoxins (*neuro* for nervous system, *toxin* for poison), some arcane, but many—like alcohol, lead, and even viruses—quite well known. All are capable of causing a spectrum of neurological problems, ranging from mild and transient to seriously debilitating or deadly.

Estimates on the precise number of neurotoxins in the environment vary widely, and hard data on their impact are often lacking. Of the 65,000 industrial chemicals on register at the Environmental Protection Agency (EPA), for example, one investigator projected that 2,000—between 3 and 5 percent—had neurotoxic potential; another researcher put the figure at more than 18,000—or about 28 percent. The March of Dimes estimates that 5 to 10 percent of birth defects are the result of environmental insult but does not have figures on how many neurological birth defects are specifically due to neurotoxins.

Environmental agents are known or suspected to play a role in many conditions: Lead, which tops the EPA's list of environmental health hazards, has been implicated as a cause of learning disability; certain solvents, ubiquitous in some industries, are linked to impaired mental functions, toxic mood disorders, and severe manic-depression; and many of the chemicals in pesticides are considered potent damagers of the nervous system.

Further complicating attempts to establish the extent to which environmental agents are linked to neurological ailments is that physicians may overlook the possibility of poisoning; and even when it is suspected, a definitive diagnosis can be difficult to establish.

HOW NEUROTOXINS HARM THE BODY

Neurotoxins affect the performance of the nervous system, an exquisitely tuned network of cells that processes and responds to information channeled from the sensory organs. In addition, the nervous system governs all of the body's major functions—thought, personality, mood, and sensation, to name a few. Because of this, even minor changes in its structure or ability to function can have serious consequences.

Exposure occurs in numerous ways; like other environmental toxins, neurotoxins can be inhaled; ingested; or absorbed through the skin, mucous membranes, and even the conjunctivas of the eyes.

Once in the body, the neurotoxin's specific effect depends on a host of factors. First, of course, is the neurotoxin itself. For example, cocaine has immediately apparent effects as well as substantial delayed effects; lead exposure can take months, even years, before producing noticeable neurologic symptoms. Dose, the frequency of exposure, the length of time over which exposure takes place, and whether exposure is continuous or intermittent are significant factors in how severe the effects will be. Individual variation also plays a role. Two people exposed to the same toxic chemical for the same period of time may have completely different physical responses to it.

Neurotoxins damage the ability of the nervous system to function by destroying or disrupting either the neurons, a type of nerve cell that are the basic microscopic building blocks that form nervous system tissue; the myelin nerve sheath, the protective sheath around the neuron; or the neurotransmitters, the chemical messengers that enable neurons to communicate with each other.

The Structure of the Nervous System

Neurons. There are two types of nerve cells, neurons and glial cells. Glial cells, which compose 90 percent of the brain's nerve cells, are believed to be the basic architectural structure that helps to support and nourish neurons. The remaining 10 percent of the brain's 10 trillion nerve cells are neurons, the cells that carry signals from one part of the nervous system to another.

Like other body cells, neurons consist of a nucleus and a cell body surrounded by a cell membrane. Beyond that however, they differ in several significant ways. For one, we are all born with a finite number of neurons. Once a neuron dies or is damaged, it cannot be replaced as can other cells, such as hair, skin, and blood, which are constantly replenished. For another, the structure of neurons is unique. Finally, and most importantly, neurons communicate with each other, transferring electrical and chemical information from one part of the nervous system to another. It is, in fact, this ability that most clearly distinguishes the nerve cell from all others.

Toxins can affect the ability of neurons to transmit information in a number of ways. Some neurotoxins cause structural damage to the neuron; others inflict functional damage by interfering with its ability to communicate. For example, mercury damages the cell body of neurons, destroying their ability to fire electrical signals. Carbon disulfide, used in the manufacture of rayon and cellophane, interferes with the ability of axons to send information.

STRUCTURE AND FUNCTION OF NEURONS. The basic body, or *soma*, of the neuron is surrounded

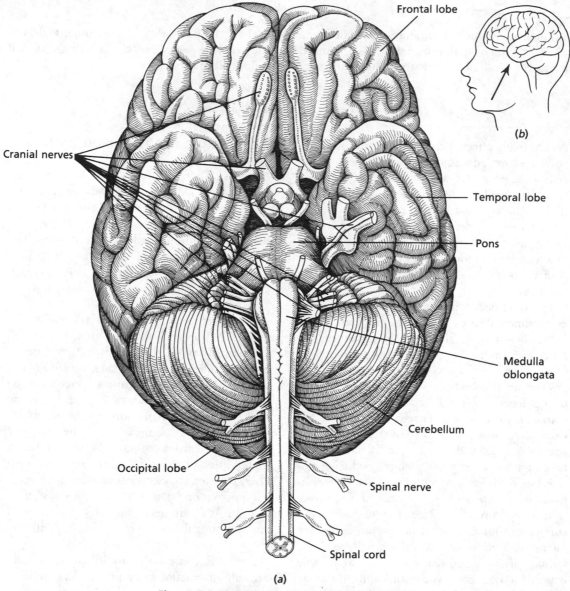

Frontal lobe

(b)

Cranial nerves

Temporal lobe

Pons

Medulla oblongata

Cerebellum

Occipital lobe

Spinal nerve

Spinal cord

(a)

Figure 5.1 THE BRAIN AND NERVOUS SYSTEM.

(a) The central nervous system is comprised of the brain, shown here from below, and the spinal cord. Twelve pairs of cranial nerves radiate from the brain to control the senses, muscles, glands, and heart. The temporal lobe and the frontal lobe, two of the "control centers" susceptible to neurotoxins, are most clearly shown here. (b) Profile of brain depicting view shown in (a). (c) The sympathetic and parasympathetic nerves, shown here, arise from the spinal cord and are part of the autonomic nervous system. They are particularly vulnerable to toxic assault. (d) Outline of thirty-one pairs of nerves that extend from the spinal cord to the muscles, organs, skin, and limbs. (e) A typical neuron. The axon with its myelin sheath forms the nerve fiber. Electrical impulses generated in the soma move from one node of Ranvier to another and reach the branching terminals of the axons; there, impulses move across the synapse via neurotransmitters, which cross to the postsynaptic membrane on the dendrites of other neurons.

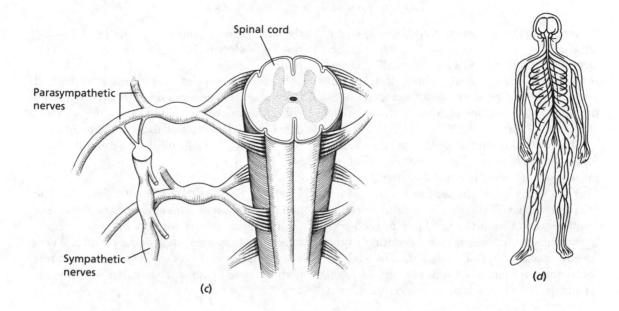

Spinal cord

Parasympathetic
nerves

Sympathetic
nerves

(c)

(d)

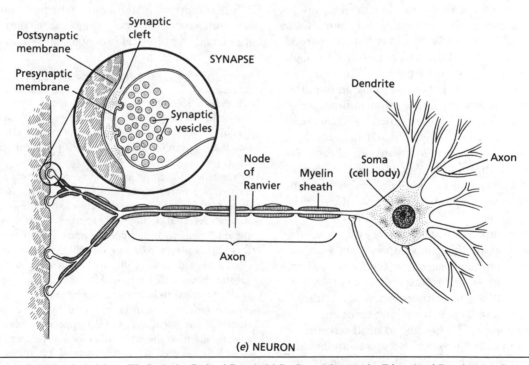

Postsynaptic
membrane

Presynaptic
membrane

Synaptic
cleft

SYNAPSE

Synaptic
vesicles

Node
of
Ranvier

Myelin
sheath

Dendrite

Soma
(cell body)

Axon

Axon

(e) NEURON

Source: Caption adapted from *The Brain*, by Richard Restak, M.D. Copyright 1984 by Educational Broadcasting Corporation and Richard M. Restak, M.D. Used by permission of Bantam Books, a division of Bantam Doubleday Dell Publishing Group, Inc. Also adapted from *The Broken Brain* by Nancy C. Andreasen. Copyright 1984 by Nancy C. Andreasen. Reprinted by permission of HarperCollins Publishers.

by long tubular projections called *axons*, which are coated by myelin sheaths that help conduct electrical impulses, and lacy, branchlike extensions called *dendrites*, along which electrical impulses travel. The length of these extensions provides a vast surface area for neurotoxins to attack (see Figure 5.1*d*).

The axon, together with its myelin sheath, forms the nerve fiber, along which electrical impulses pass. At regular intervals along the nerve fiber are areas, called the *nodes of Ranvier*, which are unprotected by the myelin sheath; electrical impulses travel from the cell body to the nerve by moving from node to node, resulting in the speedy transmission of messages. The ends of the axons can branch out into as many as 1,000 terminals, which can lead to the cell bodies or dendrites of other neurons.

Neurons communicate by firing impulses, or electrical signals, down the length of axons to the dendrites of the next cell. These signals are generated by a rapidly changing flow of charged ions, primarily sodium and potassium, through channels in the nerve membrane. When an axon receives a message that tells it to fire an impulse, sodium ions flow across the cell membrane, triggering an electrical charge called an *action potential*. The speed at which this charge travels is increased by the insulating myelin sheath. (If the myelin sheath is damaged, it can cause widespread destruction to the brain's circuitry, producing such symptoms as poor coordination or blurry vision.)

Nerve impulses usually travel away from the cell body along the axons and interact with the dendrites of other neurons at the *synapse*, where *neurotransmitters* are released (see detail on Figure 5.1). When neurotransmitters are released, they flow across the extracellular space and enter the receiving cell by binding to small cell-surface molecules called *receptors*. Receptors are exquisitely selective: They will only accept the specific neurotransmitter that fits their molecular shape.

Electrical impulses that reach the synapse cross the juncture to be picked up by dendrites, which then convey the signal to the cell body of the next neuron, and the whole lightning-fast process of electrical charging and signaling is repeated.

Because the type of neurotransmitter released helps to determine the action that a receiving cell will generate, many of the symptoms of toxic damage are the result of the specific toxin's impact on one or more of the neurotransmitters (see Table 5.1).

The Two Parts of the Nervous System. The potential impact of a toxin depends on which of the two distinct parts of the nervous system—the central nervous system or the peripheral nervous system—it affects. Some toxins may affect both systems simultaneously but in different ways.

THE CENTRAL NERVOUS SYSTEM (CNS). The CNS is comprised of the brain, which is organized into several distinct regions that control both mental and physical functions, and the spi-

---

Table 5.1
THE MOST COMMON NEUROTRANSMITTERS

Acetylcholine. Secreted by neurons in many areas of the brain but especially in the *basal ganglia*. Acetylcholine is believed to have an enhancing effect on the neuron's ability to transmit electrical impulses.

Norepinephrine. Norepinephrine-secreting neurons are located in an area of the midbrain called the *locus ceruleus*; they help to control emotion and mood.

Dopamine. Secreted by neurons in the *substantia nigra*, the midbrain, and the hypothalamus, dopamine is thought to play a role in controlling movements. (Parkinson's disease is due to loss of cells in the substantia nigra that release dopamine.) Dopamine is also believed to help regulate emotions.

γ-Aminobutyric acid (GABA). Secreted by nerve terminals in the *spinal cord*, GABA appears to play a role in inhibiting the action of other neurotransmitters. It is believed to help in controlling anxiety.

Serotonin. Serotonin is released by the *brain stem* and is diffused throughout many parts of the brain. It acts as an inhibitor of pain and helps to control mood and sleep.

nal cord, which is a two-way conduit for messages between the brain and the rest of the body (see Figure 5.1*a* and *c*).

The brain is divided into several control centers, each responsible for a certain function. The *hypothalamus*, for example, regulates hormonal function and governs such drives as appetite and sexual desire. The *basal ganglia* modulate movement and help interpret sensory information. Each function has an inborn tendency to become localized in one side of the brain or the other. For instance, for most of us speech is located in the left hemisphere of the brain while our organizational skills exist in the right hemisphere.

The brain is a wonderfully intricate organ. To try and describe the way it works, scientists have compared it to a computer, which, like the brain, stores and retrieves information, or to a sophisticated electrical circuit board. However, perhaps no one has described it better than the early twentieth-century physiologist Sir Charles Sherrington, who once called the brain "an enchanted loom" that weaves life's experiences into a shifting harmony of patterns.

The ability of the brain to organize information rests on the interaction of specialized control centers too numerous and beyond the scope of this chapter to describe in detail. It should be said, however, that each control center regulates a different function, such as the ability to speak, see, touch, or think. Respiration, digestion, motor coordination—anything we normally do without thinking—also can be altered by environmental toxins that attack the nervous system.

Depending on what control center they damage, neurotoxins can produce such effects as changes in memory or emotions, or physical damage, such as swelling of brain tissues. For example, exposure to mercury, a metal that damages many different sites in the brain, has been shown to cause irritability, anxiety, and even hallucinations and delirium.

An important feature of the CNS is the blood–brain barrier, a layer of tightly packed cells lining the walls of the blood vessels of the CNS. This unique barricade acts to partially protect the brain and spinal cord from chemicals that would adversely affect their ability to function. For a toxin to affect the CNS, it must have a specific chemical structure that allows it to pass through this safeguarding screen.

THE PERIPHERAL NERVOUS SYSTEM (PNS). The PNS is made up of the nerves that extend to every part of the body, for example, connecting skin surface and muscle to the CNS.

The part of the PNS that controls involuntary movements is called the *autonomic nervous system*, which is divided into two groupings, the *sympathetic* nerves and *parasympathetic* nerves (see Figure 5.1*c*). These nerve groupings work in opposition to each other and can be primarily distinguished by the types of chemicals their neurons release; these chemicals, called neurotransmitters, act as messengers and allow one cell to communicate with another. For example, a toxin that primarily affects the sympathetic nerves connected to the heart might raise blood pressure; one that affected the heart's parasympathetic nerves would cause blood pressure to drop. The nerves of the autonomic nervous system are especially vulnerable to toxic assault. Because the PNS lacks the protective screening of the blood–brain barrier, many toxins have stronger adverse effects on its tissues and cells than on those of the CNS.

Box 5.1 HEADACHES

Physicians now believe that nearly all headaches, whether migraine or tension headaches, develop out of the same physiological syndrome—an imbalance in the neurotransmitters serotonin, norepinephrine, and dopamine. What exactly causes

(continued)

Box 5.1   HEADACHES (continued)

the neurotransmitter imbalance is unclear, but in some cases, the cause may be exposure to a neurotoxin.

When should you see a physician about your headaches? If you find yourself not being able to leave home without pain medication, if you find that headaches are interfering with your life and draining your energy, if you experience a new type of headache, or if a headache persists for more than a day, it is time to seek professional help. Most importantly, see a doctor immediately if you begin to experience numerous headaches but have never had them before or if the headache is more severe than any you have previously experienced.

WHO IS AT RISK?

Those most likely to be affected by neurotoxins are the very young, including developing fetuses; the elderly; and individuals who work with neurotoxic chemicals or deliberately abuse drugs or alcohol. In truth, however, we are all at risk to some degree.

The Fetus

The developing fetus is particularly vulnerable to environmental insults since its nervous system is in the formative stage; the nerve cells are actively growing, dividing, migrating, and making synaptic connections, and the blood–brain barrier is not yet fully formed. During this stage, damage to the nervous system can be caused by a number of different toxins. In later stages of fetal development especially, and even after birth, exposure to a substance such as alcohol or lead can cause motor and sensory deficits, lowered intelligence levels, learning disabilities, and various behavioral problems that become easily assessed only years after birth (see Chapter 11, "Reproductive Effects and Prenatal Exposures").

Infants and Young Children

Infants and young children may be more vulnerable to toxins of all sorts, since their nervous systems are still rapidly developing, making them more susceptible to the effects of many common neurotoxins. Their natural curiosity and their penchant for exploring the world by tasting it also put them at risk. Children with pica, an eating disorder in which a person seeks out nonfood substances to eat, such as dirt, pebbles, and plaster, are at even higher risk than other children (see Chapter 12, "Of Special Concern: Infants and Children").

The Elderly

The elderly may become more susceptible to the effects of neurotoxins due to a number of structural and chemical changes that usually occur starting at about age sixty. Because aging causes a natural attrition of nerve cells, the number of cells in "reserve" gets smaller as time goes by. Exposure to neurotoxins can accelerate the attrition process, as well as act on mechanisms that do not result in cell loss. Aging also changes the body's ability to metabolize drugs and chemicals; a toxin that causes only slight or no symptoms in a young adult might have a much more or much less severe impact on someone who is seventy.

Box 5.2 AGE AND MEDICATION

Those most at risk for developing neurological problems as a result of medication use are the very young and the very old. Physicians know that at some stages children require much smaller doses of drugs to achieve the desired result and they prescribe accordingly. The metabolic changes that occur in old age also affect the amount of medication needed. For example, the proper therapeutic dose of an antidepressant medication at age forty-five may cause dementialike symptoms at age seventy.

An older person is twice as likely to have adverse reactions to a drug as a young person. This occurs for several reasons: the changing body composition and function of the excretory system with age (allowing a drug to stay in the body longer) and the drug reacts with nerve receptors in a different way. As a general rule, given the same dose, the amount of medication that circulates in the blood at age seventy is twice as much as at age thirty-five, and it will stay in the body twice as long. Given this, at times the unintended side effects of a medication can be stronger than the intended therapeutic effects. Both prescription and over-the-counter medications can result in age-related effects.

If you suspect that the medication you are taking is the cause of diminished mental alertness, consult your physician. He or she may decide that the dose can be lowered or prescribe a substitute medication. Do not stop taking the drug without your physician's approval; withdrawal from any drug (and especially one taken for a long period of time) should be carefully monitored.

Workers Exposed to Neurotoxins

People who work with neurotoxic chemicals are especially vulnerable to neurological disease if they do not take proper precautions (see Table 5.2 for neurotoxic chemicals and their effects; see also Table 5.3). To prevent excessive levels of exposure to certain metals, industries must, by federal regulation, provide protective systems (such as proper ventilation) and possibly special personal protective equipment and clothing. However, protective systems may fail and some employers may ignore the law. Moreover, there

Table 5.2 SELECTED INDUSTRIAL CHEMICALS THAT CAUSE PERIPHERAL NERVOUS SYSTEM DISORDERS

Toxin	*Effects*
Lead	Peripheral neuropathies; historically wrist and ankle weakness
Acrylamide	Sensorimotor peripheral neuropathy
Arsenic	Painful limbs, calf cramps, and leg weakness
Methyl *n*-butyl ketone and *n*-hexane	Peripheral neuropathy, weight loss, fatigue, and muscle cramps
Mercury	Sensory impairment

Table 5.3   OCCUPATIONS AND ACTIVITIES AT RISK FOR NEUROTOXIC CHEMICAL EXPOSURE

Occupation	Chemicals
Agriculture	Pesticides, herbicides, insecticides, and solvents
Chemical/pharmaceutical industries	Industrial and pharmaceutical chemicals
Degreasers	Trichloroethylene
Dentists/dental work	Mercury and anesthetic gases
Dry cleaners	Perchloroethylene, trichloroethylene, and other chlorinated hydrocarbons
Electronics workers	Lead, methyl ethyl ketone, methylene chloride, organotins tin, trichloroethylene, glycol ether, xylene, chloroform, freon, and arsenic
Hospital workers	Alcohols (such as ethanol, methanol, and isopropyl), anesthetic gases, ethylene oxide, toluene, and xylene
Laboratory workers	Solvents, mercury, and ethylene oxide
Painters	Lead, toluene, xylene, mixture of mineral spirits, methylene chloride, and other solvents
Plastics workers	Formaldehyde, lead, styrene, toluene, vinylchloride (PVCs), n-hexane, and methyl n-butyl ketone
Printers	Lead, methanol, methylene chloride, toluene, trichloroethylene, and other solvents
Rayon workers	Carbon disulfide
Steel workers	Carbon monoxide, chromium, copper, lead, nickel, tin, zinc, and other metals
Transportation workers	Lead, carbon monoxide, gasoline, and other solvents
Hobbyists	Lead, toluene, adhesives, methylene chloride, xylene, n-hexane, and other solvents

are many more substances in use whose neurotoxic properties have not been adequately studied. The National Institute of Occupational Safety and Health (NIOSH) lists neurological disturbances as one of the ten major forms of occupational hazards (see Chapter 21, "The Workplace," for a discussion of occupations and risk).

Alcohol and Drug Abusers

People who abuse alcohol or drugs, such as cocaine or heroin, risk varying degrees of neurological damage to themselves and their developing fetuses or infants (the risk to the latter occurs during breast feeding). Drinking during pregnancy is associated with fetal alcohol syndrome (FAS). FAS is thought to be the most common toxicological cause of neurological damage and, after birth, results in lowered IQ and behavioral problems (see Chapter 11, "Reproductive Effects and Prenatal Exposures"). The effects on the adult nervous system of these substances depend upon how much is taken, how often, and the overall health of the person taking them.

WEIGHING THE REAL THREAT

Exactly how much at risk is the general population? The answer is that no one really knows. Most commercial substances have not even been tested for neurotoxicity, which means that permissable exposure limits (PEL) have not been established (see p. 359). (PELs set the level of exposure that is not expected to result in adverse neurologic effects for the majority of people.) Lead is a notable exception: As more and more is learned about the effects of this metal, it is becoming increasingly clear that the PEL set by the Occupational Safety and Health Administration (OSHA) should—and is—being lowered; along these lines, the Centers for Disease Control and Prevention have continuously lowered the levels at which lead becomes a concern. In the final analysis, there may be no threshold at which exposure to lead is safe. Unfortunately, the treatment options for persons at these lower levels are severely restricted because of the limitations and toxicity of the existing chelating medications.

The list of neurotoxins common to the modern environment is long and changing. Although lead additives in gasoline have been phased out, we are now recognizing the neurotoxic properties of other constituents, including the solvents benzene, toluene, and xylene. Carbon monoxide, the second largest air pollutant, is a potent neurotoxin released from automobile and truck exhausts. Organophosphate pesticides, such as parathion, are widely available and are commonly used on lawns and in agriculture. Although they don't linger in the environment, such as other pesticides like DDT (dichlorodiphenyltrichloroethane), they can be acutely toxic. In fact, exposure to these chemicals has been linked to chronic central and peripheral nervous system abnormalities.

NIOSH recognizes that neurotoxicity is a major cause of occupational disease but has only established safety standards for seventy-two substances specifically related to neurotoxicity. The EPA has issued very few regulations specifically limiting the use of chemicals for their neurotoxic potential; most of its efforts in banning chemicals relate to the dangers of carcinogens. This lack of regulatory vigor may be due, in part, to the fact that the science of neurotoxicology is still emerging; it did not exist as a formal field of study until the early 1970s.

Much remains to be learned and scientifically proven about specific health threats to the nervous system posed by specific substances. However, a growing body of scientific studies is making it increasingly clear that neurotoxic substances, like carcinogens, pose a serious and probably widespread health risk.

Box 5.3 NUTRITION AND NEUROTOXICITY

Besides taking the obvious precautions when using toxic chemicals and medications, the most important thing you can do to prevent excess exposure or lessen the effects of neurotoxins is to eat a varied, nutritionally sound diet.

About twenty years ago, a group of cases of mercury poisoning occurred in the Midwest among people who ate canned tuna fish with a high mercury content. Although thousands of people had eaten the fish, only those who ate the tuna daily became ill.

(continued)

Box 5.3 NUTRITION AND NEUROTOXICITY (*continued*)

This example illustrates the importance of a varied diet. Not only are most fad diets lacking in certain nutrients, they may also unwittingly result in a dependence on a food that may contain toxins.

The most important vitamins for optimal nervous system functioning are the B vitamins, such as B_1, B_6, and niacin. As they are not stored in the body, it is mandatory that these vitamins be replenished frequently; they are readily found in meat (particularly organ meats), beans, and fresh vegetables.

Although vitamin B_{12} is stored for many years in the body, a lack of it can cause pernicious anemia, a condition that affects the healthy development of the nervous system, particularly nerve cells. If B_{12} is lacking, the myelin sheath, or outer coating of a nerve cell, cannot develop properly. The lack of vitamin B_{12} has also been implicated as a contributing factor in some forms of Alzheimer's disease.

A deficiency of vitamin B_1, thiamine, causes peripheral nerve dysfunction, numbness in the hands and feet. Severe deficiency of this vitamin coupled with alcoholism causes Wernicke–Korsakoff syndrome, a serious neurologic disorder characterized by severe memory loss and an inability to learn new information.

A number of "health-food" advocates recommend megadoses of vitamin B_6 to treat a variety of illnesses, from premenstrual syndrome to asthma to kidney stones. Although the daily requirement of B_6 is estimated to be 2 to 4 milligrams, some people take 4 to 6 grams a day, believing that such self-medication will prevent or relieve these disorders. Not only is scientific proof lacking that these doses are helpful, but vitamin B_6 can cause a severe neuropathy and impair the senses of touch, pain, and temperature.

Whether or not you should take vitamin and mineral supplements for protection against neurotoxins is still being studied. It is clear, however, that a balanced, varied, nutritious diet contributes to the optimal health of the nervous system (see Chapter 17, "Food Safety" for further information).

SOME COMMON NEUROTOXINS

Although hundreds of chemicals have neurotoxic effects, the ones most likely to be encountered are heavy metals, solvents, and pesticides. In addition, many drugs have direct neurologic effects, including alcohol, drugs of abuse such as cocaine, and even some prescription medications.

Box 5.4 WHY CHEMICALS FIND THE NERVOUS SYSTEM AN EASY TARGET

The nervous system is particularly vulnerable to toxic substances because of the following reasons:

(*continued*)

> ## Box 5.4 WHY CHEMICALS FIND THE NERVOUS SYSTEM AN EASY TARGET (*continued*)
>
> - Unlike other cells that make up the body, neurons normally cannot regenerate once they are lost, and cannot be replaced if destroyed by toxic damage.
> - Nerve-cell loss and other regressive changes in the nervous system occur progressively in the second half of life; therefore, toxic damage may occur simultaneously with aging.
> - Certain regions of the brain and nerves are directly exposed to chemicals in the blood, and many neurotoxic chemicals cross the blood–brain barrier with ease.
> - The nervous system depends on a delicate electrochemical balance for proper communication of information throughout the body; this provides numerous opportunities for foreign chemicals to interfere with normal function.

Metals

Several examples of heavy metals include arsenic, manganese, mercury, and thallium; however, one of the most widely distributed environmental neurotoxins is lead. Found in the air we breathe, the food we eat, and in our water, lead is found at many industrial work sites and in a countless number of homes. Lead toxicity is a significant problem for children as well as a potential hazard for adults (see Chapter 12, "Of Special Concern: Infants and Children").

The presence of lead in the blood or soft tissue is of greatest concern because it has access to the nervous system. Lead can be found in circulating blood and in soft tissue, where it is stored typically for less than a month. In bones and teeth, lead can be stored for twenty years or more; however, it cannot gain access to the nervous system. The length of storage time that lead remains in the body is a concern for women of childbearing age; several studies have shown that in pregnancy stored lead can be mobilized, entering the blood, crossing the placenta, and affecting the fetus.

Children have less bone tissue than adults, therefore, a higher percentage of lead may end up in their blood and soft tissue. Children also absorb a higher percentage of ingested lead than adults. Whereas the body of an adult will absorb about 10 percent of ingested lead, for example, a small child may absorb as much as 40 percent. The most sensitive years for exposure probably are from conception to six years. Chronic lead exposure can be devastating, irreversibly damaging a child's ability to learn (see Chapter 12, "Of Special Concern: Infants and Children").

Although lead may not be as damaging to adults as it is to children at equal doses, it can still cause serious neurological problems in adults including cognitive changes, such as loss of memory, problems with concentration and abstract thinking, fatigue, and other symptoms of toxic mood disorders (see Box 5.5 and p. 101). At high concentrations, it can cause encephalopathy, convulsions, and coma. It can also cause anemia and damage to the kidneys and contribute to painful joint diseases such as gout; lead exposure has also been associated with high blood pressure.

Cognitive changes can come on so gradually that those who are exposed to lead may not be aware that anything is wrong until the symptoms become serious. Depending on age and the length of exposure, most people will recover from mood disorders caused by lead but not from cognitive damage due to encephalopathy.

Box 5.5   ADULT LEAD POISONING: A CASE STUDY

Fran Wallace had been diagnosed with a rare genetic blood disease called porphyria. Her body was painfully sensitive to every touch, she had severe stomach cramps, and even a sip of water brought on vomiting.

When her symptoms started two years earlier, her doctor thought it was a severe case of the flu. Fran took solace in drinking tea from a treasured ceramic tea set brought back from her travels in Italy. However, her symptoms worsened.

Then as she and her husband, Donald, a member of the air force, prepared to move from California to Santa Domingo, she started to recover. During the first few months in their new location, before their household goods were unpacked, she felt fine. Then the aches and pains started to set in again. At the same time, Donald was feeling enormously pressured by his new job and was drinking vast amounts of coffee. He became very irritable, so much so that he eventually resigned from the air force.

The Wallaces moved back to their hometown of Seattle, and Fran's illness became progressively worse. Donald began reading everything he could about porphyria. He was intrigued when he read that sometimes lead poisoning was misdiagnosed as the fatal blood disorder.

He then insisted that Fran's blood be tested for lead even though she did not work in a lead-related industry, and they discovered she had a blood lead concentration of 74 micrograms per deciliter—well over the 15 micrograms per deciliter considered dangerous. Donald's own blood tested at 144—high enough possibly to cause permanent brain damage.

The source of their near-fatal bout with lead poisoning? Their ceramic cookware and serving dishes from Italy. Apparently the lead-containing glaze was fired improperly, allowing toxic doses to leach out with every use.

Ceramic ware is the top source of lead in the diet. If you are concerned about the possibility of lead in your home, there are products on the market that allow you to perform your own lead tests. The kits usually contain swabs dipped in a chemical solution, which the user rubs on the surface to be tested (for example, ceramic ware or painted walls); the swabs change color according to the lead concentration. The cost of these kits ranges from about seven dollars for a package of two to more than forty dollars for a package of 100. Some hardware and department stores have begun to carry the kits; they can also be ordered by phone. For more information about the kits and their effectiveness, contact your regional poison control center (see list, Appendix B) or your city department of health. Some local health departments and water departments also perform tests on lead in the home and in water supplies.

Box 5.6   THE MAD HATTER: MERCURY POISONING

One of the best-known cases of mercury poisoning was immortalized in literature by author Lewis Carroll in *Alice in Wonderland*. The Mad Hatter personified a

(continued)

<hr>

Box 5.6 THE MAD HATTER: MERCURY POISONING (*continued*)

nineteenth-century felt worker whose occupation caused him to develop what was called hatter's shakes. The mercury used in the manufacture of felt was then described as producing neurological symptoms and, in its advanced stages, hallucinations and psychotic symptoms. Another well-known case was the outbreak known as Minamata disease (see Box 1.2, p. 25).

A U.S. Public Health study conducted in 1941 found that more than 10 percent of felt workers in this country had chronic mercury poisoning. After scientists were able to document the toxic effects of mercury poisoning in felt workers, its use in felt manufacturing was banned in most nations.

<hr>

Solvents

These are volatile liquid organic compounds that easily vaporize when exposed to air and dissolve other organic compounds. Solvents, such as benzene, carbon disulfide, methylene chloride, methyl *n*-butyl ketone, and *n*-hexane, to name a few, are extremely useful in many kinds of industrial processes. Cleaning fluids, glue, plastics, and gasoline are among the many products that contain solvents. Some 49 million tons of solvents are produced annually in the United States, and 9.8 million workers are exposed to these chemicals daily. They are contained in an amazing array of household products, as well as everything from nail polish removers to rubber cement to furniture polish.

Solvents can be absorbed through the skin, inhaled, or ingested. Exposure is fairly common. In the home, fumes from paint and paint remover can cause headaches, nausea, and respiratory problems, as can the adhesives used by hobbyists to construct model boats. People considered at the highest risk for exposure, however, are those who work with solvents in such industries as the manufacturing of paint, adhesives, plastics, and pharmaceuticals, as well as painters, janitorial and construction workers (see Chapter 21, "The Workplace").

The short-term effects of exposure to certain solvents include light-headedness, loss of balance, impaired work performance, and a drunk-like "high" feeling. Long-term effects of chronic exposure include bouts of headache and dizziness, as well as depression, fatigue, weakness, and other symptoms of toxic mood disorders (see p. 101). Chronic prolonged exposure can impair mental function.

Deliberate exposure to solvents—solvent abuse—is a widespread problem among young people in the United States: Studies show that about 18.7 percent of high school seniors have abused solvents, with most solvent abuse occurring among boys aged seven to seventeen. Not only can this abuse result in neurological effects, there are at least one hundred deaths a year nationwide among teens while inhaling solvents. Because solvents are ubiquitous, getting rid of the sources of abuse is an impossible task. Parents should be alert to the possibility of abuse if their children have sudden changes in behavior and mood, lose interest in school or recreational activities, and have the smell of solvents on their breath.

Pesticides

Despite their ability to raise the ire and concern of an entire nation, pesticides are considered by many to be an important component for the growth and development of the food supply. Unfortunately, the use of these toxic chemicals may create the problem of exposure to pesticides as well as their residues in the air, water, soil, and food supply.

One of the many ways a pesticide can affect the nervous system is its ability to damage and inhibit the enzyme cholinesterase, which is located at the nerve ending and is essential for proper neuromuscular functioning.

Of the many kinds of pesticides commercially available, a class called the organophosphates (originally developed as nerve gases in World War II), including the chemicals malathion, mevinphos, disulfotan, and demeton, are the most commonly used. (For an overview of the types of pesticides available, see Box 17.5, p. 614.) Organophosphates are still potent neurotoxins. Even minute amounts may cause toxic mood disorders and neuropathy (see pp. 101 and 103); concentrated exposure can be potentially lethal. Most, but not all, neurological damage is reversible over time once exposure has ended.

Pesticides can enter the body in a variety of ways, but the most common route of exposure is by absorption through the skin. Those most at risk for exposure are agricultural workers and individuals who work in pesticide manufacturing plants. Many people are also exposed at home, after using pesticides in gardens or spraying the house to prevent termite or other bug infestations. Pesticides can also contaminate groundwater and food: A study by the National Resources Defense Council of the San Francisco area found one of nineteen different pesticides in 44 percent of the produce sampled (see Chapter 17, "Food Safety," and Chapter 15, "Soil," for more information).

Gases

Numerous gases also can wreak havoc on the nervous system. For example, carbon monoxide is a colorless and odorless gas that results from incomplete combustion, the burning of organic matter, including tobacco smoke. Its presence in the environment is unavoidable and widespread; carbon monoxide can affect the health of a city dweller, agricultural worker, even an unborn fetus.

Inhalation or absorption of carbon monoxide can produce numerous symptoms. For instance, long-term exposure to carbon monoxide may result in poor memory and mental deterioration. Acute exposure to this gas can lead to headache, lethargy, irritability, chest pain, confusion, nausea, impaired judgment, and shortness of breath; death may result when an individual inhales this gas in an enclosed space. Ongoing carbon monoxide exposure can have profound neurotoxic effects, possibly resulting in hyperactivity, bizarre behavior, and convulsions (see Carbon Monoxide information sheet, p. 370).

THE ABUSE OF DRUGS

Drugs of abuse—primarily those used for their ability to create a euphoric, or "high," feeling—include alcohol, opium, cocaine, heroin, and marijuana. Most were developed to treat common complaints and have a long history. For example, opium was used in medical practice in China 4,000 years ago, and its derivatives are still extremely useful in controlling severe pain. Heroin, which was developed at the beginning of the twentieth century, was so named because it was supposed to be a "heroic" treatment for morphine addiction. However, the dark side of these substances—addiction—led to the elimination, monitoring, or substitution of other substances.

Alcohol

Although most people are aware of the damage that chronic drinking does to the liver, little thought is given to the damage it can cause to the central nervous system. The short-term neurologic effects of alcohol consumption occur almost immediately after a drink or two. Inebriation adversely affects concentration and motor control, slows reaction time, and impairs the ability to make decisions; in high doses, it can lead to death.

Whether moderate social drinking (defined as not more than one or two drinks a day over a period of years) is permanently harmful to the nervous system is a matter of scientific debate. Most physicians agree, however, that there is no reason to avoid alcohol absolutely (unless you are an alcoholic) as limited quantities of alcohol do not usually produce nerve cell damage.

Alcoholics are individuals who develop a psychological and physical dependence on alcohol. Alcoholics drink more than moderate amounts daily (three or four drinks), although some drink in binges, following weeks of abstinence with days of heavy drinking. Chronic drinking and alcoholism can lead to a variety of neurologic problems, including intellectual deterioration and muscle damage. Alcohol withdrawal can cause symptoms ranging from minor tremors (the "shakes") to delirium tremens (the DTs), a potentially fatal syndrome characterized by extreme agitation, hallucinations, and a very high fever (see Box 22.9, p. 743, for a list of alcoholism warning signs).

Depending on several factors, once chronic drinking stops, there may be a gradual improvement in most neurological functions, but this is not always the case. Some alcoholics (particularly the elderly and those who are poorly nourished and may have additional risks to their neurological function) may have some level of impairment due to depletion of the nutrient thiamine and other water-soluble vitamins.

Drinking alcohol during pregnancy may be particularly harmful because alcohol easily crosses the placenta and can enter the nervous system of the developing fetus, which is particularly vulnerable to its toxic impact. Alcohol can cause a wide range of effects on the developing embryo and fetus, from mild to severe. Heavy drinking can cause FAS, in which numerous systems, including the brain, are damaged. Recent studies have shown that even moderate to light alcohol consumption may affect the developing fetus. Many authorities, such as the March of Dimes, advise pregnant women not to drink at all, since it is possible that even a few drinks at a crucial moment in fetal development could cause slight but measurable mental deficits (see Chapter 11, "Reproductive Effects and Prenatal Exposures," and Chapter 12, "Of Special Concern: Infants and Children").

Box 5.7 ALCOHOL STATISTICS

According to the National Council on Alcoholism and Drug Dependence, Inc., a nonprofit educational organization:

- Ten and one half million people in the United States show signs of alcohol abuse or dependence; an additional 7.2 million individuals show persistent, heavy drinking problems that affect or impair their health. By 1995, this group estimates approximately 11.2 million adults will be alcohol-dependent.
- Ten percent of the population consumes 50 percent of the alcohol.
- Fifty to seventy percent of alcoholics display neurological abnormalities.

(continued)

Box 5.7 ALCOHOL STATISTICS (*continued*)

- Alcoholics have thirty times the suicide rate of nonalcoholics.
- Half of the drivers involved in fatal accidents are legally drunk.
- Two-thirds of people who drown had been drinking before the accident.
- One half of the people who die from falls had been drinking before the accident.
- Alcohol is responsible for an estimated 200,000 deaths—including those resulting from cirrhosis of the liver—a year in the United States.

Cocaine

Cocaine is the most widely used illicit drug of abuse in the United States. An estimated 3 million people use it regularly, more than five times the number of those who abuse heroin. Cocaine and its smokable derivative, crack cocaine, are powerfully addictive. Although its first effects are euphoria along with heightened levels of alertness and energy, it can cause psychoses (mental illnesses characterized by lost contact with reality) including paranoia. As the drug wears off, these feelings are replaced by irritation, restlessness, and depression. Use may cause seizures, paranoia, and loss of motivation and memory. It can also cause bleeding within the brain, strokes, heart attacks, and death.

Marijuana

Marijuana (pot), another intoxicant first used in ancient China, was the most popular illicit drug in the 1960s and 1970s, but its use has declined somewhat in recent years. In addition to making the user "high," marijuana can have a number of neuropsychological effects, including tremor, brief periods of muscle rigidity, brief memory loss, and slowed reaction time. These effects may last as long as six hours after smoking pot. Studies on the long-term effects of marijuana are inconclusive as to the possibility of permanent damage.

NEUROLOGICAL SYNDROMES AND ENVIRONMENTAL AGENTS

Environmental agents are known or suspected of playing a role in many conditions. For example, lead clearly has been implicated as a cause of learning disability. Mercury, which has been found in certain varieties of fish, may adversely effect the health of a pregnant woman and her unborn child. The sweet pea plant, a hardy, drought-resistant legume that is commonly eaten by the poor, contains a neurotoxic amino acid.

However, unless there is clear-cut evidence of exposure, toxins are often overlooked as a possible source of symptoms. This is because many of the symptoms of neurotoxicity are similar to those of other diseases or psychological disorders. For example, in *The Fumigation Chamber,*

the book in which he tells the story of Dr. Page (see p. 84), Berton Roueche describes another episode of pesticide exposure that affected boys from four different families. One youngster was correctly diagnosed as suffering from organophosphate poisoning. The other children, treated by different doctors in different hospitals, were variously diagnosed as having a brain tumor, polio, and encephalitis.

Why is it so difficult to diagnose neurotoxicity? There are no pain cells in the brain; hence, there is no warning of brain injury. In particular, symptoms due to low-level exposure to neurotoxins go unnoticed because the nervous system is responsible for such a large number of bodily functions that symptoms of toxicity can manifest themselves in many different ways. Often the effects are subtle, and the function deteriorates gradually, not overnight. When mental, behavioral, or nervous symptoms are detected, they are often attributed to aging or psychological problems. The public is not aware that commercial products can affect brain function. An affected person is progressively less aware of his or her condition as neurotoxicity continues because of the toxin's cumulative effect. Ascertaining whether or not a toxin is causing a set of symptoms often requires a physician trained to evaluate and test for certain toxins. It should be noted that while there are specific blood and/or urine tests for neurotoxins, testing for most toxins via hair samples is considered an experimental technique that is not clinically useful. It has been proven to be an unreliable tool although some practicing physicians and commercial laboratories continue to use it.

Toxic Mood Disorders

Personality and mental changes are the hallmark of neurotoxicity to the CNS. These symptoms of toxic mood disorders are the first noticed and most pervasive effects of exposure. Other symptoms include sleeplessness, fatigue, and lack of energy; loss of interest in sex, food, and work; and impaired reaction time and coordination (a serious side effect because it can lead to industrial or motor vehicle accidents).

Substances capable of causing mood disorders are legion. *Any* neurotoxin can provoke mood changes, but the most common sources include metals such as lead and mercury, certain solvents and gases, and pesticides. For example, carbon disulfide, a solvent now used primarily in the rayon and cellophane industries, can cause severe manic-depression, and rates of suicide and homicide were once high among rayon workers. Today, ventilation in industries using carbon disulfide keeps exposure levels low. However, even regulated levels, those that are purportedly safe, may cause toxic mood disorders and symptoms such as depression, irritability, and insomnia.

Symptoms can be overt or subtle, depending upon the intensity and duration of exposure to the toxin. A person with toxic mood disorders may be aware that something is wrong but is unable to pinpoint the problem, or the symptom may be so debilitating that continued normal functioning is difficult.

Many of the symptoms of toxic mood disorders are identical to those of depression, which can make a correct diagnosis difficult. When no life event, such as a death in the family or loss of a job, has precipitated symptoms of depression, other possibilities, including exposure to neurotoxins, should be investigated. Remember, though, that many illnesses have depressive symptoms; a careful history and physical including a neuropsychological evaluation and standardized testing by a certified neuropsychologist, as well as various laboratory tests (including specific toxicological assessments), are necessary to attempt to definitively determine if the symptoms are being caused by a toxin or a disease or are a functional psychological disorder.

Toxic mood disorders can abate within days once exposure to the source has ceased, but symptoms can reoccur if further exposure occurs. If exposure continues, the symptoms can continue to worsen.

Box 5.8 SYMPTOMS OF TOXIC MOOD DISORDERS

How can you tell if you are suffering from exposure to a neurotoxin? Often, the first symptoms are subtle and can be mistaken for moodiness or simply overlooked.

(continued)

Box 5.8 SYMPTOMS OF TOXIC MOOD DISORDERS (*continued*)

The first sign is often a change in behavior, similar to that experienced after drinking alcohol—slower speech, foggy thinking, lack of coordination. You may also not feel "yourself" or have mood swings greater than what is usual. Here is a list of what to look for:

• *Personality changes.* Irritability, expressed in many different ways, is the most common personality change. For example, a previously pleasant person may begin to have arguments with friends, families, and co-workers. Another symptom is social withdrawal; as functional difficulties increase, a person suffering from neurotoxicity may not have the ability to cope with the minor problems that attend all relationships.

• *Mental changes.* There may be problems recalling recent events, or concentration may be impaired. The person may demonstrate mental slowness and have difficulties following a conversation, understanding what is read, or following directions.

• *Sleep disturbances.* Toxin-caused disturbances in the hormones that regulate sleep will induce some people to sleep for much longer periods than in the past, others for shorter periods. (This symptom should also be corroborated with neuropsychiatric testing.)

• *Chronic fatigue.* In order to attribute chronic fatigue to neurotoxic exposure, a person will also have impaired neuropsychiatric function that might only show up in specialized testing.

• *Motor incoordination.* This symptom may be manifested by difficulty in walking or in reduced manual dexterity. Toxic-related muscle weakness has been misdiagnosed as multiple sclerosis.

All of these symptoms can be objectively tested by a trained neuropsychologist using standard batteries of tests.

Adapted from *Neurotoxicity Guidebook* by Raymond M. Singer, 1990, Van Nostrand Reinhold, New York.

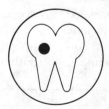

Box 5.9 DEBATE: MERCURY IN DENTAL AMALGAM

Amalgams, the most common kind of dental fillings, are composed of the heavy metals mercury and silver. It has long been recognized that mercury vapor can cause significant neurological problems, and it has been shown that chewing can release minute amounts of mercury vapor from amalgam fillings. However, there is no evidence that the amount of vapor released exceeds the acceptable OSHA standard for mercury or that it produces any adverse health effects.

In spite of this fact, it has been postulated (although the hypothesis has been highly criticized by most of the scientific community) that amalgams might play a role in toxic mood disorders and other neurological and psychological problems. Faced with growing public concern, the National Institute of Dental Research is planning a large-scale investigation to see if there is any link between dental amalgam and health problems.

In the meantime, if you have extensive amalgam fillings and are worried about possible health consequences, you can ask your physician to order a standard test for mercury in your urine. If the amount of mercury in the urine proves to be excessive (over 25 micrograms per gram of creatinine), you should investigate why levels are so high.

If you are considering having fillings removed and replaced with an alternative material, such as plastic composite, be aware that replacement with plastic composites carries its own risk—tooth structure can be damaged and the removal process can release more mercury vapor. Less is known about these plastic amalgams and they could turn out to be no better—or worse—than the old mercury ones.

Given that the risk posed by amalgam fillings is highly speculative (no one has been shown to become ill from amalgams at the time of writing) and their relatively low cost keeps dental care affordable for most families, these fillings are still the best choice for most people.

Toxic Encephalopathy

More serious than mood disorders, *toxic encephalopathy*, the term used to describe serious, generalized brain dysfunction, can occur if exposure to a neurotoxin continues. Common symptoms of toxic encephalopathy include personality changes and problems with memory and conceptual thinking. Recovery from encephalopathy can take weeks rather than days, as with mood disorders, and some people may never fully recover. For example, heavy metals such as lead or organotin can cause severe confusion as well as listlessness or, in severe cases, convulsions, coma, or respiratory arrest (see also Learning Disabilities, p. 104).

Peripheral Neuropathy

One of the most common end results of neurotoxicity is peripheral neuropathy, damage to the nerves of the PNS. This damage can occur to motor nerves, resulting in muscle weakness, or to sensory nerves, which causes diminished sensations of touch to cold, heat, pain, and pressure; damaged peripheral nerves may also be painful. Often, exposure to neurotoxins causes both motor (muscle) and sensory problems.

Like toxic mood disorders, neuropathies can develop slowly and subtly or come on quickly with intense symptoms. Often, the first telltale signs of motor neuropathy are cramps in the legs, difficulty with climbing stairs, and an inability to grasp heavy objects. Symptoms of sensory neuropathy include numbness and tingling in the feet that does not go away. The symptoms are similar to the transient sensation that occurs when a nerve is compressed and the leg or foot feels "asleep." The most severe cases of peripheral neuropathy may result in motor paralysis.

In 1930, at the height of Prohibition, solvent contamination of a popular drink caused a widespread outbreak of peripheral neuropathy paralysis. Ginger-Jake was a medicinal tonic sold as a cure for the flu and digestive and menstrual problems. (Although it did contain ginger and castor oil, Jake owed most of its popularity to a generous alcohol content.) One enterprising bootlegger substituted varnish containing the substance triorthocresyl phosphate, a colorless or pale yellow plasticizer found in lacquers or varnishes, for the more expensive castor oil. Individuals who drank this tainted concoction developed peripheral neuropathies with symptoms that ranged from temporary numbness to permanent paralysis. Estimates vary, but some 100,000 people may have been affected by peripheral neuropathies—which came to be known as the Ginger-Jake syndrome— before the bootlegger was stopped.

In addition to solvents, likely environmental causes of neuropathies are pesticides and alcohol abuse. Some toxins cause more severe symptoms than others, for example, arsenic neuropathy can cause a feeling of severe burning on the soles of the feet and create excruciating pain at the touch of any object, including the weight of bedclothes.

As with mood disorders, it is important to note that many diseases can cause neuropathy, not just environmental toxins. For example, two common illnesses, hypertension (high blood pressure) and diabetes, which impairs blood circulation to the limbs, can cause serious peripheral neuropathy. Again, careful medical evaluation, including a complete history and, when appropriate, testing, is necessary to attempt a diagnosis of toxic neuropathy.

In mild cases of toxic peripheral neuropathy, there is no specific treatment except for avoiding exposure to the cause. If symptoms come on suddenly, suspect severe toxic poisoning and seek medical assistance.

In many cases, people may have a substantial recovery from peripheral neuropathies. Unlike nerve cells of the CNS, if the nerve cell is not completely killed and the myelin sheath isn't distrupted beyond repair, the axons of peripheral nerve cells can, to a limited extent, regenerate or sprout extra connections to make up for damage.

Learning Disabilities

Learning disabilities affecting children exposed to lead, cocaine, and alcohol are the most common environmentally related neurological disorders.

Learning disabilities take many forms. They can involve mild difficulty with reading skills or trouble in memorizing spelling or math problems. They can also encompass more serious problems with speech and language problems or poor overall academic performance. Some children are burdened with attention deficit disorder, a behavioral problem characterized by poor attention span and often accompanied by hyperactivity. A child with this disorder cannot focus on one activity or toy long enough to learn from it.

Although not the only cause—and probably not even the major cause of learning disabilities—a child exposed to a neurotoxin may display some or all of these symptoms. (Heredity, environment, and many childhood diseases can contribute to the same spectrum of symptoms.)

Among the most potent environmental neurotoxins associated with learning disabilities are lead; alcohol; medications and other drugs; and drugs of abuse, such as cocaine and heroin. The effects of all of these substances on the growth and development of infants, children, and developing fetuses are discussed in Chapter 12, "Of Special Concern: Infants and Children."

Parkinson's Disease

In the United States, nearly half a million people have Parkinson's disease, with about 50,000 new cases diagnosed each year. Scientists have now begun to investigate whether environmental toxins play a role in causing this troubling disorder.

Parkinson's disease occurs when nerve cells in the area of the brain called the substantia nigra are destroyed. These cells produce dopamine, a neurotransmitter that helps to control movement; Parkinson's disease occurs when some 80 percent of the dopamine-producing neurons are lost (see Figure 5.2).

No one knows for certain what causes Parkinson's disease, although theories abound. Heredity is strongly suspected of playing a role, although no studies to date have shown a conclusive genetic contribution. Several researchers have speculated that age-related deterioration of the cells in the substantia nigra are responsible, while others have suggested that a series of environmental insults, perhaps from viruses or toxins, coupled with aging destroys enough neurons

in the substantia nigra for Parkinson's disease to occur. There is no conclusive evidence for either of these hypotheses.

The strongest substantiation that environmental toxins may play a causative role in Parkinson's disease comes from epidemiological observations. For instance, numerous individuals developed Parkinson's disease after suffering from a widespread influenza outbreak in the 1920s. Miners of manganese, a metal used in dry-cell batteries, fertilizers, and antiseptics, have developed a Parkinsonlike syndrome in as little as six months, although usually it takes much longer. In rural areas where pesticides are used, it is possible that well water, which primarily comes from pockets of groundwater that might contain accumulated toxins, may play a role in the development of Parkinson's disease (if an association is eventually and clearly documented).

Another clue in the puzzle of the causes of Parkinson's disease comes from Guam. Physicians in the U. S. Navy stationed there during and after World War II were intrigued by a very high rate of Parkinsonlike dementia and amyotrophic lateral sclerosis, a relatively rare neurological disor-

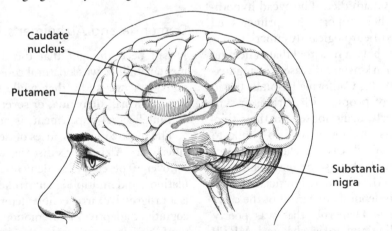

Figure 5.2 AREAS OF THE BRAIN AFFECTED BY PARKINSON'S DISEASE.

Caudate nucleus

Putamen

Substantia nigra

The symptoms of Parkinson's disease arise when an insufficient amount of dopamine, a neurotransmitter produced in the substantia nigra (highlighted), causes defective transmission between the substantia nigra and the striatum (composed of the caudate nucleus and putamen), the area of the brain that controls movement and balance.

Box 5.10 SYMPTOMS OF PARKINSON'S DISEASE

The classic symptoms of Parkinson's disease are stooped posture, shuffling gait, and trembling hands. In the initial stages, symptoms of Parkinson's disease are more subtle—perhaps a mild shaking in the thumb and index finger or of the foot when sitting. Then, as the disease progresses, the postural reflexes, which help us maintain our bodies upright in space, are damaged. With these lost, a person with Parkinson's disease can fall without feeling faint or dizzy in advance. For some people, falling without provocation is the first noticeable, frightening sign of the disease.

As symptoms progress, activities formerly performed without thought become an effort—tying shoes or buttoning a shirt. Extraordinary effort must be put into such actions as inserting a door key, eating, and brushing teeth. Movements are no longer spontaneous: People with Parkinson's disease can no longer swing their arms when they walk, and their handwriting becomes smaller and tends to trail off.

Although Parkinson's disease cannot be cured, it can be treated with medication to relieve the worst symptoms and enable a person to have a fairly normal life for a number of years. For this reason, it's important to get medical help as soon as possible.

der, among the native people. Eventually, scientists traced the source of these neurological conditions to the ingestion of cycad seeds, a mainstay of the Guam diet. The cycad hypothesis received further support when primates fed cycads developed neurological dysfunction.

Now scientists have a new tool that is helping them search for Parkinson's disease–causing toxins. In the late 1970s, California hospitals began to get an influx of people with Parkinson syndrome, particularly drug abusers in their thirties. Because it is rare for anyone so young to develop Parkinson's disease, a cluster of cases strongly suggested that some environmental toxin was causing the disorder. Physicians found that the common denominator in all of the cases was a "homemade Demerol" that was poorly produced, yielding the toxic chemical MPTP (1-methyl-4-phenyl-1,2,3,6-tetrahydropyridine). Interestingly, MPTP is structurally similar to the pesticide Paraquat, which may epidemiologically be associated with Parkinson's disease.

Because laboratory animals injected with MPTP also develop Parkinson's disease, scientists have been able to use animal studies to more selectively test new drugs to treat and study this debilitating disease.

Dementia and Alzheimer's Disease

It had been thought that the deterioration of mental abilities was a natural consequence of aging. Now we know that while some memory loss is normal, dementia, or severe memory loss and intellectual impairment, is not.

The most common causes of dementias in the elderly are Alzheimer's disease, which accounts for over 50 percent of all dementias in some populations, and multiple small strokes. Alzheimer's is a progressive, irreversible deterioration of the cognitive, adaptive, and emotional functions of the CNS. In many cases, the deterioration begins so gradually that people who have it do not notice that a problem is developing, although spouses and friends often do.

Physical illnesses that can cause dementialike symptoms are numerous. They include hypothyroidism, brain tumor, stroke, subdural hematoma, encephalitis, and meningitis to name but a few.

Several kinds of dementia clearly have environmental roots. Chronic overusers of alcohol often do not eat properly and can suffer from the thiamine-deficiency-related ailment Wernicke–Korsakoff syndrome, characterized, in part, by a severe loss of memory. Years of excessive occupational exposure or abuse of solvents, such as toluene (a paint and lacquer thinner and an additive in fuels), can cause dementia.

Now scientists are attempting to determine if Alzheimer's disease, the most common form of dementia and generally thought to be genetic in origin, is associated with aluminum, a heavy metal.

For example, individuals whose renal disease was treated by dialysis fluid that contained extremely high doses of aluminum had a high rate of "dialysis dementia." Once aluminum was removed from the dialysate, the syndrome no longer occurred. A noteworthy, but controversial, British study reported in the medical journal *Lancet*, in January 1989, demonstrated that adults who live in areas with water with high concentrations of aluminum have a 50 percent greater risk of developing Alzheimer's disease than people living in areas where the water contains virtually no aluminum. The study tested 4,100 people in eighty-eight English counties.

Scientists and the popular press are hotly debating the issue.

The only thing that can be said definitively about the issue is that upon autopsy accumulations of aluminum are found in brain lesions of people who had Alzheimer's disease. It is not known if these aluminum deposits are either a cause or a result of the disease, however, and research suggests that their presence may simply be an artifact of the way the specimens used in research are prepared.

Does this mean you should or can eliminate aluminum from your life? Most scientists discount the value of halting the use of aluminum products such as pots and pans (which may leach small amounts of aluminum into food), antiperspirants, buffered aspirin, and antacids. Even the strongest supporters of the aluminum hypothesis have made few changes in their habits to eliminate contact with aluminum through such sources.

If a grandparent, parent, or sibling has Alzheimer's disease, avoiding voluntary exposure to aluminum can do no harm. However, no proof exists that Alzheimer's disease can be prevented or delayed by doing so. Similarly, no evidence exists that chelation therapy, a process involving the use of potentially toxic drugs to promote the removal of metals such as aluminum from the body, is effective.

Box 5.11   IS IT NORMAL FORGETFULNESS OR IS IT DEMENTIA?

Everybody forgets things now and then, and even healthy people over forty-five are more forgetful than younger people. What kind of forgetting means that something is really wrong?

Let's say your spouse goes to the supermarket to buy five items. Forgetting one or two would not be at all unusual, and if he were particularly distracted, he might even forget all five. However, if he returns home and did not remember he had ever been to the supermarket or if he got lost on the way home from the supermarket it would indicate a serious problem.

In addition to memory loss and forgetfulness, people with Alzheimer's disease misuse words, have difficulty performing the tasks of daily living, and lose interest

(continued)

Box 5.11   IS IT NORMAL FORGETFULNESS OR IS IT DEMENTIA? (*continued*)

in social and recreational activities. Although many of these behavioral and cognitive changes also occur with other disorders, they occur in a unique and predictable *pattern*, or stages, in Alzheimer's disease. Recognizing and identifying this pattern is an important part of confirming a diagnosis. Also important to keep in mind is that other possible organic illnesses, such as Parkinson's disease or chronic meningitis, should be ruled out before Alzheimer's disease is the diagnosis.

Because Alzheimer's disease is an untreatable condition, it is important to eliminate every other etiology of dementialike symptoms. Certain drugs, as well as drug interactions, or overdoses can also cause dementialike effects, as can some toxic substances. It is important that the physician know about every medication being taken by a person suspected of having Alzheimer's disease, or if it is possible that toxic exposure has occurred. If the symptoms of dementia come on rapidly, which usually happens with drugs or toxins, the problem is probably not Alzheimer's disease.

After other organic causes of memory loss have been ruled out, the possibility of functional psychiatric illness should be considered—particularly because many forms of psychiatric illness are treatable. In an older person, for example, depression can easily be confused with dementia, especially if symptoms include inattentiveness to dress and grooming or interfere with communication.

There are predictable stages of decline in mental, cognitive, and other functions in the progressive deterioration of Alzheimer's disease. Table 5.4, which lists these stages, is based upon the global deterioration scale (GDS), developed by Dr. Barry Reisberg and colleagues at the NYU Medical Center. The GDS outlines the progression of decline characteristic of this disease. It should be noted that if the stages of deterioration of an individual do not match the given order, the problem may be dementia associated with conditions other than Alzheimer's disease.

The young science of neurotoxicology is still in the process of determining which substances could possibly harm the nervous system and how much exposure to any substance could possibly be dangerous. The first tantalizing hints that toxins may play a role in such devastating disorders as Parkinson's and Alzheimer's diseases have intrigued scientists a great deal. In the future, it may indeed be possible to take steps that will help prevent the development of those diseases, just as research in the relationship between smoking and lung cancer has allowed so many people to avoid having that disease.

In the meantime, steps to take to maintain a healthy nervous system include taking proper precautions when using pesticides and solvents; avoiding abuse of drugs and alcohol; following all precautions when using toxic substances at work; and eating a nutritious, varied diet.

Table 5.4   STAGES OF ALZHEIMER'S DISEASE

Stage	Symptoms
Stage 1: Normal (no cognitive decline)	The person appears normal and does not consciously note loss of memory.
Stage 2: Normal-aged forgetfulness (very mild cognitive decline)	Common complaints of memory loss in this stage include forgetting where familiar objects have been placed and forgetting names that they formerly knew very well.
Stage 3: Early confusional (borderline Alzheimer's disease)	Decline in some abilities becomes evident to others, particularly co-workers. This is the stage at which persons may begin to forget important appointments for the first time in their lives. Persons may experience difficulty in traveling to new locations, may immediately forget what is read or said to him/her, and may find it difficult to locate the right word in conversation.
Stage 4: Late confusional (mild Alzheimer's disease)	There is a clear-cut decline in cognitive abilities, and it becomes readily apparent to others. Deficits manifest in many areas, including impaired concentration, a decreased knowledge of recent events in his/her life as well as world events, and a decline in the ability to perform complex tasks accurately and efficiently. The person may have difficulty handling finances (balancing a checkbook), marketing, planning a dinner party, or traveling alone, particularly to an unfamiliar place. However, the person often remains well oriented to time and to person.
Stage 5: Early dementia (moderate Alzheimer's disease)	The person can no longer function socially without assistance. When interviewed, he or she may be unable to recall a major relevant aspect of current life, such as his/her telephone number or address of many years, or names of close family members, such as grandchildren (generally, the name of spouse and children are recalled), or name of the college or high school from which he/she graduated. Often, the person is disoriented in time (day, date, season) or place. The person can generally toilet and eat without assistance but may have some difficulty choosing the proper clothing to wear. He/she may require coaxing to bathe.
Stage 6: Middle dementia (moderately severe Alzheimer's disease)	The person becomes entirely dependent upon the spouse (or others) for survival. They may occasionally forget the name of the spouse but can distinguish familiar from unfamiliar persons in the

(continued)

Table 5.4   STAGES OF ALZHEIMER'S DISEASE (*continued*)

Stage	Symptoms
	environment and generally recall their own name. The person is largely unaware of recent events and experiences in his/her life and has only a very sketchy knowledge of past personal life. Generally unaware of the year, the season, etc. He/she may have difficulty counting backward from one to ten. He/she requires assistance with activities of daily living and requires a travel escort. His/her diurnal rhythm is frequently disturbed. Functional abilities deteriorate in the following progression: the person has difficulty putting on clothes and requires assistance bathing (may develop fear of bathing); then becomes unable to handle mechanics of toileting; then suffers urinary and then fecal incontinence.
Stage 7: Late dementia (severe Alzheimer's disease)	The brain appears to lose the ability to distinguish basic physical activities. Verbal abilities are lost; first, the ability to speak is limited (one to five words a day), then all intelligible vocabulary is lost and the person frequently only grunts. The person is incontinent and requires assistance with toileting and feeding. Basic psychomotor skills are lost: first, the ability to walk; then to sit up independently; then, to smile; and, finally, to hold his/her head up. In the final phases of this stage, stupor and coma occur.

CHAPTER 6

Respiratory Ailments

Of the three major barriers that separate the environment outside the body from that within, the lungs are perhaps the most fragile and the most vulnerable to assault by the external environment.

Even as you sit quietly reading this book, you have no choice but to breathe. The average adult inhales a pint of air twelve to sixteen times a minute. Whatever is in that air, if it is small enough, can ride along in these wisps of inhalation, potentially finding a portal of entry inside the body. Dusts and sprays, fumes and smokes, chemicals and particles—all may contain dangerous substances from which you cannot escape.

Box 6.1 SOURCES OF RESPIRATORY DISTRESS

Tobacco smoke: Tobacco smoke is the most widespread indoor air pollutant, a major cause of serious respiratory ailments and lung cancer, as well as heart disease, and the single most important preventable cause of death in our society. Both direct exposure to tobacco smoke and environmental tobacco smoke (passive smoke) are harmful to the body (see Chapter 22, "The ABCs of Staying Healthy").

Airborne biologic agents: Disease-causing viruses and bacteria, such as those that cause colds, influenza, sinusitis, and pneumonia; molds; and fungi, as well as other biological allergens such as pollens, dust mites, and animal dander, are all "natural" agents carried in the air. Air-tight buildings with poorly maintained ventilation systems often foster the growth of some of these biologic agents (see Chapter 14, "Air"). Certain workers, such as farmers and health care workers, can be exposed to other airborne biologic agents that cause a variety of pulmonary and other infections (see Chapter 21, "The Workplace").

Outdoor air pollutants: The majority of the criteria pollutants and substances classified as air toxins can affect the respiratory tract as well as other organs of the body (see Chapter 14, "Air"). Outdoor air pollutants may be irritating to some people but are especially troublesome to people who already suffer from asthma, emphysema, and other chronic respiratory ailments.

Indoor air pollutants: In addition to tobacco smoke, other indoor pollutants, such

(continued)

Box 6.1   SOURCES OF RESPIRATORY DISTRESS (*continued*)

as formaldehyde and other volatile organic chemicals, can irritate the respiratory tract. Airborne asbestos can damage the lungs causing asbestosis or two types of cancer of the lung and lining of the lungs. Exposure to high concentrations of radon indoors can contribute to the development of lung cancer and is considered a top environmental hazard by the Environmental Protection Agency (EPA) (see Chapter 14, "Air").

Workplace exposures: The oldest occupational diseases on record, dating back to the Greeks, are respiratory ailments that result from exposure to coal and silica. Today, numerous airborne irritants and toxins encountered at work sites cause countless respiratory disorders. Some of these substances are "natural," such as wood dusts, cotton fibers, and mineral dusts such as silica. Some are synthetic, such as dusts and fumes of various chemicals. Many have profoundly damaging effects.

The effects of these exposures on the respiratory system are widespread and evident: In 1990, chronic respiratory conditions, such as bronchitis, asthma, hay fever, sinusitis, and emphysema, affected 83.6 million Americans, according to the American Lung Association; acute respiratory ailments, such as colds, influenza, viruses, and acute bronchitis, affected approximately 210 million people; and respiratory ailments related to harmful occupational exposures lead the list of work-related illnesses (a conservative estimate is that more than 65,000 workers each year in the United States develop a job-related respiratory disease). Beyond these respiratory illnesses are other ailments, including damage to liver, kidney, and the central nervous system and cancer of the lungs and of other organs, all of which can arise as a result of exposure to toxic substances carried in the air.

THE RESPIRATORY TRACT AS A ROUTE OF EXPOSURE

The Gas-Exchange Process

The respiratory tract, which begins at the nostrils and mouth and extends deep into the lungs (see Figure 6.1), is a major pathway to the body's complex interior environment. Respiration, or the inhalation and exhalation of air, is a complex activity that extracts oxygen from the air for the body to use and removes carbon dioxide from the bloodstream.

Incoming oxygen is vital to every cell in the body. With each breath, oxygen is transported inside a cell, resulting in oxidation, a series of chemical reactions that allow the substance to burn food and release energy. After a cell uses the oxygen, it releases carbon dioxide, a waste product, that leaves the body with each exhalation. This activity is known as the *gas-exchange function* of the lungs.

Because the lungs are an organ of exchange between the internal and external environment, they are especially vulnerable to airborne toxins. During this gas-exchange process, harmful microscopic particles that are suspended in the incoming oxygen can become trapped in the lungs or injurious gases can make their way into the bloodstream.

The respiratory tract has numerous defense mechanisms, such as coughing, to filter out airborne toxins and protect its delicate structures. When these defenses are injured, a person is more susceptible to developing a respiratory disease or aggravating any existing lung condition.

Whether or not a substance will actually lead to a respiratory condition depends on several factors, including the toxicity of the substance, the amount used, the length of exposure time, and an individual's personal risk factors for respiratory disease. For example, a smoker may be more vulnerable to developing certain respiratory ailments than a nonsmoker. Workers who continuously handle potentially dangerous substances on the job without adequate protection also may eventually damage their lungs' defense mechanisms.

Box 6.2: THE RESPIRATORY TRACT: AERIAL GATEWAY TO THE BODY

The typical adult breathes in a pint of air twelve to sixteen times a minute while at rest (when exercising, an individual requires much more air). With each breath, incoming air enters the nose and is warmed or cooled to the appropriate temperature, humidified, and filtered before moving on to the lungs. Small hairs located just inside the front of the nose remove dust and other particles, making the nose the first line of defense in the protection of the lungs. The filtration process continues as inhaled air moves along the mucous membranes lining the nasal passages.

Hairlike cells called *cilia* line the mucous membranes, constantly and rhythmically beating and operating much like an escalator that moves in one direction—away from the nose. Dust and other impurities get carried along the membrane's surface, toward the back of the throat, where the mucous is swallowed. This defense mechanism is known as the *mucociliary escalator* (see Figure 6.1c).

After the air has been moistened and filtered for entry into the lungs, it moves down the *trachea*, or windpipe, into the chest. The trachea then divides into two *bronchial tubes* (*bronchi*) that form more intricate subdivisions with even finer branches of smaller airways, which are called *bronchioles*, deep inside each of the two lungs.

The millions of bronchioles in each lung lead to elastic air sacs called *alveoli*, each of which is surrounded by tiny blood vessels called *capillaries*. The microscopic alveoli and the capillaries have walls so thin that the delicate membrane separating them allows incoming oxygen to be exchanged for outgoing carbon dioxide.

Each lung contains about 300 million tiny, bubblelike alveoli. If these tightly packed alveoli were stretched out, their surface area would measure about ninety-six square yards.

The oxygen that enters the air sacs moves into the blood through the capillary wall and is then dissolved in the blood. A protein in the red blood cell, called *hemoglobin*, binds to a large percentage of the dissolved oxygen and then transports the oxygen to tissues all around the body. Hemoglobin is capable of carrying a large amount of oxygen, which it releases according to the body's needs. The outgoing carbon dioxide from the body's cells is dissolved in the bloodstream, and exits at the alveoli for exhalation through the lungs.

Deep inside the lungs, there is no mucus or cilia to waft away impurities. But cells called *macrophages* identify, trap, and dispose of foreign bodies that threaten to penetrate the thin walls of the alveoli. After destroying bacteria and particles, the residue from the macrophages works its way to the mucociliary escalator, which extends into the bronchioles, for clearance from the lungs.

THE LUNGS AND RESPIRATORY SYSTEM

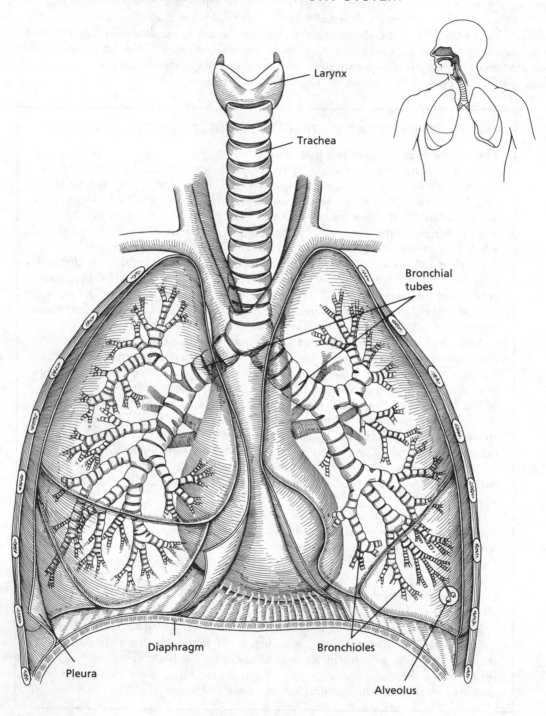

Larynx

Trachea

Bronchial tubes

Diaphragm

Pleura

Bronchioles

Alveolus

(a) LUNGS AND ASSOCIATED STRUCTURES

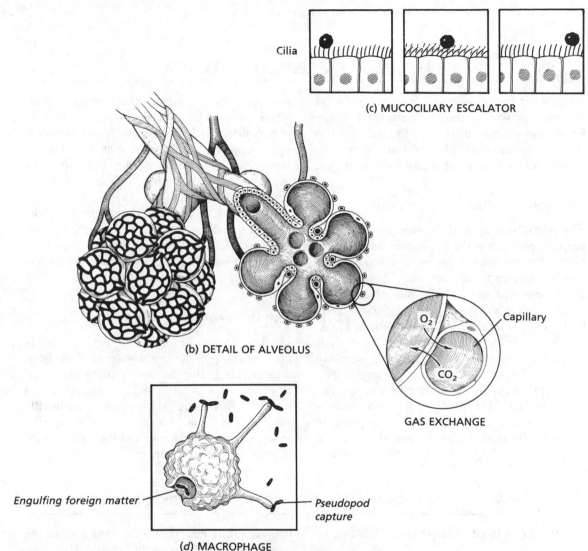

Cilia

(c) MUCOCILIARY ESCALATOR

(b) DETAIL OF ALVEOLUS

O₂

Capillary

CO₂

GAS EXCHANGE

Engulfing foreign matter

Pseudopod capture

(d) MACROPHAGE

Figure 6.1 THE LUNGS AND RESPIRATORY SYSTEM.

(*a*) The lungs and associated structures. The lungs are considered the most important—and most vulnerable—route of exposure to environmental toxins. Air moves from the nose and nasal passages through the trachea, or windpipe, into the chest. There the trachea divides into the two bronchial tubes. These divide into millions of fine branches called bronchioles. At the end of the bronchioles are the alveoli, microscopic elastic air sacs. (*b*) Detail of an alveolus, the site of gas exchange, where oxygen and carbon dioxide gases diffuse from the lungs to the blood-stream via capillaries. Inhaled agents can enter the bloodstream via the exchange. (*c*) The mucociliary escalator. The cilia that line the mucous membranes of the trachea and bronchial passages beat constantly and rhythmically, moving dust and other impurities like a one-way escalator toward the back of the throat, where the mucus is swallowed. (*d*) A macrophage. Macrophages in the alveoli engulf foreign matter that may have penetrated the lung's defenses, trapping and destroying it and conveying it to the mucociliary escalator for clearance.

DEFENSES OF THE RESPIRATORY SYSTEM

When air in the environment is clean and free of microbes or toxins, the respiratory tract's defense mechanisms quietly stand guard. Yet this complex system naturally possesses several defensive reactions to combat any harmful toxins.

The Role of Mucus Production

The rate of mucus production is just enough to keep the passages of the respiratory lining moist. Normally, the nose replaces its mucous secretions once every twenty minutes. Many bacteria and viruses that attach to the cilia are destroyed by enzymes released by the nasal mucous membrane and are transported away from the lungs.

When a foreign substance, such as dust, is inhaled and makes its way past the defensive cilia, the respiratory tract reacts by stepping up mucus production in order to clear the particles from the lungs. The ability of the mucous membrane to increase its secretions in response to inhaled substances varies in individuals. Some people may be highly sensitive to irritants and produce a lot of mucus; others, such as those who spend long hours in overheated homes, tend to have drier nasal passages and less resistance to upper respiratory infections such as colds and influenza. Smoking also irritates the respiratory tract, hampering an individual's respiratory defense mechanisms.

Illnesses, such as a respiratory tract infection, also can spur increased mucus production. When the infection has run its course and the bacteria or virus has been destroyed, the level of mucous secretion returns to normal.

Mouth Versus Nose Breathing

During vigorous exercise, a person usually breathes through the mouth instead of the nose, thus increasing the chance of pulling larger particles into the airways and prompting mucus production. Although these particles are usually exhaled, some may actually reach the smaller airways of the bronchioles and the alveoli, areas that are difficult to clear.

HEALTH EFFECTS OF POLLUTANTS AND RESPIRATORY IRRITANTS

Health Effects of Hazardous Gases

When hazardous gases—often called *vapors* in the work setting—are present in high concentrations, they can irritate or damage the lungs. There are many types of gases, and the extent of injury depends on a number of factors: whether the gas is soluble (dissolves in water) or insoluble; the type of chemical it contains; and how far down it advances in the respiratory tract, to name a few.

Water-soluble gases such as sulfur dioxide, ammonia, chlorine, and bromine quickly dissolve in the mucus that lines the nose, throat, and the upper airways. Low levels of exposure to these substances irritate the tissues below the mucous membrane, possibly causing burning. In cases of accidents where the exposure is intense, inhalation of a large amount of these gases may be life-threatening.

Insoluble gases, including nitrogen dioxide and phosgene, bypass the areas of the respiratory tract that are lined with mucous membrane and head directly to the tiny air sacs deep inside the lungs. Thus, neither of these gases produces an irritating sensation when inhaled. Instead, they seep into and damage the deep lung tissues that lack pain sensors. Hours after exposure, the gas produces edema, the accumulation of fluid in the lungs.

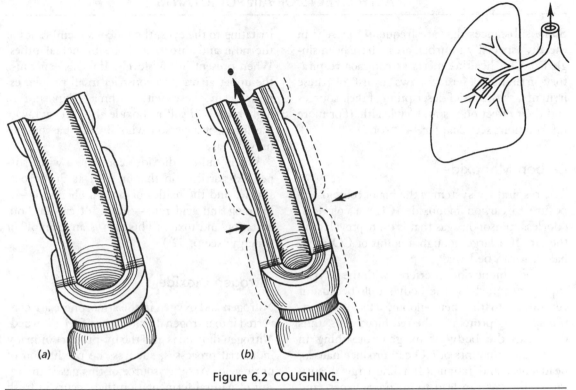

Figure 6.2 COUGHING.

(*a*) An irritant contacts the wall of the larynx, the windpipe, or the lungs and prompts the cough, (*b*) a rapid contraction of chest muscles, which usually succeeds in dislodging a foreign body. A persistent cough may signal a more serious respiratory disorder.

Some gases can cause cancer when inhaled. For example, mustard gas, used in chemical warfare during World War I, is a known carcinogen. Nickel carbonyl, a product of some nickel furnace operations, causes lung cancer. Bis(chloromethyl)ether, used in chemical manufacturing, and ethylene oxide, used in the process of cold sterilization in health care facilities, have been associated with lung cancer. Radioactive gases have been associated with lung cancers in miners. The latency period for most occupational carcinogens is quite long—typically twenty to forty years.

Occasionally, two substances that are not especially harmful alone interact together in such a way that their combination poses a much greater risk of serious injury or disease, a phenomenon known as *synergy*. For instance, the presence of a trace of sulfur dioxide and a trace of nitrogen dioxide may not cause discomfort to an individual, but if these oxidants combine to form smog, then the synergism created could produce a more hazardous effect (see Chapter 14, "Air").

Another example of synergism is cigarette smoking, which alone and in combination with other cancer-causing substances, can cause a dramatic rise in the incidence of lung cancer. For instance, researchers have found that asbestos workers who smoke have ninety-two times the chance of developing lung cancer in comparison to workers who neither smoke nor work with asbestos.

HEALTH EFFECTS OF AIR POLLUTANTS

Some substances that are frequently present in the air, especially in urban areas, have been singled out by health experts as common respiratory irritants. Here follows a list of these irritants, with a brief description of their sources and their effect on respiratory health. (For more information, see Chapter 14, "Air.")

Carbon Monoxide

The respiratory system is the major route of exposure to carbon monoxide (CO), a colorless, odorless, poisonous gas that is quite prevalent in the air. If a large enough amount of CO is inhaled, it can be lethal.

Carbon monoxide interferes with the oxygen supply destined for the body's cells because it combines with hemoglobin, the oxygen-transporting protein in the red blood cells, thus depriving the body of oxygen. Breathing in even small amounts of CO can produce nausea, headaches, and fatigue. Inhaling large quantities of the gas can lead to unconsciousness and death.

A primary outdoor source of CO is automobile and truck exhaust. Indoors, although CO exposure occurs from a number of sources, tobacco smoke and gas ranges are among the most common. Leaving a car idling in a garage that is attached to a house can unwittingly lead to a potentially lethal accumulation of CO in the home. Similarly, to avoid CO buildup indoors, space heaters that burn fuel and oil, gas-fired home furnaces, and clothes dryers must be properly vented to the outside. Charcoal-burning grills and hibachis are CO producers and should never be used indoors unless there is a strong vent to pull the smoke outside.

Sulfur Dioxide

When sulfur-containing coal or oil is burned, sulfur dioxide is formed. Sulfur dioxide is highly irritating to the eyes, the mucous membranes of the nose and throat, and the bronchial tubes. When present in low levels, this gas can cause the upper airways to constrict in all people, especially in those with asthma. Exposure to higher levels of sulfur dioxide also can aggravate the lungs of a person who already has pulmonary disease.

When sulfur dioxide combines with suspended particles in the air such as dust, soot, smoke, and the oxides of certain chemicals—as in smog and acid rain—the result can be both irritating and toxic. (This also is an example of synergy; see p. 52.)

Nitrogen Dioxide

Nitrogen and oxygen in the atmosphere are converted into nitrogen dioxide when fuel is burned. Nitrogen dioxide is also the by-product of many industrial processes, such as the production of nitric acid. Another source of this gas is the result of natural fermentation that occurs in fresh silage, such as alfalfa or grass, that is placed in poorly ventilated farm silos (see Chapter 21, "The Workplace").

The severity of the reaction to nitrogen dioxide varies with the amount of the gas that was inhaled. A small amount of the gas can cause increased mucus production, shortness of breath, cough, and headaches that disappear after several hours. In some cases, these symptoms may last for days.

Exposure to a high concentration of the gas can lead to an accumulation of fluid in the lungs, called *acute pulmonary edema*. Another potential disabling complication is *bronchiolitis obliterans*, in which the bronchioles become inflamed and stiff from the growth of fibrous tissue, typically several weeks after an initial insult. Exposure to high levels of nitrogen dioxide require emergency treatment. If left untreated, the symptoms can worsen and even become life-threatening.

Ozone

Ozone, a colorless, irritating gas that is a major component of smog, is formed by the chemical reaction of nitrogen dioxide and organic compounds in the presence of sunlight (see Figure 14.1, pp. 544–545).

The health effects of this respiratory irritant vary from person to person. Low levels of ozone may produce mild symptoms, such as coughing during light to moderate exercise (see p. 552). When the amount of ozone in the air is higher, it can trigger a dry cough, chest pain or discomfort, painful deep breath, nasal congestion, shortness of breath, and nausea. The symptoms usually disappear within several hours after exposure.

People with asthma may be highly sensitive to ozone and suffer more severe respiratory symptoms. Ozone exposure also may worsen the symptoms of such lung disorders as bronchitis and emphysema.

People who spend a great deal of time outdoors in poor air quality, including children, outdoor workers, and athletes of any age or level, are likely to have a higher amount of exposure to ozone.

RESPIRATORY PROBLEMS LINKED TO ENVIRONMENTAL EXPOSURES

Although the respiratory system has various defense mechanisms to protect it from occasional encounters with irritant pollutants and toxins in the environment, ongoing, repeated exposure to dusts, gases, vapors, fumes, and sprays can eventually damage the lungs. In some cases, the reaction to an irritating substance is immediate, but more often respiratory diseases develop slowly and insidiously for years.

For example, a worker who has lingering colds, suffers more severe respiratory infections than others, experiences breathlessness after light exertion, and coughs more frequently than normal may be experiencing the early symptoms of lung disease. It may take years before these symptoms cause permanent damage in the form of inflamed, thickened, and inelastic tissues that severely impair breathing.

The most common warning signs of lung disease are chronic cough, shortness of breath (dyspnea), chronic sputum production, wheezing, coughing up blood, and frequent chest colds. These symptoms should be discussed in detail with a physician as soon as possible.

Any number of respiratory problems can result from countless environmental situations. Some of the most common include the following disorders.

Upper Respiratory Infections

Common respiratory complaints such as colds and influenza are maladies that affect virtually everyone at one time or another. The common cold usually stays within the boundaries of the nose and throat, but when the complications of a secondary infection set in, bacterial or viral organisms may spread into the neighboring airways or passages. In this situation, the cold may evolve into an acute infection of the sinus (sinusitis), bronchial passages (bronchitis), or an inflammation of the lung itself (pneumonia).

Some people tend to catch more colds than others. For example, those who spend a great deal of time indoors in areas with poor ventilation seem to be more vulnerable. Respiratory irritants found in the work or home environment have been found to aggravate cold symptoms. An excellent example of this is formaldehyde, a very irritating substance released into the air from many products, such as from urea formaldehyde found in foam insulation.

Upper respiratory infections have been known to instigate asthma attacks, a sometimes frightening disorder in which the person's small bronchial tubes (bronchioles) suddenly narrow, making it difficult to breathe. In fact, evidence suggests there may be a relationship between acute viral infections and bronchiolitis in childhood and sensitivity of the upper airways or asthma in adulthood.

Chronic Obstructive Pulmonary Disease

Chronic obstructive pulmonary disease is a group of disorders characterized by persistent obstruction of air flow in the lungs. Among these disorders are chronic bronchitis, emphysema, and asthma.

Chronic bronchitis. This persistent condition results from an inflammation of the mucus lining in the bronchial passages.

The major cause of chronic bronchitis is cigarette smoking, although it frequently results from repeated exposure to irritants. Symptoms of chronic bronchitis include persistent coughing, shortness of breath during exertion, and excessive production of mucus, which tends to accumulate in the throat and obstruct normal breathing. A diagnosis of the illness is made when sputum is frequently coughed up for three consecutive months in two consecutive years.

When bronchitis reaches the chronic stage, it can represent permanent damage to the breathing passages. Frequently, an individual plagued with chronic bronchitis also has emphysema (see below) or tends to suffer from at least two bouts of bacterial or viral infections of the lungs each winter.

Airborne toxic substances that are present in some work environments may produce chronic bronchitis. Certain occupations carry a higher risk of developing this disorder: Miners exposed to coal dust and workers who regularly handle grain dusts are at particularly high risk (see Chapter 21, "The Workplace"). Smokers who work in such occupations further increase their risk; when tobacco smoke combines with dusts and gases in an occupational setting, it can accelerate the development of the disease.

Quitting smoking and reducing exposure to pollutants obviously can improve symptoms for bronchitis victims.

Emphysema. Emphysema is a serious, irreversible disease in which the walls of the air sacs (alveoli) lose their elasticity. As these walls become less elastic, they cannot successfully exchange oxygen for carbon dioxide in the bloodstream, so air becomes trapped inside the tiny sacs. The lungs distend as emphysema progresses, leaving the sufferer with a constant feeling of breathlessness.

Emphysema is a condition that commonly results from continued irritation by smoking; however, air pollution and occupational exposure to irritating fumes and dusts are also believed to be possible causes. In addition, there is an inherited form of emphysema, which develops early in life.

Chronic smokers invariably develop emphysema. The disease tends to progress slowly: An early sign of the illness is shortness of breath during activity; eventually, even minor exertion produces difficulty breathing. As it becomes harder to inhale oxygen, less oxygen is bound to hemoglobin and dissolved in the blood; therefore, less oxygen is transported to the body's tissues, and the skin may take on a bluish tinge (cyanosis). When the blood supply is low in oxygen, the blood pressure in the lungs increases. This condition, called pulmonary hypertension, forces the heart to pump harder to compensate for the reduced blood supply. The additional workload can enlarge the right side of the heart (cor pulmonale), resulting in a barrel-chested appearance and creating a situation that increases the risk of heart failure.

Asthma. This respiratory disorder is characterized by episodes of labored breathing due to inflammation and muscle spasms in the breathing passages that cause the bronchial tubes to suddenly narrow. Tissues in the area become swollen, and the asthma sufferer may be able to take in air but cannot easily exhale it. The labored breathing produced by this kind of episode produces wheezing or coughing.

From 1968 through the 1970s, death due to asthma declined in the United States. In the last decade, however, there has been an alarming increase in mortality rates due to this illness, especially among younger children, aged five to fourteen years, and among African-Americans.

An asthma episode may be triggered by a variety of situations and factors. A major offender is exposure to substances called allergens that produce an allergic reaction when inhaled. Among the most common allergens are pollen, dust, animal hair, mold spores, feathers, and chemical irritants. Cold air, cigarette smoke, pollutants and their odors, and exercise also can spur an episode of asthma. (Occupational asthma is the name given to asthma that results from exposure to materials handled in the work environment; see Chapter 21, "The Workplace.")

There undoubtedly is an emotional component to asthma, but it is not a psychological disorder. The myth that people get asthma because they have psychological problems became popular in the 1940s. In reality, the psychological impact a person with asthma has is a result, rather than a cause, of the disease. The physical sensation of being unable to breathe can create overwhelming panic, which in turn increases tension. A person whose life is restricted by asthma can become anxious or depressed. Sorting out the physical symptoms from their emotional impact is an important aspect of treatment. Yet once a person with asthma learns how to control his or her illness, he or she can live a normal, active life.

Box 6.3   AVOIDING ASTHMA TRIGGERS IN EVERYDAY LIFE

To bypass an asthma attack, consider the following:

- If feathers trigger an asthma attack, substitute pillows made of foam or other synthetic materials.
- Restrict pets to certain rooms or place them in adoptive homes.
- Make sure rooms are well ventilated when painting or using chemicals.
- Take prescribed medications before exercising.
- Stay indoors in extremely cold weather.
- Make sure the home and workplace are smoke-free.
- When using a vacuum cleaner, which stirs up dust and allergens in the air, wear a dust mask.
- Use air conditioners and air filters to keep the home and office clean and comfortable.

Dust mites are microscopic insects found in house dust. Despite their tiny size, they can cause a great deal of trouble. They are frequently triggers for asthma attacks. To combat these pests:

- Seal mattresses and pillows in dust-tight covers; tape over the length of the zippers.
- Wash all bedding weekly in hot water, at least 130 degrees Fahrenheit.

(continued)

Box 6.3   AVOIDING ASTHMA TRIGGERS IN EVERYDAY LIFE (*continued*)

- Don't lie down or sleep on upholstered furniture.
- Remove carpeting in the bedroom. Vacuum all carpets or rugs in the home frequently.
- Clean surface dust frequently; use a damp mop or cloth to clean.
- Don't use aerosols or spray cleaners in the bedroom.
- If you have asthma, don't vacuum, or only do it while wearing a dust mask.
- Use washable material for window coverings.
- Keep stuffed furniture and stuffed animals (except the washable kind) out of the bedroom.
- Don't overstuff closets, and keep clothing in plastic garment bags.
- Because dust mites like moisture and high humidity, cut down on the humidity in the home with a dehumidifier. An indoor humidity range between 35 and 50 percent seems to be the best level for comfort.

THE WORK ENVIRONMENT AND RESPIRATORY HEALTH

Despite their varying work situations, both blue-collar and white-collar workers share a common bond: the air they breathe. Countless substances that are in the air on the job may be hazardous or questionable in terms of safety.

Several categories of respiratory disease have traditionally affected men and women in the work environment. Toiling amid coal dust has long been associated with the dreaded *black lung disease*, a term that refers to one of a group of disorders known collectively as *pneumoconioses*. The term *pneumoconiosis* literally means "dust in the lungs" in Greek and is now used to describe a disease that is caused by the inhalation of dust in an occupational setting. The pneumoconioses include the oldest occupational diseases known to humankind, those that result from exposure to coal and silica, as well as diseases discovered in the last century, such as asbestosis (see Chapter 21, "The Workplace").

Other occupational lung diseases include occupational asthma and byssinosis, a disease that affects people who work in the cotton industry. Lung cancer also can occur as the result of ex-posure to known occupational carcinogens. Cigarette smoking, by itself and when combined with occupational carcinogens, can increase a smoker's susceptibility to lung cancer.

Pneumoconioses

When the ancient physician Hippocrates wrote of lung diseases that were common among metal diggers of ancient Greece, the symptoms he described were strikingly similar to those that we now attribute to the pneumoconioses, diseases characterized by dust in the lungs.

At the beginning of the Industrial Revolution, virtually all lung diseases—with names like miners' asthma and grinders' rot—that developed as a result of occupational exposure were classified as pneumoconioses. Later, the pneumoconioses were redefined to include ailments caused only by those accumulations of dust that cause a reaction in the lung tissue and impair the normal function of the lungs.

Silicosis, coal workers' pneumoconiosis, asbestos-related lung diseases, and mixed-dust pneumoconiosis are among the most prevalent diseases that can afflict workers who handle various minerals.

Silicosis. Worldwide, silicosis is the most commonly occurring pneumoconiosis. This illness results from the routine inhalation of large amounts of silica dust that then permanently deposit in the lungs.

Soil, granite, and sandstone are the major sources of exposure to silica, the most abundant mineral in the earth's crust (see information sheet, p. 411). Although workers in a wide range of industries are likely to encounter silica, sandblasters, foundry workers, miners, and those who work in drilling and blasting operations are at highest risk of inhaling silica dust. Pottery makers and people who make chinaware also tend to have high levels of exposure (see Chapter 20, "Art and Hobbyist Materials").

The extent of damage that occurs from inhaling silica dust on the job depends on the amount of silica in the air and the length of time a worker was exposed to the dust.

Silicosis is characterized by the formation of small, roundish nodules scattered throughout the lung tissue, primarily in the upper lobes. The disease occurs in three different forms: acute, chronic, and complicated.

Acute silicosis can affect workers who are exposed to highly concentrated amounts of silica dust even for a fairly short time span (a few weeks or up to several months). Sandblasting and rock drilling are occupations that carry a high risk of acute silicosis. This form of the disease progresses rapidly and can result in severe disability; difficult breathing, weight loss, and coughing are among its earliest symptoms.

Chronic silicosis is the most common and the mildest form of the disease. Workers who have been exposed to silica dust for at least ten years have the characteristic nodules in their lungs. Their only symptom may be breathlessness during exercise.

About 20 to 30 percent of workers with this simplest form of the disease eventually develop complicated silicosis, which is marked by the progressive enlargement and expansion of nodules in the lung tissue. Along with breathlessness, weakness, chest pain, cough, and increased production of sputum are common symptoms. At this stage of silicosis, fibrosis, or a condition in which fibers of scar tissue form in the lungs, may occur. Fibrosis severely hampers respiratory functioning and may eventually lead to heart disease.

Any form of silicosis is subject to complications from microorganisms, like mycobacterium tuberculosis, that aggravate the lung tissue and set the stage for other problems, such as tuberculosis, bronchitis, and pneumonia.

Silicosis can be prevented by wetting down the stone or rock that has to be drilled and by wearing protective respiratory equipment. Proper ventilation also can help reduce dust levels.

Coal Workers' Pneumoconiosis (Black Lung Disease). In the early nineteenth century, the medical literature of the time described the black lungs of coal miners at autopsy. Today, that term has been replaced with *coal workers' pneumoconiosis* (CWP), a disease resulting from repeatedly inhaling carbon (the main component of coal dust), which accumulates and darkens the lungs so that the tissues turn gray-black.

Often simple CWP is a condition that is almost without symptoms, although practically all miners have a slight cough and a blackish color to their sputum. As long as a miner with simple CWP has no other form of chronic obstructive lung disorder, shortness of breath is not usually a problem. However, the simple form of CWP can develop into progressive massive fibrosis, a variant of the disease in which the damage continues (even after exposure to the substance is stopped) and is characterized by a buildup of scar tissue in areas of dust deposits. Eventually, one clump of scar tissue spreads into another until the lungs become filled with stiffened tissue that can barely function.

It is not entirely clear whether the continued inhalation of coal dust increases a miner's risk of death from lung cancer. Several studies have shown that the death rate from lung cancer in coal miners has been less than what was expected from this group of workers. The decreased incidence of lung cancer is probably related to the fact that the number of miners who smoke tends to be 5 to 10 percent less than the general population, and that miners who do smoke tend to smoke fewer cigarettes per person.

Asbestos-Related Lung Disease. The word *asbestos* literally means inextinguishable, and asbestos is a catchall name for a group of virtually indestructible mineral fibers that naturally occur in rocks.

When tightly bonded in its natural form or in a commercial material, asbestos is harmless to the human body. Asbestos fibers released into the air are minute, odorless, and invisible unless viewed through a microscope. (A strand of hair is 1,200 times wider than an asbestos fiber.)

When these extremely fine fibers are allowed to float freely in the air, however, they pose a serious health hazard. Although no one knows for sure, some believe that asbestos can linger and float invisibly in the air for an indefinite amount of time.

Asbestos fibers are so light and narrow, they can elude the protective defense mechanism in the nose designed to trap incoming particles. Once these fibers enter the lungs, they remain there permanently and can result in any one of the different forms of asbestos-related diseases: asbestosis, lung cancer, mesothelioma, and other cancers.

Asbestos-related illnesses can progress over many years. The average period between first exposure to asbestos and lung cancer is estimated to be generally fifteen years or longer. Asbestosis and mesothelioma may not develop for forty to forty-five years.

Box 6.4 TYPES OF ASBESTOS

The word *asbestos* actually refers to *a group* of naturally occurring fibers that are durable, strong, and heat resistant—characteristics that makes them ideal for many industries. Asbestos fibers are mined and then used in the manufacture of textiles, plastics, insulation, shingles, tiles, and brake and clutch linings, to name a few.

Asbestos can be subdivided into two groups: serpentine and amphibole fibers. The most common type of asbestos, accounting for about 95 percent of the world's production, is the curly shaped chrysotile (white asbestos)—a member of the serpentine family. Crocidolite (blue asbestos), amosite (brown asbestos), anthophyllite, tremolite, and actinolite make up the amphibole family of asbestos.

Each type of asbestos varies in many ways, primarily in its chemical composition and durability. Therefore, when inhaled, each type will have a different effect on the lungs. For example, the rod-shaped amphiboles may make their way into the peripheral lung more easily than the bundlelike chrysotile fibers. Studies dating back as early as the 1960s linked crocidolite and mesothelioma in miners and their families. Insulation workers who frequently come in contact with amosite, chrysotile, and crocidolite also have a higher incidence of mesotheliomas, lung cancer, and other tumors.

ASBESTOSIS. In this disease, the inhaled fibers become lodged at the ends of the bronchioles, triggering the body to surround the fibers with tissue in an attempt to isolate the asbestos particles. Early symptoms of asbestosis include coughing and shortness of breath.

As asbestosis advances, chest pain and fatigue occur after even slight exertion. The air sacs in the lungs slowly break down, making it difficult for the body to take in sufficient oxygen. About ten to twenty years after the first exposure to the asbestos, a condition known as pulmonary fibrosis, or a thickening and scarring of lung tissue, and respiratory failure can occur. Sufferers of asbestosis also have an increased risk for tuberculosis, lung cancer (especially if they smoke), and mesothelioma (see below).

LUNG CANCER. The incidence of lung cancer in workers who use products containing asbestos varies with the level of exposure and the duration of asbestos-related work. However, asbestos is a known carcinogen that is responsible for at least 20 percent of all deaths among workers who have been exposed to heavy amounts of the material.

Asbestos dramatically enhances the carcinogenic capabilities of tobacco smoke and when the two are present, the combination can be extremely hazardous to the lungs (see Box 3.2, p. 52). A relatively brief exposure to asbestos may be sufficient to cause lung disease. Even family members of asbestos workers face an increased risk of exposure because asbestos fibers cling to clothing, shoes, skin, and hair.

Inhaled asbestos fibers also can lead to cancer of the larynx and gastrointestinal tract.

MESOTHELIOMA. Mesothelioma, a rare form of cancer, manifests as a tumor that develops in the pleura and the peritoneum, the thin membranes lining the chest and abdominal cavity, respectively. Normally, there is a very thin layer of fluid between the two-ply membrane that makes up the pleural lining. When asbestos fibers penetrate the soft tissues of the lung and settle in the chest lining, the stage is set for the development of mesothelioma.

It may take thirty years after exposure to asbestos for mesothelioma to develop. The early symptoms are cough, chest pain, and shortness of breath, or the illness may be asymptomatic. One of the later signs of this incurable cancer is the buildup of fluid in the thin pleural lining (pleural effusion). Cells from the mass that develop in the chest lining may metastasize or travel to other parts of the body.

Although mesothelioma rarely occurs among the general population, it is responsible for about 10 percent of cancer deaths among asbestos workers, especially smokers.

WAVES OF ASBESTOS-RELATED DISEASES. Since the late nineteenth century, American industry has been enamored with asbestos, using it extensively for a variety of commercial purposes. Asbestos use in the United States reached its peak between the 1930s and the late 1970s. This material was highly popular because its tiny strands are not affected by heat or chemicals and the fibers do not conduct electricity.

Shipbuilders used asbestos to insulate boilers and pipes. Construction materials manufacturers found asbestos useful in wall and ceiling materials. Roofing and siding manufacturers put asbestos into roofing felts, tiles, shingles, coatings, and rigid panels. Industrial and automotive manufacturers employed asbestos in brake and clutch linings, sealants, and gaskets.

Epidemiologists have identified three waves of occupationally related asbestos disease. The first wave occurred in the early 1930s and 1940s among workers who mined and milled asbestos. The second wave affected shipyard and insulation workers from around World War II into the 1950s and 1960s. At this time, the scope of the third wave remains unknown: In the United States, approximately 10,000 deaths each year until the year 2000 are expected as a result of exposure to asbestos before 1980. Those affected probably will consist of a wide range of people including construction workers, school and building custodians, firefighters, maintenance workers, demolition workers, and many others who have been exposed to hazardous concentrations of asbestos fibers.

There is growing evidence of a high rate of disease as a result of this final wave. For instance, a study of New York City firefighters found a "surprising" rate of abnormal scarring in the chest X rays of 226 veterans of the department that was described as being "consistent with prior asbestos exposure." The abnormal scarring occurred in 14 percent of the firefighters with no known previous exposure to asbestos. Similar scarring of the lungs or their lining was found in 35 percent of the sixty workers who were known to have worked in asbestos-insulated buildings. The actual level of asbestos to which the firefighters were exposed is unknown.

This unusual rate of asbestos-related scarring in the so-called never-exposed group was startling to researchers who said they would expect to find this kind of abnormal lung scarring in less than 2 percent of the overall population.

Box 6.5   THE LANDMARK CASE OF NELLIE KERSHAW

Nellie Kershaw will be remembered more for her death than her life. Born in 1891, she went to work at the age of twelve in Rochdale, England. In 1922 she became too ill with lung disease to work at her job in an asbestos factory. Her claim for National Health Insurance benefits was refused. Her physician had diagnosed her ailment as asbestos poisoning, and the government-approved Friendly Society—to which she paid premiums—did not compensate for occupational illnesses. When she applied for benefits under the Workmen's Compensation Act, this claim too was denied, because asbestos poisoning was not on the government's list of occupational diseases. Her employer, the Turner Brothers Asbestos Company, vigorously disclaimed any liability.

When Mrs. Kershaw died in 1924 at the age of 33, the *Rochdale Times* reported the event under the headline "Married Woman's Death: Tired of Going to See Doctors." Three years later her death became the first reported in the medical literature attributed to pulmonary asbestosis. Despite this documented case, no action was taken to prevent further deaths among workers. Only in the 1960s was the link between occupational exposure to asbestos and respiratory disease fully exposed. Only in the 1970s were there attempts to implement control measures.

REGULATING ASBESTOS. Since the 1970s, regulatory changes have significantly reduced the use of asbestos. Many consumer uses of asbestos, such as sprayed-on insulation and pipe coverings, were banned in the 1970s; this material no longer can be used in clothing, wallboard and plaster patching compounds, and gas heaters. The manufacturers of electric hair dryers voluntarily withdrew asbestos from their products in 1979. By 1996, use of almost all asbestos will be eliminated. However, houses built between 1900 and 1970 still contain areas with asbestos (see Box 6.6 for information on protecting yourself from asbestos exposure).

The Asbestos Hazard Emergency Response Act of 1986 required that public and private schools be inspected for asbestos hazards. It is not always desirable or necessary to remove the asbestos; more harm may be caused in the process by releasing asbestos fibers into the air than "managing" the substance. In most cases, an area containing asbestos must be managed properly through restricting access to asbestos by enclosing or encapsulating it (see Box 6.6) and by having a program of regular inspections and upkeep.

In 1990, the EPA reported that 94 percent of the nation's public school districts and private schools had complied with the law. The law would have to be expanded, however, in order for public and commercial buildings inspections to take place.

Box 6.6   PROTECTING YOURSELF FROM ASBESTOS EXPOSURE IN THE HOME

If you suspect there is asbestos in your house, there is no need for panic: Remember that asbestos is not dangerous unless the fibers break, tear, or crumble and become airborne.

Call a professional to identify sources of asbestos. Plumbers, furnace servicepeople, and building contractors can often visually determine the presence of asbestos as well as whether or not its condition presents a danger.

Other resources include your regional EPA office or state department of health, which can provide information on how to identify asbestos in the home, as well as abatement methods and names of contractors certified to perform this dangerous work.

The Consumer Product Safety Commission also has a hotline for information about asbestos removal procedures, laboratories certified for testing, and how to take asbestos samples. Call 1-800-638-2772 for more information.

If asbestos is found, unless it is deteriorated and crumbling, it may be safer to leave it in place. *Do not* try to remove it yourself; you can do more harm than good if you release the asbestos fibers into the air. Alternatives to removing asbestos insulation, for example, include enclosing it within airtight walls and ceilings, or encapsulating it with a sealant to prevent disintegration of the substance.

If you must take your own sample, do so with care. Follow the guidelines offered by the EPA or state department of health. Wear rubber gloves and a protective mask.

If the asbestos must be removed, this is a job for a professional contractor. Check his or her experience, training, and references with your regional EPA office or state department of health. Ask for a detailed account of how he or she plans to contain asbestos fibers during the removal process and make certain it follows the guidelines suggested by these agencies.

After the work is completed, the air will need to be tested to make sure no asbestos fibers remain.

Other Pneumoconioses. A large number of dusts can enter the respiratory system in the occupational environment and pose a variety of health effects ranging from the benign to the serious.

Barium, iron, tin, antimony, and titanium dusts tend to deposit in the lungs without producing any kind of fibrosis, or tissue scarring. These dusts are inert and are not dissolved and broken down by the lungs; they cause only mild irritation and are considered "nuisance dusts."

Silicates, which include kaolin, mica, and talc, can result in varying degrees of pneumoconiosis in people who work with these substances. Exposure to mica occurs primarily to workers in the electrical and furnace industries and paint and paper manufacturing.

Kaolin is ground into a fine powder and used in ceramics, paints, paper production, and the pharmaceutical industry. Some workers who handle this clay mineral may develop kaolin pneumoconiosis, which may not create any clinical symptoms until more than fifteen years after exposure. Many handlers of this substance also develop progressive massive fibrosis.

Occupational exposure to talc, which is often contaminated with silica and asbestos, also can produce the nodules and fibrosis that are typical of silicosis. Workers at a high risk of talc inhalation include those employed in the cosmetic, paint, pottery, asphalt, and rubber industries.

Fibrous glass, better known as fiberglass, is often used as an asbestos substitute in insulating materials. Fiberglass can irritate the skin as well as the mucus membranes of the respiratory tract. In fact, tests on laboratory models have suggested that fiberglass in certain fiber (particle) sizes can cause fibrosis of the lung and the lining of the chest.

The substance beryllium was once used in fluorescent light tubes, but its use was discontinued when its toxicity was recognized. Inhalation of beryllium dust—resulting from the light but strong metal used in metallurgy, some machine tools, ceramic production, and the nuclear power industry—can cause an acute or chronic form of beryllium disease. Exposure to beryllium also has been associated with increased rates of cancer of the lung, liver, and gall bladder.

Other metals that may be inhaled in the workplace include aluminum, carbon black, graphite, and tungsten. A condition called mixed-dust pneumoconiosis can arise when a worker is exposed to a mixture of dusts, which is a common occurrence in the foundry, steel, and iron industries.

Other Lung Diseases in the Workplace

Three lung disorders, characterized by hypersensitivity to substances in the work environment, are diseases known as hypersensitivity pneumonitis, occupational asthma, and byssinosis.

Hypersensitivity Pneumonitis. Also known as allergic alveolitis, hypersensitivity pneumonitis is a disease that affects the air sacs deep inside the lungs, classically as a result of inhaling fine organic dusts. Fungal spores that grow in wet hay, animal dander and proteins, feathers and bird droppings, and organisms that grow in commercial and home humidifiers are among the causes of this disease. Chemicals such as diisocyanates and epoxy resin also cause hypersensitivity pneumonitis (see Information Sheets, p. 376 and p. 379).

Typically, a person can inhale the dust several times and have no noticeable reaction. Unlike asthma, which produces immediate symptoms, hypersensitivity pneumonitis does not produce symptoms until four to six hours after an attack begins. Coughing, shortness of breath, and tightness in the chest accompanied by flulike symptoms including fever, chills, and fatigue are the telltale signals.

Inside the lung, the alveoli become inflamed and fluid may fill the air sacs. Continued exposure to the dust and repeated attacks of hypersensitivity pneumonitis produces fibrous scar tissue in the lungs, impairing normal breathing.

The condition farmer's lung is a well-known example of this disease. The same organism that causes farmer's lung also thrives in the water of poorly maintained humidification systems. Because moist conditions are necessary for the growth of this organism, farm workers can prevent the disease by drying and then storing the offending substance, for example, hay. (See Profile of a High-Risk Occupation: Agriculture, p. 708.)

A worker may be in contact with the offending substance for a period of months or years and then develop immunological reaction and damage to the lungs.

Box 6.7 PREVENTING OFFICE HUMIDIFIER DISEASE

To prevent outbreaks of "office humidifier disease" (see Box 14.7, p. 557), hypersensitivity pneumonitis, and other respiratory syndromes caused by microbes that enter an office environment through humidifiers, air washers, and contaminated filters in air-conditioning units, the Centers for Disease Control and Prevention (CDC) recommends the following measures:

- Promptly and permanently repair all external and internal leaks.
- Maintain relative humidity below 70 percent in occupied spaces.
- Prevent the accumulation of stagnant water under cooling-deck coils of air-handling units through proper inclination and continuous emptying of drain pans.
- Use steam rather than recirculated water as a water source for humidifiers in heating, ventilation, and air conditioning systems.
- Replace filters in air-conditioning units at regular intervals.
- Discard rather than disinfect carpets, upholstery, ceiling tiles, and other porous furnishings that are grossly contaminated.
- Provide outdoor air into ventilation systems at minimum rates of at least 20 cubic feet per minute per occupant in areas where occupants are smoking and at least 5 cubic feet per minute in nonsmoking areas.

Occupational asthma. Workers with occupational asthma usually notice that their characteristic wheezing, coughing, and shortness of breath improve or disappear over weekends, vacations, or periods away from the office, only to recur upon returning to work. When a worker is diagnosed with occupational asthma, extensive efforts to make the workplace safe should be employed first before the individual is reassigned in order to avoid further contact with the irritating substance.

Several agents are capable of causing occupational asthma in a wide range of industries and jobs. A number of chemicals that induce asthma are routinely used in the plastics industry, including toluene diisocyanate, a substance used in the manufacture of polyurethane foams. Woodworkers, carpenters, and sawmill workers exposed to certain types of wood dust are susceptible to occupational asthma. Cedar, oak, mahogany, and western red cedar dusts can provoke job-related asthma.

A study of workers in the detergent manufacturing industry found that more than 20 percent of those who were exposed to powdered enzymes used in the detergent product developed asthma after they inhaled the substance.

Box 6.8 THE DETECTION OF OCCUPATIONAL TRIGGERS FOR ASTHMA

According to the Centers for Disease Control and Prevention (CDC), occupational asthma is an increasingly important cause of respiratory impairment that can persist long after workplace exposures cease. More than 200 agents have been associated with workplace asthma, including microbial products, animal proteins, plant products, and industrial chemicals.

(continued)

Box 6.8   THE DETECTION OF OCCUPATIONAL TRIGGERS FOR ASTHMA
(*continued***)**

In 1987 the National Institute for Occupational Safety and Health (NIOSH), along with the CDC, began the Sentinel Event Notification System for Occupational Risks (SENSOR), a pilot project to improve the reporting and surveillance of work-related health conditions. Of the ten states participating in the SENSOR program by 1990, six (Colorado, Massachusetts, Michigan, New Jersey, New York, and Wisconsin) targeted occupational asthma for surveillance.

After increased physician education and case follow-up, the number of occupational asthma cases reported increased sharply—in Michigan from 18 during 1984–1986 to 101 cases from September 1988 through August 1989. As a result of follow-up investigations, at least one new setting was recognized for occupational asthma—sugar beet pulp processing. For example, in New Jersey, from June 1988 through October 1989, the SENSOR program received reports of sixty-six cases of possible occupational asthma. Seven of the first eight worksites investigated had inadequate engineering controls. In these workplaces, thirty-five co-workers of the reported patients also had respiratory symptoms.

Important findings from programs like SENSOR indicate that occupational risk factors for illness are probably more important in the overall health of a population than are generally recognized. Because too few physicians ask their patients about their occupations and work histories, it is mandatory for the patient to inform the physician of his or her situation, detailing any potentially toxic substances and the overall work environment in general.

Byssinosis. Byssinosis, or brown lung disease, affects cotton textile workers and those who inhale cotton dust, flax, or soft hemp.

In many ways, byssinosis resembles occupational asthma, but the pattern of this disease is different enough to merit its own status as a work-related illness. The classic symptoms of byssinosis are coughing and tightness in the chest upon returning to work after a weekend off. This "Monday symptom," as it has come to be known, may develop after a few months of employment in the textile industry or after several years.

With continued exposure to cotton dust, the Monday symptom may persist longer into the workweek. Eventually, an affected worker develops a chronic cough and breathlessness and may not have any relief from symptoms even during time away from the job. The continued

inhalation of cotton dusts can set the stage for the development of chronic bronchitis and emphysema.

Although the actual agent that causes byssinosis remains unknown, this disease can be prevented by adopting dust control measures in the workplace and steam-washing cotton bales before workers handle them.

Lung Cancer. Since the 1950s, lung cancer has been the leading cause of cancer deaths in men and now has replaced breast cancer as the number one cause of cancer deaths in women.

Because cigarette smoke contains a large number of carcinogens, the risk of lung cancer in heavy smokers is twenty or more times higher than the risk for people who have never smoked. In addition, cancers elsewhere in the body, including the larynx, oral cavity, esophagus, pancreas, and the bladder, also have been associated with smoking. Smokers who quit can reduce their risk of lung cancer as well as heart disease (see Chapter 22, "The ABCs of Staying Healthy").

Cigarette smoking and asbestos exposure have traditionally been the major causes of lung cancer. Today, radon, a radioactive gas that occurs naturally in soil and rock formations, has the dubious distinction of being the second leading cause of lung cancer in the United States (see Chapter 14, "Air"). Studies by the EPA and the National Research Council have shown that prolonged exposure (about the average lifespan, or seventy years) to high radon levels causes as many as 20,000 of the 136,000 annual deaths from lung cancer in this country. It has been estimated that 85 percent of these deaths are due to a combination of radon and smoking.

Increasingly, environmental and occupational exposure have been recognized as contributors to the development of lung cancer (see Chapter 7, "Cancer"). In 1993, after two years of reviewing an expert panel's findings, the EPA reclassified secondhand smoke, an important component of environmental tobacco smoke, as a carcinogen; they concluded that exposure to secondhand smoke is responsible for 3,000 adult deaths each year.

Increased levels of air pollutants, especially in urban and industrial areas, enter the respiratory system and may adversely affect lung function, possibly leading to lung cancer. In fact, the rates of lung cancer are higher in urban areas (see Chapter 14, "Air").

On-the-job exposure to carcinogens is believed to be a significant cause of lung cancer. Occupations that require the use of hazardous chemicals have been linked with an increased risk of the illness. Workers employed in the aluminum industry, and those employed in foundries, coke plants, carbon black processing facilities, man-made mineral fiber production plants, and the rubber industry are among those whose work carries a higher risk. Exposure to such agents as arsenic, bis(chloromethyl)-ether, coal tar and pitch volatiles, petroleum, mustard gas, coal carbonization products, chromates, asbestos, X rays, radium, uranium, nickel and nickel carbonyl, and isopropyl oil have been linked with above-average rates of lung cancer.

The first symptom of lung cancer most frequently is a persistent cough. Other symptoms may include coughing up blood, shortness of breath, chest pain, and wheezing. The cancer may only involve immediately affected tissue, which can result in a collapsed lung, pneumonia, or pleural effusion (a collection of fluid between the lung and chest wall). The lung cancer eventually may spread to other sites in the body, particularly the liver, brain, and bones.

Lung cancer is difficult to treat for many reasons: It often reaches an advanced stage by the time a person seeks medical attention and the cancer can spread easily, making surgery an inadequate treatment. It is possible to significantly reduce the rate of most lung cancers by not smoking and by avoiding or safely handling carcinogenic substances in the workplace.

CHAPTER 7

Cancer

Of all of the possible adverse health effects of environmental hazards, perhaps the most dreaded is cancer. In America, the incidence of cancer in the population is relatively high; almost everyone has a friend, relative, or acquaintance who has had some form of this illness.

The reactions to learning that one has cancer are legion. Anger, fear, and depression are common. It is also common to ask, Why me? Often, people assume that something in the environment—chemicals, food additives, or perhaps pollutants in the air or water—must have caused the cancer to develop. While this most certainly can be the case, for the most part we still do not know exactly what induces a cancer to begin, or why, given the same set of variables, some individuals contract the disease and others do not.

In this chapter, we will examine what is currently known about how cancers arise and the role that environmental agents play in causing cancer. It is a complex topic that requires a careful review.

WHAT IS CANCER?

Although cancer is generically referred to as a single illness, there are actually over one hundred different forms of cancer, each with its own provoking causes, prognosis, and treatments. However, all forms of the disease share some common biological features.

The common denominator of all cancers is that they start when normal cells begin to grow abnormally. The human body is composed of hundreds of billions of individual cells. Although we are born with a set number of cells in the nervous system and heart, virtually all other types of cells in the body are created, grow, die, and are replaced by new cells throughout our lifetimes. New cells are created when existing cells divide in half, thus duplicating themselves. This process is regulated by the body's internal control mechanisms; normally, the body creates only enough new cells to replace the cells that have died.

Cancerous cells, however, do not behave normally. They do not die when they are supposed to and they continue to divide without stopping, creating more cells than the body needs. They don't necessarily grow faster than normal cells (often they grow more slowly), but they continue growing inexorably.

The ability of cancer cells to reproduce unceasingly is a phenomenon clearly evident when cells are grown for study in a test tube. In a petri dish, healthy human cells multiply until they form a continuous flat layer one cell thick, then they stop. Cancer cells, however, are radically different. They continue to grow, piling on top of one another, forming rounded mounds of cells. This shows a basic property of cancer cells: They have lost what scientists call *cell-contact growth regulation*.

The mass of extra cells forms a growth, or tumor, which invades space needed by other organs as it grows. It also interferes with the supply of oxygen and nutrients that these organs need to function efficiently. Eventually, a growing tumor will destroy healthy tissue and organs.

There are two types of tumors—benign and malignant. A benign tumor grows only at its site of origin and does not invade neighboring tissues. Even though it can cause serious problems or even death, it can usually be excised by surgery. A malignant (or cancerous) tumor invades adjacent tissues and spreads to other areas of the body. This spreading is called *metastasis*. In many common cancers such as colon and breast cancer, death is generally caused by tumor cells that travel to other parts of the body and establish secondary cancerous outgrowths.

In addition to abnormal growth, one other property distinguishes cancer cells. Most of the body's cells perform special functions. Some cells form the structures of bone or blood, for example, whereas others secrete hormones and still others make antibodies. This is called *cell differentiation*. When cells become cancerous, they frequently lose their differentiation and stop performing their specialized functions or perform them in an abnormal manner.

Because of these two features of the disease, scientists often describe cancer as normal growth and differentiation gone awry.

How Does a Cell Become Cancerous?

It is not a simple process for a cell to become cancerous. Scientists believe that a cell becomes cancerous through a chain of intricate steps.

Substances in the environment play a role in this complex process and the mechanism underlying this transformation to unrestrained growth is the focus of much cancer research.

The Initiation–Promotion Hypothesis. One theory of how cancer begins, proposed in the 1940s, has gained wide recognition. It is called the *initiation–promotion hypothesis*.

INITIATION AND INITIATORS (CARCINOGENS). In this theory, initiation is considered to be the first of two steps in the growth of cancers. Initiators (chemicals, viruses, or radiation) affect a cell's genetic material, or DNA, in such a way that the cell then becomes susceptible to the effects of other substances called promoters. Initiators do not cause cancer themselves; in effect, they prime a cell to *become* cancerous, given the right set of circumstances.

Initiators share several characteristics. The changes they effect in a cell's DNA are irreversible. The effects of initiators can be cumulative (one exposure to a substance may not prime a cell to become cancerous, but repeated exposures might). There are no known thresholds for initiators (a threshold is the amount or dose of a substance that will cause an effect), so *any* amount of an initiator may increase the chances that a cell will become cancerous.

The term commonly used for a cancer initiator is *carcinogen*. Some carcinogens act directly on a cell's DNA; others must be broken down, or metabolized, by the body before they can react with DNA to exert effects. Known carcinogens include a number of chemicals, such as benzene, polycyclic aromatic hydrocarbons (chemicals released by burning fuel or other combustible substances), and tobacco smoke, as well as ionizing and ultraviolet radiation. (See Table 7.1 for EPA classification of carcinogens; see also Table 7.3.)

PROMOTION AND PROMOTERS. Promotion is the second step in the development of cancers. Promoters are substances that act on cells that have

ENVIRONMENTAL CAUSES OF CANCER DEATHS

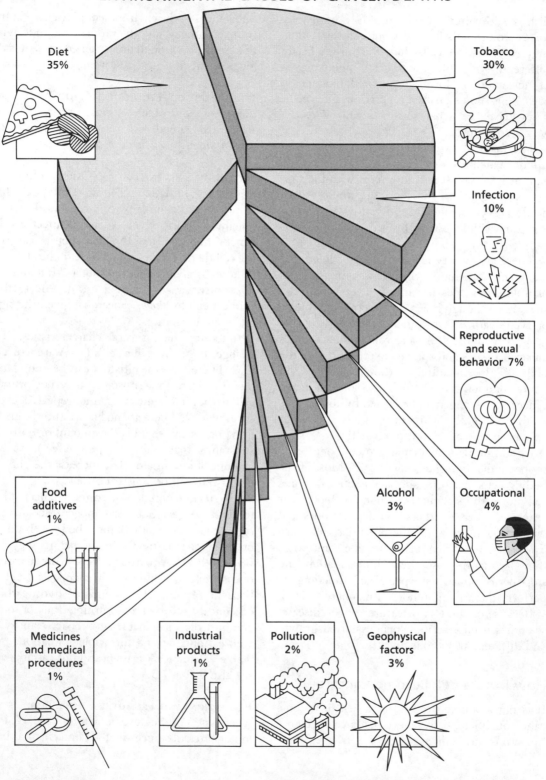

Diet 35%

Tobacco 30%

Infection 10%

Reproductive and sexual behavior 7%

Occupational 4%

Alcohol 3%

Geophysical factors 3%

Pollution 2%

Industrial products 1%

Medicines and medical procedures 1%

Food additives 1%

Table 7.1 EPA CLASSIFICATION OF CARCINOGENS

Group	Category	Scientific Evidence
A	Human carcinogen	Sufficient human epidemiologic studies
B1	Probable human carcinogen (high probability)	Limited human epidemiologic studies; sufficient evidence in animals
B2	Probable human carcinogen (low probability)	Inadequate human epidemiologic studies; sufficient evidence in animals
C	Possible human carcinogen	Absence of human data; limited evidence in animals
D	Not classified	Inadequate evidence in animals
E	No evidence of carcinogenicity for humans	At least two negative animal studies *or* one negative animal and one negative human study

More than 400 chemicals have been shown to cause cancer in animals; only 30 have been *proven* as causing cancer in humans.

been "initiated." In and of themselves, promoters do not cause cancer. However, they promote cancer by stimulating cells that have been initiated to undergo further changes, multiply, and form a tumor.

The characteristics of substances that are cancer promoters are very different from those of initiators. Initially, the effects of promoters can largely be reversed. The impact of promoters varies and can be moderated by life-style factors. Unlike initiators, there are probably definable thresholds for promoters, that is, a person must be exposed to a large enough amount of a promoter before cancer will develop.

A number of environmental substances are likely to be cancer promoters. Some substances, such as cigarette smoke, asbestos, and radiation, are potent carcinogens because they are simultaneously both initiators and promoters. Other substances, including dietary fat, nitrosamines, hormones such as estrogen, and alcohol are believed to be only promoters of cancer.

The theory of initiation and promotion has been around since the 1940s. It is only since the recent advent of powerful new techniques in molecular biology that health professionals have had the tools to understand more precisely how carcinogens in the environment might initiate and promote cancer (see Box 7.1).

Unraveling the Mysteries of Cancer: Genetic Studies. The theory of initiation–promotion has now received support from sophisticated studies of how the inner workings of cells are controlled by genes.

Genes are sequences of DNA that make up the chromosomes and carry the instructions that tell a cell what to do. They are the basis of inheritance. Most people know that genes control such things as height and eye and hair color, but genes also control how cells function. For exam-

Figure 7.1 ENVIRONMENTAL CAUSES OF CANCER DEATHS.

This chart is based on the landmark 1981 Doll and Peto study, still considered the best estimate to date of the relative frequency of environmental cancer causes in the U.S. (The study gave an estimated percentage range for each cause, so the figures do not add up to 100 percent.) Estimates of the percentage of cancers caused by environmental factors run from 70 percent down to 10 percent and less. While the relative proportions suggested by the study are widely accepted, the total percentage of cancers caused by environmental factors remains a matter of debate.

(*Source for statistics: Journal of the National Cancer Institute* 66[6]:1256 [June 1981].

Box 7.1   ADVANCES IN MOLECULAR BIOLOGY AND CANCER RESEARCH

Traditionally, the determination that a substance is a cause of cancer has rested on animal and epidemiologic studies. Within the past ten to fifteen years, however, advances in molecular biology have led scientists to search for laboratory tests that may better predict the potential cancer risk of various agents in the environment.

Molecular biology examines the structure of cells at their genetic level, probing into secrets of nucleic acid—the substance of life itself—to understand the chemical, electrical, and physiologic functioning of cells. In recent years, a number of new techniques for studying the cell, such as immunoblotting, polymerase chain reaction, gene amplification, and gene mapping, have been developed, allowing scientists to understand cell function with ever-greater precision.

Scientists are now attempting to develop tests that will yield information on damage done to DNA by chemicals and other substances. The ultimate goal of these studies will be to develop biologic "markers" (substances in the blood or genetic screening tests) that can be used to identify those at risk for developing cancer, to determine if early-stage cancer exists, and/or to differentiate malignant conditions from nonmalignant disease. To date, no biologic test has been developed that is of wide clinical use, but it is fairly certain that such tests will be developed in the future.

---

ple, genes govern the preprogrammed life cycle of a cell and the rate at which cells divide and reproduce. Because cancer is the result of uncontrolled cell growth, substances that affect the genes that control growth can have a direct bearing on the development of cancer.

A cancer may begin when a cell is exposed to a substance that causes an irreversible change in its genetic material. These changes are called *mutations*, and the substances that cause them are called *mutagens*. Many substances cause mutations in the genetic material of cells. Not every mutation, however, causes a cell to become cancerous.

Cancers are believed to arise only if the mutation affects the genes that control the cell's growth. These genes fall into two classes, *oncogenes* and *tumor suppressor genes*. Both of these types of genes control how a cell grows but in different ways.

Normal oncogenes, or proto-oncogenes, are believed to play an essential role in regulating how cells grow. If these genes become altered, they have the capacity to stimulate the abnormal growth that is associated with malignant transformation.

There are two primary routes by which proto-oncogenes can become activated to oncogenes and cause abnormal growth. First, they can be modified or altered in such a way that unregulated growth is stimulated. Second, they may be moved to different chromosomal locations, causing protein abnormalities that lead to an excess of growth. For example, this could happen if exposure to a chemical agent caused a break in a chromosome. Carcinogens may exert their damaging effects by "turning on" or activating oncogenes or by mutating a normal proto-oncogene.

Tumor suppressor genes work the opposite way, by inhibiting growth and thus preventing the formation of tumors. If a cell's tumor suppressor genes are "turned off" or lost (deleted), the cell loses its ability to regulate growth. The loss of tumor suppressor genes has been implicated in a number of cancers, including retinoblastoma, lung cancer, osteosarcoma, and colon cancer. Although scientists do not know precisely how these genes are inactivated, they surmise that it may result from interaction with environmental agents.

In addition to the differences in their routes of action, tumor suppressor genes differ from proto-oncogenes in another important way. Whereas proto-oncogenes are inherited, their cancer-causing actions are not. Proto-oncogenes cause cancer only through acquired changes in a cell's DNA after birth. With tumor suppressor genes, on the other hand, defects that could dismantle their protective action can be passed from one generation to the next. A child who is born with a defective tumor suppressor gene would have a greater risk of cancer than a child born with these genes intact.

Although scientists still do not fully understand how oncogenes and tumor suppressor genes work or precisely how environmental agents switch them on or off, it is probable they will learn more in the future. What is known is that the steps that lead to cancer are not simple, but complex and multiple. The activation of an oncogene or deactivation of a tumor suppressor gene does not in and of itself appear to be sufficient to cause malignant change. A number of factors must converge before a cell becomes cancerous.

Can Cancer Be Inherited? People often ask whether or not cancer is inherited. This is a complicated issue and not one to which a simple answer is possible.

There are a few cancers in which susceptibility is clearly inherited as opposed to acquired from genetic changes after birth; these include retinoblastoma, familial polyposis, and some colon cancers. Other cancers appear to "run in families," meaning that the families appear to have a predisposition to develop them, although the linkage from one generation to the next is not such that the cancer could actually

be described as "inherited." In this case, a person may be born with a specific gene pattern that renders him or her susceptible in some way to cancer. Some cancers appear to have strong familial linkages in some families but, for the most part, strike individuals with no seeming link to heredity. For example, there is a family tendency toward breast or ovarian cancer in a minority of people, yet no link to heredity has yet to be found for the majority of others who develop these same malignancies.

For the most part, it is very difficult to distinguish cancers arising from environmental causes from those of hereditary origin.

Translating Theory into Practicality: Studies of Carcinogens

How many of the cancers that arise are actually due to exposure to environmental substances? In general, it is very difficult to pin down a particular substance as causing cancer. The clues come from epidemiological and laboratory studies and a fine-tuned combination of the two.

Proving a Link Between Cancer and a Suspected Carcinogen. How are suspected carcinogens linked to cancer in humans? There are two main ways: epidemiologic studies, which trace disease trends in the general population, and animal research. A third route, just now beginning to receive wider use, is laboratory test tube studies. (See Chapter 2, "Illness and the Environment: Finding the Links," for a more complete discussion of these methods and their drawbacks.)

Epidemiologic studies analyze the relationship of risk factors, such as life-style habits or exposure to chemicals, to cancer incidence. They determine broad patterns of cancer incidence. The link between smoking and lung cancer (as well as head and neck, bladder, and esophageal cancers) was clearly demonstrated through epidemiologic studies. This type of study has also been able to point to specific cancer-causing substances in specific work environments, such as asbestos and benzene.

Epidemiologic studies have several drawbacks, however. They allow researchers to make generalizations about cancer but only *after* it occurs. Because there is often a long latency period (the amount of time between when a person is exposed to a carcinogen and when cancer actual develops), epidemiologic studies are not good predictors of what *new* chemicals or substances may cause cancer.

Scientists also rely upon animal tests to investigate the potential carcinogenicity of a substance. In most animal studies, high doses of test chemicals are administered to the animals; if they develop cancer, the test chemical is assumed to also be a human carcinogen.

However suggestive, animal studies cannot tell with absolute certainty that a particular substance will cause cancer in humans. Although all mammals are broadly similar biologically, differences do exist between species. For example, thresholds—the amounts of substances that will cause an effect—vary between humans and animals because of differences in body weights. Organ systems also function differently from animal to animal.

Because of these dissimilarities, animal studies have to be interpreted, that is, their applicability to human beings must be surmised. It is not uncommon for studies of the same substance to yield conflicting surmises and lead to disputes. Chemical manufacturers, for example, often argue that people are exposed to small doses of chemicals compared to those administered to animals. (Industry critics, for example, argued that to equal the amount of saccharin given to animals in a cancer study, a person would have to drink some 400 cans of diet soda daily.)

Decades of testing on animals, however, have shown that a chemical that causes cancer in multiple species can be strongly suspected of also doing so in humans. Of the thirty-plus agents that are definitely known to cause cancer, almost all have been found to cause cancer in animal tests. Furthermore, the determination of carcinogenicity usually comes from multiple studies and sources of evidence that repeatedly demonstrate malignant change.

Such arguments pose a problem for the ordinary person concerned about health and cancer. How does one assess personal risk? How does one know what to believe and what measures to take for protection?

Assessing the Risk of Cancer. We all live with risk. In an environment pervaded with natural and manufactured substances, as well as viruses, any of us could be exposed to something that has the potential to cause cancer. The issue for most people should be not whether or not they come into contact with carcinogens, but rather, given exposure, what is the individual's risk? Unfortunately, there is no clear answer.

Scientists project risks on the basis of epidemiological and animal studies. These types of studies have suggested, for example, that about one in every ten heavy cigarette smokers will develop lung cancer and that about one of every nine women will develop breast cancer in the course of a lifetime. However, such studies cannot tell us who specifically will develop which cancer, under what circumstances, and at what time.

Susceptibility to cancer varies from individual to individual. A number of different factors can affect susceptibility, including internal factors, such as age and overall health, and external and environmental factors, such as where one lives or works. Genetic predisposition also plays a role. However, studies of populations that have migrated demonstrate that what was once thought to be ethnic or racial predisposition to specific types of cancers is in fact due more to environmental factors. For example, although the Japanese in Japan show lower incidences of breast cancer and higher incidences of stomach cancer than Americans, Japanese who have migrated to Hawaii show higher breast cancer and lower stomach cancer rates than those in Japan (much the same as Hawaiian Caucasians).

The issue of what percentage of cancers are

caused by toxic substances in the environment is also a subject of much debate. Some health experts claim that as many as 30 percent of all cancers are caused by chemicals in the environment, including tobacco smoke. Others suggest that if dietary fat and sunlight are included as environmental carcinogens, perhaps as many as 60–70 percent of all cancers are environmentally stimulated. (See Figure 7.1, p. 134.)

Still other health experts claim that extremely few cancers are caused by the environment. The Environmental Protection Agency (EPA) and the National Institutes of Health (NIH) take a middle view between these two extremes. Their data suggest that perhaps 10 to 20 percent of cancers are the result of environmental exposure.

Although the causes of most cancers remain an enigma, individuals *can* take steps to protect themselves. Although we can't do much about our genetic heritage, we can avoid or reduce environmental risks. Research has shown that at least two of the major cancer killers—lung cancer and colorectal cancers—may be preventable through changes in life-style and diet. In the following section, we report on some of the most common carcinogens as well as provide information on how to protect yourself.

CANCER-CAUSING SUBSTANCES OF CONCERN

There are a number of specific chemicals and substances that have been identified as being carcinogenic (see Table 7.3). Exposure to a carcinogen does not mean that a person will develop cancer, but it does mean that the RISK of cancer will increase.

For the most part, the risk of cancer from occupational exposures to a carcinogen is potentially greater than from an environmental exposure to the same carcinogen (see Chapter 21, "The Workplace"). This is because, in general, people who work with carcinogenic agents are exposed to them in higher concentrations and for more extended periods of time. Similarly, artists, hobbyists, and gardeners may be exposed to high concentrations of substances for extended periods of time, 365 days a year. (See Chapter 20, "Art and Hobbyist Materials.")

Although, in general, the risk of developing cancer from a chemical in the environment is quite small, precautions should be taken wherever feasible. (See Table 7.2.)

Tobacco Smoke: The Most Widespread Carcinogen

Among all identified carcinogens, tobacco stands out as one that is extremely widespread.

If you wanted to design the ultimate mixture of carcinogens, you might well come up with cigarette smoke. It contains more than 3,600 complex chemicals, among which are at least 43 substances known to be carcinogens. These include benzo[a]pyrene, aromatic amines, benzene, and nitrosamines. Both initiators and promoters of cancer are found in cigarette smoke, making it a complete, self-contained carcinogenic stew.

The single most important thing that individuals can do to prevent cancer is not to smoke and not to expose others who are close to them—their spouses and children—to smoke. Exposure to tobacco smoke is the greatest preventable cause of cancer. This includes smoking tobacco directly as well as through passive smoke; passive smoke consists of *sidestream smoke* (smoke from the burning tip of the cigarette, which is not filtered either by the cigarette or the smoker's lungs) and *mainstream smoke* (smoke exhaled by the smoker). The American Cancer Society and the National Cancer Institute (NCI) estimate that tobacco smoke causes about one-third of *all* cancer deaths in the United States—more than all other carcinogens added together.

Tobacco smoke is most closely associated with

Table 7.2 TYPES OF CANCER AND ENVIRONMENTAL FACTORS THAT MAY CAUSE THEM

Type of cancer	Risks
Biliary tract (gallbladder, biliary duct)	Chemicals used to process rubber; high-fat, low-fiber diet
Bladder	Cigarette smoking, coke oven emissions, dye manufacture (i.e., aromatic amines and benzidine), rubber manufacture, diesel exhaust, ionizing radiation
Bone	Therapeutic radium exposure
Brain and central nervous system	High-dose X rays, specific (and rare) familial conditions
Breast	High doses of therapeutic radiation; high-fat, low-fiber diet; obesity; inheritance and family history.
Uterine cervix	Human papilloma virus infection, cigarette smoking, multiple sex partners
Colon and rectum	Preexisting inflammatory bowel disease such as ulcerative colitis; high-fat, low-fiber diet; low intake of fruits and vegetables; family history of this type of cancer and familial polyposis syndromes; prior benign polyps
Esophagus	Cigarette smoking, alcohol, smokeless tobacco, low-fiber diet, low intake of fruits and vegetables
Kidney	Cigarette smoking, coke oven emissions
Larynx	Cigarette, pipe, and cigar smoking; alcohol; smokeless tobacco
Leukemia	Ionizing radiation, benzene (i.e., chemical and rubber manufacturing and gasoline), human T-cell leukemia virus infection, some anticancer drugs
Liver	Hepatitis B virus infection, alcohol, plastics industry (vinyl chloride)
Lung	Cigarette smoking, ambient cigarette smoke, ionizing radiation, industrial exposure to asbestos (especially in smokers), industrial exposure to arsenic (a by-product of copper refining), exposure to cadmium, chemical and plastic manufacture [bis(chloromethyl)-ether], chromium plating and alloy making, chromate pigment manufacture, coke oven emissions, occupational exposure to soot and tars (roofing), radon gas (i.e., underground mining and tightly sealed homes), refining of nickel, low intake of fruits and vegetables (particularly β-carotene)
Mouth (oral) (includes tongue, lips, cheek, gums, and throat)	Cigarette, cigar, or pipe smoking; smokeless tobacco; alcohol (even very low levels); ionizing radiation

(continued)

Table 7.2 TYPES OF CANCER AND ENVIRONMENTAL FACTORS THAT MAY CAUSE THEM (*continued*)

Type of cancer	Risks
Pancreas	Cigarette smoking, methylene chloride
Prostate	Occupational exposure to cadmium (welders)
Skin	Excessive exposure to the sun, workers with coal tar or pitch, arsenic, ionizing radiation
Stomach	Cigarette smoking, preserved (pickled, salted, or smoked) foods, ionizing radiation, low intake of fruits and vegetables
Thyroid gland	Ionizing radiation (medical), I^{13} radioactive iodine (as was released at Chernobyl)
Uterus (endometrium)	Prolonged unopposed estrogen therapy, obesity, ionizing radiation

lung cancer, and particularly with one type, small cell carcinoma. Only about 13 percent of all diagnosed lung cancer patients survive five years after diagnosis. (The survival rate is much better—about 37 percent—if the cancer is detected early, before it metastasizes. However, only about 20 percent of all lung cancers are caught this early.)

Tobacco smoke is also associated with cancers of the larynx, oral cavity (mouth, tongue, lips, and throat), and esophagus, and for 30 to 40 percent of all cancers of the urinary bladder, as well as some cases of kidney and pancreas cancer.

Tobacco in all of its forms can cause cancer. Although cigarette smoke is the most common source of tobacco-caused cancer, smoke from cigars and pipes and "smokeless" tobacco (snuff and chewing tobacco) are also potent carcinogens.

New studies also demonstrate the dangers for nonsmokers of breathing in the sidestream smoke given off by cigarettes (also called passive or secondhand smoking). People exposed in this way also have an increased risk of developing cancer. A 1990 study of lung cancer in nonsmokers estimated that about 1,700 cases of lung cancer each year are due to exposure to secondhand smoke during childhood and adolescence. Nonsmoking spouses of smokers are also at increased risk.

These findings are not surprising. Sidestream smoke has greater concentrations of several known carcinogens—three times more benzo[*a*]-pyrene, six times more toluene, and much more nitrosamine—than directly inhaled smoke (see also Chapter 22, "The ABCs of Staying Healthy").

Box 7.2 SMOKING STATISTICS

The statistics documenting the interrelationship of cancer and cigarette smoking are grim. Cigarette smokers have a much higher risk of developing lung cancer than nonsmokers. One smoker in ten will develop the disease, as compared to about one in one hundred nonsmokers. In 1991, 161,000 new cases of lung cancer were reported and another 143,000 individuals died from the disease. Some 90 percent of lung cancers and lung cancer deaths are attributed to smoking.

Radiation and Cancer

There is a long history of cancer from radiation exposure. Historically, the discovery that exposure to ionizing radiation can increase the risk of cancer came from the observation that radiologists and patients who received high doses of X rays had subsequently increased rates of cancer. (See Chapter 16, "Radiant Energy," for a discussion of radiation terminology, including the difference between ionizing and nonionizing radiation, as well as information on the carcinogenic effects of radiation.)

Studies of survivors of the atomic bombs dropped in Japan have also contributed greatly to our understanding of the carcinogenic effects of ionizing radiation. More than 100,000 Japanese living in Hiroshima and Nagasaki survived the atomic bomb blasts over those cities. The most heavily irradiated survivors have shown increases in both leukemia and solid tumors (including cancers of the thyroid gland, breast, and gastrointestinal organs) as long as two to three decades after exposure. The Radiation Effects Research Foundation, set up to study these survivors, has estimated that 1 percent of deaths among bomb survivors between 1950 and 1984 was due to the carcinogenic effects of atomic bomb radiation (see p. 582).

Estimates of radiation-caused cancer vary, but it may conceivably account for some 10,000 cancer fatalities annually, or roughly 2 percent of all cancer deaths. Most of these deaths are thought to result from natural background radiation, including radon, with many resulting from medical and occupational exposures (see Figure 7.1).

Medical and occupational exposures are typically lower today than earlier in the century and are spread out over years. Today's chest X rays, for instance, involve such a low dose that it would take one hundred of them to deliver 1 rad (or radiation absorbed dose) to the chest. In contrast, some victims of Hiroshima are estimated to have received 300 rads in one dose.

At present, there is no definitive evidence of increased cancer risk from either contemporary *low-dose* medical X-ray exposure or from working in nuclear installations. Epidemiologists at the NCI are investigating whether repeated low-dose medical X rays delivered over many years increases cancer rates. To date, they have not found any relationship between such low doses of radiation and the rates of leukemia or lymphoma (cancers that are believed to be radiation sensitive). Although we simply do not know if there is a "safe" or threshold dose for radiation, the NCI findings are reassuring.

A potent cause of lung cancer is radon, an inert gas that is released during the decay of uranium. Inhaled radon can damage the cells lining the airways, leading to lung cancer. Radon is ubiquitous—it is found in both indoor and outdoor air, as well as in soil, water, and building materials. In houses that are located over geologic formations containing uranium deposits, radon in soil can seep into the air in basements, reaching unacceptably high concentrations (see Chapter 14, "Air"). The risk of radon-caused lung cancer is dose dependent—the higher the exposure, the greater the risk. Smokers are believed to have a greater risk of lung cancer due to radon than nonsmokers.

Ultraviolet light from the sun is another source of radiation strongly linked with cancer. There is a direct link between exposure to ultraviolet light and the subsequent development of skin cancers some ten to twenty years later (see Chapter 4, "Skin Ailments").

Carcinogens in the Workplace

The first identification of a carcinogen-linked cancer was related to occupational exposure. In 1775, British surgeon Sir Percival Pott observed that young boys who were chimney sweeps, whose work involved being smeared with soot from chimneys, in young adulthood developed an unusually high incidence of scrotal cancer (a disease known at that time as "soot-wart"). Drawing the connection between the conditions under which sweeps labored and their subsequent development of illness led to the first cancer prevention strategy: using daily baths and clothing changes. Although rudimentary, the intervention worked. In Denmark, where these measures were adopted, the rate of scrotal cancer in chimney sweeps dropped. In England, where sweeps continued to work without improving hygiene measures, the rate of scrotal cancer remained high.

Nearly a century and a half later—in the 1930s—scientists began to categorize industrial causes of cancer more formally. Drawing upon Pott's observation and the then recently developed tool of spectroscopy, scientists identified the carcinogen in tar, soot, and carbon products as the class of chemicals *polycyclic aromatic hydrocarbons* (PAHs). Today, scientists know that a broad range of cancers are related to PAHs and carbon-based compounds.

When it comes to chemical carcinogenicity, industrial workers have been described by the NCI as the "flagmen" of society. If a substance used in the workplace is a carcinogen, reports the NCI, the cancers it can cause will most likely be seen first in workers. Scientific evidence points overwhelmingly to the work environment as the place where Americans are most likely to be exposed (and exposed for prolonged periods) to chemicals that increase the risk of cancer. In fact, the EPA cites exposure to workplace chemicals as one of the leading environmental hazards.

Many of the chemicals discussed below, which are significant carcinogens found in the work environment, have entered the general environment as well, often through pollution. Although this can be a cause for concern, in most instances, the concentrations disseminated may not be sufficient to cause serious cancer threats to the general public.

Since 1971, the International Agency for Research on Cancer, an agency of the World Health Center, has been reviewing and cataloging data on the carcinogenicity of chemicals. To date, they have identified twenty-three chemicals and groups of chemicals as capable of causing cancer, with another sixty-one identified as

probable carcinogens. The EPA classifies thirty chemicals as *proven* human carcinogens (see Table 7.1). It is possible, if not probable, that many more chemicals have carcinogenic properties; however, evidence is insufficient at present to label them as such. Chemical carcinogens are not limited solely to the blue-collar factory; they can be found in a variety of settings, from offices and hospitals to artists' studios.

Arsenic. Arsenic is a naturally occurring element that is a common ingredient in insecticides, but it is also used in smelting processes, wood preservatives, and the electronics industry. Trace amounts of arsenic (not necessarily in its most dangerous chemical forms or amounts great enough to cause cancer) have been measured in air, water, and food. In industrial settings, research has shown that inhaling arsenic can cause lung cancer; dermal contact can cause skin cancer. Because of its potency, arsenic in consumer insecticides is strictly regulated by the EPA.

Epidemiologic studies have shown that people who live close to ore smelters, and thus experience chronic, long-term exposure to arsenic, may have an elevated risk of lung cancer (see Arsenic information sheet, p. 364).

Benzene. A chemical derived from petroleum and coal, benzene is an ingredient found in a variety of products, including gasoline, paint and paint removers, pesticides, plastics, and many other products. Cigarette smoke also releases benzene into the air. Because it is used in so many products, it is widely distributed in air and water.

There is a clear association between exposure to benzene and leukemia, as well as to aplastic anemia, an irreversible depression of the production of red blood cells in the bone marrow (see Benzene information sheet, p. 366).

Cadmium. Cadmium is a naturally occurring element used as a pigment in paints and a preservative in plastics. It is also used in fertilizers. Like arsenic and benzene, cadmium is widely distributed in air, water, and food. Concentrations of it have been found in seafood (including flounder, mussels, scallops, and oysters) and plants taken from polluted areas and in water supplied through pipes soldered with cadmium-containing materials. It is also a chemical released by cigarette smoke; heavy smokers show twice the concentration of cadmium in their blood as nonsmokers. The EPA classifies cadmium as a probable human carcinogen (see Cadmium information sheet, p. 368, and Table 7.3).

Dioxin. Dioxin is a chemical that is produced in minute amounts as a contaminant by-product in the production of other chemicals. Dioxin is formed as the result of manufacturing processes that bleach wood pulp to make white paper (which means that trace amounts of dioxin have been found in such products as milk carton containers, disposable diapers, tampons, and toilet paper) and that incinerate chlorine-containing waste products; fish in streams into which dioxin-containing wastes have been discharged have been found to contain measurable levels of dioxin. It also can be found in automobile exhaust.

Dioxin is most notorious as a contaminant produced in the manufacture of herbicides, especially Agent Orange, the herbicide used during the Vietnam War. The form of dioxin that contaminated Agent Orange is 2, 3, 7, 8-tetrachloro-dibenzo-*p*-dioxin (TCDD), and has been described as "the most toxic chemical known." However, although it has been shown in animal studies to cause cancer and to have numerous side effects in humans, including headaches, peripheral neuropathy, ulcers, and immune system dysfunction, its carcinogenicity to humans has not been firmly established.

Although numerous studies have suggested an association between TCDD and non-Hodgkin's lymphoma, a cancer of the lymph glands, and stomach, nasal, and liver cancer, other studies have been inconclusive. However, in 1990, a study of 5,000 individuals who worked in the herbicide industry between 1942 and 1984, many of whom were exposed to high levels of dioxin, among other chemicals, demonstrated an increased risk of soft-tissue cancers, such as sarcoma and non-Hodgkin's lymphomas. In March 1990, the Department of Veterans Affairs agreed to compensate Vietnam veterans with non-Hodgkins lymphoma, ending a long-standing debate with veterans' groups (see p. 168).

Ethylene oxide. Although classified as a probable human carcinogen, ethylene oxide is widely used to sterilize medical supplies as well as in the manufacture of products such as cosmetics and detergents, brake fluids, inks, emulsifiers, and lubricants, among others. The government estimates that 270,000 persons are occupationally exposed to ethylene oxide.

Animal studies have shown that ethylene oxide is a carcinogen. Human studies have been difficult to organize and are limited. A 1988 Swedish study found an increased rate of leukemia and stomach cancer among workers exposed to ethylene oxide, but the workers were also exposed to other carcinogens. Other studies found no increase but included smaller numbers of subjects.

Many other chemicals are found at the worksite that cause cancer, as listed in Table 7.3 and in Chapter 21, "The Workplace." (If you work with chemicals, we suggest you read Chapter 21 for a review of how to protect yourself at the worksite.)

Carcinogens in the Air We Breathe

It is difficult to make generalizations about cancer and the hazards of air pollution, because the quality of outdoor air varies so greatly from region to region, city to city, and even block to block. As mentioned earlier, depletion of the ozone layer leads to increased levels of ultraviolet radiation at the earth's surface and has increased the incidence of skin cancer. The major damage to the ozone layer comes from chlorofluorocarbons, compounds that are used in refrigerants and solvents (see p. 29).

Table 7.3 COMMON CARCINOGENS AND THEIR EFFECTS

Carcinogen	Occupational or other means of exposure	Type(s) of cancer caused
4-Aminobiphenyl	Rubber and dye manufacture, chemical manufacture	Bladder cancer
Arsenic and arsenic compounds[a]	Copper mining and smelting, pesticide manufacture, drinking water	Lung, skin, and liver cancers
Asbestos[a]	Manufacture of building materials and brake linings, installation of insulation	Mesothelioma and lung cancer
Benzene[a]	Chemical and rubber manufacturing, petroleum refining	Leukemia
Benzidine and related chemicals used in dye making (auramine, 2-naphthylamine, and 4-nitrophenyl)	Dye manufacture	Bladder cancer
Benzo[a]pyrene	Roofing materials (in hot pitch)	Lung cancer
Bis(chloromethyl)ether and technical-grade chloromethyl ether	Chemical and plastics manufacture	Lung cancer
Chlorambucil	Anticancer therapy	Leukemia
Chromium and chromium compounds[a]	Chromium plating, making chromium alloys and chromate pigments	Lung cancer
Coke oven emissions (including polycyclic aromatic hydrocarbons)	Steel making, especially coke oven operation	Lung, scrotum, kidney, and genitourinary cancers
Cyclophosphamide	Cancer therapy, immunosuppression	Leukemia and bladder cancer
Diethylstilbestrol (DES)	Therapy of female hormonal disorders	Vaginal and endometrial cancers
Dioxin (2, 3, 7, 8-tetrachloro-dibenzo-p-dioxin)	Herbicide manufacture	Lymphoma and soft-tissue sarcoma
Ionizing radiation[a,b]	Nuclear weapons industry, radiology	Leukemia
Melphalan	Anticancer agent	Leukemia
Nickel and nickel compounds[a]	Nickel refining	Nasal, sinus, and lung cancers
Polycyclic aromatic hydrocarbons	Truck exhaust, tar distilling	Bladder, lung, and skin cancers
Radon (exposure from iron and uranium mining)	Miners	Lung cancer

(continued)

Table 7.3 COMMON CARCINOGENS AND THEIR EFFECTS (*continued*)

Soots, tars, and mineral oils (probably due to polycyclic aromatic hydrocarbons)	Roofing, chimney cleaning, manufacture of coal tar and creosote, lathe operators, metal working, printing press operation	Malignant neoplasms of the scrotum; lung, skin, gastrointestinal, oral, and colon cancers
Vinyl chloride[a]	Manufacture of plastics	Angiosarcoma of the liver
Wood dust (hardwoods) (see also information sheet on nuisance dusts)	Woodworking, cabinet/furniture making	Cancer of nasal cavities

[a] See also information sheet.
[b] See Chapter 16, "Radiant Energy."

Other than tobacco smoke, the percentage of cancers (and specifically lung cancers) caused by air pollution is the subject of much debate. At present, there are very few studies that equate specific cancers to air pollution. Some health professionals estimate the percentage of cancers caused by air pollution to be negligible, perhaps about 1 percent; others estimate that it is higher.

Air analyses do show that both polluted indoor and outdoor air contain traces of chemical carcinogens, including benzo[a]pyrene, dioxin, asbestos, arsenic, cadmium, trichloroethylene (TCE), and the gas radon. In animal studies, cancer has been induced in animals subjected to polluted air; epidemiological studies have found increased cancer rates in urban areas (where air pollution is higher than in rural areas) and in areas surrounding factories. Whether or not this increase can be attributed to pollution is questionable, however; two more likely factors are higher workplace exposures and the greater incidence of cigarette smoking among those who live in cities.

Outdoor air pollution. Most health experts consider the risk of cancer being caused by outdoor air pollution to be minimal, mainly because the carcinogens released into the air are not concentrated. Even from toxic spills (for example, when railroad cars have overturned, releasing toxic gas into the atmosphere) the danger of cancer is limited. Wind disperses the concentration of chemicals, so that—except in the immediate vicinity of the spill—the dose of a carcinogen that people receive tends to be quite small.

Individuals who live near factories that improperly and/or illegally vent carcinogens into the outside air may be at higher risk, as may individuals who live near smelters and foundries.

Indoor air pollution. Polluted indoor air is a greater potential source of exposure to carcinogens and people spend an estimated 70 percent of their time indoors (see Chapter 14, "Air"). Some of the common airborne carcinogens include:

BENZO[A]PYRENE. Benzo[a]pyrene is a polycyclic aromatic hydrocarbon (PAH). It is produced as a by-product of inefficiently burned fuel, including coal, wood, and oil. (Benzo[a]pyrene is also found at worksites that use coke ovens, in meat-smoking factories, and in trash incinerators.) Benzo[a]pyrene attaches to dust particles in the air, which then enter the lungs and lodge in the lung tissue. The release of benzo[a]pyrene by cigarette smoke is one of the reasons that smoking is so carcinogenic.

Animal studies show a clear association of benzo[a]pyrene to cancer. Although many people sustain low but frequent exposure to benzo[a]pyrene, there are no good statistics on the resulting cancer risk. On the basis of animal data, however, the EPA has classified benzo[a]pyrene as a probable human carcinogen (see Table 7.3).

Box 7.3   HOW TO PROTECT YOURSELF FROM BENZO[*A*]PYRENE EXPOSURE

- Keep the home ventilated. Make sure that air circulates.
- Make sure cooking stoves are equipped with exhaust fans, and use them.
- Install only furnaces or wood stoves that burn fuel efficiently. Buy wood stoves that are the right size for a room space.
- Make sure rooms that have wood stoves or fireplaces also have ventilation.
- Do not allow fires to smolder.
- Burn only well-seasoned wood. Do not use wood that has been treated with chemicals.
- Inspect and clean the chimney yearly. Have an expert confirm that it is venting properly.
- Reduce consumption of smoked foods.
- Stop cigarette smoking and avoid breathing secondhand smoke.
- If cooking with gas, make sure that the burning flame is uniformly blue. If the tip is yellow, it means that combustion is incomplete. Have the stove adjusted.
- Do not use a gas stove to heat a room.

ASBESTOS. There is a strong correlation between exposure to asbestos and both lung cancer and mesothelioma, a rare cancer of the membranes lining the chest and abdominal cavities, as well as a noncancerous lung disease known as asbestosis (see Chapter 6, "Respiratory Ailments," and Asbestos information sheet, p. 365.) When a cigarette smoker is exposed to asbestos, the risks multiply (see Box 3.2, p. 52).

Although asbestos is found in many areas of the home (i.e., floor, tiles, walls, and insulation around furnaces and pipes), it is dangerous only if its airborne fibers are inhaled. This can happen if the fibers are released from asbestos-containing materials when they are disturbed or damaged, as can occur in the process of removing them (see Box 6.6, p. 127).

Where asbestos fibers settle in the lungs is related to their size. Fibers that are over 10–20 micrometers long tend to be filtered out in the lung's upper airways, where they are removed by the lung's filtration system or trapped in respiratory mucus, which is coughed up or swallowed. Fibers that are not filtered out are thought to be most likely to initiate lung cancer.

Tumors that are caused by asbestos fibers usually start in airway walls, eventually blocking airways and penetrating blood vessels. It is common for lung cancer to metastasize to other parts of the body. All three types of asbestos fiber (amosite, chrysotile, and crocidolite) are associated with lung cancer, although the crocidolite is the most likely to cause it.

Asbestos has also been found in drinking water as a result of deteriorating asbestos-containing concrete water pipes. The risk of cancer from drinking water that contains asbestos is considered to be extremely low, however, as is the risk from asbestos in outdoor air, although there have been documented cases of asbestos-caused lung disease in individuals who live next to shipyards where asbestos was once heavily used.

Asbestos-related disease has a long latency: It can take thirty years from exposure to asbestos before the disease is apparent. Many persons now living are at risk even though they may not currently be exposed to asbestos. Some health experts suspect that there is no safe dose of asbestos exposure—that is to say, they suspect that *any* exposure may cause some increase in the risk of lung cancer.

(For information on what to do if you suspect that there is asbestos in your home, see Box 6.6, p. 127.)

Carcinogens in the Water We Drink

The water we drink comes from two sources: surface water (lakes and rivers) and groundwater (water percolating into the ground and collected through wells). Although cancer-causing compounds can be found in both, the levels are typically so small that there is probably very little, if any, risk associated with most drinking water supplies.

In surface water, which usually comes through our taps after being processed by municipal water plants, it is not unusual to find traces of nitrates, chloride, arsenic, and cadmium. Groundwater can be contaminated by pesticide and fertilizer residues as well as chemical runoff from factories or even toxic waste dumps.

It has not been possible to establish any definite relationship between carcinogens in water and the incidence of cancer. However, it is reasonable to assume that some risk may exist for people who live near toxic waste sites and draw their water from ground sources, because chemicals from such sites may leach into the local groundwater. Although the risk of cancer from chemically contaminated water is considered low, it is not certain exactly how low. (See Box 13.2, p. 521, for information on having water supplies tested.)

Chlorine. Municipalities add chlorine to drinking water to disinfect it and kill naturally occurring bacteria. Although doing so confers great benefits to society—chlorinating the water supply is responsible for wiping out many waterborne illnesses such as typhoid and cholera—chlorine can also produce toxic by-products called trihalomethanes (THMs) if mixed with certain pollutants. The best-known THM is chloroform.

A few studies have suggested an association between chlorinated drinking water and gastrointestinal and bladder cancers. However, because the results of these studies are inconsistent, a causal relationship between THMs and these cancers has not been firmly established. Nevertheless, the EPA regulates the amount of THMs in drinking water to minimize potential risks and has established a limit of 100 parts of THM per billion parts of drinking water (see Chapter 13, "Water").

Carcinogens in the Food We Eat

Food can contain intentionally added chemicals, such as preservatives and appearance-enhancing colors, as well as unintentionally added substances, such as residues from pesticides. Many of these substances, including polychlorinated biphenyls (PCBs), are considered to be cancer promoters (see p. 623).

In theory, food additives are strictly regulated. The Delaney clause of the Food, Drug, and Cosmetics Act expressly prohibits the addition of chemicals to food if either human or animal studies show that the chemical can induce cancer (see p. 607 for a discussion of the Delaney clause). In practice, the Food and Drug Administration (FDA) does not regulate some additives that some animal studies have shown to have induced cancer, because the risk posed by these chemicals is considered too slight to merit action. Most of the chemicals used in food are used in very small quantities.

Chemicals that are unintentionally added to food include pesticide residues directly sprayed onto plants. Pesticides polluting groundwater can also be absorbed directly into the fibrous bodies of plants. To date, only three chemicals used in pesticides—arsenic, methyl bromide, and vinyl chloride—have clearly shown an increased risk of cancer in humans. This does not mean that pesticides as a class of chemicals are *not* carcinogenic; it may simply mean that the appropriate tests or studies that would determine if specific pesticides pose a cancer threat have not been conducted. (See Chapter 12, "Of Special Concern: Infants and Children," and Chapter 17, "Food Safety," for a further discussion of pesticides and cancer.)

Among those pesticide chemicals *suspected* of having the capacity to cause cancer are alachlor (a herbicide used primarily on corn and soybeans), aldrin, dieldrin, and DDT (organochlorine insecticides).

An infamous incident involving chemical contamination of food occurred in Michigan in 1973. Polybrominated biphenyl (PBB), a chemical used in fire retardants, was inadvertently mixed in animal feed and given to several herds of cows. Humans who subsequently ate meat or drank milk from these cows were exposed to PBBs. However, as of 1989, 4,000 people who consumed PBB-contaminated products were found not to have suffered any adverse health effects. (Although the 1989 study is the most informative study to date on the long-term effects of PBB contamination, it remains conceivable that health effects could develop over a greater period of time after exposure.)

In addition to synthetic chemicals added to food, naturally occurring carcinogens also contaminate food. The most potent of these is aflatoxin, a cancer-causing substance caused by the mold *Aspergillus flavus*, which grows on grains and nuts. In general, this mold grows only in hot, humid climates, but it can also grow on harvested crops that are left to dry in the field after rain or stored in moist areas.

Aflatoxin is more of a problem in developing countries with hot, humid weather and few regulatory controls. In the United States, all susceptible crops are subject to routine testing for aflatoxin, and the chemical is not considered to be a major source of cancer risk in this country. However, feed crops for animals are not as well regulated, and aflatoxin can contaminate meat and milk from animals fed aflatoxin-contaminated feed—albeit the levels of aflatoxin in these products is low, and the risk of cancer to humans via animals is not considered particularly high (see Chapter 17, "Food Safety").

Can Your Diet Cause Cancer? Of all the associations between a specific dietary habit and a specific cancer, the one most strongly supported by scientific evidence is that a lower fat intake reduces the risk of colon cancer. Biochemical studies have shown that a high intake of fat increases the secretion of bile acids and converts these into chemicals that can act as cancer promoters.

A diet high in fat also may promote breast cancer. It is true that breast cancer rates are much lower in parts of the world where diets are low in fat, such as China and Japan. However, these countries are different from the United States in many other ways as well. To date, some studies have shown an association between breast cancer and fat, whereas other studies have shown no association. Of the studies that do link breast cancer to fat, some have suggested that the strongest association occurs with saturated fatty acids—the type of fat found in milk, meat, and some vegetable oils—although other studies have shown an association with dietary levels of fat in general.

There is also some evidence that increasing the amount of fiber in the diet can reduce gastrointestinal cancer. Again, studies have been mixed, and there is currently no absolute proof that this is so. Fiber, however, taken in moderate amounts is safe for most people. Keep in mind, when considering how to increase fiber intake that the people described in studies that suggested that fiber decreased colon cancer got their fiber from grains, fruits, and vegetables—not artificial fiber supplements. These foods contain many other nutrients and even nonnutrients thought to be protective against cancer. It is not clear whether the observed decrease in cancer is due to increased fiber intake or to some other protective substance. This is why the NRC report recommends increasing the intake of foods high in both fiber and other substances, not merely increasing the intake of fiber alone (see Chapter 22, "The ABCs of Staying Healthy").

Fruits and vegetables occupy a central role in any cancer-reducing diet strategy. They provide high-fiber nutrition, as well as a broad spectrum of chemicals that may be *protective* against cancer, such as vitamins C and E, selenium, and β-carotene (a substance that is converted to vitamin A in the body).

More than a dozen studies have shown a high intake of vegetables and fruits is associated with lower rates of cancer (most consistently the lung, but also the colon, stomach, bladder, esophagus, mouth, larynx, pharynx, and cervix). The evidence suggesting that β-carotene, as part of foods, has protective power against cancer is quite strong. A fifteen-year prospective study was begun in 1986 following more than 20,000 American physicians who are taking either β-carotene or placebo pills on a daily basis.

A number of other dietary substances are also believed to confer anticancer benefits. These include isothiocyanates, found in cruciferous vegetables such as broccoli and cauliflower; tannins, found in Chinese green teas; and triterpenoids and isoflavones, found in licorice-root extract and cruciferous vegetables. To what extent these substances and vitamins confer anticancer benefits is under study; present data are very limited and insufficient to allow strong statements to be made about their protective effects.

These dietary compounds are thought to block the action of cancer-causing chemicals. For example, triterpenoids may inhibit the action of estrogens, which promote cancers of the breast and uterus. Flavonoids, found in many higher plants, appear to inhibit how carcinogens interact with DNA. Because of this, it is possible they could disarm cancer-causing chemicals that form during the cooking of meat or fish (see Chapter 22, "The ABCs of Staying Healthy").

Dietary Recommendations

In 1982, the Committee on Diet, Nutrition and Cancer of the National Research Council (NRC) released its landmark study on the relationship between diet and cancer. Based on animal and epidemiologic studies, the NRC concluded that there is a link between fat intake and colon cancer and that dietary fiber can reduce the risk of colon and other digestive system cancers.

The NRC updated its report in 1989, emphasizing that the amount of red meat and animal fat in the American diet should be substantially reduced and the intake of fruits, vegetables, and grains be substantially increased. These recommendations may sound like simple common sense, but they are actually based on a large and varied body of scientific evidence (see Chapter 22, "The ABCs of Staying Healthy").

Adopting the NRC's dietary recommendations would drastically change American eating habits. On a given day, only one in five Americans eats cruciferous vegetables or fruits and vegetables high in vitamin A; only one in six eats high-fiber breads and cereals. Nearly half of all Americans eat no fruit on a given day and nearly a quarter eat no vegetables, and half the population eats red meat or nitrite-containing foods such as bacon and lunch meat daily.

Achieving the goals of the report requires a new way of thinking about food: We will have to treat meat as a condiment, with rice, beans, and pasta as the core of the meal and fruit and vegetables as staples (see Figure 17.1, p. 737, for the new food pyramid).

How much would such a diet benefit us? In 1981, the renowned British epidemiologist Sir Richard Doll (one of the first scientists to recognize the association between cigarette smoking and cancer) estimated that dietary modifications could prevent 35 percent or more of fatal human cancers, including almost all deaths due to stomach and colon cancer.

Box 7.4   CANCER SCREENING TESTS

The earlier that cancer is detected, the more likely that it can be effectively treated. Here are some guidelines on cancer screening tests:

Colon and Rectal Cancers

The American Cancer Society recommends three tests for the early detection of colon and rectum cancer in individuals without risk factors:

- A digital rectal examination, which is performed by a physician during an office visit, should be done every year after the age of forty.
- A stool blood test is recommended annually every year after fifty.
- A proctosigmoidoscopy examination should be carried out every three to five years after the age of fifty following two annual exams with negative results.

Do-it-yourself (at-home) stool blood tests generally are not reliable enough to replace this recommended regimen.

Prostate Cancer

An examination for prostate cancer should be done as part of the part of the digital rectal examination performed for colorectal cancer. As noted above, this should be done every year after age forty. In addition a blood test for prostate-specific antigen (PAS) is recommended.

Cervical Cancer

About 13,000 new cases of cervical cancer are diagnosed each year in the United States. When detected early, these cancers are eminently treatable. To increase the chances of early detection of cervical cancer, women who have reached age eighteen or who are sexually active should have a Pap test and a pelvic examination annually.

After three or more consecutive normal annual examinations, the American Cancer Society advises that less frequent Pap tests can be considered. However, the American College of Obstetrics and Gynecology recommends continuing with yearly Pap smears, even after a series of normal examinations.

Breast Cancer: Mammography Screening and Safety Guidelines

Mammography, the radiographic examination of the breasts, has been demonstrated to be an effective way to detect early-stage breast cancers and to prolong survival.

The American Cancer Society recommends a baseline mammogram between ages thirty-five and thirty-nine, and a mammogram every one to two years for women between ages forty and forty-nine. Women age fifty and over with no symptoms should have an annual mammogram. Women under fifty who have a strong family history of breast cancer should discuss with their physicians whether to start having yearly mammograms earlier.

There has been concern about increased cancer risk from X rays used in a mammogram. Women need to be sure that they get a mammogram at a facility with

(continued)

Box 7.4   CANCER SCREENING TESTS (*continued*)

equipment that produces a high-quality image at the lowest possible radiation dose. With a poor-quality image, the benefit of mammography may be lost. Repeating the examination because of poor quality doubles the radiation dose.

Modern equipment produces a high-quality mammogram at a dose as low as 0.1 rad (see p. 577 for definition of rad). A mammogram delivering 0.2 rad given to 100,000 women at age forty-five might lead to the loss of about one life from radiation-induced cancer, but between twenty and fifty lives would be saved in this group from early detection of breast cancer.

The number of mammography units in the United States increased from 184 in 1982 to 10,000 in 1990, not all of which operate at the lowest possible dose or are of optimal quality. According to an inspection program conducted by the FDA in 1985, 36 percent of units produced "substandard" images. This figure improved to 13 percent by 1988. The American College of Radiology (ACR) conducts a voluntary accreditation program for mammography facilities. Call 1-800-4-CANCER for the names of facilities in your area that have passed this program.

Fewer than half of mammography facilities subscribe to ACR's accreditation program. In some parts of the country, there are no accredited facilities. In these situations, the FDA's inspection results suggest that imaging tends to be better at hospital-based facilities and those that specialize in mammography. Pick a facility that does fifty or more mammographic examinations per week. Also, ask whether the person taking the X ray is a registered technologist, such as a member of the American Registry of Radiological Technologists. Find out whether the equipment has recently been examined by the state or calibrated by a radiological physicist.

BREAST SELF-EXAMINATION

The American Cancer Society recommends that women twenty years and older practice monthly breast self-examination. A three-step method is suggested:

1. Palpation of the breasts in the shower or bath to check for any lump, hard knot, or thickening.
2. Standing in front of a mirror, raising arms to check for any changes in the breast contour or in the nipple or for dimpling of the skin.
3. Palpating each breast with circular motions while lying on the back.

Women who have no prior history of breast cancer or breast cysts should have their breasts examined by a health professional at least every three years from ages twenty to forty. Women over age forty should have a physical examination of the breast every year.

Skin Cancer: The ABCDs of Melanoma

Malignant melanoma is an invasive and potentially deadly form of skin cancer. More than 30,000 cases of melanoma are diagnosed each year in the United States.

(*continued*)

Box 7.4   CANCER SCREENING TESTS (*continued*)

If detected early, malignant melanoma can be surgically excised, which offers an excellent chance of cure.

To detect malignant melanoma before it has spread beyond the skin, be alert to changes in a mole or pigmented spot on the skin. Consult a dermatologist immediately if any of the warning characteristics appear in a mole or pigmented spot (see Figure 4.3, p. 77).

Box 7.5   CANCER PREVENTION

To prevent cancer, each person must reduce or eliminate his or her exposure to carcinogens. Because not everything causes cancer, such a strategy is reasonable and workable. Here is an approach to cancer prevention formulated by the American Cancer Society:

- Don't smoke cigarettes, pipes, or cigars. Don't chew tobacco or dip snuff.
- Vary your diet to include foods low in fat and low enough in calories so that you will stay trim. Include fresh fruits, vegetables, whole grains, and whole grain bread and cereals in your daily diet.
- Drink only in moderation, if at all, particularly if you smoke. (One or two drinks a day is considered moderate.)
- Avoid too much sunlight, particularly if you are fair skinned; wear protective clothing and use effective sunscreens.
- Don't ask for an X ray if your doctor or dentist does not recommend it. If you need an X ray, be sure X-ray shields are used if possible to protect other parts of your body.
- Regulatory agencies, industries, and organized labor have developed health and safety measures to reduce hazardous exposures in the workplace. Industries can take a number of steps to reduce or eliminate risks to workers. Individuals also can take steps. Health and safety rules of the workplace should be known and followed.
- Take estrogens only as long as necessary and discuss their use with your physician (see Box 10.2, p. 203).

Precancerous Conditions and Susceptibility to Cancer

Scientists believe that a tendency to develop cancer is enhanced by several biological factors. Some of these are inherited; others develop during a person's life as a result of viral infection or as a side effect of medical therapy. Some suspected predisposing conditions are listed here:

DNA Repair Defects. As noted on p. 133, one theory on cancer is that it originates from the action of mutagens on DNA. Normally, repair systems correct much of this genetic damage. However, there are certain inherited conditions in which repair enzymes are dysfunctional.

One of the most studied of these hereditary diseases is *xeroderma pigmentosum*, in which the type of DNA damage caused by ultraviolet light (thymidine dimers) is not normally repairable. In people with xeroderma, exposure to even low doses of sunlight leads to a multiplicity of skin cancers at an early age.

Immunodeficiency. An intact immune system has the ability to ward off infectious diseases and to detect and destroy cancerous cells before they multiply and form a tumor. Any defect in immunity has the potential to lead to infections with bacteria, viruses, and fungi, as well as an increased cancer risk. For instance, higher incidences of both lymphoma, a cancer of the blood vessels, and Kaposi's sarcoma are observed in people in whom immune function is impaired, including transplant patients treated with immunosuppressive drugs (such as azathioprine, cyclophosphamide, and corticosteroids) and persons infected with human immunodeficiency virus. Several inherited immune deficiency diseases are associated with an increase in non-Hodgkin's lymphoma and acute leukemia.

Leukoplakia. Literally "white plate," leukoplakia is the development of white, thickened patches on the mucous membranes of the cheeks, gums, or tongue, which cannot be rubbed off. It is common in cigarette smokers and persons who chew smokeless tobacco. Leukoplakia can be a precursor to cancer of the oral cavity.

Polyps of the Colon. A polyp is a protruding outgrowth of the mucous membrane in the lining of the large bowel (colon), often as the result of the hereditary condition *polyposis coli*. In this familial disease, hundreds of polyps may grow on the wall of the colon, some of which turn cancerous by the time the person is forty years old. *Polyposis coli* has been traced to a defect in a tumor suppressor gene.

Papilloma. Papillomas of the lining of the urinary bladder are superficial bladder tumors that appear after exposure to carcinogenic chemicals.

Chronic Cystic Disease. Chronic cystic disease of the breast, also called proliferative breast disease, is a benign condition in which excessive growth of epithelial cells occurs in the terminal portions of the breast ducts. Because this is the site where breast cancer most often originates, chronic cystic disease is considered to be a possible precursor of breast cancer. Women with chronic cystic disease have a two- to fivefold increased risk of invasive breast cancer.

Drugs. Three classes of drugs increase the risk of cancer: estrogenic hormones, anticancer drugs, and immunosuppressive drugs (for the last one, see Immunodeficiency).

Hormones. Estrogenic hormones, including estrogen and the nonsteroidal estrogen diethylstilbestrol (DES), are known to promote cancer in women.

Between 1940 and 1971, an estimated 6 million pregnant women at risk of miscarriage were treated with DES. It was subsequently determined that this compound raised the incidence of a certain type of vaginal cancer in women who had been exposed to it in the womb (see Chapter 11, "Reproductive Effects and Prenatal Exposures").

Hormone replacement therapy (HRT) is now widely used to treat postmenopausal symptoms and to prevent osteoporosis. Many women still fear estrogen replacement therapy because of studies, in the mid-1970s, that reported a higher incidence of breast and uterine (endometrial) cancer in women who had taken estrogen. Today, this type of HRT combines estrogen with another hormone, progesterone, and the combination appears to decrease the risk of uterine (endometrial) cancer (see Box 10.2, p. 203, for more information on estrogen replacement therapy). Whether HRT increases the risk of breast cancer is subject to debate. The more recent studies indicate that HRT does not increase the incidence of breast cancer, but that if breast cancer is present, it is likely to grow more quickly in the presence of estrogen.

Anticancer Drugs. Most drugs used to treat cancer are cytotoxic, that is, they kill growing cells. Many of them do so by attacking DNA. In the process, sometimes mutations are produced in the cells that are not killed. As a result, anticancer drugs can increase the risk of new cancers. For example, in patients treated with certain chemotherapy regimens (involving alkylating agents) for Hodgkin's disease, so-called second cancers, particularly acute leukemia, can appear many years after therapy.

CHAPTER 8

Immunological Alterations

The immune system can be thought of as our set of defenses against the small enemies of the environment, microorganisms that prowl about the world looking for ways to make a biological profit at the expense of the human body. It is a collection of tissues, cells, and mediators working together to recognize and attack those enemies.

When the immune system works properly, it is because of a complex, intermeshed set of activities by specialized cells and the molecules they produce. Like any other complex mechanism, the immune system can malfunction, and many of these immunological effects are provoked by environmental agents.

Immunological alterations can be grouped in four general classes. First is the most common—*allergy*. An allergy is an adverse immune response to a usually harmless substance, such as ragweed pollen or milk. Second is *immune deficiency*, such as that induced by chemotherapy drugs or by AIDS, in which the immune system loses part of its defenses. Third is *autoimmune disease*, such as rheumatoid arthritis, which occurs when the immune system mistakes the body's own cells and tissues for enemies and attacks them. Fourth, there is *malignancy*, or cancer, a major aspect of which is that the immune system is overwhelmed by the uncontrolled proliferation of cells.

Each of these four alterations—allergy, autoimmunity, immune deficiency, and malignancy—can be triggered by environmental factors. These factors can range from viruses to by-products of human activity, such as air pollutants, industrial chemicals, or medications—all of which can alter the delicate balance of the immune system. Although in a few cases an altered immune response can be beneficial, such as when drugs are given to suppress the immune response in order to prevent the rejection of a transplanted organ, much of the time these alterations have adverse effects.

This chapter will examine not only the environmental aspects of these four immunological alterations but also the issue of chemicals in the environment and the controversial subject of multiple chemical sensitivity, which attributes a large number of physiological and psychological ills to low levels of synthetic chemicals.

COMPONENTS OF THE IMMUNE SYSTEM

An essential building block of the immune system is the basic stem cell that is made in the marrow, the spongy substance found in the center of bones. Stem cells and their offspring migrate to different parts of the body to perform many functions. Some stem cells evolve into macrophages, cells that are in the front line of defense against viruses and other microbes. One function of a macrophage is to ingest foreign proteins that are found on the outer walls of viruses and bacteria. These proteins are called *antigens*. The cells of the body display their own antigens, but a properly functioning macrophage singles out only foreign antigens for attack by the immune system. Other immune cells, a group of white blood cells called granulocytes, do the same thing.

Sometimes granulocytes can destroy an invader such as a virus. When they cannot, macrophages engulf the virus and display the viral antigens on the outer surface of their cell membrane. That display attracts two other kinds of immune system cells, which are both lymphocytes, or white blood cells: T cells and B cells (see Figure 8.1). These cells work in concert to activate the immune system's defenses and produce the complex proteins called antibodies that attack antigens.

T Cells, B Cells, and Antibodies

B cells are responsible for the production of antibodies, a function called *humoral immunity*. B cells recognize foreign entities, such as an invading cell, by the antigens—protein, carbohydrate, or lipid molecules—found on the cells' surface. This recognition causes the B cell to multiply and change into an antibody-producing factory, called a *plasma cell*. The antibody molecules combine with the antigens and inactivate them either directly or by calling into play other cells of the immune system, the *macrophage* and *killer cells*, which attack and destroy the invaders.

When this encounter ends, the antibody-producing plasma cells become inactive, but the immune system retains a memory of the invasion in the form of sensitized B cells, called *memory B cells*. If the same virus invades the body again, it can be overwhelmed before it can do great damage. Another group of immune system cells, the *T cells*, play several roles in this process.

"Virgin" (unspecialized) T cells sense the antigen, and this initiates the activation of a variety of specialized subsets of T cells, including *memory T cells* (which like memory B cells, retain a memory of the antigen and can be called into action should the same antigen enter the body in the future), *T helper cells*, *T suppressor cells*, and *cytotoxic T cells*.

T helper cells activate the immune system by secreting *lymphokines*, molecules that modulate and control immune activity by "turning on" various cells of the immune system. These cells include antibody-producing B cells, macrophages and killer cells, and another specialized T cell, the cytotoxic T cell, all of which destroy invading cells.

This response is regulated by the T suppressor cells to ensure that the immune system does not continue to react once the invader has been dealt with.

An antibody molecule consists of four protein chains, two heavy (or long) and two light (or short) chains, joined in a Y shape. In the fork-shaped part of the Y are *hypervariable regions*. Alterations in the hypervariable region allow the immune system to produce a nearly infinite variety of antibodies to attack any antigen that enters the body.

Antibodies belong to a group called the immunoglobulins, so named because they have a globular shape. Five classes of antibodies have been identified, each with a different function. Immunoglobulin G (IgG) is the major class, accounting for 75 percent of all the immunoglobulins in the body. Immunoglobulin E (IgE) is responsible for immediate-type allergic reactions. The other immunoglobulins are IgA, IgM, and IgD, which have specialized roles.

Figure 8.1 THE IMMUNE SYSTEM: T CELLS AND B CELLS.

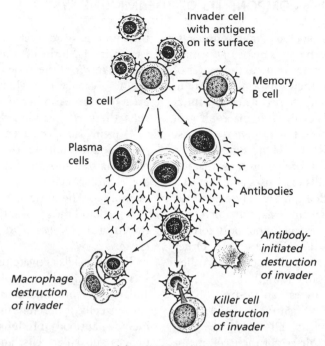

(a) HUMORAL IMMUNITY

(*a*) Humoral Immunity. B cells recognize an invader by an antigen on their cell surface, causing them to multiply and change into *plasma cells*, which manufacture antibodies that attack invaders directly or signal other cells to attack, such as *killer cells* and *macrophages*. *Memory B cells*, primed to recognize the agent, remain in the bloodstream afterward.

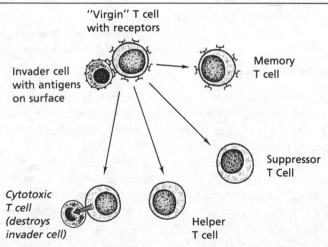

(b) RISE OF SPECIALIZED T CELLS

(*b*) The Rise of Specialized T cells. When "virgin" T cells sense an antigen, they initiate the activation of various specialized subsets of T cells, including *memory T cells* (which, like memory B cells, remain in the bloodstream), *T helper cells*, *T suppressor cells*, and *cytotoxic T cells*.

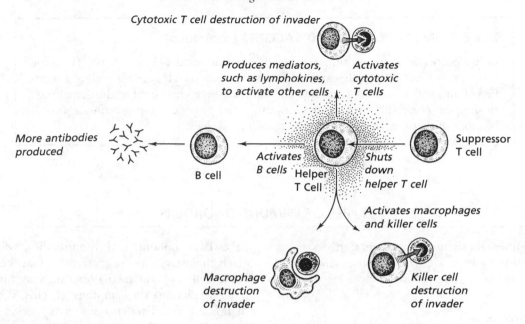

(c) FUNCTION OF SPECIALIZED T CELLS

(c) Function of specialized T cells. T helper cells secrete lymphokines, which "turn on" various attack cells, including the cytotoxic T cell. T suppressor cells regulate this response, ensuring that the immune system does not continue to react once the invader has been dealt with.

Box 8.1 IMMUNIZATION AND VACCINES

Vaccines protect against infection by exposing the immune system to the antigens of viruses and bacteria in a modified or harmless form. When the virus and bacteria appear, the immune system is ready to respond because it has been sensitized to the antigenic components of the microorganisms. The first vaccine was made by Edward Jenner, a British doctor who, in the late eighteenth century, discovered that exposure to a harmless virus called vaccinia could protect against smallpox. It was more than a century before a scientific basis for vaccination was established and researchers could systematically develop vaccines.

There are different kinds of vaccines. One contains a weakened or altered form of the infectious agent. Another uses a killed virus or bacterium. The Salk vaccine for polio uses a killed virus, whereas the Sabin vaccine uses live, but weakened, polio viruses.

New kinds of vaccines developed by genetic engineering are now being tested. Some experimental acquired immune deficiency syndrome (AIDS) vaccines use

(continued)

Box 8.1 IMMUNIZATION AND VACCINES (*continued*)

only a portion of a surface antigen of the human immunodeficiency virus (HIV), the virus that causes AIDS. Researchers also have discovered that genes coding a number of antigens can be inserted into the same vaccinia virus used against smallpox, raising the possibility that a single injection can provide the protection against a number of diseases that now require multiple vaccines.

TYPES OF IMMUNE DISORDERS

When we talk about environmental attacks on the immune system, we can often describe which component of the immune response is affected.

Allergies

Allergy is the most widespread environmentally caused adverse immune response. An estimated 40 million Americans suffer from allergic conditions, including asthma. One of every eleven visits to a doctor's office in the United States is due to an allergy. The most common allergic condition is popularly called hay fever and is an allergic reaction to an inhaled substance, such as pollen or mold. However, many people have allergic reactions to other environmental agents, including food, house dust, metals, cosmetics, medications, and animals. (See Box 6.3, p. 121, for details on combatting some of the respiratory allergens.)

The type E immunoglobulins (IgE) play a central role in allergy. Many of the same symptoms that occur during a common cold occur when someone has an allergy, except that a cold usually is accompanied by fever and generalized aching, whereas an allergy is not. The mechanism is quite different in the two disorders. Cold symptoms are caused by the body's response to a viral infection. In an allergy, for unknown reasons, the immune system reacts against something that usually is harmless. When an allergic person is first exposed to an allergen, he or she makes large amounts of IgE antibodies, which attach themselves to the surfaces of mast cells. These cells contain mediators, such as histamine, which cause the symptoms of colds. When the IgE antibody later encounters its specific antigen, it triggers the release of mediators, causing the symptoms of allergy (see Figure 8.2).

Hay Fever. Despite its name, this allergy is not directly caused by hay per se but by a mold that grows on hay. Hay fever symptoms start when a sufferer breathes in any of a variety of airborne pollen; tree, grass, or mold spores; or other allergens.

In this kind of reaction, the immune system mistakenly reacts to the allergen in the same way it would to an actual harmful agent, such as a virus or parasite.

Normally, the immune system releases chemicals called *histamines* to destroy these invaders. In the process, they cause the coughing, sneezing, and mucus production that we associate with colds and flu. In a hay fever allergy reaction, histamines are triggered by the allergen and released, even though there is no harmful invader present.

The development of the allergy is a two-step process (see Figure 8.2). An allergic individual's first contact with the allergen results in *sensitization*. The allergen encounters plasma cells, causing them to produce IgE antibodies, which can "recognize" the particular allergen by binding

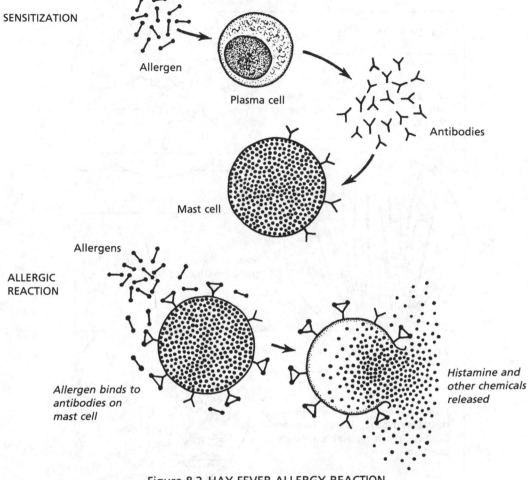

SENSITIZATION

Allergen

Plasma cell

Antibodies

Mast cell

Allergens

ALLERGIC
REACTION

Allergen binds to
antibodies on
mast cell

Histamine and
other chemicals
released

Figure 8.2 HAY FEVER ALLERGY REACTION.

The first time an allergen enters the blood-stream, the immune system is *sensitized*, creating mast cells primed to release invader-fighting chemicals, including *histamines*. These chemicals are released on subsequent contact, causing coughing, sneezing, runny nose, and, possibly, asthma symptoms.

with it chemically. The antibodies then attach to immune system cells called *mast cells*, which, now primed to identify the allergen, remain in the bloodstream for years.

When the allergen enters the system again, it encounters the mast cells and binds to the allergen-specific antibodies attached to them. This binding cues the mast cells to release histamines, triggering coughing, sneezing, teary eyes, and runny nose. By constricting respiratory passages, histamines can also produce the symptoms of asthma.

Each region of the country has its unique assortment of allergens that are released at different times of the year.

Anaphylaxis. This is the most severe, often life-threatening allergic reaction. It results from

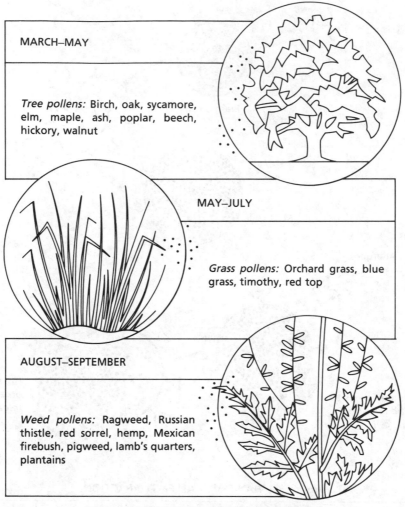

MARCH–MAY

Tree pollens: Birch, oak, sycamore, elm, maple, ash, poplar, beech, hickory, walnut

MAY–JULY

Grass pollens: Orchard grass, blue grass, timothy, red top

AUGUST–SEPTEMBER

Weed pollens: Ragweed, Russian thistle, red sorrel, hemp, Mexican firebush, pigweed, lamb's quarters, plantains

Figure 8.3 THE SEASONS OF THE SNEEZE.

The seasons for allergy-causing pollens in the northeastern United States. Pollen almanacs that chart hay fever plants by month and region are available.

an immediate reaction to exposure to a usually harmless allergen. Common allergens include drugs (such as local anesthetics or penicillin); an insect venom; or a food, such as shellfish, milk, eggs, fish, or peanuts. Although the initial exposure to the allergen may not have produced a reaction or produced only mild allergic symptoms, the immune system becomes sensitized to the allergen. A later exposure can result in an unusually violent immune response in which a flood of mediators produces devastating symptoms that affect the entire body.

The symptoms of anaphylaxis can include a rapid heartbeat or palpitations, hives, intense itching, headache, nausea and vomiting, diarrhea, a sudden drop in blood pressure, cardiovascular collapse, and severe respiratory distress caused by constriction of the airways. In some cases, breathing can become so impaired that a tube must be put in the trachea to open a pathway and prevent death from asphyxiation. Persons who are known to be vulnerable to this violent reaction—for example, people with insect allergies—often carry kits that include epinephrine, an injection of which can be life-saving by reversing the reaction. Corticosteroids, antihistamines, and intravenous fluids are also used to treat anaphylaxis.

Technically, allergists distinguish between anaphylaxis, in which the release of mediators is triggered by IgE, and anaphylactoid reactions, caused by such things as sulfites or radiological dyes, in which a non-IgE mechanism directly causes the release of mediators. In practical terms, the effects are the same—a sudden reaction affecting the entire body.

There are several ways to detect persons who are vulnerable to anaphylaxis. Doctors routinely question patients about prior exposure before administering antibiotics or other potentially allergenic drugs. There are several tests that can diagnose the existence of an allergy to insect venom or foods. Especially for drugs and food, these tests are far from perfect and are risky in and of themselves, and so cases of anaphylaxis cannot be predicted with complete accuracy.

Contact Dermatitis. This allergic inflammation of the skin can be caused by exposure to, among other things, poison ivy and its relatives, cosmetics, metals, and drugs (see Chapter 4, "Skin Ailments"). The symptoms, red and itchy skin and blisters that may form and break, are produced during the response to the allergen by immune system cells.

Poison ivy and plants in the Rhus family—poison oak and poison sumac—are the most common triggers of these skin reactions. The sap (resin) of these plants contains a potent allergen called urushiol. Up to 70 percent of Americans will develop contact dermatitis when exposed to large amounts of urushiol for prolonged periods of time. An individual becomes sensitized to urushiol upon first contact with the oily sub-

stance. A second contact causes sensitized white blood cells to release mediators that cause swelling; itching; a red, warm papular rash; blistering; and other painful, annoying symptoms, which reach their peak in five days and then gradually disappear. Symptoms can be reduced or prevented by washing the skin thoroughly soon after exposure.

The sap of other plants, such as the pencil cactus, creeping spurge, and ginkgo, can cause contact dermatitis. The best defense is to avoid the offending plants and to wash the skin and clothes vigorously when contact is made. An allergic reaction can be prevented if the sap is washed off within a few minutes of exposure.

Cosmetics ingredients can cause contact dermatitis in certain people; they are found in hair dyes, sunscreens, perfumes, and lipsticks. They include coloring agents in lipsticks, plastics in nail polish, and ethylenediamine and *para*-phenylenediamine (chemicals used as preservatives in hair dyes and many cosmetics) (see pp. 65 and 655).

Among drugs, the antibiotics neomycin and penicillin and antihistamines such as diphenhydramine (Benadryl) in salves can cause contact allergies. Some drugs, including the tetracycline antibiotics, can cause photosensitivity, which results in a rash after exposure to sunlight. The metals that most often cause contact dermatitis are nickel and chromates (chromium compounds) (see p. 64).

Food Allergy. Although there is no controversy that certain foods can cause allergic reactions in certain people, up to and including anaphylaxis, some practitioners maintain that food "allergies" can cause a wide range of physical and psychological disorders that range far beyond the usual symptoms of allergy. These claims are met with extreme skepticism by the majority of physicians (see Multiple-Chemical Sensitivities, p. 170).

Food-induced allergy is sometimes missed as a diagnosis because its symptoms are mimicked by other conditions that cause gastrointestinal upset, nausea, diarrhea, and bloating. For example, gluten, a protein in wheat, corn, and barley, causes a gastrointestinal disorder called celiac disease, which can result in some individuals having symptoms such as diarrhea and failure to grow. Celiac disease is not generally regarded as a true allergy (although it is felt to have autoimmune characteristics), but its symptoms persist unless gluten is excluded from the diet. Lactose intolerance, a condition that occurs in individuals who lack the enzyme needed to digest lactose, the chief sugar in milk, is characterized by bloating, diarrhea, and other symptoms that resemble those of an allergy but is not an allergy itself.

Among other foods whose side effects mimic those of allergy are beans and onions, which can cause digestive symptoms, and tomatoes, avocados and cheeses, which contain natural chemicals that can cause allergylike symptoms.

Nevertheless, allergic reactions to foods do occur. Most of the time, symptoms occur in the digestive tract, usually in the form of nausea and vomiting, but a food allergy can also cause skin reactions—rashes (hives), itching, and swelling—and even anaphylaxis. Among the more common foods that cause allergic reactions are milk and wheat products, chocolate, nuts, citrus fruits, eggs, beans and other legumes, herbs, spices, and shellfish.

To further complicate the issue, allergic reactions can be caused not only by foods themselves but also by colorants, preservatives, residues of antibiotics, insecticides, and molds that they contain. Some food additives have been linked to allergic reactions. One such group is the sulfites, antioxidants that are used to keep fruit, vegetables, and fish looking fresh and are found in some wines, dried fruits (i.e., raisins and apricots), processed foods, and baked goods. Sulfites have been linked to deaths from anaphylaxis, and some people with asthma suffer severe attacks when exposed to sulfites. The use of sulfites to retain the fresh appearance of restaurant salad bars or produce in supermarkets has been reduced by the food industry, and the Food and Drug Administration (FDA) requires wine labels to note the presence of sulfites.

The incidence of food allergy appears highest in children; estimates of its prevalence range from 1 to 7 percent. Adults, however, can develop allergies to foods that they have previously eaten for years without reactions.

DIAGNOSING FOOD ALLERGIES: The most reliable way to diagnose a food allergy is by a double-blind challenge. A person is given the suspected food and another substance, usually in capsules, without the subject or the person administering it knowing which is which and is then observed for symptoms. (Because there is the potential for severe reactions, this should be done under medical supervision.)

Another diagnostic method is to eliminate the suspect food or foods from the diet and to see if the symptoms stop and then to reintroduce them in the diet and observe if symptoms resume.

Skin testing for food allergy may not be clinically relevant. Someone who is allergic may have a positive reaction to a food antigen yet not manifest symptoms when the food is ingested. Depending on many variables, including the quantity of the food allergen, a positive skin test has very little predictive value for symptomatic food allergy. A negative skin test is more reassuring in excluding immediate food sensitivity.

Once the diagnosis is certain, so is the remedy: Keep the food out of the patient's diet permanently. The only effective treatment for a food allergy is avoidance.

Immune Deficiency Diseases

Immune deficiency conditions can be caused by underactivity of specific components of the immune system. One example is Wiscott–Aldrich syndrome, an inherited condition that causes a deficiency in antibody production. Until the sudden appearance of acquired immunodeficiency syndrome (AIDS) in the early 1980s, immune deficiency conditions were relatively rare diseases, the majority of which were caused as a by-product of chemotherapy drugs used to treat cancer. Similarly, drugs used to prevent rejection of transplanted organs intentionally suppress the immune system, and unless the body's ability to fight infection is preserved, immune deficiency disorders can arise.

Viral infections and other diseases, including tuberculosis, leprosy, and coccidioidomycosis, can cause immune deficiency, as can malnutrition, radiation, and old age.

Immune deficiency also weakens the body's defenses against certain malignancies. For example, an increased incidence of leukemia and lymphomas (cancers of the blood cells or lymphoid organs) is seen in people who have transplants and undergo treatment to prevent rejection of transplanted tissue, and in persons who survive for prolonged periods with AIDS.

AIDS. The immune deficiency disorders that are seen in people with AIDS occur due to the direct infection with human immunodeficiency virus, or HIV. This one virus is responsible for most, if not all, of the immune system defects seen in AIDS.

HIV does so much damage because it attacks a white blood cell that is at the center of the immune system's activity, a lymphocyte variously called the helper T cell or the CD4 cell. The CD4 cell is important in regulating the response of other cells of the immune system. When CD4 cells die, the immune system loses its ability to respond to microbial invaders.

The result is "opportunistic" infections, so called because the microbes take advantage of the crippled immune system. Many opportunistic infections are caused by microbes that often routinely reside harmlessly in the bodies of people with normally functioning immune systems, such as pneumonia caused by the microbe *Pneumocystis carinii*. Some cancers also flourish under these conditions, most commonly Kaposi's sarcoma and leukemia (see p. 154).

AIDS also opens the way for other infectious agents that do not affect persons with intact immune systems. For example, the rapid increase in tuberculosis infections that began in the late 1980s is attributed in large part to the weakened resistance of HIV-positive individuals.

HIV is not spread by casual contact, a fact established by long-term studies of family members who lived in the same house, used the same dishes, and frequently came in contact with HIV-infected individuals. The risk of family members contracting HIV infection from household exposure is minute to nonexistent. HIV spreads from person to person by direct transfer of body fluids, such as blood and semen. (Tiny amounts of HIV have sometimes been detected in saliva, but saliva has not been shown to be a means of transmitting infection.)

The two major means of HIV infection are sexual intercourse and reuse of hypodermic needles contaminated with the virus. HIV can also be transmitted by the transfusion of infected blood or blood products, such as the clotting factor given to persons with hemophilia to prevent bleeding. A number of cases of HIV infection were caused by contaminated transfusions in the 1980s. In the United States, testing of donated blood as well as intensive interviewing of blood donors and exclusion of blood from donors in certain risk groups has now reduced the risk of infection to less than 1 in every 250,000 transfusions. Some infected blood escapes detection because the test measures the presence of antibodies to HIV, which do not appear for some time after infection occurs. There are tests that can detect HIV itself in blood, but they are too complex and costly for use in mass screening.

Autoimmune Diseases

In autoimmune diseases, the immune system somehow regards the body's own tissue as foreign and attacks it. The list of autoimmune diseases that are possibly linked to environmental factors includes rheumatoid arthritis, multiple sclerosis, and myasthenia gravis.

Many autoimmune conditions are known to involve an interplay of genetic and environmental factors in which exposure to an environmental agent, such as a virus, triggers a condition in genetically susceptible individuals. Such conditions include the rare, fatal disease subacute sclerosing panencephalitis (SSPE), which results from a delayed autoimmune response to the measles virus (in perhaps one person in a million, the immune system responds to this infection months or years later by attacking and killing brain cells). Similarly, progressive multifocal leukoencephalopathy, a disease in which the protective coating of myelin is stripped away from nerves in the central nervous system, causing death in months, is related to an infection by the JC papovavirus. Studies show that about 85 percent of American adults have been infected by this virus at one time or another. As in the case of SSPE, it is not known why the virus causes a fatal autoimmune disease in a few individuals.

Other environmental factors may ultimately be implicated in autoimmune ailments. For example, a current and controversial issue is the relationship between autoimmune disorders and silicone, which is used in breast implants and in some cosmetic surgery procedures to reduce wrinkles. About 2 million American women have had breast implants, and several thousand have reported a number of medical problems including rashes, swollen joints, hair loss, and severe fatigue, which scientists attribute to an autoimmune response to the silicone. Scientifically, the issue is not resolved. In early 1992, the FDA called for a moratorium on silicone implants until it could more fully evaluate evidence on their safety.

The general assumption is that an interplay of genetic, environmental, and hormonal factors is involved in a number of autoimmune disorders. Some clues are offered by Graves' disease, the thyroid condition that achieved notoriety when it struck both former President George Bush and his wife, Barbara. Graves' disease is presumed to be an autoimmune condition that causes overactivity of the thyroid gland. A number of European studies related high iodine intake to the incidence of Graves' disease. A link to hormone levels comes from studies of pregnancy. Graves' disease and similar thyroid conditions improve during pregnancy and worsen after delivery, apparently because of the dramatic hormonal swings that accompany childbirth. The exact interplay of these factors that triggers the condition remains unclear.

Other diseases in which the same sort of autoimmune response is believed to occur include rheumatoid arthritis, in which the target is the tissues of the joints; systemic lupus erythematosus, which is a general autoimmune attack on many of the body's tissues; scleroderma, in which the target is the skin and connective tissue; and multiple sclerosis, in which progressive destruction of the protective coating surrounding nerves causes progressive neurological deterioration. Insulin-deficient diabetes, in which the body fails to produce insulin, may also be an autoimmune disease.

Rheumatoid arthritis affects perhaps 5 million Americans. The autoimmune attack is against the joints and surrounding soft tissues. Rheumatoid arthritis can occur at any age; one form, Still's disease, strikes children under the age of four. The destruction of joint tissue is unpredictable, sometimes occurring quickly and sometimes stopping completely for a period of time. The unpredictable pace of the disease makes it difficult to assess proposed treatments.

The autoimmune attack in multiple sclerosis is against myelin, the protective coating of nerve cells. As cells lose their protection, the patient experiences symptoms ranging from numbness to paralysis. Multiple sclerosis is more common in northern latitudes, where its incidence is about 1 in 1,000 individuals. It is more common in women (the ratio of female to male patients is 3 to 2) and usually starts in the early adult years. Its progression is unpredictable. In some cases, remissions last for years; in others, the disease progresses swiftly.

Lupus erythematosus attacks the body's connective tissue. A more common form, discoid lupus erythematosus, affects the skin. A second form, systemic lupus erythematosus (SLE), affects many organs of the body and can be fatal. Hormonal factors, genetics, and infections are believed to play a role, since 90 percent of the cases occur in women. People who have SLE have an unusual butterfly-shaped rash on the face, and suffer general malaise, joint pain, weight loss, loss of appetite, arthritis, and many other conditions. SLE can cause kidney failure, pleurisy (inflammation of the tissue that lines the lungs), and pericarditis, inflammation of the tissue around the heart.

All these diseases are puzzles waiting to be solved. Most researchers believe these diseases are caused by agents in the environment, most likely infectious organisms, and occur in persons whose genetic makeup somehow produces an inappropriate immune response. The nature of the genetic vulnerability is not known, nor is the relationship between genetics and environmental factors. In some cases, there has been limited success against one or another of these diseases using treatments that act on the immune system. For example, treatment with cyclosporine, a drug used to prevent organ transplant rejection, has delayed the onset of diabetes in some children in clinical studies. Cyclosporine has reversed a rapid decline in insulin production in these children, presumably by aborting the autoimmune attack on the insulin-producing cells of the pancreas.

CHEMICALS THAT CAUSE IMMUNE SYSTEM ALTERATIONS

Numerous substances, many of them industrial chemicals, can cause allergic reactions, immunological abnormalities, or toxic effects of one kind or another.

For example, between 2 and 15 percent of allergic problems in the United States are due to exposures in the workplace, and on-the-job exposures to some agents also can cause asthma (see Chapter 6, "Respiratory Ailments"). However, it's not necessary to work in a factory to encounter a problem. Persons living near a plant may be exposed as well, and develop an adverse effect. Consumers can be exposed to products containing industrial chemicals, and all of us come in contact with air pollutants, some of which have been implicated in immunological abnormalities.

Chemicals of Concern. Some chemicals implicated in adverse and allergic reactions and other immunological abnormalities are the following:

• *Formaldehyde*, found in insulation, disinfectants, deodorants, paper, dyes, textiles, inks, and many other products, causes contact dermatitis (see Chapter 4, "Skin Ailments").

• *Benzene*, found in various products such as gasoline, paint and paint removers, pesticides, and plastics, is known to increase the risk of cancer in occupationally exposed workers. Benzene has been found in animal studies to inhibit antibody production and reduce the number and activity of white blood cells.

• *Toluene diisocyanate*, used in production of plastics and resins, causes both contact dermatitis and asthma arising from sensitized lung tissue and, in some cases, can cause chronic lung scarring.

• *Polyhalogenated biphenyls* is a chemical family whose members include polychlorinated biphenyls (PCBs), polybrominated biphenyls (PBBs), and dioxin. PCBs were widely used for decades in a number of industrial applications, including as insulating fluids in electric system transformers. Their use has been halted, but large amounts remain in old equipment. Animals exposed to large concentrations of PCBs have lowered antibody production. In some tests, cellular immunity also has been found to be reduced, but to a lesser extent. Studies of some humans who have ingested PCB-contaminated foods have shown immune alterations. For example, in 1979, residents of Taiwan who consumed rice oil contaminated with PCBs were found to have reduced levels of IgA and IgM (but not IgG) and a reduction in numbers of T cells (but not B cells). The clinical significance of these findings has not yet been established. However, some exposed individuals developed a toxic syndrome called Yusho disease, whose symptoms include increased susceptibility to respiratory infections.

PBBs are used as flame retardants. There is scant human evidence on the effects of PBBs; however, there have been reports of immune system effects. (In 1973, cattle in Michigan ingested large amounts of PBBs when they ate contaminated feed, and widespread pollution of meat and dairy products resulted. Tests on persons in the area found lowered counts of white blood cells and widespread white-cell abnormalities.)

Dioxin, the most intensively studied of these compounds, appears to affect humoral and cellular immunity. Dioxin occurred as a trace element in such herbicides as Agent Orange, which was used to destroy vegetation during the Vietnam War. Agent Orange has been accused of causing several forms of cancer and birth defects, but studies of the military personnel exposed to it have been logistically impossible to perform (see p. 144). The information on Agent Orange that was available and reviewed was found to be inconclusive. In animal studies, exposure to dioxin reduced cell-mediated immune response and other immune system functions; however, there are significant differences between humans and laboratory animals in the way this chemical is metabolized and stored in the tissue.

Human studies of children living in Seveso, an Italian community contaminated with dioxin after a factory explosion, found a high incidence of a form of chloracne, a skin disease, but no changes in most major immunological functions. Studies of British chemical workers exposed to dioxin on the job, however, found several alterations in immune functions as well as an excess of cancers, but the workers were exposed to other chemicals as well. More research on the mechanisms by which dioxin affects humans is needed to establish the medical importance of immune system changes that may occur due to dioxin exposure.

• *Urethane*, another industrial chemical, suppresses killer cell activity sharply in animals, an action that probably helps make it a potent cancer inducer. No such activity is reported for polyurethane, a widely used polymer made of urethane.

• Animal studies on immune system effects have been done on three classes of *pesticides:* organochlorine compounds, such as DDT; carbamates, such as carbaryl (Sevin); and organophosphates, such as malathion and parathion.

There is convincing evidence that high doses of organophosphates can suppress the immune response, although the immune effects are hard to separate from the other overwhelming toxic effects of these chemicals. Carbaryl and other carbamates have been tested in the United States and Europe, with mixed results; they are not believed to have serious immune system effects (see p. 607). DDT and other organochlorine pesticides consistently depress immune responses in animal tests, but the clinical significance of these effects has not been established.

Heavy Metals. Metals can affect the immune system, altering the immune response to infection and producing other immunological abnormalities. Among the metals known to cause these effects are beryllium, cadmium, lead, manganese, and mercury, although the mechanism by which these metals affect the immune system is unknown. Although some animal studies suggest that routine exposure to heavy metals may result in being more vulnerable to infectious diseases of the lung, the results in animal tests have not been consistent.

Beryllium is an industrial metal used in alloys and a number of processes and is also released when coal is burned. It has been linked to a number of immune disorders in workers exposed to it on the job, including contact dermatitis, lung inflammation, and the lung condition chronic pulmonary granulomatosis (or berylliosis).

Mercury, lead, and cadmium have reduced antibody production in some animal studies and have inhibited cell-mediated responses in others. Mice that were fed mercury-containing food had an increased death rate when infected with a disease-causing virus.

Cadmium and manganese also have been shown to alter the immune response of laboratory animals exposed to the metals by inhalation. (In animal studies, airborne cadmium reduced the number of functioning macrophages in the lung fluid, making the animals more susceptible to bacterial infections, although we have no human studies on this effect). Manganese depressed macrophage function in the same kind of studies, as did airborne nickel. Lead inhibited the development of antibody-producing cells and lowered antibody levels in animal studies. Children with high blood concentrations of lead who were immunized with tetanus toxin were found to have lower than normal levels of antibodies to the toxin, while workers exposed to lead on the job had lowered levels of IgA antibodies.

The nickel in costume jewelry and garment fasteners often causes allergic skin reactions. Gold and silver also have been reported to cause contact dermatitis in some people (see Chapter 4, "Skin Ailments").

Air Pollutants. A multitude of air pollutants, both gases and particles, can affect immune function.

The principal pollutants in the air of a city such as Los Angeles are oxidants, compounds produced by the action of sunlight on hydrocarbons and nitrogen oxides that are emitted primarily by automobiles (see Box 14.2, p. 547). The major oxidant is *ozone*, a three-atom species of oxygen that is highly reactive with almost anything it touches. Ozone is known to worsen respiratory conditions such as asthma and bron-

chitis. Studies have shown that exposure to ozone has adverse effects on the immune system much like any irritant, including the release by macrophages of enzymes that damage lung cells and depressed production of immune system cells (see p. 553).

Nitrogen oxides seem to damage the immune system. Several studies of nitrogen dioxide have seen the same immune system effects produced by ozone, namely a depression of both the number of macrophages and their activity, and depression of the antibody response to pulmonary infection caused by both bacteria and viruses.

Sulfur dioxide, a pollutant released by industrial processes and power plants that burn coal and oil, appears to be less damaging to the immune response, mostly because it does not get deep into the airways. Most sulfur dioxide is absorbed in the nose and upper throat. Very high concentrations of sulfur dioxide depress macrophage function, but the animals in these tests had little increased vulnerability to infection. The same is true of sulfuric acid, which is formed when sulfur dioxide reacts with water in the air.

Polycyclic aromatic hydrocarbons are the product of incomplete combustion of many products, including wood, paper, coal, and petroleum products, and so are common air pollutants. Animal tests have found a variety of depressed immune responses on exposure to various polycyclic aromatic hydrocarbons.

Factories and powerplants can also emit complex particles containing many chemical elements. One major element is carbon, a basic ingredient in coal and oil, which is emitted in a number of forms, including fly ash. There have been animal studies of fly ash and carbon, sometimes in combination with sulfur dioxide or sulfuric acid. In laboratory studies, a variety of effects were seen, but most of them seemed to have little clinical effect. One of the more fascinating studies was done after the 1980 eruption of Mount Saint Helens in Washington, which exposed animals to very high levels of airborne volcanic ash. That exposure did not have a significant effect on the immune defenses of the respiratory tract of the animals that were studied.

The difficulty of determining exactly what happens in humans who breathe polluted air was demonstrated by animal tests of the combined effects of ozone and sulfuric acid. Animals that were exposed first to ozone and then to sulfuric acid were more likely to be infected by streptococci. Animals in which the sequence was reversed had no such response. At this stage of research, what can be said is that air pollutants certainly harm the respiratory system and probably harm the respiratory immune system, although not much is known about the nature of the immunological damage.

Workplace air pollutants are a different story, because they often are found in very high concentrations. For example, asbestos has been an occupational hazard in a number of industries (including construction and shipbuilding) as is the case with silica. Animal studies show that airborne asbestos and silica dust cause irreversible lung fibrosis. (Contact with airborne asbestos, especially by people who also smoke, also causes cancer.) In animal studies, asbestos also seems to lower immune defenses both by damaging macrophages and by affecting T-cell function. Silica dust, common in sandblasting and mining, is associated with an increased incidence of autoimmune disease (see Chapter 6, "Respiratory Ailments," for further information on asbestos and airborne dusts).

Multiple-Chemical Sensitivities

Multiple-chemical sensitivities is a description used to characterize a syndrome in which a number of medical symptoms involving many organ systems are reported and attributed by clinical ecologists to exposure to many different chemical compounds at doses far lower than those known to cause harmful effects. The very existence of this syndrome is a subject of controversy, as are some of the techniques used to treat the condition of people thought to have the syndrome.

Clinical ecology is based on the belief that people can develop severe, incapacitating, yet poorly documentable illnesses from exposure both to foods and to even small amounts of synthetic chemicals in the environment. These reported symptoms are hypothesized as being mediated by a variety of physiological mechanisms, one of which results from the weakening of the immune system by exposure to pollutants and industrial and household chemicals. However, this hypothesis is as yet unproven.

Clinical ecologists diagnose multiple-chemical sensitivity by examining the patient's daily routine and medical history, concentrating on the relationship between ingestion of food and exposure to airborne substances and the occurrence of symptoms. They also employ provocation testing, in which the patient is exposed to substances suspected of causing symptoms, either by injection, by oral application, or in environmental control units, whose air is supposedly treated to be free of all fumes and contaminants and which have no furnishings made of synthetic material. Substances are judged on the basis of the appearance of symptoms following provocation testing.

Three typical methods of treatment are used in clinical ecology. One is the use of elimination diets that are free of any food to which a patient has shown a positive response. Another is avoidance of all synthetic chemicals that have been linked to symptoms. In extreme cases, some patients move to rural areas and live in homes built without any synthetic materials. Many patients also are prescribed neutralization therapy, in which small amounts of a variety of food extracts, chemicals, hormones, or drugs are given to reduce symptoms.

Every aspect of multiple-chemical sensitivity—from its existence to its diagnosis and treatment by the methods of clinical ecology—is a subject of controversy. Many physicians regard multiple-chemical sensitivity as a psychiatric rather than a physical condition. Others, who are in a small minority, regard it as a very real syndrome that is often missed by conventional methods of diagnosis.

Some physicians acknowledge that chemical sensitivity may be a real problem for some patients and that it could be a physical condition with a strong psychological component. The controversy is fed by some recent court cases that have begun to accept a diagnosis of environmental illness for some workers' compensation cases (on a case-by-case basis). For example, the Social Security Administration in 1988 rewrote its manual on disability claims to include a section on chemical sensitivity. Although the agency said there is no evidence of immune malfunction in persons diagnosed with the condition, it said that disability claims based on multiple-chemical sensitivities should be judged on a case-by-case basis. Currently, disability is given for impairment due to a demonstrated inability to function in the workplace. The cause of the inability, however, is not clearly defined.

Clearly, more research on this topic is needed. At this writing, however, multiple-chemical sensitivity remains a concept without merit for the vast majority of the scientific community. After prolonged studies of the subject, expert panels appointed by the California Medical Society and the American College of Physicians reached essentially identical conclusions, that clinical ecologists have not identified specific, recognizable diseases caused by exposure to low-level environmental stressors, that it is unlikely that the diagnostic and therapeutic methods of clinical ecology can uncover and relieve disease. The American Academy of Allergy and Immunology says it considers the approach of clinical ecologists "unproven and experimental methodology."

CHAPTER 9

Heart and Circulatory Ailments

We speak of the heart as the seat of our emotions, the center of our feelings, the core of ourselves as spiritual beings. Personalities are described as full-hearted or hard-hearted; decisions can be heartfelt; situations can be heartbreaking; and when we sit down to talk to one another seriously, we try to get to the heart of the matter.

Just as our hearts lie at the center of our individual sense of ourselves, our personal choices about many external and environmental factors are crucial to the health of the heart and for the circulatory system that supports it. Decisions about life-style—about what we eat and drink, whether or not we smoke, if and how often we choose to exercise, how angry or relaxed an attitude we attempt to cultivate—all have bearing upon the well-being of our hearts and whether we are prone to cardiovascular disease.

Many of us seem to acknowledge this and have made significant changes: Since the late 1970s, there has been an astonishing decline in death rates from heart attack, stroke, and other cardiovascular diseases. Fatalities due to heart attacks are down almost 30 percent, deaths attributed to strokes are down over 33 percent, those due to hypertension are down over 20 percent, and those due to rheumatic heart disease are down over 40 percent.

Some of the credit for this good news goes to advances in medical treatment and prevention of such diseases as rheumatic fever. However, much of it squarely rests on *personal* environmental factors, such as adopting healthier diets, regular exercise programs, better control of high blood pressure, and giving up cigarette smoking.

Unfortunately, cardiovascular disease remains the number one killing disease in the United States. In 1988, the deaths of nearly 1 million Americans were attributed to heart and blood vessel diseases, almost as many deaths as cancer, accidents, pneumonia, influenza, and all other causes combined. More than one in four Americans suffer some form of cardiovascular disease, and almost one in two Americans die of it—one person every thirty-two seconds.

Environmental factors may be responsible for some of the bad news: The American diet is still too high in cholesterol and fat, too many people are still overweight, not enough people exercise, and cigarettes are still a problem. Other environmental factors, such as exposures to certain chemicals in the workplace, may also play a role in triggering any latent risks for cardiovascular disease.

For although heredity—the genes you are born with—determines the underlying level of risk of developing cardiovascular disease, environmental factors may determine how soon and how intensely these risks are expressed.

Box 9.1 A LESS THAN PERFECT POPULATION

Change does not come easily, even in the face of overwhelming evidence that certain behaviors are detrimental to health.

- One-fifth of the population exceeds acceptable weight levels.
- About one-quarter of the adult population (46 million people) still are addicted to cigarettes.
- Over one-quarter of the adult population (48 million people) have blood cholesterol levels of 240 milligrams per deciliter and above.
- Over half of the adult population (101 million people) have blood cholesterol levels of 200 milligrams per deciliter and over.
- Of those people with high blood pressure, it's estimated that almost one-half don't know that they have it.
- Of all people with high blood pressure, approximately two-thirds are not on any therapy (special diet or medication). Almost one-quarter are on inadequate therapy, one-tenth on adequate therapy.
- One-half of all heart attack victims wait more than two hours before calling for help.

ATHEROSCLEROSIS: A MAJOR FORM OF CARDIOVASCULAR DISEASE

Cardiovascular disease—often referred to as heart disease—is actually many different kinds of diseases, disturbances, and defects that affect the heart's individual parts, as well as its ability to function (see Box 9.2).

When most people speak of cardiovascular disease, they frequently are referring to hardening of the arteries, medically known as arteriosclerosis. This process—in which the inner walls of arteries leading to the heart become thickened and somewhat stiffened—is, to a certain extent, considered a normal part of aging.

One type of arteriosclerosis—atherosclerosis—is not normal. It is the slow, stealthy progressive disease that most scientists believe originates in childhood, ultimately resulting in angina pectoris, heart attack, stroke, or sudden death (see Box 9.2).

In order to understand the atherosclerotic process, it is important to know how the heart functions in a normal state.

The heart is a pump of extraordinary efficiency. Every minute, it circulates 22 pints (5 liters) of blood through 75,000 miles (120,000 meters) of blood vessels. Although only as big as a closed fist, it can force blood from the heart to the big toe and back again in under 30 seconds. The heart is a muscle, not very thick, and shaped only vaguely like the heart symbol used to represent our strongest emotion. Like any muscle, it is capable of contracting and then relaxing, when it lengthens to its full size. The heart, in fact, is the most active, hardest working muscle in the body.

The heart is hollow and divided into four chambers: the *atria* (upper sections) and the *ventricles* (lower sections). Blood is pumped through them, aided by four valves that open and close to let blood flow whenever the heart contracts (see Figure 9.1).

When blood is dispersed, it delivers life-giving oxygen to every part of the body. Blood then

---

Box 9.2 MAJOR TYPES OF HEART DISEASE

Some 130 abnormal conditions of the heart and blood vessels are listed by the New York branch of the American Heart Association in its classic reference book, *Nomenclature and Criteria for Diagnosis of Diseases of the Heart and Blood Vessels*. In addition to heart attack, hypertension, and stroke, here are the seven others that affect the majority of the population:

1. *Angina pectoris*, or chest pain, results from a lack of oxygen to the heart muscle when blood flow is insufficient during times of physical or emotional stress.
2. *Arrhythmias*, also called dysrhythmias, are abnormal rhythms or rates of heartbeat. They are usually caused by a disturbance in the electrical impulses to the heart.
3. *Congestive heart failure* is an inability of the heart to maintain its normal workload of pumping blood to the lungs and the rest of the body; the heart continues to work, but not as efficiently.
4. *Heart valve disease* occurs when one or more of the four valves of the heart becomes defective, thus disrupting normal blood flow.
5. *Heart muscle disease*, or cardiomyopathy, has many causes and is associated with abnormal and unusually decreased function of the heart. It may affect young people more than coronary artery disease.
6. *Rheumatic heart disease* is a condition in which one or more of the heart valves is damaged by a disease process that begins with a strep throat (streptococcal infection).
7. *Congenital defects of the heart* are malformations that can either obstruct or cause abnormal blood flow through the heart or its major vessels. They often are present at birth but often not recognized until adolescence or adulthood.

---

comes back "blue" (from its relative lack of oxygen) into the right side of the heart, where it is quickly pumped into the lungs to pick up fresh oxygen. Next, blood flows into the left side of the heart. Now bright red because it is loaded with oxygen, it is pushed into the *aorta*, the main artery leading to other tissues of the body.

The two sides of the heart beat in synchrony. The ventricles create the pulse you can feel in your wrist, pumping when they contract, then relaxing and refilling—100,000 times a day.

A built-in pacemaker—a specialized nerve tissue—automatically adjusts the pulse rate, depending on how much blood and oxygen you need: faster for exercise, tension, fear, pain, or sexual activity; slower for sleeping, resting, meditating, or reading.

Atherosclerosis (from the Greek word *athero*, meaning gruel or paste, and *sclerosis*, meaning hardness) is characterized by deposits of mostly fatty substances like cholesterol, cellular waste products, calcium, and fibrin (a clotting material in the blood) in the inner lining of an artery. The resulting buildup is called *plaque*. (See Figure 9.1 for an illustration of the inside of an artery seriously narrowed by plaque buildup.)

Although the process is insidious, sooner or later it can create enough blockage in the coronary arteries so that the heart muscle lacks the proper amount of oxygen, creating a condition known as cardiac ischemia. Sometimes, the first and only signal is heart attack or sudden death, but usually there are earlier signs, notably the pressurelike sensation of angina pectoris. Usually described as an uncomfortable sensation of squeezing, constriction, tightness, or heaviness in the center of the chest, rather than a pain, it is brought on by exertion and relieved by rest or nitroglycerin. This sensation feels very much like indigestion, and many heart patients, unaware of their disease and experiencing angina for the first time, easily overlook the symptom.

Box 9.3   WHEN YOUR HEART "ATTACKS" YOU

A heart attack, or myocardial infarction, is the end result of a drastically reduced supply of oxygen-rich blood to the heart muscle (myocardium), usually caused by a blood clot lodged in an artery (coronary thrombosis or occlusion). This reduced blood supply to the heart causes the affected heart muscle cells to suffer irreversible injury and die unless the blockage is opened rapidly.

When a portion of the myocardium is infarcted, it dies and no longer contributes to the pumping function of the heart. A mild heart attack might kill about only 10 to 20 percent of the muscle; a major heart attack, 40 percent or more.

The sudden constriction, or spasm, of an artery may also deprive the heart of its needed blood supply, causing chest pain or heart attack. Why spasms occur is not entirely clear; blockage by atherosclerosis might be one trigger. Spasms occur both at rest and during exertion; if the spasm is severe and sustained, a heart attack or sudden death may result, although this is a much less common cause of heart attack than a blood clot.

THE ROLE OF RISK FACTORS

Unlike infectious diseases that can be traced to a specific organism and then treated, there is no simple strategy for coronary artery disease. In part, it can be understood in terms of *risk factors*, personal behaviors and characteristics that predispose people to heart attacks.

Extensive clinical and statistical studies have confirmed these risk factors, which the American Heart Association groups into three classifications:

1. *Major unmodifiable risk factors*: Age, gender, and heredity.
2. *Major modifiable risk factors*: Elevated blood cholesterol, hypertension, and cigarette smoking.
3. *Contributing risk factors*: Diabetes, obesity, physical inactivity, and stress.

The way these risk factors interrelate is a good example of the whole being greater than the sum of its parts. People who smoke at least a pack a day are twice as likely to have a heart attack than nonsmokers. In addition, the Framingham study, one of the largest and longest-running studies of risk factors in carefully followed population groups, found that the increased risk doubles again for a smoker with high cholesterol. A smoker with high cholesterol levels and high blood pressure has an eight- to tenfold increased risk of heart attack.

In addition, people with high blood pressure are four times as likely to have a stroke than people with normal blood pressure. In people who have diabetes and high blood pressure, the risk of stroke increases about six times.

THE HEART AND CIRCULATORY SYSTEM

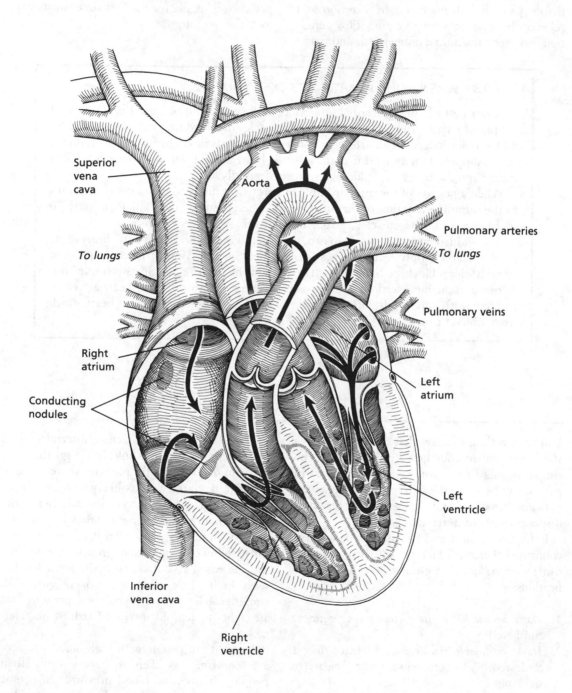

Superior vena cava

Aorta

Pulmonary arteries

To lungs

To lungs

Pulmonary veins

Right atrium

Conducting nodules

Left atrium

Left ventricle

Inferior vena cava

Right ventricle

(a)

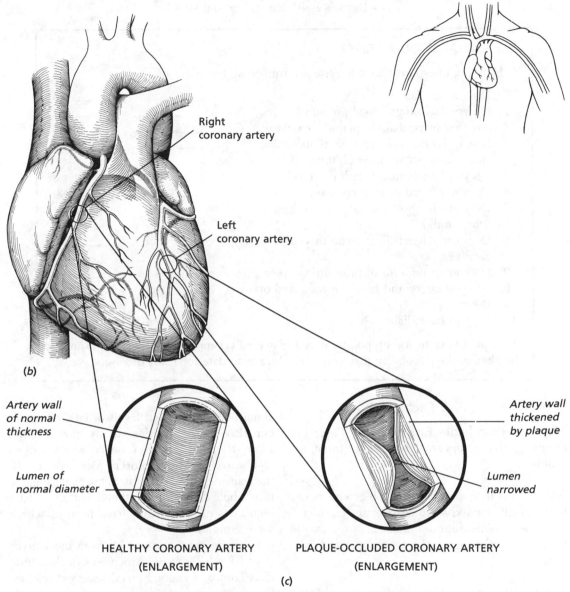

Right coronary artery

Left coronary artery

(b)

Artery wall of normal thickness

Lumen of normal diameter

Artery wall thickened by plaque

Lumen narrowed

HEALTHY CORONARY ARTERY
(ENLARGEMENT)

PLAQUE-OCCLUDED CORONARY ARTERY
(ENLARGEMENT)

(c)

Figure 9.1 THE HEART AND CIRCULATORY SYSTEM.

(*a*) A cutaway view of the heart showing all four chambers, all four valves, and the conduction system. Because of the perspective, the left and right chambers are reversed.

(*b*) The three coronary arteries curl around the heart and branch into the heart's muscle (myocardium), bringing in a supply of blood. They are especially prone to damage and atherosclerosis. The right and left coronary arteries are visible (reversed because of perspective); not visible is the circumflex artery on the opposite side of the heart.

(*c*) In a healthy coronary artery (*left*), the channel, or lumen, through which blood flows is of normal thickness and diameter. The plaque-occluded artery (*right*) has a wall thickened by plaque, blocking the flow of blood. This condition can cause ischemia and/or heart attack.

Box 9.4   ARE YOU AT RISK?

Here are questions that will raise a warning flag for you.

1. Do you smoke? _____ YES _____ NO
2. Do you have high blood pressure? _____ YES _____ NO
3. Are you more than 20 pounds overweight? _____ YES _____ NO
4. Is your blood cholesterol level above 200 milligrams per deciliter (200 mg/dL)? _____ YES _____ NO
5. Do you love (and eat) rich desserts? _____ YES _____ NO
6. Do you eat red meat every day? _____ YES _____ NO
7. Do you eat eggs, use butter, and drink whole milk? _____ YES _____ NO
8. Does early heart disease run in your family? _____ YES _____ NO
9. Do you spend a lot of time sitting down? _____ YES _____ NO
10. Are you angry and hostile a good deal of the time? _____ YES _____ NO
11. Do you have diabetes? _____ YES _____ NO

You don't have to add up points. If you answered yes more than twice, you should be alert to the possibility that you might be a candidate for heart disease.

A Look at the Risk Factors

Major Unmodifiable Risk Factors. Three of the major risk factors are "given" and cannot be changed.

AGE. More than half of all people who have heart attacks are sixty-five years of age or older. Of those who die, four out of five are over sixty-five. For women, age is the most important risk factor.

GENDER. Before age fifty, men are more likely to have heart attacks than women. After menopause, women's and men's death rates from heart attacks are quite comparable.

HEREDITY. A tendency toward heart disease or atherosclerosis appears to be hereditary; children of parents with cardiovascular disease are more apt to develop it themselves (see Box 9.6).

One important inherited genetic trait that has been well-defined is that which produces abnormally high blood levels of fats, which accumulate in the arteries. In its most extreme form, this can cause coronary artery disease and heart attacks in children. More commonly, the trait manifests itself by abnormally high serum cholesterol in adulthood, often causing high rates of early death from heart attacks in some families.

Fourteen years of research from the University of Utah shows that members of the immediate family of young heart disease victims have five to ten times the risk than the rest of the population of dying early (before age fifty-five) from coronary heart disease. These statistics suggests a strong hereditary link.

In addition to genetic susceptibility toward coronary heart disease, which simply sets the stage, there is another factor, or most likely a number of risk factors in collaboration, that actually triggers the disease process.

Figure 9.2 depicts a family at high risk. This illustrates the fact that detecting coronary heart

---

Box 9.5 NOT FOR MEN ONLY: EQUAL FATALITIES

Much of the research into the relationship between the various risk factors and heart disease has, until very recently, involved mostly men. With government urging and support, newer research projects involve women and children also.

Women and Heart Disease

- Coronary artery disease is the number one killer of women, accounting for nearly 250,000 deaths each year.
- Cholesterol level is second only to age as the most important risk factor. At least nine different studies have demonstrated that women develop coronary heart disease at higher cholesterol levels than men. Women also are at particular risk of heart disease if they have elevated levels of low-density lipoproteins, which carry cholesterol to the blood vessels (see p. 181).
- Although women tend to develop coronary heart disease later than men, nearly as many women die from it. Heart attacks are more often fatal in women than in men; women are twice as likely as men to die within sixty days of a heart attack.
- Heart and blood vessel diseases in women tend to go undiagnosed until much later in life.
- Women who use oral contraceptives have at least three or four times the heart attack risk of women who don't. However, women who have taken birth control pills have no additional risk of heart disease once they stop taking them.
- The incidence of heart disease for women may rise since teenage girls are smoking more. Female smokers are up to six times more likely to have a heart attack than female nonsmokers.
- Evidence suggests that estrogen replacement therapy (ERT) after menopause may lower a woman's risk for heart attack. This may be because estrogen is associated with increases in blood levels of high-density lipoproteins, or that estrogen protects against heart disease by triggering a mechanism that keeps arteries from constricting. ERT is also protective against stroke. However, women and their doctors must carefully weigh these benefits against other effects of ERT treatment (see Box 10.2, p. 203).

---

disease in one family member almost always signals the need to test, diagnose, and probably treat all members of the family.

Major Modifiable Risk Factors. Having a genetic predisposition for cardiovascular disease does not mean you are fated for a fatal heart attack. Quite the contrary; it is especially important that people from families with a known tendency to develop cardiovascular disease be alert to the modifiable life-style factors and do their best to change potentially dangerous habits. They are the following:

BLOOD CHOLESTEROL LEVELS. The risk of coronary heart disease increases as blood cholesterol levels rise. When other risk factors, such as high blood pressure, are present, the risk increases even more.

Blood cholesterol is not the same as cholesterol in foods, but they are related. Cholesterol is a soft, fatty substance found in all body cells

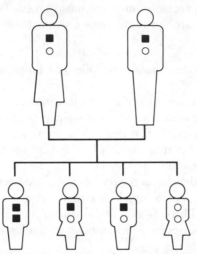

■ Hypercholesterolemia variant gene

○ Normal gene

Figure 9.2 FAMILY TREE (IT'S IN THE GENES).

Each parent in this family has one hypercholesterolemia variant gene. A person who has two such genes has an elevated chance of suffering from high cholesterol. Because each parent contributes one gene to the offspring, this couple has a one in four chance during each pregnancy of producing a child with this condition (bottom left child).

Box 9.6   CHILDREN AND HEART DISEASE

- Children may be born with the gene(s) that predispose them to cardiovascular disease later in life. How much later depends on cultural and environmental factors (see p. 725).
- More than 50 percent of children exceed the recommended intakes of fat and cholesterol.
- Children who overeat foods that are high in saturated fat tend to have higher cholesterol levels, which contribute to arteriosclerosis.
- The American Heart Association recommends that parents should limit fat intake for healthy children ages two and older to 30 percent of their daily calories and that they should eat no more than 300 milligrams of cholesterol per day. The American Academy of Pediatrics puts the recommended percentage of fat between 30 and 40.
- The American Academy of Pediatrics as well as the National Heart Blood and Lung Institute suggests that children whose families have a history of heart disease

(continued)

Box 9.6   CHILDREN AND HEART DISEASE (*continued*)

should have their blood cholesterol levels tested. Many pediatricians, however, recommend screening even when a child is not thought to be at high risk. Screening a child has, on occasion, turned up a potential problem that can be traced back to a parent who was unaware of the presence of a cardiovascular risk.

- Children who eat a lot of salty foods and are overweight are more likely to have high blood pressure.
- Despite the well-documented dangers of smoking, more than 10 percent of third-grade (eight-year-old) children have tried cigarettes. More than half of those who start smoking before the age of thirteen report that their first cigarette was shared with a family member or an older friend. In the third grade, about 2 percent are steady smokers.
- Children experience stress-related physical problems just as adults do, especially resulting from peer pressure, school demands, and family problems.
- Children who exhibit certain personality traits, such as hostile and aggressive behavior and a constant sense of time urgency, are more likely to smoke, use alcohol, and have high cholesterol levels.

---

and necessary for the production of sex hormones, cell membranes, vitamin D, and certain digestive salts. It is made in the liver each day, then released into the bloodstream where it charts a course to the cells.

Cholesterol travels through the bloodstream to get to the various cells; it does not travel alone, however. It is insoluble in blood, so it attaches to substances called *apolipoproteins* in order to be transported through the body. The cholesterol/apolipoprotein package is called a *lipoprotein*. One type of lipoprotein, called low-density lipoprotein, delivers cholesterol to cells where it is used to build cells' membranes. An excess of low-density lipoproteins may cause cholesterol to collect in the arteries. A second type of lipoprotein, called high-density lipoprotein, removes the fatty, potentially artery-clogging substance from the tissues for disposal by the liver.

About 93 percent of the body's cholesterol is inside the cells. The remaining 7 percent circulates in the bloodstream. This would probably not pose a problem were it not for the additional 400 to 500 milligrams or more each day that can come directly from dietary sources. Foods from animals, especially egg yolks, meat, and whole-milk dairy products, contain it; foods from plants don't. A diet high in animal products rich in fat and cholesterol will overload the body with it.

Testing Blood Cholesterol Levels. Certain parameters have been set up for "healthy" and "unhealthy" levels of blood cholesterol. Ideal values of cholesterol (CHOL), high-density lipoproteins (HDLs), and low-density lipoproteins (LDLs) are:

CHOL: Less than 200 milligrams (one-fifth of a gram) per deciliter (one-tenth of a liter) of blood (200 mg/dL).

HDLs: More than 40 milligrams per deciliter of blood (40 mg / dL).

LDLs: Less than 130 milligrams per deciliter of blood (130 mg/dL).

Heart specialists agree that healthy adults should have their blood cholesterol tested (it involves taking a small amount of blood). If the reading is high, steps should be taken to bring it under control and the test should be repeated in six months.

Because LDL is the type of cholesterol that can cause arterial blockage, it can be a good idea to have a cholesterol test that includes a "lipid profile," which is a breakdown of the different HDL and LDL levels. You should order a lipid profile if your total cholesterol is "high" (over 240), or if it is "borderline high" (200–239) and you belong to two or more of the following risk groups: males, cigarette smokers, people with a family history of heart disease, people with high blood pressure, obese people, and diabetics. (*Important:* Although LDL is identified as "bad" cholesterol, *no* cholesterol that you eat is good; HDLs are manufactured in the body.)

How to Modify Blood Cholesterol Levels. Fats in food—especially saturated fats—have a subtle but detrimental effect on blood cholesterol. A diet providing a maximum of 30 percent of all calories as fat—a reduction of about 15 percent from the diet most American adults consume—was recommended by the National Cholesterol Education Program, in February 1990, in a report endorsed by thirty-eight federal agencies, organizations of health professionals, and health organizations. Here is how that breaks down:

- Limit intake of saturated fats to no more than 10 percent of calories. (Saturated fats are solid at room temperature and come mostly from animal sources including meat, poultry, dairy products, chocolate, lard, and the tropical oils coconut and palm.) On the average, people now get 13 percent of their calories from these fats.
- Limit intake of polyunsaturated fats, such as corn, sunflower, and safflower oils; mayonnaise; and fish oils, to another 10 percent of calories consumed.
- Limit intake of monounsaturated fats (contained in avocados, peanuts, almonds, olives, and peanut and cottonseed oils) to no more than 10 percent of calories consumed.
- Limit cholesterol to less than 300 milligrams a day, a decrease of 125 milligrams from what men are now eating (women are nearly on target).

To figure acceptable fat intake, you must learn to translate the numbers into foods and determine how to readjust your eating patterns with new choices (see Chapter 22, "The ABCs of Staying Healthy"). Everyone over age two should follow this type of diet—not only those persons who are considered at highest risk.

Box 9.7 HEART-HEALTHY DIET: HOW TO CHOOSE FOODS LOW IN CHOLESTEROL AND SATURATED FAT

The American Heart Association and the National Cholesterol Education Program Adult Treatment Panel offer these suggestions:

- Eat a variety of foods.
- Choose a diet that allows maintenance of desirable weight.
- Avoid too much fat, saturated fat, and cholesterol.
- Eat foods with adequate starch and fiber.
- Avoid too much sugar.
- Avoid too much sodium.
- If you drink alcoholic beverages, do so in moderation.

Consult Table 9.1 to choose foods low in cholesterol and saturated fat. (See Table 22.1, p. 739, for more low-fat alternatives.)

HYPERTENSION (HIGH BLOOD PRESSURE). Blood pressure is the force created by the heart as it pushes blood into the arteries and arterioles or small arteries. The walls of the arterioles can contract or expand, altering the amount and resistance of blood flow. When the arterioles expand, blood flow increases, while resistance decreases. When the arterioles contract, the opposite effect occurs. If arterioles are constricted, the condition of high blood pressure (hypertension) may develop. Everyone has blood pressure—without it, blood wouldn't circulate in the body. When pressure is excessively high—defined as 140/90 and above—there is cause for concern (see Box 9.8). The higher pressure damages the endothelial layer, or inner lining, of arteries and arterioles, which causes the entire vessel wall to develop atherosclerosis. These vessels become scarred, hardened, and less elastic and cannot supply the amount of blood the body's organs need, which can result in organ malfunctioning.

High blood pressure can damage blood vessels throughout the body. It raises the risk of stroke, because it accelerates clogging of arteries and reduces normal blood flow to the brain. The increased pressure also can put an added strain on an already weakened blood vessel in the brain, causing it to "blow out" like a ruptured automobile inner tube.

It can lead to heart failure, a condition in which the pumping action of the heart simply becomes overwhelmed by the task with which it is faced. Blood cannot be moved as effectively about the body and its fluid component "backs up," leaks out of the blood walls, and begins to accumulate in the ankles and elsewhere. This makes it even more difficult for the heart to function and perpetuates a vicious cycle.

When high blood pressure damages blood vessels in the eye's retina, it can result in some loss of vision. When it affects the kidneys, it may interfere with removal of wastes from the blood and lead to chronic kidney failure.

How or why high blood pressure develops to begin with is still not known. In only 5 to 10 percent of the cases in the U.S. are specific causes found, such as kidney or hormonal diseases. In the vast majority of the cases, there is no detectable cause, and the condition is *essential hypertension*.

A diagnosis of high blood pressure (over 140/90) usually means continued careful monitoring and, possibly, lifelong treatment. For a substantial number of people with borderline or mild hypertension, diet and weight loss may be sufficient. Even if such therapies don't lower blood pressure to a normal range, they are important; people who adopt these life-style changes may need lower doses of antihypertensive drugs (see Box 9.9).

CIGARETTE SMOKING. According to a 1989 report from the surgeon general's office, smoking is responsible for more than one of every six deaths in this country. Smoking remains the single most important preventable cause of death in our society.

Cigarette smoking is the number one risk factor for sudden cardiac death. A smoker has two times the risk of having a heart attack than a nonsmoker. Smokers are more likely to die from their heart attacks and more likely to die suddenly within an hour.

Smoking is the major risk factor in peripheral vascular disease, a condition that results in the narrowing of blood vessels that leads to impaired delivery of blood and nutrients to the legs. Peripheral vascular disease is seen almost exclusively among smokers and people with diabetes.

Nicotine in cigarettes makes the heart beat faster and increases the resistance to blood flow by constricting tiny blood vessels, the arterioles, in the body. This puts an added strain on the heart. A normal heart has extraordinary reserve powers and can probably withstand the effects of smoking for a period of years.

Approximately 4,000 substances have been identified in cigarette smoke, including some toxins that can either affect the development of a fetus (teratogens), cause genetic mutations (mutagens) or cancer (carcinogens), or trigger an im-

Table 9.1 FOODS LOW IN SATURATED FAT AND CHOLESTEROL

Food	Acceptable	Avoid or Use Sparingly
Meat, poultry, fish, dried beans and peas, nuts, eggs	Chicken and turkey (without the skin), veal (except the breast), fish, shellfish[a] (clams, crab, oysters, scallops), lean meats, egg whites	Duck, goose, heavily marbled meats, luncheon meats, bacon, sausage, ham, frankfurters, organ meats, such as heart, kidney, sweetbreads, and liver
	Dry beans and peas, such as kidney beans, lima beans, vegetarian-style baked beans, pinto beans, lentils, chick peas, split peas, and navy beans	Egg yolks (limit to four times per week, including yolks used in cooking)
	Soybean curd (tofu), peanut	
Vegetables and fruits (canned, fresh, or frozen)	All varieties	Avoid if fried, served in cream, butter, or cheese sauces
Breads and cereals	Bread made with a minimum of saturated fat, such as whole wheat, enriched white, French, Italian, oatmeal, rye, pumpernickel, English muffins, pita	Pastries, butter rolls, commercial biscuits, muffins, donuts, cakes, egg breads, cheese breads, commercial mixes containing dried eggs and whole milk; many of these products are made with saturated fat (lard, butter, suet, palm oil, palm kernel, coconut oil, hydrogenated vegetable oil, etc.)
	Pasta, cereal, rice, melba toast, water crackers, matzos, pretzels, popcorn with polyunsaturated oil, water bagels	
Milk products	Ones that are low in saturated fat: skim milk and milk powder, low-fat products, buttermilk (from skim milk), low-fat yogurt, evaporated milk	Whole milk and whole-milk products, including ice cream, cheese made from whole milk or cream, butter; all creams (sour, half and half, whipped)
Fats and oils	Liquid oil shortenings, salad dressings, and mayonnaise made from polyunsaturated oils, vegetable oils (canola, corn, cottonseed, olive, sesame, partially hydrogenated soybean, sunflower, safflower)	Butter, lard, salt pork, meat fat, coconut oil, palm oil, palm kernel, completely hydrogenated margarines and shortenings; use peanut oil occasionally for flavor
Desserts, beverages, snacks, and condiments	Fresh fruit and fruit canned without sugar, cocoa or carob powder, fruit ices, sherbet, gelatin, fruit whip, angel food cakes, cakes made with polyunsaturated oils	Coconut; cream products; fried food snacks (potato chips, corn chips, etc.); chocolate pudding; ice cream; and most commercial cakes, pies, cookies, and mixes
	Vinegar, mustard, herbs, spice	

Note: New, acceptable versions of standard products are appearing on the market. Be sure to read product labels on any items you are interested in purchasing.

[a] Shrimp and lobster are moderately high in cholesterol, although low in fat.

Box 9.8 MEASURING YOUR BLOOD PRESSURE

Over 60 million Americans have high blood pressure. In most instances, they are symptomless and only become aware of the disease through a routine medical checkup. A blood pressure check is a painless process requiring about three and a half minutes.

Blood pressure is a measure of the force that the blood exerts against the walls of the arteries. Each time your heart contracts, or beats—some seventy to ninety times a minute—blood pressure in the arteries goes up, resulting in an "upper," or systolic, blood pressure; each time the heart relaxes between beats, blood pressure goes down, resulting in a "lower," or diastolic, blood pressure.

Blood pressure is recorded with the systolic number placed over the diastolic (120/80, for example, which is read "120 over 80"). Pressures are expressed in terms of millimeters of mercury, that is, the height to which a vertical column of mercury would be lifted by the pressure in the arteries (120 millimeters is approximately 4.8 inches). Both numbers provide important information.

Blood pressure figures are not absolute. Your reading may vary at different times of the day. Pressure may rise after eating a heavy meal and fall significantly several hours later, especially in the elderly. It may also rise during times of excitement or nervousness. One such time, in fact, is during your medical examination; an unexplained rise in blood pressure may be a case of "white coat hypertension."

Although 120/80 is considered healthy and "ideal," blood pressure readings by themselves are not enough to assess your overall health.

At birth, blood pressure is typically about 80/46 and goes up gradually with the passage of time. For ages twenty to twenty-four, the average pressure·for men is 122/76; for women, 116/72. At ages thirty-five to thirty-nine, it's up to 127/80 and 124/78, respectively. By age fifty to fifty-four, the trend of women to have lower pressure reverses, with men averaging 134/83 and women, 137/84. High blood pressure is considered anything over 140/90.

---

mune response (antigens). In the body, some of the substances behave like drugs. Carbon monoxide, one of the gases that comes out of the exhaust pipe of an automobile, is also plentiful in cigarette smoke. It can combine with the hemoglobin of red blood cells more readily than does oxygen, leading to a reduction in the supply of oxygen to the heart muscles, thus increasing the effect of atherosclerosis. In people who have heart disease, exposure to carbon monoxide can lower their tolerance threshold for angina.

The U.S. Public Health Service calls cigarette smoking a medical problem of epidemic proportions, maintaining that it can affect the heart in three ways: (1) by prompting repeated injury of an artery's endothelial layer, (2) by increasing the tendency to form blood clots, and (3) by causing an imbalance between supply and demand of oxygen, impairing its transport and use.

How to Modify Cigarette Smoking: There is only one way to change the smoking habit: Stop! If you stop smoking today, the benefits begin to accrue almost immediately. The benefits are most notable for those who have smoked fewer than a pack of cigarettes a day; two years after

---

Box 9.9 HOW TO MODIFY HIGH BLOOD PRESSURE

- *Lose weight if necessary*. The Framingham offspring study of the 5,000 children of the original Framingham group showed that overweight women were seven times more likely to develop hypertension than women who were not overweight.
- *Limit intake of salt in daily diet*. Only certain people with hypertension—those sensitive to salt—will benefit from reduction of salt in the diet. Most Americans, however, use far too much of this condiment, by some estimates twenty times what the human body needs. Excess salt in the diet can interfere with some medications for high blood pressure.
- *Maintain potassium intake*. Studies in England and Japan link low potassium diets with high blood pressure. About 3 grams a day of potassium is sufficient; a medium sweet potato and a banana a day will provide more than the necessary intake.
- *Increase aerobic exercise*. Aerobic activity seems to protect against hypertension, and can also help achieve weight loss, another way to bring down blood pressure.
- *Limit (or eliminate) alcohol intake*. Some studies suggest that more than 4 to 6 ounces of 80 proof alcohol (the equivalent of about four to six glasses of vodka) a day will raise blood pressure. In any case, alcohol insidiously adds calories and can cause liver disease.
- *Stop smoking*. Cigarette smoking is linked with elevated blood pressure and with a higher risk of strokes and heart attacks.

---

giving up the habit, their risk of having a heart attack is no greater than that of a person who has never smoked (see Box 22.5, p. 732, for tips on how to quit smoking).

The good news is that the prevalence of smoking among adults decreased from 40 percent in 1965 to 29 percent in 1987. Nearly half of all living adults who ever smoked have quit. The bad news is that the incidence of smoking among teenage girls in the United States is alarmingly high (see Box 9.5).

Contributing Factors. In addition to the major risk factors, other factors strongly suggestive of an increased risk of cardiovascular disease are the following:

PHYSICAL INACTIVITY. Despite the exercise boom of the 1980s, surveys reveal that more than half of all Americans, in all age groups, do not exercise for at least twenty minutes three times a week. Ironically, during that same decade, researchers discovered that exercise does directly lessen the chances of a heart attack and premature death over a lifetime—even for people who have already suffered one heart attack.

Although one large study of 17,000 Harvard alumni demonstrated that people who are active and fit can expect to live a year or so longer than their sedentary counterparts, the evidence is still inconclusive. Nonetheless, exercise does appear to have these several benefits for the heart.

- *Efficiency*. The heart of a fit person simply works better than that of a sedentary individual. Fit persons have slower heart rates, which means their hearts can accomplish the same amount of work with considerably less effort or oxygen expenditure.
- *Cholesterol*. There is considerable evidence now

showing that those who participate in regular, sustained aerobic exercise have higher blood levels of HDLs, which is thought to protect against heart disease.

- *Weight loss.* Physical activity is an important factor in overall control of obesity, which in turn may diminish the development of hypertension and exert a positive effect in diabetes management.
- *Clot dissolution.* Regular physical activity may increase the amount of activity of tissue plasminogen activator (t-PA), a natural clot-dissolving protein produced by blood vessel cells. By elevating t-PA activity, regular exercise may better enable people to clear blood clots on their own and avoid heart attacks. (t-PA is the same compound now given to people who have heart attacks to dissolve the clots that caused the attacks.)
- *Other benefits.* Exercise may provide a possible antidiabetic effect, offsetting another coronary artery disease risk factor. Physical activity also has been shown to be effective in alleviating stress responses, which in certain respects are linked to cardiovascular disease (see below).

How to Modify Physical Inactivity: One need not take up triathalon training in order to protect against heart disease. Health benefits of exercise, such as reducing risks of cardiovascular disease and osteoporosis (see p. 201), can begin to accrue with just moderate levels of activity. It also is not necessary to reach your "target" heart rate, although fitness benefits, such as boosting aerobic capacity and muscle mass, do require that higher level of exercise intensity (see Chapter 22, "The ABCs of Staying Healthy").

If you are sedentary and forty years old or older, you should consult your personal physician to determine a safe starting level of exercise. Stress tests are necessary for those who have had a heart attack and are beginning a workout program. A complete history and physical examination is recommended for young and older athletes in training, because underlying heart problems may be detectable.

OBESITY. People who are more than 30 percent over ideal body weight are considered obese and more likely to develop coronary artery disease and stroke, because obesity influences blood pressure and blood cholesterol and may lead to diabetes.

Some research suggests that the way fat is distributed on the body is important, but unfortunately there is little we can do to change this except keep weight within acceptable limits.

How to Modify Obesity: Although quick weight loss programs may be enticing, they are a sure route to subsequently regaining lost pounds. What's more, very low-calorie diets (800 calories a day or less) can lead to serious health problems such as gallstones, kidney stones, psychological changes, and other complications. Lose weight slowly and steadily—one to two pounds weekly is best—until your goal weight is reached.

One pound of body fat contains 3,500 calories. To lose 1 pound of fat in a week, 3,500 calories need to be burned. By eating 500 calories less a day or burning it through exercise, 3,500 calories will be used over the course of seven days.

DIABETES. Middle-aged and overweight people can develop diabetes, the inability of the body to metabolize or use glucose (sugar) properly; this is usually referred to as type II, or insulin-independent, diabetes. (Type I diabetes usually occurs in young people.) Heredity is also a factor in developing this condition.

Diabetes greatly increases the risk of developing cardiovascular disease, and more than 80 percent of people with it have some form of heart or blood vessel disease.

How to Modify Diabetes: Type II diabetes can be controlled via diet, weight control, exercise, and medication to keep blood sugar levels under control.

STRESS. Every person is under stress at times. Although early research into the effects of stress on cardiovascular disease implicated the hard-driven, workaholic behavior as a precursor to cardiovascular disease, later research suggested that it is not necessarily fast-talking, fast-walking people who are likely to suffer a coronary event, but rather those who do not control their workplace environments and have two key personality components: anger and hostility.

How to Modify Stress: Research suggests that when stress management techniques, such as stretching, breathing, meditation, yoga, and relaxation exercises, are included in a program that minimizes other risk factors, coronary artery disease may be halted or reversed. Although such data are encouraging, they are preliminary, and the number of patients studied is relatively small. However, incorporating such stress management techniques into your life-style won't produce any negative side effects.

Another way to reduce risks is to modify or eliminate the stressor. One particularly potent stressor is absence of control. Sociologists correlating incidence of past heart attacks with characteristics of men's jobs found the most heart disease in low-echelon jobs—high-strain occupations involving high demand and low control.

Although stress can come from job demands, the key factor is the degree of freedom in deciding how to meet the demands. In short, having no control over decision making seems to pose a risk (see Chapter 22, "The ABCs of Staying Healthy," for more on stress).

Another potent stressor is the *lack* of a job or imminent threat of its loss. Studies have demonstrated that economic downturns causing unemployment are often accompanied by an increased incidence in illness. A long-term study monitored the physical and emotional health of workers in two plants that were being shut down and documented an increase in hypertension and, using laboratory tests, an increase in risk factors for coronary heart disease, diabetes, and gout.

THE ROLE OF OTHER ENVIRONMENTAL EXPOSURES

Researchers are now looking at the effects of a variety of chemical and physical environmental factors in causing heart disease, largely those listed in Table 9.2. While all have been implicated in the development of cardiovascular disease, large, well-defined studies are needed to clarify the role of each agent.

Angina, heart attack, abnormal heart rhythms, blood clots (claudication) in the legs, and sudden death are all conditions that can occur when the heart is ischemic (deprived of oxygen), and all have been associated with exposure to a variety of environmental substances that are mainly found in the workplace.

Chemicals

There is good evidence that exposure to carbon monoxide, carbon disulfide, and nitrates can cause ischemic events. For most Americans, these substances do not present a serious threat except through exposures related to occupation, cigarettes, or from drinking beer that contains cobalt additives.

Some evidence points to arsenic (as well as stress and noise) as causing ischemic heart disease. There are also reports and small studies that link ischemic heart disease to temperature extremes, radiation, cadmium, halogenated hydrocarbons, and ethanol or phenol used as industrial solvents.

Table 9.2 ENVIRONMENTAL AGENTS AND HEART DISEASE

Environmental Agent	Route of Exposure	Workers Possibly at High Risk	Cardiovascular Manifestations or Diseases	
			Acute	*Chronic*
Antimony	A heavy metal found in basic steel and metalworks and foundries	Bronze workers, drug makers, pewter workers, typesetters	Changes in EKG[a]	
Arsenic	Chronic poisoning is caused by exposure to fumes or dust of pure arsenic; water may also be contaminated	Alloy makers, insecticide makers, smelters	Changes in EKG Higher death rate	
Cadmium	Poisoning can occur when cadmium-coated metals are fired or welded or when cadmium is present as an impurity in other metals	Alloy makers, jewelry makers, and hobbyists and artists using cadmium-containing paint		Possible link to higher death rate and to high blood pressure
Carbon disulfide	A volatile liquid used in manufacture of viscose rayon, both liquid and vapor are highly irritating	Ammonium salt makers, bromine processors, carbon tetrachloride makers, degreasers, dry cleaners, electroplaters, fat processors, iodine processors, oil processors, paint workers, preservative makers, putty makers, rayon makers, resin makers, rocket fuel makers, rubber cement makers		Higher death rate, increased atherosclerosis

(continued)

Table 9.2   ENVIRONMENTAL AGENTS AND HEART DISEASE (*continued*)

Environmental Agent	Route of Exposure	Workers Possibly at High Risk	Cardiovascular Manifestations or Diseases	
			Acute	*Chronic*
Carbon monoxide	A colorless gas produced by combustion; anything that will burn contains carbon and, therefore, will produce carbon monoxide (methylene chloride is metabolized in the body into carbon monoxide)	Blast furnace workers, boiler-room workers, brewery workers, coke oven workers, diesel engine operators, garage mechanics, steelworkers, miners, organic chemical synthesizers, pulp and paper workers, water gas workers (also found in wood paint strippers)	Heart attack, angina, arrhythmias, sudden death	Possible link to increased atherosclerosis, may exacerbate underlying heart disease
Cobalt	A heavy metal usually found as an alloy and in cemented tungsten carbide	Alloy makers		Congestive cardiomyopathy
Cold	Condition prevalent in winter, early spring, and late fall months; low temperatures are considered dangerous	Outdoor workers, refrigeration workers, packinghouse workers	Does not cause cardiovascular disease, but extremes can trigger heart attack, angina, sudden death	May exacerbate underlying heart disease
Halogenated hydrocarbons		Aerosol bomb workers, ceramic mold makers, dry cleaners, drugmakers, fire extinguisher workers, heat transfer workers, metal conditioners, plastic makers, refrigeration makers,	Arrhythmias	

(continued)

Table 9.2 ENVIRONMENTAL AGENTS AND HEART DISEASE (*continued*)

Environmental Agent	Route of Exposure	Workers Possibly at High Risk	Cardiovascular Manifestations or Diseases	
			Acute	*Chronic*
		pressurized food makers, rocket fuel makers, solvent workers		
Heat	Condition prevalent in summer, late spring, and early fall; high temperatures are considered dangerous	Bakers, boiler-room workers, furnace workers, foundry workers, kiln workers, smelter workers	Does not cause cardiovascular disease, but extremes can trigger heart attack, angina, sudden death	May exacerbate underlying heart disease
Lead	Inorganic form is found in paint or grinding operations and usually enters the body when dusts and fumes are inhaled, the organic form is the antiknock component in gasoline and is easily absorbed through the skin as well as through the lungs	Smelters, battery makers, brass foundry workers, bridge painters		High blood pressure
Nitrates		Explosive makers, drugmakers	Angina, heart attack, sudden death	May exacerbate underlying disease
Radiation (ionizing)	Exposure to X rays during radiation therapy (not diagnostic procedures) is the most common incident; also can occur by exposure to alpha, beta, and gamma rays and neutrons; radioactive	Not usually an occupational problem; exposure more usual due to radiation therapy; atomic energy plant workers, uranium workers, dentists and assistants, X-ray technicians		Very high doses specifically aimed at particular body sites, increased atherosclerosis

(*continued*)

Table 9.2   ENVIRONMENTAL AGENTS AND HEART DISEASE (*continued*)

Environmental Agent	Route of Exposure	Workers Possibly at High Risk	Cardiovascular Manifestations or Diseases	
			Acute	Chronic
	materials emit radiation but different metals emit different energy			
Vibration		Workers who use vibratory tools such as chain saws, pneumatic drills, etc.		Peripheral vascular disease, Raynaud's phenomenon

a Electrocardiogram.

Noise

Noise has long been suspected of causing a stress reaction that increases adrenaline, changes heart rate, and causes blood pressure to rise. For example, studies in Sweden have found higher blood pressure levels among workers exposed to high levels of noise. Studies of grade-school children exposed to aircraft noise in school and at home showed they had higher blood pressure readings than those who lived in quieter areas. More troubling in this research: Even after the noise stimulus was removed, blood pressure levels tended to remain high (see Chapter 18, "Noise").

Vibration

Vibration can be related to noise. Workers who use tools that transmit vibrations vertically through the body through the soles of the feet, the palms of the hands, or through the seat are at risk for a circulatory disorder called Raynaud's phenomenon.

A study from the 1970s estimated that approximately 8 million Americans were exposed to occupational vibration, often a by-product of sources of noise (see Table 9.3). About 6.8 million workers were exposed to whole-body vibration, most while operating vehicles such as trucks, tractors, helicopters, buses, and construction equipment. The remaining 1.2 million workers used chain saws and hand tools that vibrated their arms and hands.

Subsequent studies of workers exposed to whole-body vibration revealed a variety of physical effects that are not necessarily dangerous but may be indicative of trouble. These effects include:

- Increases in oxygen consumption.
- Changes in bone structure, such as decalcification.
- Blurred vision.
- Changes in blood chemistry.
- Nausea and weight loss.
- Insomnia.
- Back pain and spine deformities.
- Motion sickness.

Table 9.3   OCCUPATIONS WITH VIBRATIONAL HAZARDS

Farm equipment operators
Helicopter pilots
Truck drivers
Barbers and hairdressers
Construction workers
Loggers
Road workers

Although some of these effects may be attributed to factors other than vibration, such as poor posture and diet, vibration is still considered a significant cause.

Temperature Extremes

Although environments that are very hot or very cold do not increase the incidence of atherosclerosis or cardiovascular disease, either extreme may trigger the onset of symptoms of heart disease. This is due to the physiologic changes that the temperature causes.

Exercising in hot weather forces the heart to pump a large volume of blood to the skin in order to dissipate body heat and provide active muscles with their metabolic needs. If the heart cannot supply the blood flow needed, it increases the risk of heat-related disorders, such as heat exhaustion and heat stroke.

In a cold environment, the body conserves heat by closing down the supply to blood vessels close to the skin, where heat would be dissipated into the environment, moving it to warm internal organs. The skin may turn bluish because smaller amounts of oxygenated blood are being pumped to these vessels. For people without heart disease, exercise on a cold day helps to maintain the body's normal internal temperature because heat is generated by the contracting muscles. However, for people with heart disease, it is not advisable to go beyond reasonable exertion when exercising in cold environments as the low temperatures may constrict arteries, raise blood pressure, and possibly lead to chest pains (angina) or a heart attack.

It's also important to note that those with cardiovascular conditions, such as high blood pressure or heart disease, should not visit altitudes 10,000 feet or more above sea level. At higher altitudes, less breathable oxygen is available, thus creating a greater burden on the heart as well as the lungs.

THE ROLE OF LIFE-STYLE

When it comes to looking at the factors that contribute to the development of cardiovascular disease, what seems to be key is the *pattern* of the way we live—the interaction of diet, work, stress and activity levels, and behaviors such as smoking. A great deal of research suggests that this overall tapestry of behavior plays a very important role in helping to determine who will develop heart disease, who will survive, and who will succumb to it.

For example, scientists have observed that people living in different parts of the world and regions of the same country have different rates of developing heart disease. Most telling, when people from countries with a low incidence of heart disease move to another area in which heart disease is more prevalent, their risk of developing this illness rises toward that in their new homeland. This higher risk may be due to their adoption of new and detrimental life-style behaviors.

Frequently, risk factors coexist in the same person. For example, 40 percent of the people with high blood cholesterol also have high blood pressure.

As we design individual programs to reduce our risk of developing cardiovascular disease, it is essential to keep this whole picture in sight. Although it may help to alter a particular risk factor, the most effective programs will likely be those that modify many risk factors, altering our overall behaviors toward more heart-healthy life-styles.

CHAPTER 10

Musculoskeletal Ailments

B ones, muscles, ligaments, tendons, and joints are natural marvels of engineering and construction, evolved over millions of years to provide strength, control, and flexibility. Evolution, however, has not caught up with human invention; our bodies are simply not designed to handle many of the physical stresses of modern life. Activities such as plucking chickens, typing at a word processor, or gliding cans and bottles through the supermarket checkout counter for eight hours each day can tax the human body's musculoskeletal system beyond its capacity to absorb stress, resulting in damage.

Ailments of bones and muscles due to environmental stresses are extensive. Back pain affects 5.4 million Americans each year, costs $16 billion annually for treatment, and is cited in 30 to 40 percent of all workers' compensation claims, according to the Office of Ergonomics at the Occupational Safety and Health Administration (OSHA). Overuse disorders—wear and tear on joints and tendons that comes from repeating the same motion hour after hour, day after day—affect six out of every one-hundred workers; in some industries, such as meat packing and automobile assembly, more than one-third of the employees complain of these ailments.

THE BASIC ANATOMY OF THE MUSCULOSKELETAL SYSTEM

We may think of bones and muscles as different from inorganic materials, such as steel or glass, but in many ways they are very similar. Just as excess stress causes glass to shatter, a sudden force can break a bone. Just as the cumulative effects of rust and vibration will cause a steel girder in a bridge to fail, so can a lifetime of small injuries add up to produce osteoarthritis in a joint.

We do have a built-in advantage over bridges and buildings because our bones and muscles can adapt to stress. They can remodel their structures, heal when at rest, and be trained to respond more effectively to environmental demands. The bones, joints, muscles, tendons, ligaments, cartilage, and bursas of the human body have evolved sophisticated strategies to respond to varying stresses while supporting us and providing protection for other body organs.

All the musculoskeletal disorders in this chapter can be seen as responses to overloads on the body, caused in varying degrees by unhealthy levels of physical stress in the environment. Looked at in this way, prevention of these injuries comes down to reducing the amount of stress to which the system is exposed and/or increasing the amount of stress each system can tolerate through such interventions as exercise, better diet, and improved habits.

Bones

The skeleton is a living scaffolding that gives the body structure and strength. The 206 *bones* of the human skeleton not only give the human body its shape and form, but protect delicate organs, such as the heart and the brain; act as reservoirs for essential elements, such as calcium and phosphorous; provide a site for the production of important blood cells; and provide the levers, articulation, and locations for attachment of muscles that allow movement.

The bones of the skeletal system are divided into four classifications: long, short, flat, and irregular. The shape of each type of bone suits it to respond to different environmental stresses. For example, the round shape of the skull gives it extra strength to protect the brain, while the bones of the spine thicken as they progress down the back, enabling them to support extra weight.

The Spine. The spine consists of thirty-three bones called *vertebrae*, classified into five separate regions: the *cervical spine* (neck area), seven vertebrae that support the head and protect the spinal cord on its way up to the head; the *thoracic spine*, twelve vertebrae, each connected to rib bones; the *lumbar spine*, five lumbar vertebrae, which are slightly larger than the other vertebrae because they are designed to bear much of the weight of the body (the lower back is the most common site of back pain); the *sacrum* or *sacral vertebrae*, five fused bones at the base of the spine; and the four *coccygeal vertebrae* that comprise the *coccyx*, or tailbone (see Figure 10.1).

In their stacked alignment, the vertebrae surround a central canal containing the spinal cord, the major nerve trunk for the body and the seat of reflexes. Also passing through the vertebrae are nerves leading from the spinal cord to the limbs and other organs. The openings between verte-brae that these nerves pass through can become injured, a common cause of pinched nerves.

Joints

The *joints*, which connect two moving bones together to allow motion and provide stability, have evolved into three types, each with its own biomechanical advantage.

There are three types of joints: *Fibrous joints*, such as those in the skull, which have very limited motion and provide stability; *cartilaginous joints*, such as those between vertebrae, which allow some motion in the spine; and *synovial joints*, such as those found in the elbow, wrist, and knee, which are the most common type and allow the greatest degree of movement.

Muscles

The more than 600 *muscles* in the human body make possible movement and such crucial functions as pumping blood and inhaling and exhaling air. They also generate heat, enable us to sit and stand, and protect bones by absorbing impacts to the body.

The *skeletal muscles*, the best-known and most common type, make up about 40 percent of body weight; they are also called voluntary muscles because they are under conscious control. The other two types of muscles—*visceral* and *cardiac*—are involuntary muscles that work without conscious control. Visceral muscles are involved in the function of internal organs, such as the stomach, intestines, uterus, and blood vessels; they are not attached to bone, act slowly, and can remain contracted for long periods of time. Cardiac muscle, found only in the heart, makes up much of the heart wall.

Ligaments

Ligaments are made up of long bands of collagen fibers arranged in parallel bundles, that hold bones to other bones and give a joint stability, allowing movement in some directions while re-

Figure 10.1 THE MUSCULOSKELETAL SYSTEM.

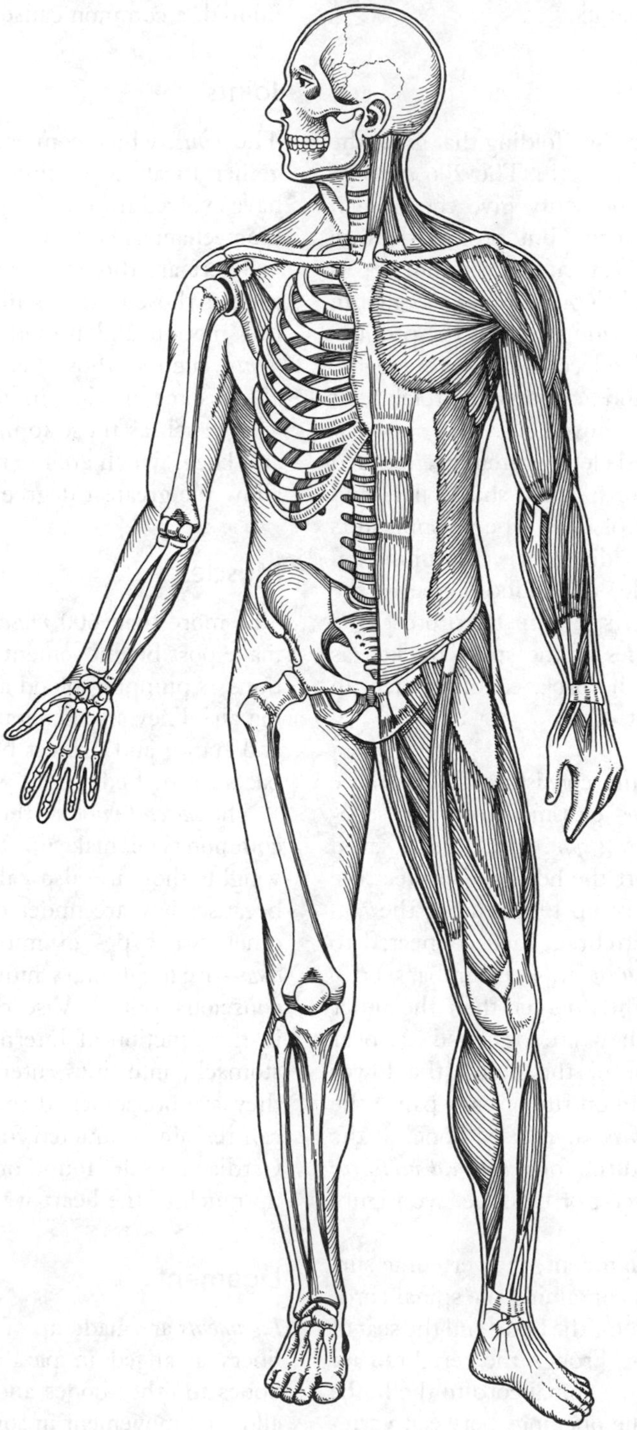

THE HUMAN MUSCULOSKELETAL SYSTEM, SHOWING BONES AND MUSCLES

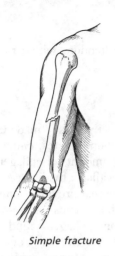

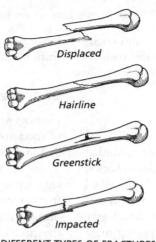

Displaced

Hairline

Greenstick

Impacted

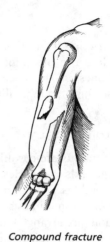

Simple fracture

Compound fracture

DIFFERENT TYPES OF FRACTURES

Simple fracture, a "clean" break of the bone, with little damage to surrounding tissue. Compound fracture, surrounding tissue is damaged and the bone punctures the skin. Displaced fracture, the ends of the broken bone are moved out of position. Hairline fracture, a "crack" across the bone. Greenstick fracture, the bone is splintered but not completely severed. Impacted fracture, the ends of the broken bone are intermeshed.

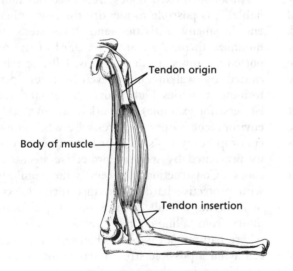

Tendon origin

Body of muscle

Tendon insertion

MUSCLE-BONE ARRANGEMENT

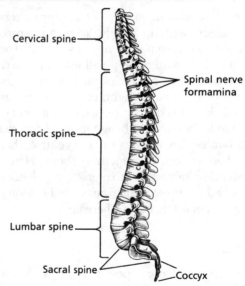

Cervical spine

Spinal nerve formamina

Thoracic spine

Lumbar spine

Sacral spine

Coccyx

BONES OF THE SPINE

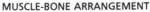

Tendons unite a muscle with another body part and transmit the force that the muscle exerts. Note the origin and insertion points of the tendon in this arrangement of bones and muscles.

The vertebrae, which comprise the spinal column, form five general regions: the cervical (seven vertebrae), thoracic (twelve vertebrae), lumbar (five vertebrae), sacral (five fused vertebrae), and coccyx, or tailbone (four fused vertebrae). Nerves connect to the spinal cord through openings called the spinal foramina.

stricting it in others. They can be found encircling the hip joint and parallel to the ends of bones in the knee joint, where they provide strength and stability.

Tendons

Tendons are cordlike bundles of fibers found at the ends of muscles and attach muscles to bones. Tendons enable muscles to move the attached bone (sometimes at a distance). The cells in tendons are arranged in parallel bundles, which give them high tensile strength while allowing them to transmit force from muscle to bone without getting damaged. The length of tendons ranges from less than 1 inch to more than 1 foot, the longest being the Achilles tendon, which runs from the heel to the calf.

Cartilage

Cartilage is a type of connective tissue made up of specialized cells called chondrocytes, embedded in a matrix of varying amounts of collagen. There are three types of cartilage: hyaline cartilage, a tough, smooth tissue that provides a low-friction coating for the bony ends of joints; fibrocartilage, a solid, strong collagen found in the intervertebral disks between the bones of the spine; and elastic cartilage, a soft and rubbery substance found in such places as the outer ear and the epiglottis.

INJURIES AND AILMENTS OF BONES AND JOINTS

A tiny broken bone in the foot can turn a traveling salesperson's life upside down. A fractured wrist can put a computer operator out of work for weeks. A shattered hip will leave an elderly person bedridden and helpless. Few of us give our bones a second thought; only once they are injured do we suddenly realize how important and fragile they are. Although many factors that lead to injury are often out of our control, there are others we can do something about. Here is an overview of the most common problems of bones and joints resulting from a combination of environmental factors and heredity.

Fractures

There are two basic types of fractures. A low-energy fracture, such as that experienced by a skier who breaks a leg, tends to be less serious because the soft tissues surrounding the bone can absorb some of the shock. A high-energy fracture, such as that caused by a bullet or being hit by an automobile, tends to cause more serious damage to a bone and to the soft tissues around it. Most fractures in the workplace are of the low-energy variety.

Although broken bones are sometimes inevitable, it is possible to identify the risks inherent in many activities and take steps to minimize them. As many as a third of the reported fractures are due to slips, falls, or trips caused by walking on uneven surfaces, performing activities high above the ground (on ladders, for example), or working in an untidy environment. Other fractures arise when workers drop heavy tools on their feet—injuries easily prevented by wearing protective steel-toed shoes. Construction workers who regularly wear protective hard hats reduce their chances of incurring a skull fracture and critical brain injury from falling debris. Even an avid walker whose natural gait is biomechanically incorrect can avoid a possible stress fracture by modifying his or her shoes or orthotics (supportive shoe cushions).

Similarly, fractures are more likely when engaging in risky recreational pursuits, such as skiing, mountain climbing, white-water rafting, hang gliding, skydiving, and horseback riding. However, people can lower their chances for injuries by training properly, using the best possible equipment, following standard procedures, and—most importantly—understanding and respecting their limits.

In all activities, the chances of breaking a bone are higher if the muscles are tired. Fatigued muscles lose some of their capacity to absorb shock; this can lead to abnormal compression of the joints, altered stress patterns, and fracture.

Osteoporosis

According to the National Center for Health Statistics, over 24 million Americans, most of them women, have osteoporosis, a serious condition in which the mass of bone declines literally to the breaking point. As we age, the balance between bone breakdown and buildup starts to fail, and there is more bone destruction than bone rebuilding (see Box 10.1). Osteoporotic bones become so frail and weakened that a minor fall, a jarring movement, or an attempt to pick up a moderately heavy object can lead to fracture.

While weight-bearing bones are primarily affected, leading to loss of height as we age as well as to "dowager's hump" (technically known as *kyphosis with cervical lordosis*) (see Figure 10.3), those of the hip, pelvis, and the long bones of the arm and leg may be affected as the disease progresses. For this reason, osteoporosis raises the specter of dangerous hip fractures. This is a particular danger among the elderly, for whom hip fracture is the leading cause of hospitalization from injury; 5 percent of elderly patients hospitalized for hip fracture die during hospitalization from such complications as blood infections (septicemia) and pneumonia.

Box 10.1 BONE BUILDUP AND BREAKDOWN

Bones are constantly being built up and broken down throughout life; as much as one-fifth of the body's bone content is turned over annually. Studies have found that the destruction and synthesis occur simultaneously, but at different locations on the bone.

The structure of bone is somewhat analogous to reinforced concrete. The core is a framework of *collagen fibers* which gives the bone some flexibility, embedded with minerals that provide strength and rigidity. However, unlike a piece of chalk, which is pure calcium, bone is not brittle.

Bloodborne cells, called *osteoclasts*, destroy old bone tissue and create little cavities in the bones. Other cells, called *osteoblasts*, then arrive and fill the tiny holes with fresh collagen. A third type of cell, the *osteocytes*, are believed to play a role in mobilizing calcium into new bone tissue.

Calcium is an important factor in regard to bone strength and the development of osteoporosis. If proper levels of calcium are available through the diet, the calcium is embedded in the collagen for strength. If calcium levels are insufficient, the bone will continue to break down but will fail to regenerate; this is believed to cause the bone weakness seen in osteoporosis.

Osteoporosis is the result of a complex interplay of factors, some inherited, some environmental. The current medical view is that osteoporosis can be prevented to some degree and does not have to be an inevitable consequence of aging if several important life-style changes are implemented.

Risk Factors. Some risk factors are inherited and unmodifiable, including the following.

GENDER. Women are considered to be at higher risk for osteoporosis, because the level of the female hormone estrogen is key in the development of this disease.

EARLY MENOPAUSE. Estrogen does not build up bone, but normal levels can prevent further bone loss. The decline in estrogen levels that accompanies menopause leads to a loss of this protective effect. Researchers are still not sure how estrogen influences bone density; it may affect another hormone or work directly on bone tissue, which does have estrogen receptors. An estrogen drop also can occur when ovaries are surgically removed, or when certain drugs, such as steroids and heparin, are taken.

RACE. Caucasians and Asian females are at higher risk than blacks. One-fifth of Caucasian women have lost enough bone mass after menopause to pose a significant risk of fracture.

NATURAL BONE DENSITY. Heredity sets the baseline for bone density with thin-boned people at greater risk because their bone density levels rapidly can fall dangerously low. Women generally have thinner bones than men; as they age, they lose one-half of their bone mass, compared with men, whose naturally larger bones lose one-quarter of their mass.

Prevention. There are major risk factors that we can modify to stave off osteoporosis, including the following.

CALCIUM LEVELS. When sufficient calcium is not available through diet, this mineral is released into the bloodstream from bones, depleting its reservoir and weakening the bones. This process also leaves less stored calcium available for future bone rebuilding.

Calcium deficiencies can arise due to malnutrition, poor diet fads or "crash diets," or anorexia; it also may occur during pregnancy and breastfeeding when increased demands for calcium are needed for the developing fetus. As we age, calcium deficiencies can result because our ability to absorb calcium from food decreases.

The diet should meet recommended daily allowances of nutrients that help bones stay strong, such as vitamin D, calcium, and protein. A person should consume at least 1,000 milligrams of calcium each day—the equivalent of four 8-ounce glasses of milk. Dairy products need not be the only source of calcium, as there are several calcium-rich foods available, as well as calcium supplements. Some good calcium sources are listed in Table 10.1.

Table 10.1 SOURCES OF DIETARY CALCIUM

Food Group	Calcium Content (mg)
Dairy	
Yogurt (plain low-fat), 1 cup	452
Yogurt (plain nonfat), 1 cup	415
Milk (skim), 1 cup	302
Milk (1% lowfat), 1 cup	300
Milk (whole), 1 cup	291
Buttermilk, 1 cup	285
Cheese (Swiss), 1 oz	275
Cheese (American), 1 oz	176
Cheese (Parmesan), 1 tbsp	86
Vegetables	
Spinach (fresh, boiled), ½ cup	122
Turnip greens (fresh, boiled), ½ cup	99
Broccoli (fresh, boiled), ½ cup	89
Collard greens (fresh, boiled), ½ cup	74
Dandelion greens (fresh, boiled), ½ cup	74
Mustard greens (fresh, boiled), ½ cup	52
Kale (fresh, boiled), ½ cup	47
Fruit	
Figs (dried), ¼ cup	72
Orange (one)	52
Others	
Sardines (canned, with bones)	326
Tofu (with calcium sulfate), ½ cup	258
Salmon (canned with bones), 3 oz	181
Almonds, 1 oz	75
Beans	
Small, white, ½ oz	66
Baked, canned, ½ cup	64

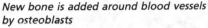

New bone is added around blood vessels by osteoblasts

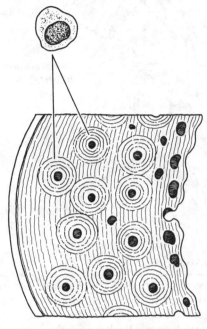

Bone is removed in cavities by osteoclasts

(b) Bone with osteoporosis

(a) Section of dense bone

Figure 10.2 BONE BUILDUP AND BREAKDOWN.

In the section of healthy, dense bone (*a*), new bone is added by osteoblasts around the blood vessels while bone is removed in cavities by osteoclasts (*b*). Note the higher concentration of cavities in the section of bone with osteoporosis (*b*).

LEVELS OF PHYSICAL ACTIVITY. Studies have shown that regular exercise, such as walking, jogging, swimming, or bicycling, throughout one's lifetime strengthens bones and prevents osteoporosis.

Because bone strength and density peak between ages twenty-five and forty, regular physical activity early in life (before age twenty-five) will help bones to reach their maximum density. During adulthood, exercise plays an important role in preventing or reducing further bone loss.

Especially important exercises are ones that stress and, ultimately, strengthen bones; weight-bearing workouts, such as running, walking, and aerobics, and court sports, such as tennis, are good choices for those who want to promote bone density. Regular exercise is particularly important for women, who are more likely to develop osteoporosis.

ESTROGEN LEVELS. Because estrogen helps maintain bone density, it may be advisable for premenopausal women who have low estrogen levels to be given hormone replacement therapy. After menopause, estrogen may be appropriate to strengthen bones in women who have not developed osteoporosis or to lessen further decline of bone mass in those in the early stages.

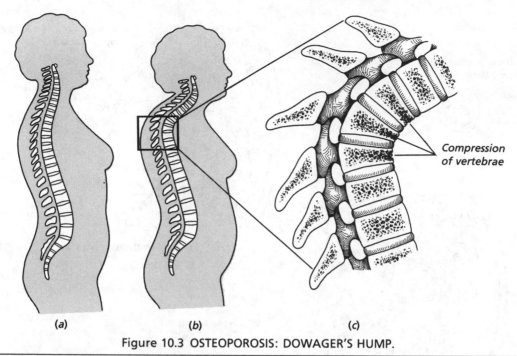

(a)   (b)   (c)

Figure 10.3 OSTEOPOROSIS: DOWAGER'S HUMP.

The mineral loss that results from osteoporosis thins the bones in the spine, making them more fragile. Instead of the normal curves seen in the healthy spine (*a*), vertebrae in the spine of the woman with osteoporosis (*b*) are weakened and compressed (*c*). In later stages, vertebrae in the lower back may collapse completely causing "dowager's hump." This condition is usually associated with severe back pain and further loss of height.

OTHER FACTORS. Consuming excessive amounts of alcohol (more than two drinks daily) or caffeine (five or more cups per day) increases the likelihood of developing osteoporosis. Smoking can contribute to the degenerative bone loss that leads to osteoporosis.

When osteoporosis is present, several environmental and life-style changes can be made to prevent or reduce the likelihood of a potentially bone-splitting fall (see Box 10.3 for some suggestions). Some type of exercise regimen may also be advised, although it must be carefully balanced in order not to stress already-fragile bones (swimming or exercising in a pool may be preferable to jogging, for example). It is best to work out such a program with your physician.

Osteoarthritis

Osteoarthritis, the most common form of arthritis, is a condition in which the cartilage and surrounding tissues of joints become inflamed and either deteriorate or form new, dysfunctional bone.

Some degree of osteoarthritis is considered a normal part of aging; by age seventy-five, most people have developed osteoarthritis in one or more joints. However, certain environmental stresses, activities, and occupations are worse at wearing and tearing.

Repetitive activity, particularly if it impacts or vibrates the joints, increases the risk of developing osteoarthritis. Impact on the joint appears to initiate the degenerative cycle that leads to

---

Box 10.2   ESTROGEN REPLACEMENT THERAPY

Research indicates that estrogen replacement therapy, the use of estrogen to prevent osteoporosis, can slow the loss of bone if given before or within three years of menopause. Estrogen has been credited with reducing osteoporotic fractures by half.

While estrogen has been found to stop bone loss, this effect only lasts while the drug is being taken and seems to wear off with time. Some doctors recommend giving estrogen after menopause to all high-risk women—women with a slight build and a family history of osteoporosis. Others feel that each person must be evaluated individually to weigh the risks of treatment versus the possible benefits. Treatment should begin soon after menopause (within at least five years) and last for at least five years.

There is a good deal of controversy over whether or not some women should take estrogen for osteoporosis. Studies in the mid-1970s reported a higher incidence of breast and uterine (endometrial) cancer in women who had taken estrogen. Today's estrogen replacement therapy—actually hormone replacement therapy—is quite different. Most doctors now recommend a regimen that combines low doses of estrogen (1.25 milligrams or less per day) with another hormone, progesterone, unless the woman has had a hysterectomy. Incorrect doses of estrogen can cause excessive buildup of cells of the uterine lining, a condition that can increase the risk of cancer of the uterus (endometrial cancer) in some women; progesterone promoted the shedding of the uterine lining, thus preventing this excess proliferation of cells. The incidence of uterine cancer has been found to be significantly lower.

Studies have demonstrated that estrogen replacement therapy can also help offset the development of heart disease in menopausal women. However, estrogen replacement therapy is not for everyone. Women who have a history of breast cancer, thrombophlebitis, and abnormal vaginal bleeding should be wary of estrogen because it causes such side effects as uterine bleeding and an increased risk of uterine and breast cancers. (While estrogen does not appear to increase the risk of breast cancer per se, if a breast cancer is present it appears to be likely to grow more quickly in the presence of estrogen.) If the uterus is still present, some doctors recommend taking estrogen with progesterone because this combination appears to be safer with regard to future uterine cancer than estrogen taken alone.

The bottom line is that all women need to discuss the estrogen issue with their doctors.

---

osteoarthritis (see Figure 10.4 and Box 10.4); this is why the feet and ankles of ballet dancers, the hips of farmers, the elbows of miners, and the fingers of cotton pickers and boxers are all prone to this disease.

Subjecting the body to vibration continually can also initiate the degenerative cycle, which is why train operators, truck drivers, and pneumatic drill workers are so often affected.

Athletes, such as football players and runners, often put a terrible strain on their joints. For example, the pressure of the kneecap against the femur during running is equal to *four to six times* the body weight with every strike of the foot. For a 150-pound person, this is equivalent to putting 600 to 900 pounds of pressure on a kneecap for 1,000 steps a mile.

The early symptoms of osteoarthritis begin

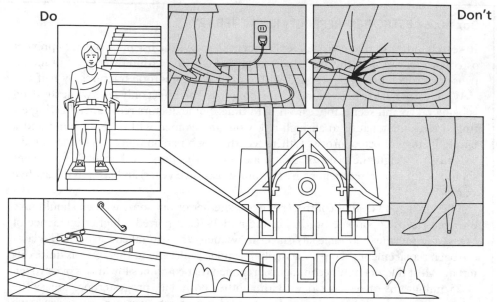

(Clockwise from lower left) **Do** install handrails on bathtubs and chair lifts on stairs where possible. **Don't** leave loose wires on the floor, use slippery throw rugs, or wear high heels.

Box 10.3   MAKING THE HOME ENVIRONMENT SAFER

- Eliminate hazards that can cause preventable slip-and-fall accidents, such as throw rugs placed on highly polished floors.
- Eliminate anything that can catch the feet, such as loose wires or settings between rooms. Even thick carpeting can sometimes cause falls since elderly people with arthritis or other problems may not lift their feet as high as they used to.
- Proper footwear is essential. High heels can cause falls, soles with too much traction can cause elderly people to stop suddenly and lose their balance, and slippery soles can lead to sliding and falling.
- If a person with osteoporosis or arthritis lives in your home, be sure the bathtub has rails and a seat that allows easy access, and that the bathtub or bathroom floors are not slippery. Perhaps move all of the person's things into one area, so he or she doesn't have to go upstairs or travel around the home as much. If the affected person needs to use the stairs, install a chair lift to avoid falls.
- To reduce the possibility of injuries, a person with osteoporosis should be given only minimal amounts of medications that may make them dizzy and thus prone to falling.

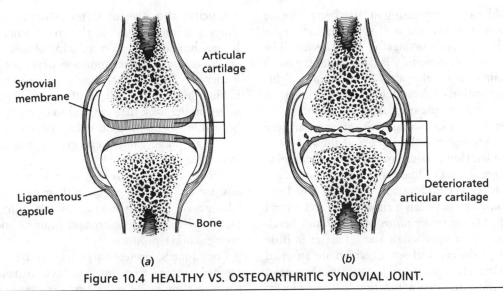

Figure 10.4 HEALTHY VS. OSTEOARTHRITIC SYNOVIAL JOINT.

Synovial joint. Healthy joint is shown in (*a*) in cross section; osteoarthritic joint is shown in (*b*).

Box 10.4   FORMATION OF AN OSTEOARTHRITIC JOINT

Synovial joints have a smooth covering called the *articular cartilage* at the point where the two bones of the joint meet. A joint is lined with a *synovial membrane*, which contains a fluid that lubricates the two opposing bones during movement. Surrounding the synovial joints are ligaments, muscles, and tendons, which strengthen and stabilize the joint.

To reduce friction, many joints have two additional structures: *bursas* and *tendon sheaths*. Bursas are sacs lined with synovial membranes that are filled with synovial fluid, found between tendons and bones. Tendon sheaths wrap around the tendon and cushion it where it crosses the joint.

Repetitive compression of a joint can lead to microfractures in the bones which meet at the joint. The bone responds to these tiny fractures by adding new bone tissue, which places additional stress on the cartilage in the joint, causing it to break down, thus resulting in osteoarthritis.

In joints, osteoarthritis is caused by a gradual erosion of the smooth cartilage; this erosion starts with the appearance of small "pits" in the cartilage which spread to form large areas of missing cartilage, primarily at those points where the pressure is greatest.

Although the cartilage is not rubbed away or thinned in nonstressed areas, it can become undernourished and unhealthy. At the same time, there is often growth of new bone and cartilage tissue in the joint, resulting in the formation of obstructive spurs, called *osteophytes*, that can limit the mobility of the joint.

in middle age, progressing in later years. Fingers and toes may become red, swollen, and tender and, later, numb or lacking in dexterity. The most common symptom is deep, aching pain in the joints, especially after exercise or weight-bearing activity. A sufferer can develop joint pain at night as the osteoarthritis advances.

The areas most commonly affected are the lower extremities—the knee and the hip—and the lumbar (lower back) and cervical (neck) spine (see Figure 10.1). These parts of the spine are the least protected joints in the body: The lumbar spine lies between a rigid pelvis and a rigid thorax, taking tremendous torsional and bending loads in a very small area. The seven little blocks of the cervical spine, which are attached to a relatively rigid thoracic cage (backbone and ribs), must balance a bowling-ball-like object, the head.

Reducing the Risk of Osteoarthritis. Sometimes a simple change in the environment can have a dramatic effect on reducing osteoarthritis at work. For example, someone who operates a loader may be constantly turning around to look behind him- or herself, putting an unnatural stress on the neck that can lead to osteoarthritis. Something as simple as installing a rearview mirror or a remote camera can greatly reduce the stress.

Office workers who lean over keyboards all day are also putting stress on their neck bones. Changes in the ergonomics of the office can greatly reduce discomfort and injuries and increase worker productivity.

For runners, protecting joints may be as simple as changing to a different style of running shoes or running on softer surfaces that put less stress on their joints.

DISORDERS OF MUSCLES AND TENDONS

Back Pain

Aching backs are second only to headaches in the number of people they affect. Most of us—85 percent—will experience back pain at some point in our lives.

Historically, the vulnerability of the back has been viewed as a biomechanical problem: Even when standing erect, the anatomy of our back is not well designed to absorb stress compared with the lying down position; extra pressure is placed on the vertebrae of the lower back, particularly the lumbar region where the back curves. Given this vulnerability, most of us need not look beyond behavioral and environmental factors to find the reason for our back discomfort.

However, posture is now considered to be only part of the cause. Although the specific reasons for acute low back pain are still unknown, the new thinking is that it is simply a part of the normal degenerative process of spinal disks.

This may be why back pain peaks during age thirty to thirty-five—the years in which there is a switch in the ratio of bone buildup to breakdown (see Box 10.1).

Many workplaces are not designed with an understanding of their effect on the body and the back. Occupations such as construction work, mining, and meat packing are inherently biomechanically stressful, whereas others, such as word processing or secretarial work, involve long periods of sitting—an inherently stressful activity in a different way (see Box 10.6 for general tips on good office design).

Although most people develop back pain, 90 percent of those forced to leave work return within six weeks. However, most will also have a bout of the ailment again.

Avoiding back pain is often a matter of learning to sit, stand, and move in ways that acknowledge the biomechanical limitations of the human body and respecting our individual physical limits (see Box 10.5).

Box 10.5 STEPS TO PREVENT BACK PAIN

Lift properly. Keep the load lifted close to the body and do not twist. Use the abdominal muscles to support the spine.

Stand with good posture. A properly positioned center of gravity safely and comfortably stresses the back; when off center, the muscles make unnatural and body-stressing adjustments.

Shed excess pounds. Extra weight continuously stresses and weakens back muscles.

Wear sensible shoes. High-heeled shoes distort natural good posture (see Figure 10.6).

Avoid prolonged periods of sitting. Contrary to popular belief, sitting—not necessarily chair design—is responsible for many of the musculoskeletal problems associated with office work. Move around periodically (at least five minutes every half hour). If this is not possible, move joints and flex muscles periodically and incorporate some activity at lunchtime.

Exercise to strengthen back muscles. Strengthening and lengthening abdominal and back muscles will help stabilize the spine and reduce back pain. *Anyone who has experienced back pain should investigate its causes and possibly consider working with a physical therapist to design an exercise program to increase strength, mobility, and stability.*

Sleep on a firm mattress. Soft mattresses do not support the back; for extra firmness, put a half-inch plywood board under the mattress. A habit of sleeping on the stomach allows the back and hamstrings to tighten and can lead to stress on the back.

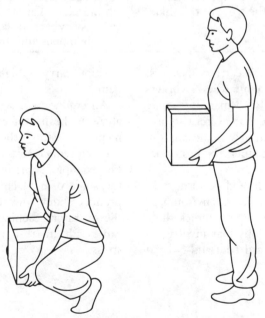

Figure 10.5 HOW TO LIFT CORRECTLY.

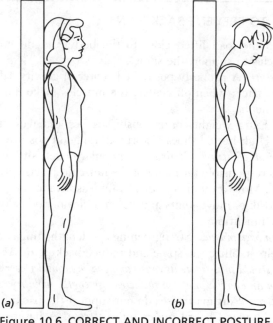

Figure 10.6 CORRECT AND INCORRECT POSTURE.

(*a*) Correct posture. A line drawn down the center of the body from ear level should cross the outer edge of the shoulder, the middle of the hip, the back of the kneecap, and the front of the ankle.

(*b*) Incorrect posture. If the center of gravity is too far forward, it can cause kyphosis (rounded shoulders and a caved-in chest), as well as shortened pectoral and rib muscles. If it is too far back, it can cause swayback, a condition in which the abdomen and buttocks protrude.

Movers, nurses aides, mail carriers, farmers, paramedics, stockroom employees—workers whose jobs are physically demanding—may need measures more drastic than exercise to protect themselves from back injury. Some employers train workers to use their bodies more efficiently and safely.

Even when workers are fit and perform tasks correctly, a poorly designed work environment can still add stress. For example, studies show that people who work in jobs that involve repetitive lifting in the forward bent-and-twisted position carry a high risk of developing back pain.

An ergonomist, a professional trained to analyze the health effects of the working environment, can study the environment and devise ways to reduce stress below the level of injury. For example, something as simple as modifying the angle of a machine in a factory so that a product slides toward the operator instead of the operator reaching forward to drag it out, can result in a significant reduction in back stress.

Figure 10.7 WILLIAMS' SIX BACK EXERCISES.

Try to do these exercises when you are not pressed for time. First, take a hot bath or shower or apply a heating pad to your lower back (lie on the pad with your knees bent as described in Exercise 1). Exercise on a hard surface, preferably the floor, and repeat each exercise twice. IMPORTANT: If you are seeing a physical therapist, please discuss your exercise program with the therapist. *Stop* if any exercise causes pain.

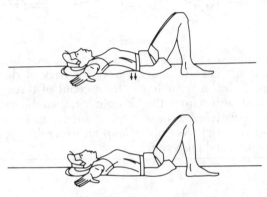

Exercise 1

Exercise 1: Lie on your back, bend both knees, and place feet firmly on the floor. Press your lower back into the floor by tightening your buttocks and abdominal muscles. Next, tuck your chin in gently to flatten the back of your neck to the floor. Hold this position for a slow count of three. *Do not hold your breath*. Relax by releasing first your neck and shoulders, then your abdomen and buttocks.

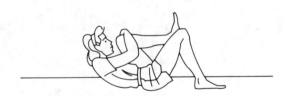

Exercise 2

Exercise 2: Repeat Exercise 1 to the hold position. Bend your *left* knee to your chest, grasp it in both hands, and draw firmly toward your chest. Tuck your chin in and attempt to touch your fore-head to your knee. Hold for a count of three. *Slowly* return the neck, then the knee to the starting position. Relax as in Exercise 1, then repeat for the right knee.

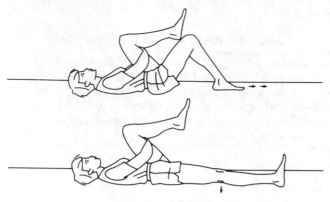

Exercise 3

Exercise 3: Repeat Exercise 1 to the hold position. Bend your *left* knee to your chest as in Exercise 2; *hold it* securely. Slide your *right* heel away from the body until the leg is flattened against the floor, then bend your right foot upward. Hold this position and push your whole right side to the floor, particularly the back of the right knee. Hold for a count of three. *Slowly* return the right leg, then the left leg to the starting position. Relax as in Exercise 1, then repeat, using the opposite legs.

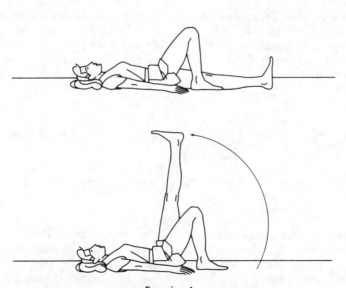

Exercise 4

Exercise 4: Repeat Exercise 1 to the hold position. Straighten the left knee and bend the left foot upward. Raise the left leg toward your head as far as you can without bending the knee, hold for a three count, and return to the starting position. Relax as in Exercise 1, then repeat, using the right leg.

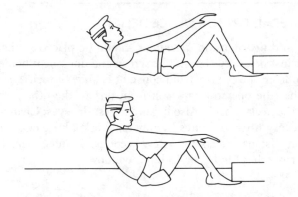

Exercise 5

Exercise 5: Repeat Exercise 1 to the hold position. Have someone press down on your ankles and feet or secure them under the edge of a couch or chair (in which case place a towel or pad on top of them). Extend both arms forward, tuck in your chin, and slowly curl into a sitting position. Hold for a count of three. Uncurl, lowering the midback to the floor first, followed by the shoulders, neck, and head. Relax as in Exercise 1.

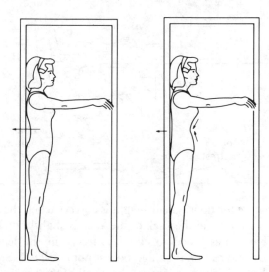

Exercise 6

Exercise 6: Stand with your back against a door frame and your heels about four inches away from the frame. Flatten your lower back into the frame, allowing your knees to bend a little. Tucking in your chin, try to flatten your neck into the frame. Press your hands against the opposite side of the frame (press *straight forward*, not down). Straighten both knees. Your entire trunk should now be pressing against the door frame; if, when straightening your knees, your back comes away from the door frame, STOP. Hold for a count of three, then relax.

Box 10.6   GENERAL TIPS FOR OFFICE DESIGN

- To ease back and neck tension, terminals should be placed so that the top of the screen is at or just below eye level. The screen and document holder should be the same distance from the eye (to avoid constant change of focus), and close enough together so that the operator can look from one to the other without excessive movement of the neck or back. Also be sure to rest the eyes: Change the focal point at least once every fifteen minutes by moving work a little closer or farther away or focusing on distant objects for a few seconds. Reduce glare by not working directly under overhead lights or facing a window.

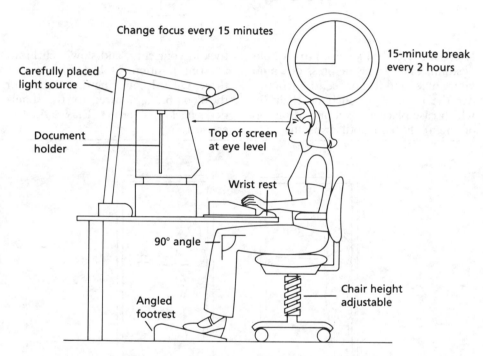

- Feet should be flat on the floor. Chair height is correct when the entire sole of the foot can rest on the floor and the back of the knee is slightly higher than the seat of the chair. This allows blood to circulate freely in the legs and feet. The worker's weight should rest on the thigh bones, not on the base of the spine. The backrest should be positioned to support the small of the back. Avoid chairs that encourage you to lean back in a leisurely posture; a plain straight-backed chair is fine for the office as long as you use seat cushions to adjust yourself to the proper height.
- When the user's hands rest on the keyboard, the upper arm and forearm should form a right angle. Fingers should just reach the keyboard; armrests should permit periodic support as needed.

(continued)

Box 10.6   GENERAL TIPS FOR OFFICE DESIGN (*continued*)

- Glare from windows or lighting should be kept to a minimum to prevent eyestrain. Some experts think screens with white backgrounds produce less glare than those with dark screens.
- For more information, write the University of California's Labor Occupational Health Project at 2521 Channing Way, Berkeley, California 94720.

Herniated Disks

The herniated, or "slipped," disk comprises less than 5 percent of all back injuries. Herniated disks occur when some of the soft, gelatinous tissue inside the spine, called the nucleus pulposus, escapes through a weakened portion of a vertebral disk and pushes against a spinal nerve, causing pain (despite its common name, there is no slippage involved).

Herniated disks can be the result of many different types of problems: trauma, such as a car accident; strain; improperly lifting something heavy; the natural, slow degeneration of disks; or, in rare instances, an inborn weakness in the back, such as a malformation of the vertebrae (spondylolisthesis). The most commonly herniated disks are those in the lumbar region, although herniation can also occur in the cervical vertebrae around the neck (see Figure 10.1).

In 90 percent of cases, the herniated disk occurs in the lumbar and lumbar–sacral areas. Symptoms include severe pain in the lower back that radiates to the buttocks, legs, and feet. When the herniated disk is in the cervical vertebrae (about 8 percent of cases), symptoms are severe pain in the upper back radiating to the arms.

Once a disk is herniated, it is wise to avoid causing further injury while pain is present; avoid sports that stress the back and switch to less stressful activities, such as swimming. Consult a doctor before resuming normal activities.

CUMULATIVE TRAUMA DISORDERS

Whether called overuse disorders, cumulative trauma disorders, or repetitive motion disorders, these injuries to muscles, tendons, or ligaments result from performing the same motion hour after hour, day in and out.

Aircraft and automobile assemblers, fruit packers and hay makers, writers, telephone operators, reporters, textile workers, housekeepers, waiters, musicians, postal workers, typists, computer operators, meat processors—even the check-out person at the supermarket—are all vulnerable to these ailments.

Cumulative trauma ailments are as common on the tennis court or jogging track as in the meat-packing plant or assembly line. In sports, an injury of this type is more likely to occur when a person is out of shape and launches into an inappropriately demanding activity or when athletes push themselves to reach new levels of skill and performance (see Box 10.9).

Back-related ailments are by far the most common on-the-job hazard; however, wrist and hand damage is now considered the fastest-growing category of cumulative trauma disorders.

Stress is believed to play a role in some cumulative trauma disorders. Work-related stress can lead to muscle tension, which can lower crucial oxygen-rich blood flow to muscles and tendons. This lack of oxygen is sorely felt and muscles become fatigued, even inflamed, increasing their risk for a trauma disorder.

Although there are steps an individual can take to minimize or prevent the likelihood of developing these problems, the cause may be a combination of work and athletic activity, and the solution may involve a series of musculoskeletal adjustments in both realms of life (see Box 10.7). Many disorders can be extremely painful and permanent, however, forcing an individual to change careers or greatly alter his or her normal activities.

Carpal Tunnel Syndrome

This disorder is caused by stressful, repetitive activity that irritates the tendons in the wrist and causes them to become inflamed. The inflammation creates swelling that painfully compresses or pinches the median nerve (the nerve with branches to the thumb, index, middle, and ring fingers) in the wrist within the cramped quarters of the carpal tunnel, the space in the wrist through which pass nerves, tendons, and blood vessels for the fingers. In severe cases, carpal tunnel syndrome can be permanently disabling. Carpal tunnel syndrome is one type of wrist and hand ailment, which are collectively considered the fastest growing category of cumulative trauma disorders.

Several physical aspects have been identified as increasing an individual's risk for developing a hand/wrist disorder. They include:

- Long-term repetition of the same movement.
- Unnatural, bent, or awkward positioning. (The correct wrist position should be with the wrist flat and straight so that the hand is level with the arm, forming a straight line.)
- Forceful or high-impact actions.
- Inadequate rest periods. (Workers should allow themselves a fifteen-minute respite at least every two hours.)

Box 10.7   STEPS TO PREVENT REPETITIVE MOTION DISORDER

- Sit with good posture in a properly adjusted chair.
- If keyboard is too high (making you bend your wrists upward), get a keyboard support that clamps onto the side of your desk or table to allow the keyboard to rest at a lower level. Ideally, your hands should rest level with your arms.
- Put a telephone book or some other spacer under a video display terminal monitor that's too low.
- To prevent repetitive motion disorder, as well as eyestrain, the National Institute for Occupational Safety and Health (NIOSH) recommends a fifteen-minute work rest break after one hour of continuous video display terminal work for operators under high visual demands and workload, or people engaged in repetitive tasks.

Occupational Setting. At greatest risk for this painful problem are people who repeatedly use poorly designed tools; engage in a great deal of grasping, twisting, or flexing of the hands (such as gardeners and seamstresses); or work on an assembly line. Most recently, the ailment has been reported increasingly by office workers who type a great deal, including secretaries, reporters, and data-entry workers.

The first symptoms are usually weakness, pain, numbness, or tingling in one or both hands. Carpal tunnel syndrome may produce pain that radiates from the wrist to the forearm or shoulders; the pain can be worse at night and in the morning possibly because blood vessels dilate when we rest, further blocking the carpal tunnel. Shaking the hands vigorously and dangling arms at the side often relieves the pain. In severe cases, carpal tunnel syndrome can be crippling and require long periods of intensive rehabilitation or corrective surgery.

Careful design of tools and the workplace environment can decrease the incidence, as can taking frequent breaks, changing position (to prevent unnatural and dangerous hand angles), using a keyboard wrist rest that prevents excessive flexing of the hands while typing, and changing the way you perform repeated tasks.

Workers in professions that are prone to carpal tunnel syndrome may need to consult with their physicians to learn ways of reducing hand and wrist stresses. Workers might ask the employer or union (if appropriate) to bring in an ergonomist to review procedures and design less taxing alternatives.

Tendinitis

One of the most common overuse syndromes is tendinitis, an inflammation or tear of a tendon or its sheath (covering). Any tendon can become inflamed, but those that are usually affected are the wrist, elbow, shoulder, thumb, and ankle.

This condition can be due to the repetitive performance of a movement or incorrectly using body parts involving that tendon; a sudden increase in activity without proper conditioning or technique; or a traumatic event, such as a partial rupture of the tendon while playing a sport. Sometimes tendinitis can be caused by an inflammatory disease process, such as rheumatoid arthritis or infection (such as gonorrhea).

Occupational Setting. According to one study, the risk for tendinitis is almost thirty times greater among people whose jobs involve highly repetitive and forceful movements; environmental stresses, such as vibration and low temperature; or require forceful blows or torque-like movements. The narrow handles of such tools as scissors or pliers fail to distribute forces over a wide enough area and can cause injury. Although often short-lived, severe cases of ten-

dinitis can become permanently disabling and interfere with the ability to continue in an occupation.

A number of measures can reduce the likelihood of developing tendinitis. By altering hand position, the amount of force required for tasks such as lifting can be reduced by up to a third. Tool design is also important: Decreasing the weight of tools, being sure they are properly balanced, and adding handles to them to further reduce the strain on tendons can help prevent tendinitis: For example, one electronics manufacturer who suffered a high rate of tendinitis among workers who used needle-nosed pliers on tasks that required them to turn their wrists in odd positions, alleviated the problem by redesigning the handles to keep the wrist in a neutral position.

People who develop "tennis elbow" (see below) may need to change their lifting habits or workplace environment so that lifting or repetitive work tasks are performed with the palm up to put less stress on the wrist. They should also evaluate whether or not sports and recreational activities may stress their bodies in similar ways, and make appropriate adjustments.

Sports Setting. A classic tendinitis occurs in the Achilles tendon, a strong and thick tendon in the body and a common area of inflammation in runners. Although it can affect anyone, it is a special problem in those who have naturally less flexible musculoskeletal profiles.

To minimize the risk of this injury, stretch and warm up the calf muscles and the Achilles tendons before and after running (see Box 10.8), run on surfaces that have some "give" (dirt paths rather than concrete sidewalks), and wear shoes that will help absorb some of the shock to the body.

EPICONDYLITIS (GOLF OR TENNIS ELBOW). Although commonly referred to as tendinitis, tennis elbow is actually an inflammation of the origin or starting point of the muscles in the forearm.

When it develops on the thumb (lateral) side

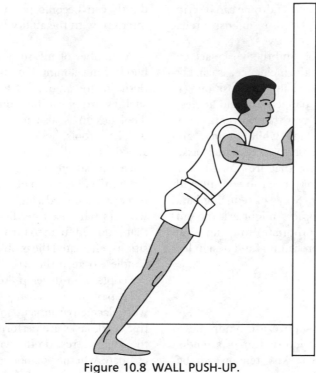

Figure 10.8 WALL PUSH-UP.

Box 10.8 PREVENTING ACHILLES TENDON INJURY

A wall push-up is recommended as a warm-up for people concerned about injuring the Achilles tendon. To do this, stand an arm's length from a wall; lean toward it while keeping your body straight, with knees locked and heels flat. Hold the stretch for fifteen to twenty seconds. Repeat several times. All stretches should be done slowly and easily without pain.

---

of the elbow, tendinitis is called tennis elbow. When it develops on the pinky (medial) side of the elbow, it is called golfer's elbow. It is common among tennis players, golf players, and factory workers—people whose activities require a forceful grip, wrist extension or flexion against resistance, or frequent rotation of the forearm. The first symptom is pain in the elbow that gradually worsens and may radiate to the forearm and the back of the hand when an object is grasped or the elbow is twisted.

Epicondylitis can be avoided by doing proper twenty- to thirty-minute warm-ups, using good performance technique, and wearing an elastic support when performing any activity that stresses the forearm or elbow.

Tennis players who develop tennis elbow may need to modify their technique and change racquet size and weight and grip size in order to avoid reoccurrence. Once symptoms have ceased, stretching and wrist-extensor strengthening exercises are recommended.

Box 10.9 HOW TO AVOID SPORTS INJURIES

Warm up properly. A ten-minute warm-up gets blood flowing to muscles and prepares them for the physical demands that they will experience.

Stretch. Stretching loosens muscles and reduces the risk of tearing an overly tight muscle.

Condition. If muscles are out of shape or weak in one part of the body, such as the back, strengthen them before engaging in more strenuous activities.

Respect your limits. Don't push too fast or too hard. Give the body time to adjust to earlier stresses.

Listen to your body. If you have injured a muscle, wait until the pain completely disappears until using that muscle again, otherwise you might seriously injure the area.

Bursitis

This inflammation of one or more of the seventy-eight bursas in the body is known by many colorful names: housemaid's knee (infrapatellar bursitis), weavers' bottom (ischial bursitis), students' or miners' elbow (olecranal bursitis), police officer's heel (subcalcaneal bursitis), even manure shovelers' hip (trochanteric bursitis). The bursas are fluid-filled sacs found in areas such as bony prominences, the shoulder, elbow, and front of knee. The bursas act as shock absorbers protecting the underlying bone or tendon. When a joint is subjected to trauma or overuse, the bursa becomes inflamed and tender, filling with excess fluid. Bursitis can occur wherever bursas are located.

Bursitis is more likely to occur in middle age. It can be found in workers at almost any job that requires movement of arms and legs, especially those that require activities that raise the pressure of the bursa, such as kneeling.

Occupationally related bursitis is not as common today as in the past, in part due to the invention of tools and machines to aid in stressful activities; these inventions reduce stress to bursas but can cause other injuries.

Knee Injuries

Knee injuries are common in sports because of the joint's design. Unlike other joints, such as the hip or the shoulder, in which a ball on the end of a bone fits snugly into a socket, the knee connects the ends of two bones: the *femur* (the long bone between the knee and the hip) and the *tibia* (the main support bone in the lower leg, along with the smaller bone, the *fibula*). The *patella* (kneecap) acts as a pulley to redirect the quadricep muscles as the knee bends and flexes (see Figure 10.9).

To allow these bones to move smoothly, the ends of the bone are covered with smooth cartilage, which rides on a fibrous pad of cartilage called the *meniscus*. The knee joint is held by four ligaments. The *collateral* ligaments run along the outside of the knee, and the *cruciates* crisscross the inside of the knee, limiting how far the knee bends.

Although the knee is built to withstand large amounts of normal pressure, it is not structurally capable of withstanding the pounding and twisting given it by professional athletes. For example, the lateral, or sideways, thrusts experienced by some football players during clip and blind-sided tackles are among the more dangerous aspects of the game, because they bend the knees in anatomically incorrect directions and result in torn ligaments or sprains. A torn ligament is a serious problem because it can lead to degeneration of the joint surfaces in a destabilized knee; as such, sprains require immediate medical attention.

Runners, tennis players, and other athletes who repetitively pound hard surfaces are also at risk for knee injuries, particularly if they do not wear the proper footwear. Ultimately, the surfaces of the joint and intervening soft tissues can deteriorate, leading to pain and joint damage. A mild sprain causes pain during movement and some swelling in the area just around the knee. More severe sprains can involve the complex cartilage of the knee (shock absorber) and result in a considerable amount of tenderness, swelling, and pain during movement.

Proper footwear, knee supports, and exercise of the muscles around the knee can reduce the chances of knee injuries. For football players, the best prevention is simply not to play the

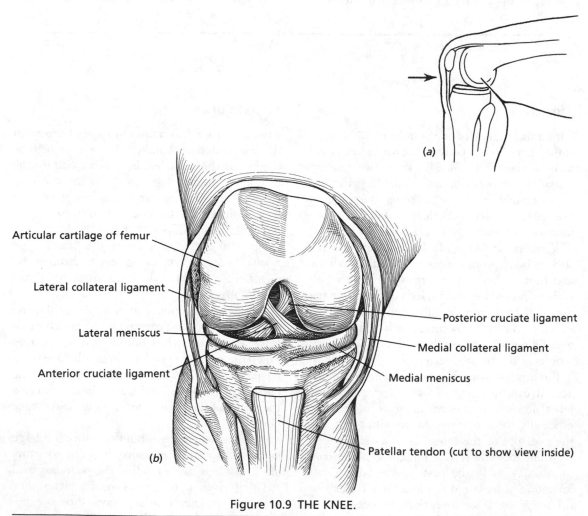

Figure 10.9 THE KNEE.

(*a*) A flexed knee joint. (*b*) The view is from the front.

game. Braces do not protect against injury, but combined with exercise, they can help stabilize the knees of athletes who have previously been injured but choose to play anyway. Other athletes, such as bikers and runners, can follow this advice, too.

OTHER MUSCULOSKELETAL INJURIES

The other major cause of bone or muscle injuries is accidents. Taking a wrong step, improperly lifting a too-heavy box, or being in a rear-end car collision can cause a broken bone, a sprained ankle, whiplash, or a hernia.

Neck Injury/Whiplash

Whiplash is the common term for a neck injury that occurs when the head is flung backward beyond its safe limits suddenly and forcefully, followed by an equally sudden snap forward. National surveys report that this type of injury occurs in one-half million people each year and costs $5 billion in medical and related expenses each year. In the majority of cases, whiplash injuries involve the soft tissues—ligaments, muscles, nerves, and blood vessels—in the neck.

Whiplash is most commonly caused by the impact of a rear-end automobile collision. Although there may be no symptoms immediately after the accident, they can appear within one to four days and range from neck pain that lasts a few days to severe and painful nerve damage that can last a lifetime. Using head restraints and shoulder harnesses (seat belts) greatly reduces the risk of whiplash.

Neck Tension Syndrome

This condition develops in people who sit for long periods in static positions, such as laboratory workers who peer through microscopes, dentists and dental hygienists, and word processors. The syndrome is characterized by neck pain, often followed by headache. It is caused by muscle contraction, which results in diminished blood flow to the muscles and the accumulation of metabolic by-products, such as lactic acid.

To avoid this ailment, take small stretch breaks one to two times an hour and practice relaxation techniques. These minibreaks will allow blood to flow back to the muscle.

Hernia

A hernia is a tear in the wide band of muscles, stretching from the groin area to the ribs, which hold internal organs in place. A sudden strain can cause these muscles to tear, creating a gap that allows organs, such as the intestines, to poke out. The symptoms are the sudden appearance of a lump under the skin along with localized tenderness and, in some cases, a feeling of heaviness in the region.

A hernia can pose a more significant danger if the intestine pushing through the muscle wall cannot properly move its contents; this condition is called *obstructed hernia*. If the blood supply to the protruding section of the intestine is obstructed, it can lead to death of these tissues and, possibly, gangrene.

People who work in occupations that pose the risk of hernia—such as movers, haulers, garbage men, and others—can be trained to perform their tasks in ways that reduce the chance of this injury occurring. Exercises that strengthen muscles in the abdomen, such as sit-ups, as well as using proper form when lifting objects can help people who have been treated for hernia in the past.

CHAPTER 11

Reproductive Effects and Prenatal Exposures

Human reproduction is a complex, fragile process of interdependent events—a complexity that allows it to respond to the impact of external influences but also renders the process of conceiving and bearing new life particularly vulnerable to toxic assault.

Agents that can cause damage to tissue can adversely affect reproduction in a number of ways. They can cause sexual dysfunction in both sexes, disrupt a woman's menstrual cycle, and interfere with the ability of women and men to conceive and bear children. These harmful agents also can affect the physical, metabolic, and eventual mental development of the fetus forming within the womb.

Our daily lives bring us into contact with hundreds of such potentially harmful chemicals and emissions—in car exhaust, food additives, tobacco smoke, and any number of chemical-containing products available in the home as well as at the worksite. Although many of us wonder about the possible threat to our health from these agents, the time prior to conception and during pregnancy are times that, rightfully, bring increased concern.

We cannot expect to completely avoid every environmental agent that can potentially affect reproductive function and pregnancy outcome, but nature does a good job. In any given year, 95 to 97 percent of all children in the United States are born without a significant birth defect. Of the 3 to 5 percent born with birth defects, some 2 to 10 percent (estimates vary) may be caused by environmental, drug, or chemical exposures. Another 2 to 3 percent of birth defects are the result of infections, such as rubella, cytomegalovirus, and hepatitis. The majority of birth defects, however, cannot be linked to a specific cause.

In most instances, even though they are exposed to a potentially hazardous substance, a mother and her developing fetus will not be adversely affected. However, when they do occur, the consequences are so great that these agents merit concern.

By knowing which substances are safe, which are dangerous, how toxins can cause fetal damage, and when exposure to some agents is most likely to cause harm, women and men can make intelligent choices to minimize the risks to their reproductive health and avoid possible harm to their children.

EFFECTS OF TOXINS ON THE REPRODUCTIVE SYSTEM

To protect reproductive health against harm from environmental agents, it is important to understand how fertility can be affected by toxins and why the fetus is vulnerable. The reproductive systems of both men and women can be affected by drugs and chemicals. However, at this point in time, scientists have expended much more effort studying female reproduction than male reproduction, and thus much more is known about the female reproductive system.

Scientists generally make a distinction between the reproductive and developmental effects of a toxic agent. Reproductive toxins affect both men and women. They can interfere with fertility, sexual functioning, or make it difficult to conceive a child.

On the other hand, developmental toxins affect the child as it develops in the womb or postnatally. When a woman is exposed to developmental toxins during pregnancy, the exposure can cause structural and functional abnormalities in organs, alter the child's growth patterns, and/or provoke miscarriages or stillbirth. Increasing evidence suggests that a man's exposure to toxins prior to conception also can have adverse developmental effects on the fetus. (See Chapter 12, "Of Special Concern: Infants and Children," for information on developmental toxins that affect infants and small children after birth.)

Reproductive Effects: How Toxic Agents Can Impair Fertility

There are a number of different mechanisms by which environmental agents or chemicals can affect fertility. Generally, infertility is caused when a drug or chemical interrupts the normal functioning of cells or organs (see Tables 11.1 and 11.2).

Fertility depends upon a number of factors. Women must be able to produce an oocyte, or egg, that is capable of being fertilized. After fertilization, the oocyte must be capable of implantation in the uterine wall. Drugs, such as cancer chemotherapy agents, and chemicals, such as benzo[*a*]pyrene, that interfere with ovary functioning and destroy oocytes can cause infertility (see Figure 11.1 for the anatomic structures of male and female reproductive systems).

Men must be able to produce sperm. The sperm must be of good quality (the right size and shape and capable of propelling itself), must be produced in sufficient quantity, and must be conveyed into a woman's body. Drugs and chemicals can affect male fertility by impacting a man's ability to achieve an erection and to ejaculate and by adversely affecting the quality and quantity of sperm produced. For example, lead exposure has been shown to have a detrimental effect on sperm count.

One way that reproductive toxins are believed to work is by producing mutations in the germ cells (the cells that become eggs and sperm) *prior* to conception. Substances that do this are called *mutagens*. Mutations can be caused by either maternal or paternal exposure to drugs and environmental agents. These mutations change the genetic information, or genetic code, that is imbedded in cells. The change may have no noticeable effect, or it may cause the developing fetus to be born with a mild or severe birth defect. Or, it may cause the developing fetus to spontaneously abort. Examples of mutagens are radiation and ethylene oxide, a sterilizing agent.

Another way that drugs and chemicals impair fertility is by disrupting the production of hormones that control the process of fertilization. Contraceptive drugs work via this mechanism; they suppress the hormones necessary for ovulation. Another drug that affects the fertility by interrupting hormone production is the estrogen drug diethylstilbestrol (DES), which inhibits the release of gonadotropin hormones from the pituitary gland. (DES gained notoriety because of its ability to cause cancer in female children many years after birth [see p. 154.])

Men's fertility can be affected by the suppres-

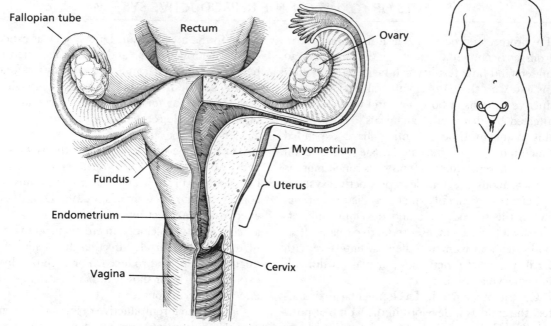

Figure 11.1 (a) THE FEMALE REPRODUCTIVE SYSTEM.

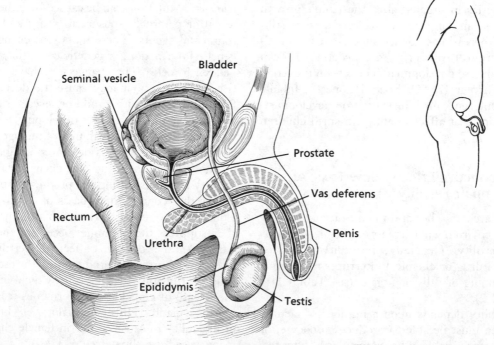

Figure 11.1 (b) THE MALE REPRODUCTIVE SYSTEM.

Box 11.1   THE DISTINCT FEATURES OF THE FEMALE AND MALE REPRODUCTIVE SYSTEMS

The distinct features of the female reproductive system include the ovaries, two walnut-size, spherical organs that secrete hormones and produce eggs, or ova; the fallopian tubes, or oviducts, tubular structures that connect each ovary with the uterus; the uterus, a small, pear-shaped organ located in the pelvic cavity that expands almost one hundred-fold in weight during pregnancy; the endometrium, the lining of the uterus in which the fertilized egg implants and to which the placenta attaches during pregnancy; and the vagina, a long muscular tube that connects the lower part of the uterus, or cervix, to the outer environment. The several muscular layers of the uterus are the myometrium, and the upper portion of the uterus is known as the fundus. The structures of the male reproductive system include the testes, two small walnut-sized structures in the scrotal sac that secrete hormones and produce sperm; the epididymis, the tube in which sperm mature and that connects each testis to the urethra; and the urethra, which, like the vagina, serves as the conduit to the outside environment. When a man ejaculates, seminal fluid flushes the sperm from the epididymis, through the urethra, and out the tip of the penis.

---

sion of hormones. For example, the fumigant 1,2-dibromo-3-chloropropane (DBCP) affects the release of the gonadotropin hormones, thus lowering male fertility. (DBCP is one of the few industrial chemicals where there is definite proof of an effect on male fertility. Both it and DES have been withdrawn from the U.S. marketplace.) It is believed, but not proven, that marijuana may have an adverse effect on fertility by lowering a man's production of testosterone.

Reproductive toxins can also impair fertility by contributing to miscarriages. (It should be noted that miscarriages are common and, indeed, a *normal* part of conception. Perhaps as many as 50 percent of all conceptions are lost in the first three weeks of development, often without a woman realizing she is pregnant; 15 percent of all confirmed pregnancies end in miscarriage.) If defects are so serious that the developing embryo could not survive even if brought to term, miscarriage typically occurs. Because of this, miscarriage is sometimes thought of as nature's way of protecting against pregnancies that are not viable.

Miscarriage can occur if a woman's reproduc-

tive system is damaged by a chemical in such a way that it cannot sustain the pregnancy. In addition, chemical exposures may cause chromosomal defects or other genetic alterations that precipitate miscarriages. However, you cannot and should not assume that a chromosome abnormality and subsequent miscarriage are caused by environmental agents. Most chromosomal defects are the result of preexisting or spontaneous genetic problems.

Developmental Toxins: How the Developing Fetus Can Be Affected

A developmental toxin is an agent that causes damage to a fetus as it develops in the womb. Scientists use the term *teratogen* to describe developmental toxins that cause birth defects or functional problems after birth, although developmental toxins also include such agents as direct abortifacients (substances used to induce abortions). Teratogens can cross the placenta and damage or kill the developing fetus (see Figure 11.2). They can affect the child's morphology (his or her shape or physical characteristics)

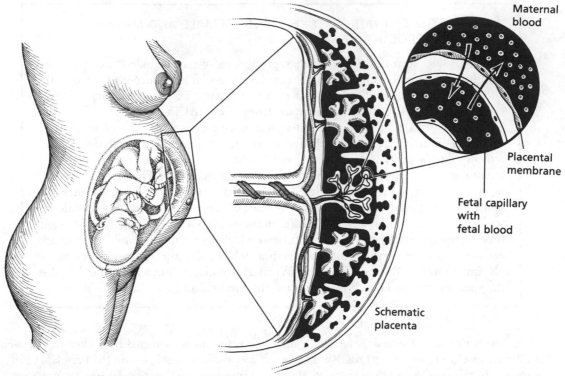

Figure 11.2 MATERNAL–FETAL CIRCULATION VIA THE PLACENTA.

The placenta acts as a conduit between mother and child. Oxygen and nutrients easily pass from the mother's bloodstream into the child's as can many potentially harmful drugs or chemicals. Blood cells do not cross the placenta, except for a small number of fetal cells that cross into the maternal bloodstream. Rather, nutrients and wastes are diffused across the placenta as they pass through tiny blood vessels within the chorionic villi. Chemicals vary in the rate at which they diffuse across the placenta.

or impact on the child's ability to function after birth by causing problems such as mental retardation. Many toxic agents, such as ionizing radiation, have both reproductive and developmental effects.

If a woman finds that she has been exposed to the substances in Table 11.3 during her pregnancy, it does not necessarily follow that her child will be born with any of the birth defects listed. There is a risk element that should be recognized, elevated, and monitored by a physician.

To determine whether a drug or chemical is a *teratogen*, that is, whether it can cause abnormal fetal development, scientists apply these criteria:

- Whether cell replication and cell differentiation, the processes by which the body grows and replaces cells, is affected. Disturbances in cell division can alter the way that cells form tissues and that tissues then form organs.
- How easily the substance crosses the placenta to enter fetal circulation (even if the mother shows no effects from exposure to the substance, it, or its metabolic by-products, may still be toxic to the fetus) (see Figure 11.2).
- When did exposure occur? The organ undergoing the greatest degree of development will

Table 11.1 AGENTS REPORTED TO AFFECT FEMALE REPRODUCTIVE CAPACITY

Steroids
Androgens (natural and synthetic), estrogens, and progestins

Antineoplastic agents
Alkylating agents and antimetabolites

Central nervous system drugs
Alcohols and anesthetic gases/vapors (halothane, enflurane, methoxyflurane, and chloroform)

Metals and trace elements
Arsenic, beryllium, cadmium, lead (organic and inorganic), lithium, mercury (inorganic and organic), molybdenum, nickel, selenium, and thallium

Insecticides
Benzene hexachlorides (lindane), carbamates (carbaryl), chlorobenzene derivatives (DDT and methoxychlor), lindane derivatives (aldrin, chlordane, and dieldrin), phosphate esters (parathion), and miscellaneous (chlordecone, ethylene oxide, hexachlorobenzene, and mirex)

Herbicides
Chlorinated phenoxyacetic acids (2,4-dichlorophenoxyacetic acid and 2,4,5-trichlorophenoxyacetic acid)

Food additives and contaminants
Cyclohexylamine, diethylstilbestrol, dimethylnitrosamines, monosodium glutamate, nitrofuran derivatives, nitrosamines, and sodium nitrate

Industrial chemicals and processes
Formaldehyde, chlorinated hydrocarbons (polychlorinated and polybrominated biphenyls, trichloroethylene, and tetrachloroethylene), ethylene dibromide, ethylene dichloride, ethylene oxide, ethylene thiourea, epichlorohydrin, aniline, plastic monomers (caprolactam, styrene, vinyl chloride, vinylidene chloride, and chloroprene), phthalic acid esters, polycyclic aromatic hydrocarbons (benzo[*a*]pyrene), solvents (benzene, carbon disulfide, ethanol, glycol ethers, hexane, toluene, and xylene), carbon monoxide, methylene chloride, nitrogen dioxide, aniline, and miscellaneous (cyanoketone and hydrazines)

Consumer products
Alcohol (ethanol), tobacco smoke, and flame retardants [tris(2,3-dibromopropyl)phosphate]

be the most severely affected (see Figure 11.3). (Because some organs, such as the brain, continue to grow and mature, even late pregnancy exposure may cause birth defects and complications.)

• The level and duration of exposure. The larger the dose at one time or multiple doses over a longer period, the more likely and severe the effects.

Of the approximately 90,000 chemicals in use in the workplace, only 3,000 to 4,000 have been tested (primarily through animal studies) for their effects on the fetus; hence, for many workplace chemicals, *no* data on their reproductive effects are available. Of those that have been tested, about 30 have been clearly associated with birth defects in humans, and another 1,000 are suspected to cause problems. Many substances are believed to have negative effects on the developing child (such as on birth weight or postnatal development) even though they don't actually cause a physical malformation. (See Table 11.3 for some chemicals that are believed to cause birth defects.) It is usually very difficult to say with certainty if a child's birth defect was in any way due to exposure to an environmental substance during pregnancy.

Table 11.2 AGENTS REPORTED TO AFFECT MALE REPRODUCTIVE CAPACITY

Steroids
  Androgens (natural and synthetic), estrogens, and progestins

Antineoplastic agents
  Alkylating agents and antimetabolites

Central nervous system drugs
  Alcohols and anesthetic gases/vapors

Metals and trace elements
  Aluminum, arsenic, boranes, boron, cadmium, cobalt, lead (organic and inorganic), manganese, mercury (inorganic and organic), molybdenum, nickel, silver, uranium, and zinc

Insecticides
  Benzene hexachlorides (lindane), carbamates (carbaryl), chlorobenzene derivatives (DDT and methoxychlor), lindane derivatives (aldrin, chlordane, and dieldrin), phosphate esters (dichlorvos and hexamethylphosphoramide), and miscellaneous (chlordecone)

Herbicides
  Chlorinated phenoxyacetic acids (2,4-dichlorophenoxyacetic acid and 2,4,5-trichlorophenoxyacetic acid, yalane), kepone (chlordecone), quaternary ammonium compounds (diquat and paraquat)

Rodenticides
  Metabolic inhibitors (fluoroacetate)

Fungicide, fumigants, and sterilants
  Apholate, captan, carbon disulfide, dibromochloropropane (DBCP), ethylene dibromide (EDB), ethylene oxide, thiocarbamates, and triphenyltin

Food additives and contaminants
  Aflatoxins, cyclamate, diethylstilbestrol, dimethylnitrosamine, gossypol, metanil yellow, monosodium glutamate, and nitrofuran derivatives

Industrial chemicals
  Chlorinated hydrocarbons (hexafluoroacetone, polychlorinated and polybrominated biphenyls, and tetrachlordibenzodioxin) hydrazines (dithiocarbamoylhydrazine), monomers (vinyl chloride, chloroprene), polycyclic aromatic hydrocarbons (benzo[a]pyrene), solvents (benzene, carbon disulfide, glycol ethers, epichlorohydrin, hexane, thiophene, toluene, and xylene), and toluene diisocyanate

Consumer products
  Alcohol (ethanol), flame retardants [tris(2,3-dibromopropyl)phosphate], and plasticizers (phthalate esters)

Miscellaneous
  Physical factors (heat, light, and hypoxia), radiation (alpha, beta, gamma, and X rays)

In order for a teratogen to produce effects, it must come into contact with the fetus, usually by crossing the placenta from the mother's blood (see Figure 11.2) (X rays are an example of teratogens that can harm the fetus by directly penetrating tissue). Depending on multiple factors, such as size or fat solubility, different drugs and chemicals have varying abilities to cross the placenta. Any drug, legal or illegal, that has a molecular weight of less than 600 will readily cross the placenta, a size that includes many industrial chemicals. (Molecular weight is the sum of all of the atomic weights of the atoms that constitute the molecule.)

The effect of a teratogen also depends on when the exposure takes place during the pregnancy.

Table 11.3 TERATOGENIC SUBSTANCES

Substance	Known or Suspected to Cause
Alcohol (ethanol)	Craniofacial and limb defects, mental retardation, microencephaly, poor coordination and muscle tone, intrauterine growth retardation, and fetal alcohol syndrome (Risk occurs at more than two drinks a day)
Anticoagulant drugs (blood thinners) (Coumadin)	Fetal Warfarin syndrome, craniofacial defects, central nervous system malformations, microcephaly, hydrocephalus, skeletal deformities, and mental retardation
Carbon monoxide	Cerebral atrophy, mental retardation, microencephaly, convulsions, spastic disorders, intrauterine or postnatal deaths (These effects occur only with severe carbon monoxide poisoning; there is no increased risk of birth defects with mild exposures)
Chemotherapy agents (bisulfan, chlorambucil, cyclophosphamide, aminopterin, cytarabine, methotrexate, and 5-fluorouracil)	Growth retardation; eye, ear, and nose defects; kidney and cardiac defects; hydrocephalus; meningoencephalocele; anencephaly; craniofacial defects including cleft palate; and skeletal abnormalities. (Cancer chemotherapy agents are potent teratogens; however, because of the seriousness of the illness that they treat, most physicians consider their benefit to outweigh their risk. The risk of these drugs causing birth defects is greatest during the period when organs are forming.)
Diethylstilbestrol (DES)	*Females:* Vaginal or cervical cancer; irregular menstrual periods; lowered pregnancy rate; increased rate of premature birth; and increased rate of miscarriage. *Males:* Cysts of the epididymis; cryptorchidism; hypogonadism; and lowered sperm count. (Risk for cancer is greatest when exposure occurs before the 18th week of gestation; perhaps 1 in 1,000 of female fetuses exposed to DES during this time period will develop cancer as adults; another 40 percent or so demonstrate changes in the cells of the vagina; because of this, DES has been removed from the market for this use).
Lead	Lowered scores on development tests, hyperactivity, and learning disabilities. (Risk for these effects is greatest when lead in a mother's blood measures above 0.01 mg/dl [see p. 537]; if the concentration is consistently above 0.025 mg/dl, chelation [removal of lead from the body via chemicals] should be

(continued)

Table 11.3 TERATOGENIC SUBSTANCES (*continued*)

Substance	Known or Suspected to Cause
	considered. However, chelation is not recommended during pregnancy unless the woman is severely symptomatic and at risk of significant health impairment.)
Lithium carbonate (an antidepressant drug)	Defects of the heart and blood vessel, hydrocephalus, and spina bifida
Mercury	Microencephaly, eye malformations, cerebral palsy, mental retardation, and fetal Minimata disease. (Risk is greatest when exposure occurs between the sixth and eighth months of pregnancy; women with children affected by mercury poisoning had blood levels of 9–27 parts per million.)
Polychlorinated biphenyls (PCBs)	Stillbirth, swollen gums, hyperpigmentation, deformed nails, acne, central nervous system damage, and developmental disabilities. (Exposure must be high before such effects are seen)
Phenytoin (an epilepsy drug)	Craniofacial defects; skeletal abnormalities, microencephaly, mental retardation, growth deficiency, neuroblastoma, cardiac defects, cleft palate, and mental retardation
Radiation	Mental retardation, microcephaly, and skeletal malformations (these effects are seen at high doses)
Retinoic acid (an antiacne drug)	Spontaneous abortions, heart and liver defects, hydrocephalus, limb deformities, and neural tube defects
Trimethadione (an anticonvulsant)	Intrauterine growth retardation, cardiac problems, and cleft palate
Thalidomide	Limb defects, hypoplasia, congenital heart defects, renal malformations, cryptorchidism, deafness, and microtia (because of its ability to cause birth defects, thalidomide has been banned from sale in the United States)
Tetracycline	Staining of teeth and destruction of tooth enamel
Tobacco smoke	Intrauterine growth retardation
Valproic acid	Spina bifida, meningomyelocele, central nervous system defects, microcephaly, and cardiac defects

Reprinted from *Maternal-Fetal Toxicology: A Clinician's Guide*, Gideon Koren, ed., pp. 20–24, by courtesy of Marcel Dekker, Inc.

If the exposure takes place before the seventeenth day after conception, it is likely that there will either be no effect or that the effect will be so devastating that the pregnancy will spontaneously abort. During the embryonic period, from the seventeenth day until the end of the tenth week of pregnancy, most of the body's major organs form. The effect that a teratogen will have depends upon what organs are forming at the time it crosses the placenta. The drug or chemical may very selectively target an organ, or it may have multiple sites of action. After the first ten weeks, the effects are more subtle. A drug or chemical exposure at this point in the pregnancy may affect the fetus's growth in the womb or the brain and developing nervous system (see Figure 11.3).

Although these teratogenic effects occur most frequently if the mother is exposed during pregnancy, in very few cases, exposure to a developmental toxin *prior* to conception can cause harm to the developing embryo or fetus. For example, lead accumulates in the body over the years and is eventually stored in the bone (see p. 242). When a woman becomes pregnant, she draws upon the reserves of calcium in the bone, a process that quite possibly may also release stored lead back into her bloodstream. The possible effect of this on the fetus depends upon a variety of factors including the amount of lead released.

In some instances, men can also expose the developing fetus to teratogens. This can happen, for example, if a man works in an industry where he is exposed to substances that have reproductive effects and he brings those chemicals home on his workclothes. (There have been cases where fetuses have been exposed to lead in this fashion.) There is also some scientific speculation that seminal fluid might transport drugs or chemical traces into a woman's body.

For the most part, however, a man's impact on reproductive outcome is limited to two pathways; either through chemical exposure lowering fertility, or through chemical mutagens causing changes in DNA, which may then genetically pass on to the child.

Evaluating Risk

Fortunately, most fetuses exposed to harmful drugs or chemicals manage to be born without any defect, let alone a serious defect. The likelihood of impact depends upon a host of factors—the timing of exposure, the amount (or dose) to which the fetus or mother is exposed, the genetic susceptibility of the mother and fetus, and the characteristics of the drug or chemical itself. It is suspected, for example, that the third week of pregnancy is the time when alcohol causes most of the effects associated with fetal alcohol syndrome (FAS) (see p. 235). Alcohol exposure after the eighth week of pregnancy, on the other hand, is most likely to cause intrauterine growth retardation (IUGR) and perhaps subtle mental and behavioral problems.

Not every exposure to a teratogen will cause a birth defect. It is for this reason that exposure to drugs and chemicals during pregnancy poses difficult choices for prospective parents. There is a risk that a child with a deformity will be born, but there is also a risk that by precipitously rushing to have an abortion, a parent will terminate a perfectly normal pregnancy. For this reason, if a woman is exposed to a developmental toxin, the risk to the fetus must be evaluated by a physician with toxicological expertise.

Scientists generally believe there is a dose–response effect between the degree (or amount) of exposure to a substance and the effects produced. Effects are generally more toxic and destructive at higher doses. What is not known for most drugs and chemicals is the *minimal* dose below which exposure is totally safe. There is general agreement, however, that harm is more likely if the mother consistently consumes large doses of drugs or is consistently exposed to hazardous chemicals.

There are relatively few chemicals that are known with certainty to cause teratogenic effects, although many are suspected of doing so

CRITICAL PERIODS IN HUMAN FETAL DEVELOPMENT

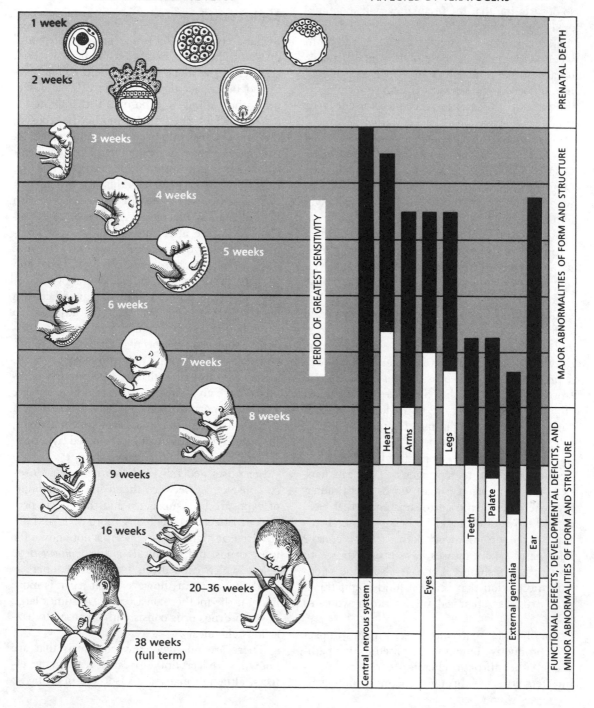

AGE OF DEVELOPING FETUS

CRITICAL ORGANS
AFFECTED BY TERATOGENS

PRENATAL DEATH

MAJOR ABNORMALITIES OF FORM AND STRUCTURE

FUNCTIONAL DEFECTS, DEVELOPMENTAL DEFICITS, AND MINOR ABNORMALITIES OF FORM AND STRUCTURE

PERIOD OF GREATEST SENSITIVITY

1 week

2 weeks

3 weeks

4 weeks

5 weeks

6 weeks

7 weeks

8 weeks

9 weeks

16 weeks

20–36 weeks

38 weeks
(full term)

Central nervous system

Heart

Arms

Eyes

Legs

Teeth

Palate

External genitalia

Ear

(some chemicals pose no risk to fetal development). As noted earlier, relatively few commercial chemicals have been thoroughly evaluated for the possible toxic effect on reproduction and development.

There are two major types of studies conducted to investigate the impact of toxins on reproductive health: epidemiological studies and studies on various animal species. Both types have limitations (see Chapter 2, "Illness and the Environment: Finding the Links").

Epidemiological studies examine the milieu in which a cluster of birth defects or other adverse outcomes have occurred and attempt to trace the cause to a specific source. In many epidemiological studies, only one or two reproductive effects are examined, leaving others open to question. Factors such as age, nutrition, alcohol consumption, or poor prenatal care must be considered or they can skew the results.

Most of the information regarding chemicals and their impact on reproductive health comes from animal studies (ethical considerations obviously prohibit testing on people). The results of these studies cannot always be directly extrapolated to humans. In many cases, the risk of a substance is exaggerated because test animals are given higher doses than a person would normally be exposed to. Also, a toxin that causes defects in one species, such as the rat, may not cause toxic effects in humans or vice versa. In some cases, risk is underestimated because humans may be *more* sensitive to the teratogenic effects of a chemical or drug than the animals used for testing purposes. For example, thalidomide, the sedative that was prescribed to pregnant women for its antinausea effects and caused an outbreak of serious birth defects in Europe and the United States in the 1960s, had no teratogenic effects in rats (see Box 11.2).

More research needs to be done to identify chemicals that pose a threat to reproductive health. At the present time, most birth defects do not have a known etiology. Yet it is certainly conceivable that elements within the environment may cause many more reproductive and developmental problems than we have identified.

Figure 11.3 CRITICAL PERIODS IN HUMAN FETAL DEVELOPMENT.

This chart shows the periods of greatest susceptibility to agents that cause birth defects. The shaded areas in the chart show the time of greatest organ susceptibilities; in the unshaded areas, the organs can still be affected, but usually not as severely.

During the first two weeks after fertilization, exposure to an environmental agent may interfere with implantation of the fertilized egg and/or cause a spontaneous miscarriage but only rarely causes congenital malformations. However, this exposure can cause chromosomal abnormalities that later lead to congenital malformations.

During the third through the eighth weeks of pregnancy—the period during which most of the major organs are formed—the developing embryo is very vulnerable to the effects of environmental teratogens. Exposure to toxic agents can result in major damage to the structure and functions of organs or in death, resulting in miscarriage.

During the fetal period, which begins after the eighth week and lasts until birth, exposure is more likely to cause minor physical defects; physiological defects; slowed growth; or, because the central nervous system is still forming, developmental deficits, such as mental retardation. It is important to remember that each organ has a critical period during which its development may be harmed and teratogens may affect different organ systems that develop at the same time.

Box 11.2   THE THALIDOMIDE DISASTER

Teratogens are agents that cause birth defects. Perhaps the worst teratogen disaster involved thalidomide, a drug widely used in Europe in the early 1960s for its ability to counteract vomiting and as a sedative.

The first case of thalidomide poisoning was reported in 1959 in Germany by a pediatrician named Weidenbach. He had delivered a severely deformed baby girl with phocomelia. The infant's hands and feet were attached to her trunk by stubby stumps resembling seal fins. At this meeting, Dr. Weidenbach surmised that the child's deformities were the result of hereditary defects. Phocomelia is extremely rare; there had not been a single incident of it in Germany in the ten years prior to 1959.

Within the year, however, several more children were born with the telltale deformities. It was not until 1961, however, after a number of children were born with phocomelia and other severe birth defects, that scientists suspected that a common element, perhaps a drug, might be at fault. The drug proved to be thalidomide.

It was immediately removed from the marketplace. However, upward of 10,000 babies, spread throughout some thirty countries, were born with deformities ranging from mild to severe. (Fortunately, the United States was spared much of the thalidomide tragedy because of the Food and Drug Administration's (FDA's) refusal to release the drug until further data proved its safety.)

Thalidomide was touted as an extremely safe drug by its manufacturer, a German pharmaceutical company. In Germany it was sold over-the-counter, and clinical tests had shown it to be a safe and effective sedative. However, it was tested only for *general* toxicity: how much of the drug could be safely taken without causing side effects. No tests for its effects on the fetus were conducted.

Even with testing, it is unclear if the thalidomide's dangers would have been detected. Although thalidomide causes severe birth defects in humans, it does not readily do so in animals. An estimated 20 percent of the children born to mothers who had taken thalidomide during the first trimester period were born with defects. Deformed children were born to some mothers who had taken minimal quantities of the drug, whereas mothers who consumed large doses still give birth to normal children. Scientists still do not completely understand how or why the drug causes such severe birth defects, why some children were affected but not others, and why it is so particularly damaging to humans but not other mammals.

As a result of the thalidomide incident, tough guidelines were passed in the United States and elsewhere that mandate testing for reproductive effects before a new drug is released on the market. These laws have helped to provide protection to mothers and infants (see p. 250).

Several new areas of investigation underscore this speculation. The ability of environmental agents to cause genetic damage is just now beginning to be intensely scrutinized, using newer molecular biological techniques. It is possible that at least some of the defects or developmental problems that are now attributed to unknown causes may actually be the result of environmental exposure. As briefly mentioned earlier, it is known that some chemical exposures can cause changes, or mutations, in a cell's DNA, and it is possible that these changes can be passed along to offspring. Scientists are now attempting to determine if childhood cancer is one effect of genetic damage that can be passed from parent to offspring. So far, there is limited but suggestive evidence that this may indeed be the case.

Another possible effect of environmental exposure is subtle disruption of the hormone systems that govern reproduction. One class of pesticides, the organochlorine compounds (which includes DDT and dioxin), as well as polychlorinated biphenyls (PCBs) may cause changes in sexual behavior or ovulation mimicking the action of hormones (see Chapter 17, "Food Safety," for further information on pesticides). So far, this effect has only been studied in rats and birds, and the scientists involved in the research refuse to speculate on whether humans could be similarly affected because there are no data to support this supposition. However, the research clearly points out one thing: There is much more that we need to know about chemical effects on reproduction.

ENVIRONMENTAL AGENTS THAT CAN AFFECT REPRODUCTION AND DEVELOPMENT

Exposures Due to Self-Administration

A common means by which a fetus is exposed to potential toxins is through a parent's self-administration of drugs, legal or illegal. In men as well as women, drug use and/or abuse can upset the delicate balance of reproductive hormones, leading to sexual dysfunction, infertility, and changes in sex drive.

Self-administered substances with known impact on reproduction and development include alcohol, tobacco smoke (including passive or environmental tobacco smoke), cocaine, opioids, marijuana, and prescription and over-the-counter medications; all can pass through the placenta to enter fetal circulation.

Alcohol. Alcohol is so widely used in our society that most people do not think of it as a powerful and potentially dangerous drug. Some 75 percent of men and 60 percent of women drink alcohol, and, according to government studies, one in ten Americans has a problem involving alcohol abuse (see pp. 741–742 for more information on alcohol abuse). Although most people are aware that heavy alcohol consumption can adversely affect the developing fetus, that it can also affect fertility is less well known.

REPRODUCTIVE AND DEVELOPMENTAL EFFECTS. One reason that alcohol is so damaging is that ethanol and its metabolite, acetaldehyde, are toxins that easily pass through the placenta into fetal circulation. Studies suggest that the more a woman drinks during pregnancy, the greater the likelihood of damage to the fetus, particularly in the first trimester, when the major organs are forming. Fetal damage may be caused directly by alcohol or indirectly by its metabolized toxic by-products. One such by-product, acetaldehyde, may cause birth defects by disrupting cell growth and metabolism.

Excessive alcohol consumption increases obstetrical complications, particularly vaginal bleeding, premature separation of the placenta, and fetal distress. Heavy or frequent drinkers double their risk of miscarriage. Some studies have shown an increased rate of stillbirth associated with heavy drinking as well. There is also some speculation that alcohol consumption contributes to premature delivery, although research in this area is not conclusive.

Box 11.3   HOW MANY DRINKS ARE SAFE?

Researchers do not yet know all the primary and secondary effects of alcohol on the fetus at various stages of its development or why some fetuses are more vulnerable to fetal alcohol syndrome (FAS) than others.

Although there is no conclusive evidence to date that light drinking (one to two drinks a day) severely impacts the fetus or causes physically deforming birth defects, many reproductive specialists believe that all alcohol consumption, however light, should be avoided. There is some indication that even light drinking may cause subtle behavioral changes such as decreased attention span or delayed reaction time. Although a woman who drinks occasionally before her pregnancy is confirmed probably does not need to be concerned, further drinking should be avoided to minimize potential consequences to the developing child.

Heavier drinking is associated with a range of serious effects. The risk of FAS is high if six or more drinks a day are consumed. The risk of fetal alcohol effects (FAE) (see p. 235) increases at two to six drinks per day. Some researchers believe that "binging" (infrequent but heavy drinking) may have as serious an impact as sustained drinking.

Because we do not know the threshold limit for alcohol (the level below which there is absolutely no effect) there is no time during pregnancy when it is completely "safe" to drink.

The most common effect of heavy alcohol intake during pregnancy, however, is lowered birth weight and intrauterine growth retardation (IUGR). These two problems are often accompanied by shorter than normal length and smaller head and chest circumference measurements. They also increase the risk of the child developing respiratory difficulties, feeding problems, infections, and long-term developmental problems, particularly if the child weighs less than 5.5 pounds at birth. The impact of alcohol on birth weight appears to be most severe when alcohol is consumed excessively during the third trimester. Some researchers suspect that a father's regular use of alcohol may contribute to lowered birth weight, although the studies on this are currently inconclusive.

Fetal Alcohol Syndrome. Alcohol abuse, particularly during early pregnancy, carries a high risk of causing FAS, a cluster of irreversible physical and mental defects. Estimates on the number of children born annually with FAS vary, from a low of some 1,200 cases a year to a high of about 7,000. Many more children—perhaps as many as 35,000 to 50,000—suffer less severe alcohol-related birth defects.

Diagnosis of FAS due to exposure to alcohol is made when a child is born with at least one feature from each of the following three criteria:

1. Prenatal or postnatal growth in the child's weight, length, or head circumference is delayed.
2. Certain physical characteristics are present.

There is a pattern of abnormal features of the face and head, including at least two of the following: small head, small eyes or short eye openings, a narrow lip without the center groove, short upturned nose, or flattened midfacial area (see Figure 11.4).

3. There are abnormalities of the central nervous system, with signs of abnormal brain functioning, delays in behavioral development, and/or cognitive impairment.

Many children exposed to excessive alcohol prenatally exhibit some, but not all, of these features. Because of this, the term *fetal alcohol effect* (FAE) has been coined to describe alcohol-related birth defects that are not as severe as those of FAS. FAE can encompass a wide spectrum of birth defects, including eye and heart defects; impairment of the lungs, kidneys, and other organs; slowed growth; musculoskeletal defects; and such behavioral problems as hyperactivity and extreme irritability. Mental retardation is the most serious and damaging of all alcohol-related birth defects.

Postnatally, the effects of heavy alcohol consumption during pregnancy have been associated with behavioral abnormalities and cognitive deficits that may be present at birth or become apparent only later in infancy or childhood. For example, infants of heavy drinkers usually sleep less than other children and are often more restless during sleep. Frequently, their mental and motor development may be slowed. Even alcohol-exposed babies born with normal intelligence, however, may learn to sit, crawl, and master hand–eye coordination later than babies whose mothers did not drink. Throughout childhood, children exposed to alcohol prenatally may show signs of attention deficit disorders, delayed reaction time, and learning disabilities.

Effects on Fertility. Alcohol can also interfere with the fertility of men and women. Although moderate drinking does not generally cause impotence, many men who are chronic heavy drinkers have difficulty achieving or maintaining an erection. Alcohol can damage cells in the testicles, causing a drop in testosterone production.

In women, excessive drinking causes hormonal imbalances that can contribute to infertility and irregularities in the menstrual cycle. Alcohol-associated reproductive problems include amenorrhea (cessation of the menstrual period) and anovulation (cessation of ovulation).

Tobacco. Like alcohol, tobacco smoke has significant and well-documented adverse effects on fertility and on the fetus, affecting a number of processes from sperm production to implantation of the fertilized egg in the womb.

REPRODUCTIVE AND DEVELOPMENTAL EFFECTS. There are links between a woman's use of tobacco and reproductive effects, including miscarriage, IUGR, premature detachment of the placenta (abruptio placenta), vaginal bleeding, abnormalities in placenta attachment to the uterus (placenta previa), and preterm delivery. The greater the number of cigarettes smoked, the higher the risk. For example, in a

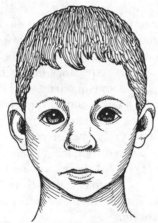

Figure 11.4 PHYSICAL CHARACTERISTICS OF FETAL ALCOHOL SYNDROME.

Note the shortened nose, flattened midfacial area, and narrowed lip.

California study, smoking a pack or more of cigarettes a day was associated with a 20 percent increase in the risk of delivering a baby prematurely.

There are also developmental effects associated with tobacco use. Maternal smoking is linked to giving birth to slightly smaller babies. Smoking ten to twenty cigarettes per day throughout pregnancy reduces birth weight by approximately 200 grams. Although the exact cause-and-effect relationship between smoking and low birth weight is still unknown, many researchers believe that it is related to reduced supply of oxygen. (Some effects of smoking are immediate: Within minutes after a mother inhales smoke, for example, fetal activity decreases and fetal heart rate increases rapidly due to exposure to nicotine and carbon monoxide in the cigarette smoke. When carbon monoxide enters the fetus's blood supply, it attaches to hemoglobin molecules, reducing the amount of oxygen available to growing fetal organs. Compounding the problem, nicotine causes the umbilical artery to constrict, restricting the flow of oxygenated blood from the mother to the fetus.) It is fairly certain that the more a woman smokes during pregnancy (especially during the third trimester), the less her baby will weigh at term regardless of whether or not it is born prematurely.

There are conflicting findings about whether smoking can cause birth defects, such as cleft palate and hernias, and central nervous system abnormalities, such as neural tube defects. Some researchers believe that there is some association, although cigarette smoking is probably not the sole cause for these abnormalities.

Recent studies have indicated that exposure to environmental tobacco smoke (also called passive or secondhand smoke) can also have harmful effects on pregnancy. In one study of 500 Danish women, pregnant nonsmokers who were married to smokers gave birth to babies that were lower in weight than babies born to women married to nonsmokers. Although this is far from conclusive evidence, additional studies seem to bear out this finding. A study of 900 nonsmoking American women exposed to environmental tobacco smoke were twice as likely to deliver a low-birth-weight baby. Infants exposed to passive smoke have more respiratory illnesses than children in nonsmoking households (see Chapter 12, "Of Special Concern: Infants and Children"; see also Chapter 6, "Respiratory Ailments," and Chapter 22, "The ABCs of Staying Healthy," for additional information on environmental tobacco smoke).

After birth, epidemiologic studies and animal research have also shown a correlation between maternal smoking and sudden infant death syndrome (SIDS). For example, a 1990 Swedish study found that moderate smokers (defined as those who consumed between one and nine cigarettes a day) doubled the risk of SIDS, whereas women who smoked more than ten cigarettes a day tripled the risk. Another estimate attributes one-quarter of all SIDS cases to cigarette smoke exposure in the womb. However, SIDS research is greatly confounded by numerous social and economic factors, any one of which may ultimately turn out to outweigh the contribution by smoking itself to the higher rates of SIDS.

Perhaps because babies born to mothers who smoked throughout pregnancy have smaller, less developed lungs, they tend to be vulnerable both to serious respiratory illnesses, such as bronchitis and pneumonia, and delayed growth. There is also some, though not conclusive, evidence that behavior and intellectual development may also be affected by prenatal exposure to cigarette smoke. There is firmer evidence that babies born to smokers have scored lower on neurological tests and seem to be more likely to be irritable and exhibit hyperactive behavior.

Can quitting make a difference? The earlier in pregnancy that a woman stops smoking, the better her chances for delivering a normal-weight, full-term baby (see Chapter 22, "The ABCs of Staying Healthy").

Effect on Fertility. Smoking can impair the fertility of both men and women. In some men, smoking reduces the secretion of testosterone, decreasing fertility; levels of this hormone rise when they quit smoking. Research also shows that some smokers tend to have low sperm counts, "sluggish" sperm, and a greater percentage of abnormally shaped sperm.

The link between cigarette smoking and female infertility is even stronger. On the average, women who smoke take longer to conceive, and those who smoke more than a pack a day are likely to have irregular periods. Women who smoke also have a higher incidence of spontaneous abortion.

Another way that fertilization may be affected is through the concentration of nicotine in the cervical mucus of women who smoke; some researchers believe that nicotine is toxic to sperm. Smoking may also interfere with the hormonal mechanisms involved with the transport of the fertilized egg from the fallopian tube to the uterus.

Finally, cigarette smoking can affect female fertility in two other ways: Studies have shown that smokers have three times the risk of developing cervical cancer in their twenties and thirties than nonsmokers, and women who smoke one or more packs a day reach menopause up to two years sooner than nonsmoking women.

Cocaine.

Cocaine, an extract of the coca plant, is a powerful stimulant that is used medically as a topical vasoconstrictor and a local anesthetic. It has become a widely used illegal drug, however, primarily for the sense of euphoria it creates. Large doses of the drug can create paranoid thinking that may result in bizarre or violent behavior. Crack is the street name for a crystalized form of smokable, rapidly acting cocaine.

REPRODUCTIVE AND DEVELOPMENTAL EFFECTS. Cocaine crosses the placenta and reaches the fetus, and its dangers are probably directly related to its effects on the cardiovascular systems of both the mother and fetus. Cocaine reduces the supply of blood and oxygen available to the fetus by causing blood vessels in the placenta to constrict; this increases the risk of miscarriage and prematurity, especially when cocaine is taken during the last three months of pregnancy. In late pregnancy, stillbirth can occur when cocaine use causes *abruptio placentae*, when the placenta suddenly detaches from the wall of the uterus.

As a result of its cardiovascular effects, using cocaine even once during pregnancy may cause lasting damage to the fetus. Although cocaine and its metabolic by-products are excreted from the adult system within twenty-four hours, they remain in the fetal system for much longer. A fetus may continue to be exposed to the effects of a single dose of the drug for up to five days.

It is well established that babies exposed to cocaine in the womb can have growth deficits. They are more likely to be of low birth weight and may suffer neurologic abnormalities as well as later learning and behavioral problems. However, it is difficult to assess the role played by cocaine in these ailments, because many other factors, including poverty, malnutrition, and multiple-substance abuse, can contribute to these effects. Cocaine-exposed infants tend to be extremely jittery, cry shrilly, and startle at even the slightest stimulation. Motor development may be delayed, and these babies may be slower to crawl and walk. Later in life, such children may exhibit behavioral disorders, such as hyperactivity and attention deficit disorders that are associated with learning disabilities, although this may be overstated because almost no studies have compared cocaine-exposed children to an unexposed cohort.

In some studies, cocaine is also associated with urinary tract birth defects, such as abnormalities in the bladder or urethra; kidney damage; and malformations of the small intestine.

Stopping cocaine use in the first trimester may reduce the risk of low birth weight and prematurity. However, neurologic impairment is still possible. The best action is to avoid cocaine altogether: This drug also threatens the life of the woman using it.

Effect on Fertility. Little information is available on the effects of cocaine on male and female fertility. However, some researchers believe that high doses may inhibit testosterone production in men, leading to infertility.

In men, epidemiologic studies have shown that using cocaine for five or more years is associated with low sperm count and abnormalities in sperm shape. However, laboratory studies of cocaine and sperm have to date failed to prove an association between cocaine use in men and specific sperm abnormalities.

Heroin and Other Opioids.
Opioids act on the central nervous system and many act at other levels of the nervous system as well. This class of drugs includes illicit drugs, such as heroin, as well as such therapeutic drugs as morphine, codeine, meperidine (Demerol), and oxycodone (constituent in Percodan and Percoset). Continuous use of opioid drugs can cause physical dependence; this is common when they are used illicitly. If drug use is stopped, withdrawal symptoms appear that include chills, rapid heart rate, high blood pressure, irritability, nausea, vomiting, goose flesh, insomnia, and muscle spasms.

DEVELOPMENTAL EFFECTS. Opioid drugs cross the placenta to reach the fetus, although it is difficult to assess the effects of opioids on the fetus because, when used illicitly, these drugs are often mixed with other substances. Also complicating the issue is the fact that opioid users, as is true of other substance abusers, are often malnourished and frequently do not receive appropriate general medical or prenatal care. Although the level of drug remains lower in the fetal bloodstream than in the mother's, some 60 to 90 percent of infants born to opioid abusers suffer withdrawal symptoms which, in some cases, can be life-threatening to the neonate. Symptoms of withdrawal range from restlessness and tremors to fever, irregular breathing, and seizures.

About 80 percent of babies born to heroin-addicted mothers have serious medical problems, including hyaline membrane disease (a serious lung disorder), brain hemorrhages, respiratory problems, and low birth-weight. Women who inject themselves intravenously are at risk for HIV infection which can be transmitted to the fetus. Children born to heroin-addicted mothers also generally exhibit irritability, caused by overarousal of the central nervous system, as well as feeding and sleep disturbances.

Research on the result of long-term effects of prenatal opioid exposure points to abnormal fetal brain growth. Animal studies have shown that heroin reduces the number of brain cells, and delays the development of biochemical systems that carry nerve impulses.

Effect on Fertility. Female heroin addicts typically experience decreased sexual desire, as well as menstrual irregularities, which may interfere with fertility. Opioid-addicted women may misinterpret early signs of pregnancy, such as nausea and tiredness, for withdrawal symptoms.

Marijuana.
Marijuana consists of the dried part of the Indian hemp plant, *Cannabis sativa*, and is taken for its ability to alter sensory perceptions. The major psychoactive ingredient is Δ-9-tetrahydrocannabinol (THC), but sometimes the leaves are coated with additional additives. Concentrations of THC in marijuana vary from 1 to 5 percent.

DEVELOPMENTAL EFFECTS. Although animal studies have demonstrated marijuana-caused abnormalities of the heart, nervous system, and urinary tract of developing animals, there is no definitive evidence that the drug causes such birth defects in humans. However, several studies have found that babies born to women who use marijuana during pregnancy are smaller than average, although this has not been a consistent finding.

Like that of tobacco, the smoke given off by marijuana can have potential effects on the fetus by increasing carbon monoxide levels in the mother's blood, thereby reducing oxygen flow to the fetus. One researcher found that newborns of mothers who consistently smoked marijuana throughout their pregnancy were more easily startled and more likely to have tremors than infants of non-marijuana-smoking mothers.

Effect on Fertility. In male laboratory animals, THC lowers testosterone concentration and creates abnormalities in the size and shape of sperm. There is conflicting evidence on whether marijuana or THC has similar effects in humans, although a number of studies do show that chronic marijuana users have lowered sperm counts. In female animals, THC appears to inhibit ovulation and disrupt the menstrual cycle.

Prescription and Over-the-Counter Medications.
Like illegal drugs, many prescribed medications pose a potential hazard to reproduction and fetal development. A pregnant woman should check with her doctor before taking *any* medication; if its use is approved by her doctor, she should follow all directions carefully. Before prescribing a drug, a doctor and the woman should carefully weigh the possible risk posed by the drug against its therapeutic benefits.

Women who must take a drug with known effects on the fetus to treat a chronic medical condition, such as anticonvulsants for epilepsy, anticancer drugs, or lithium to control manic-depression, can face an especially poignant dilemma: Although the drugs they take may increase the risk of birth defects, stopping treatment also may cause life-threatening complications for both the woman and the fetus. For example, seizures during pregnancy can temporarily interrupt blood flow and oxygen to the fetus, causing brain damage, and the risk of continuing to take anticonvulsant medication must be weighed carefully against the risk of possible damage to the fetus.

It is essential that a woman of childbearing age who has an illness that can only be controlled by ongoing drug therapy consult her doctor before planning to become pregnant (or as early as possible in the pregnancy) to determine whether risks to the fetus can be minimized. In some cases, it may be possible to suspend treatment during the first trimester.

Common prescription drugs with known adverse prenatal effects include the following:

Isotretinoin (Accutane). A vitamin A derivative that is used to treat acne, Accutane should never be used during pregnancy as its use is associated with severe mental retardation, defects of the external ear, and defects of the cardiovascular system. Any woman of childbearing age using isotretinoin or other vitamin A-derivative drugs is recommended to use birth control measures.

Antibiotics. Tetracyclines used during the latter half of pregnancy may cause permanent discoloration of a child's teeth. From all studies to date, penicillin (including amoxicillin, ampicillin, and dicloxacillin) and erythromycin, as well as the cephalosporins, appear to have no adverse effects on pregnancy.

Anticonvulsants. Phenytoin (Dilantin) and other antiseizure medications, such as primidone, trimethadione, and valporic acid, have been associated with an increase in heart defects, cleft lip and palate, cognitive deficits, and impaired growth. However, since withdrawal of medication may cause maternal- and fetal-threatening seizures, the risk of stopping treatment must be thoroughly discussed and carefully weighed by a woman and her doctor (for instance, in some cases, the doctor may actually suggest increasing, rather than lowering, the dosage during pregnancy because of an increased risk in a change of the distribution of the drug due to pregnancy).

Benzodiazepines (tranquilizers). Use of tranquilizers near the time of delivery may complicate the delivery and leave newborns lethargic, with respiratory difficulties (including episodes of not breathing, or apnea) and poor muscle tone. The use of diazepam (Valium) during pregnancy has been linked to a fourfold increase in cleft palates, lip anomalies; and malformations of the heart, arteries, and joints. Chlordiazepoxide (Librium) and Al-prazolamam (Xanax) have been linked to abnormalities in the central nervous system.

Common over-the-counter medications. Many over-the-counter drug labels carry the warning, "As with any drug, if you are pregnant or nursing a baby, seek the advice of a health professional before using this product."

Aspirin compounds and substitutes. Even a drug as commonly used as aspirin can cause problems by inhibiting blood clotting in both the mother and fetus and may increase the duration of labor. Because of these effects, the FDA now requires a warning on aspirin bottles: "It is especially important not to use aspirin during the last three months of pregnancy unless specifically directed to do so by a doctor, since it may cause problems in the unborn child or complications during delivery." Ibuprofen and other nonsteroidal anti-inflammatory agents have been required to carry this warning for years. Medications containing acetaminophen have also not been proven safe.

Cough, cold, and allergy medications. Neither antihistamines nor decongestants or cough suppressants have been proven to be safe in pregnancy. There is some suspicion that they may be associated with various birth defects.

Hair care products. Studies of hair dyes, permanent wave solutions, and bleach in animals have not demonstrated toxic fetal effects.

Laxatives. Laxatives are among the most commonly used drugs during pregnancy. No human studies have shown risk associated with laxative use. Castor oil, however, may possibly induce contractions in the uterus and its use is not recommended.

Workplace and General Environment Exposures

Overall, little is known about the extent to which occupational exposures produce adverse reproductive outcomes. Few of the thousands of chemicals used in the workplace have been evaluated for effects on reproductive health, although the National Institute of Occupational Safety and Health (NIOSH) registry lists at least 5,300 chemicals (including lead, mercury, cadmium, glycol ethers, organophosphate pesticides, organic solvents, and vinyl chloride) that are suspected to impair fertility or cause fetal damage.

Although many agents in the workplace are regulated for their health effects, typically the reproductive effects have *not* been considered when limits of exposure for these agents were set; rather, regulatory agencies have based standards on carcinogenicity and other health effects. The Environmental Protection Agency (EPA) and the Occupational Health and Safety Administration (OSHA) are currently working to address this issue.

Men exposed to worksite chemicals, metals, or solvents can potentially lose sexual desire, experience impotence, decreased fertility or sterility, and these exposures may contribute to miscarriage or structural or functional birth defects (see Table 11.2). Women can experience menstrual irregularities and, as described earlier, an increased risk of miscarriage. Children may be born prematurely, be of low birth weight, or suffer birth defects or neurologic problems. Some evidence links occupational exposure and cancer in children, although risk and incidence are poorly defined (see Chapter 7, "Cancer").

Even in the absence of conclusive proof of reproductive toxicity, however, worksite practices on handling and disposing of toxic chemicals need to be viewed with an eye toward minimizing exposures. Employees should also be made aware of potential hazards and taught safe work practices.

Employers cannot exclude women from jobs that carry a high risk of exposure to reproductive toxins. The U.S. Supreme Court ruled that such bans are considered sex discrimination under the Title VII discrimination law; therefore, employers can't simply ban pregnant women but must clean up workplaces to comply with safety regulations (see Box 11.4).

Box 11.4 SUPREME COURT PROHIBITS BANS ON WOMEN IN THE WORK- PLACE

In 1982, Johnson Controls, Inc., the United State's largest manufacturer of auto-motive batteries, adopted a policy banning women of childbearing age from working in jobs that carried a high risk of exposure to lead, which can cause adverse repro-ductive and developmental effects. Only women who could prove they were unable to have children were allowed to retain their jobs; even those who said they had no plans to have children were banned.

Johnson Controls' policy was one of many adopted throughout the 1980s by companies who argued that such restrictions were necessary both to protect poten-tial offspring and to protect the companies from possible lawsuits. In 1990, however, the U.S. Supreme Court ruled that these policies constitute illegal sex discrimina-tion under Title VII of the Civil Rights Act of 1964.

In *United Auto Workers v. Johnson Controls, Inc.*, the court ruled that it is the employers' responsibility to ensure the safety of all workers in a way that does not discriminate. The ruling did not mean that the prohibited jobs should be considered safe, but rather that employers must take steps to *make* such jobs safe for all em-ployees rather than simply enacting a ban on certain employees.

Johnson Controls based its case on the assertion that the fetus is more vulnerable to lead, and that this vulnerability justifies discrimination. However, the United Auto Workers refuted this claim by demonstrating a range of health effects on adult workers of both sexes. Besides being a teratogen, lead is also associated with impo-tence, decreased sex drive, and decreased sperm counts in men, as well as increased rates of miscarriage and stillbirth in the wives of men exposed to lead. There is evidence that the families of lead workers may be harmed by lead dust carried home on the workers' clothing.

In the case of lead and other potential reproductive toxins, there is simply too little known about the hazards to both men and women to prove or disprove a need for different exposure levels, largely because relatively little research has been done on the effects of toxins on *both* sexes. Thus, many public health officials and reproductive health professionals hailed *United Auto Workers v. Johnson Controls* as changing the fo-cus of the debate from job exclusion to the broader issues of general workplace safety and the need for employers to provide adequate protection for *all* their employees.

Agents of Concern. The following are some of the most significant substances capable of affect-ing reproductive health that are commonly found in the workplace and general environ-ment. Many toxins found in the workplace have far-ranging impact. Not only are they dangerous to the employees who handle them, they have become so widely distributed in the environ-ment that they potentially affect the health of the entire population.

LEAD. This soft gray metal is used in a variety of industries and businesses as well as being found in air, water, food, and soil (see Chapter 13, "Water"; Chapter 14, "Air"; Chapter 15, "Soil"; Chapter 17, "Food Safety"; and informa-tion sheet, p. 392).

Lead affects both the nervous and reproduc-tive systems. Exposure to it, both maternal and paternal, has been shown to affect the hormones that control the processes of fertilization, decreasing fertility. For example, battery plant workers, whose work exposes them to high lead levels show decreased sperm counts and increased number of abnormal sperm.

Although maternal high-dose exposure to lead has been proven to cause spontaneous abortion, it is also possible, though not proven, that paternal lead exposure may also cause it. A 1991 Finnish study investigated this possibility. The study found that there may indeed be an association with high lead exposure of men and miscarriage, although there were many variables confounding this result (including the wife's age, her use of alcohol, and heavy lifting during pregnancy). The Finnish study does seem to be supported by animal research, however. One researcher has found in animal studies that male exposure to lead has an effect on fertility and fetal brain development, possibly because of damage to sperm.

Carried by the bloodstream, lead is distributed extensively throughout body tissues, although most of it eventually is concentrated in bone, which acts as a reservoir for future unloading of lead to tissues and blood. Because lead concentrates in bone, as we age the level of lead in the body slowly increases. Although lead does not appear to cause any adverse effect on the bone itself, bone-stored lead released back into the bloodstream can be a continuing source of toxicity even after direct exposure has ceased. This can be a problem during pregnancy, because pregnancy is a time when maternal calcium stores from the bone are drawn upon; in the process, lead may also be mobilized. Once released from the bone back into the bloodstream, lead easily crosses the placenta, affecting the fetus. High levels of this metal have been found in the bone and liver tissue of fetuses, as well as in the blood, brain, heart, and kidney. Umbilical cord blood tested for lead levels at birth correlate with the concentrations of lead in the mother's blood. Lead is also mobilized after menopause as bone demineralization occurs.

At high doses, lead exposure can cause spontaneous abortion, stillbirth, premature birth, and increased infant mortality. The exact level of lead exposure causing miscarriage is still the subject of research. One recent study, for example, showed no association with blood lead levels up to 40 micrograms per deciliter and miscarriage.

Both pre- and postnatally, evidence suggests that lead can have serious effects on the cognitive development of a child. A number of studies have shown that there is a correlation between lead levels and a child's IQ. Infants born to mothers with high levels of lead can have poor motor reflexes and muscle tone. (For more information on the developmental effects of lead, see Chapter 5, "The Brain and Nervous System," and Chapter 12, "Of Special Concern: Infants and Children.")

Workplace Exposure. In the early years of the industrial era, workers were often exposed to high levels of lead, with correspondingly high levels of reproductive problems. In the eighteenth and nineteenth centuries, women who worked in industries using lead were known to have high rates of sterility, miscarriage, premature delivery, and stillbirth.

Lead exposure is now regulated in many large, established industries, but it still poses a major problem in some businesses, such as battery manufacturing. Many small businesses do not have adequate control measures in place, so that individuals who work in fields such as scrap recovery, radiator repair, home remodeling, or construction may still be exposed to high levels of lead. Lead is still a common ingredient in paint used in industrial settings and for exterior coatings because of its weather-resistant properties. "Red lead" is used as a rustproofer and primer for structural steel.

Exposure in the General Environment. Although lead-based paints used in residential structures were banned for use in 1977 because of the dangers of childhood lead poisoning (see p. 258), lead-containing paint chips and household dust from paint applied before the late 1970s are major sources of exposure for children and adults. Exposure via drinking water is also a major concern (one estimate holds that 20 percent of the American population consumes drinking water with significant lead concentrations). Because lead is used in printing ink, repeated burning of newspapers and magazines could be a source of inhalation exposure.

Lead has been banned from most gasoline, but it is still permitted in gasoline for some farm and marine uses and also is used in many gasoline additives (hence, auto emissions continue to be a source of lead pollution). In urban environments, a significant proportion of the lead in the environment still comes from motor vehicle emissions, possibly adding to a pregnant woman's exposure to lead.

MERCURY. There are several types of mercury—elemental (the type found in thermometers), organic (such as methylmercury), and inorganic (see Mercury information sheet, p. 394). Although each type of mercury is slightly different from the others in terms of its effects, most forms can cross the placenta and enter fetal circulation. Mercury concentrates in fetal blood cells in higher concentrations than in maternal blood cells, indicating that its effects may be more substantial on the fetus than on the mother.

Only organic methylmercury is an established human teratogen. The most common exposure to organic mercury occurs due to bioaccumulation in the human food chain: Inorganic mercury discharged into the water is converted by aquatic bacteria to organic mercury (such as methylmercury), a form that is easily stored in fish muscle. Organic mercury is taken up by and accumulates in fish and shellfish, which are then eaten by humans. Fish at the top of the food chain (those that eat other fish, such as swordfish, pike, and trout) have the highest concentration of mercury in their tissues. The EPA has estimated that people who consume more than 30 pounds of these fish a year are at higher risk for mercury exposure; pregnant women or women contemplating pregnancy should probably consume much less (see Chapter 17, "Food Safety").

Organic methylmercury. As with almost all teratogens, the effect that organic methylmercury has on a developing fetus depends upon the time of exposure and the quantity of mercury consumed, although susceptibility to this substance extends over a larger portion of the prenatal period than many other teratogens.

Organic methylmercury accumulates in various parts of the body. Because of this, it can cause maternal hormone imbalances and has been associated with spontaneous abortion, low birth weight, and birth defects. It has a particular affinity for tissue in the central nervous system, which continues to develop after the first trimester and even after birth. It can have dramatic effects on the fetal nervous system. For example, mild exposure can delay development; more severe exposure can cause structural abnormalities in the brain and impair motor and mental development.

Inorganic mercury. In men, exposure to inorganic mercury has been associated with a decreased ability to produce sperm and lowered sexual desire. One recent study found an association between paternal mercury exposure in the preconception period and miscarriage. In women, it can create menstrual disturbances and lead to spontaneous abortion.

Workplace-Related Exposures. Mercury is widely used in industry, including the manufacture of fluorescent and neon lighting, batteries, electrical equipment, pesticides, and fungicides.

Dental workers are at high risk of exposure to this metal because of mercury vapors released by the products used in dental fillings. However, there is no evidence that mercury fillings themselves cause any harm to pregnant women.

There have been several incidences of widespread mercury poisoning with dramatic reproductive and fetal effects as a result of industrial pollution. The most famous occurred in Minimata, Japan, in the 1950s when a local manufacturing plant disposed of its inorganic mercury wastes by dumping them into the nearby bay. The inorganic mercury was converted to methylmercury by aquatic microorganisms, resulting in the contamination of local seafood. A number of infants born to mothers who had eaten contaminated fish suffered severe growth and neurologic problems, although, in some cases, their mothers appeared unaffected by the mercury they had ingested. Many of these children appeared normal at birth, but by six months of age they had developed severe neurologic and anatomic deformities—deformed limbs, disturbed skeletal growth, muscle weakness (including the inability of neck muscles to support the head), convulsions, and cognitive disturbances, to name but a few. As a consequence of the poisoning in Japanese Minimata Bay, the syndrome of mercury-caused birth defects is frequently called Minimata disease (see Box 1.2, p. 25).

Although disposal of mercury is now regulated in the United States, many lakes and streams remain contaminated from past pollution. Regulation does not mean that there is no mercury released in the environment; in fact, a goal of regulation remains the further reduction of air emissions and water discharges. Fish taken from contaminated sources contain methylmercury. Seafood remains a concern in many underdeveloped countries, as the disposal of mercury wastes may not be well monitored (see Chapter 13, "Water," and Chapter 17, "Food Safety").

OTHER METALS. In addition to lead, there are many other metals that can potentially cause effects on fertility and fetal development. Adverse effects have been observed (although not necessarily considered proven) in animals and humans exposed to cadmium, manganese, arsenic, chromium, nickel, and copper, among others (see information sheets for chemical profiles). Individuals who are jewelry makers or who work in mining and smelting industries, battery plants, microelectronic firms, and plastics manufacturing may be exposed to high levels of heavy metals (see Chapter 20, "Art and Hobbyist Materials"; Chapter 21, "The Workplace"; and "The Twenty Common Symptoms and Exposures in the Workplace," p. 422.

Cadmium, which is used in electronics manufacturing and is a component of batteries, paints, insecticides and fungicides, has been observed to cause infertility in both men and women. It is also believed to interfere with implantation of the embryo in the uterine lining.

SOLVENTS. Organic solvents (liquids that are used to dissolve other substances) have many uses in industry. Organic solvents are used in paint thinners, dry cleaning fluids, and many household and industrial products. In the United States, an estimated 10 million workers are exposed to organic solvents. Most solvent exposure occurs through inhalation and may easily pass from maternal to fetal blood.

There are many animal studies documenting the teratogenic effects of solvents and suggesting that they can cause such effects in humans. For certain solvents, reproductive effects include impotence, sperm and menstrual abnormalities, spontaneous abortion, premature birth, and birth defects. A 1989 Finnish study examined the relationship between men exposed to organic solvents and the incidence of spontaneous abortions and congenital malformations among their wives and children. The study found that solvent exposure increased the risk of spontaneous abortion but, at least in this study, did not increase the risk of birth defects.

Toluene. Toluene is a widely used organic solvent. Although the main routes of exposure to toluene are through airborne pollution and skin absorption, traces of this chemical have also been found in water and soil. Toluene is considered a hazardous waste. It is found in many commercial and household products, but especially in gasoline and paints.

A number of adverse reproductive outcomes,

including IUGR, premature delivery, and postnatal neurobehavioral effects, have been associated with toluene exposure. Although it may affect the fetus, it does not appear to affect male or female fertility. (Most studies of this chemical are careful to point out that it is usually difficult to say that toluene caused a specific reproductive effect because, in most commercial uses, toluene is mixed with other chemicals.)

Pregnant women who sniff glue or gasoline containing toluene to create a euphoric, or "high," sensation have given birth to children with defects similar to those seen in FAS (see p. 234). These effects, sometimes described as fetal solvent syndrome, include craniofacial and limb deformities, central nervous system defects, and postnatal intellectual impairment. In these instances, the women absorbed doses of toluene that were very high.

Ethylene glycol ethers. The organic solvents known as glycol ethers are used in the manufacture of semiconductors and are found in products such as industrial paint, varnishes, fingernail polishes, dyes, inks, cleaners, and degreasers (see Glycol and derivatives information sheet). There are more than one hundred glycol ethers on the market; not all have been shown to be harmful, but certain ones, belonging to a group called *ethylene glycol ethers*, have been linked to reproductive effects. There are many animal studies showing an interrelationship between exposure to certain ethylene glycol ethers (2-methoxyethanol, 2-ethoxyethanol, and their acetates) and reduced sperm count; a recent study of shipyard painters demonstrated a lower sperm count in these workers as well as an increase in abnormally shaped sperm. The ethylene glycol ethers also cause birth defects in animals. OSHA is formulating tighter regulation of these ethylene glycol ethers due to their reproductive effects.

Benzene. Exposure to benzene appears to increase the risk of developing leukemia and aplas-

tic anemia; it also may be linked to an increased incidence of menstrual irregularities, spontaneous abortion, and premature births (see Benzene information sheet).

Carbon disulfide. Exposure to carbon disulfide appears to cause irregular menstrual flow and to increase the risk of spontaneous abortion (see information sheet, p. 370).

PESTICIDES. Although pesticides are potent chemicals, their effects on fertility and fetal development have not been widely studied in humans, and their reproductive hazards remain largely unknown. This does not mean that pesticides do not cause reproductive and developmental effects; it only means that they require further study in humans. In animal studies, however, insecticide and organophosphate compounds produced developmental effects including fetal death and malformations.

Two pesticides that were associated with lowered male fertility, 1,2-dibromo-3-chloropropane (DBCP) and kepone (also known as chlordecone), have been withdrawn from the market in the United States. A pesticide similar in structure to DBCP and also known to cause reproductive effects, ethylene dibromide (EDB), has not yet been completely withdrawn from commercial uses.

DBCP was once used to fumigate citrus crops, grain, and soil; it was widely used because it did this effectively without damaging plants. In the late 1970s, this chemical was found to damage the testes and therefore lower the sperm count. The effect was discovered by workers in a California pesticide company, who noted that relatively few children were conceived by those who manufactured the chemical. After submitting semen samples for analysis, the men were found to have lowered sperm counts. This finding was confirmed by studies of DBCP-exposed workers at other sites. The reproductive effects of this chemical on women are virtually unknown.

DBCP has been banned for use in the United States. However, a number of water wells in California and Arizona are contaminated with DBCP. Although it is not known whether the level of this contamination is sufficient to constitute a serious health risk, residents with contaminated well water have been advised to use alternate sources of potable water.

EDB is a soil fumigant formerly used to control insect infestations of grain, fruit, and vegetables. Because of its toxicity and cancer-causing potential, its use was strictly limited in 1984, although unlike DBCP and kepone, it is still on the market. EDB can be found in "antiknock" additives in gasoline (although its use has been declining with the phaseout of leaded gasolines); in several other commercial products, including some fire extinguisher products; and in pharmaceutical manufacturing.

Plant and animal studies have shown that EDB appears capable of inducing changes in DNA structure and, thus, is classified as a mutagen. However, to date, it has not been linked to specific birth defects. Animal and some human studies have shown that it affects spermatogenesis and reduces fertility in males. It is not known to affect women's fertility.

CARBON MONOXIDE. This colorless, odorless gas is widely found in the environment as a by-product of any type of incomplete combustion, such as cigarette smoke, automobile exhaust, and faulty heating systems and furnaces.

Carbon monoxide easily crosses the placenta, where it binds to hemoglobin in fetal blood with such high affinity that it is found in higher concentrations in fetal blood than in maternal blood. The effect of this binding is to reduce the supply of oxygen in fetal blood, possibly causing fetal tissue damage and death.

Acute carbon monoxide poisoning is associated with stillbirth. Chronic low-level exposure is associated with IUGR, which is also seen in fetuses exposed to cigarette smoke (see Carbon Monoxide information sheet, p. 370, and p. 118).

POLYCHLORINATED BIPHENYLS. This group of one hundred plus chemicals were used for commercial insulation in electrical equipment, such as transformers, and in hydraulic fluids and lubricants. PCBs accumulate in the fatty tissues of animals, including humans (see Figure 17.1, pp. 600–601). Birth defects related to high-dose PCB exposure include low birth weight, premature delivery, and small head circumference.

In the late 1970s, manufacturers in the United States voluntarily stopped sales of PCB-containing chemicals for uses that might have environmental consequences. However, years of improper disposal of PCB-containing chemicals have made this chemical a major environmental threat. Disposal of industrial fluids in lakes and rivers have contaminated fish in both fresh and coastal waters; the ground of many industrial sites is saturated with PCBs (see Chapter 13, "Water").

ETHYLENE OXIDE. Ethylene oxide is a colorless, odorless gas that is widely used as a sterilization agent for medical equipment and hospital supplies, such as syringes, gloves, catheters, and a number of surgical instruments. It is also an ingredient used in the manufacture of other chemicals, including ethylene glycol (see information sheet, p. 380).

Because it is highly flammable, use of ethylene oxide is, for the most part, strictly controlled and exposure to it is infrequent. Those most likely to be exposed to this gas are hospital workers who sterilize equipment. (Portable ethylene oxide sterilizers are easily available and are often used in dental offices and other medical settings. The design of these units makes it almost impossible to restrict exposure.)

The gas has been associated with leukemia. Its reproductive effects include damage to DNA and chromosomal abnormalities. In animals, it has been shown to produce lethal mutations. In humans, epidemiologic studies have suggested an association with spontaneous abortions, but the data are inconclusive. Nevertheless, the evidence suggests that pregnant women working in areas where equipment is sterilized with ethylene oxide should be sure that exposures are well controlled. OSHA has established strict regulations for control of ethylene oxide in sterilizing areas, and badges are available to monitor worker exposures.

RADIANT ENERGY. Radiant energy is a broad term that describes the transmission of energy through space. There are two types of radiation: (1) ionizing radiation, which includes X rays and gamma rays, and (2) nonionizing radiation, which includes ultraviolet radiation; visible light; and the electromagnetic waves transmitted by power lines, microwaves, and radio and television transmission (see Chapter 16, "Radiant Energy").

Ionizing Radiation. This form of radiation easily penetrates human tissue and can damage or kill cells. The degree of damage is determined by a numbers of factors, including the type of radiation, the dose absorbed by tissue (usually expressed in terms of rad), and where in the body the dose is absorbed. Because of this, tissues out of the radiation field are customarily shielded (usually by lead aprons) from the effects of high doses of ionizing radiation.

The environment naturally contains low-dose background ionizing radiation from sources such as cosmic rays and radionuclides in soil, rock, and air. Hence, we are all exposed to low doses of such radiation. Nonnatural sources include diagnostic X rays, radioactive fallout from atmospheric weapons testing, and nuclear power plant operations.

Rapidly dividing cells are particularly sensitive to radiation; because of this, radiation can damage the growing embryo. During the first trimester, exposure of the embryo to high doses of radiation may cause birth defects, including microcephaly (an abnormally small head), stunted growth, mental retardation, eye and vision abnormalities, and skeletal malformations.

Exposures later in pregnancy are less likely to cause fetal death or malformation, but delayed or slowed growth can still occur.

Ionizing radiation also has reproductive effects. It can damage the formation of sperm in men, leading to temporary or permanent sterility, depending on the dose. In women, low-dose exposure probably does not cause sterility, but high doses (600+ rads) may do so by destroying eggs (oocytes).

Although ionizing radiation has been observed to cause genetic defects in laboratory animals, studies have so far failed to document a corresponding pattern of genetic disorders in humans whose parents were exposed to high levels of radiation. (See pp. 579–582 for a discussion of the effects of radiation exposure on survivors of Hiroshima.)

Although pregnant women should avoid unnecessary exposure to radiation, there is no medical justification for terminating a pregnancy if a woman is exposed to diagnostic radiation. (Various diagnostic X rays expose a person to a dose anywhere from 0.02 to 5.0 rads.) Where possible, alternative sources of diagnostic imaging, such as ultrasound, are generally used. Women undergoing therapeutic pelvic radiation (e.g., for treatment of cervical cancer) during pregnancy are exposed to much higher doses that may have adverse fetal effects.

Nonionizing radiation. This term describes a wide variety of electric and magnetic waves, including radio frequencies, ultraviolet rays, and microwaves, that may interact with biological tissues (see p. 593 for a description).

Video display terminals. After a 1988 study by researchers at Kaiser-Permanente Medical Center in California suggested that a cluster of miscarriages and birth defects might be linked to video display terminals (VDTs) (the screens used with computers), concern was raised about the effects of these devices on reproductive health.

VDTs produce both ionizing and nonionizing radiation. Ionizing radiation can be potentially hazardous to fetuses; however, in VDTs, ionizing radiation is absorbed by the glass screen and only negligible amounts reach the viewer. The amount of nonionizing radiation emitted by VDTs is comparable to that given off by most electrical appliances and consists of frequencies that are not thought to be harmful. Studies subsequent to the California investigation indicate that VDTs do not pose an increased risk to pregnant women or fetuses. For example, a study by NIOSH of 730 female telephone operators found that the proportions of live births, stillbirths, and miscarriages were similar for both those who worked with VDTs and those who did not. Most experts now believe that the amount of nonionizing radiation given off by VDTs is not dangerous to either the mother or her fetus.

Microwave ovens. Microwave ovens are usually safe at the power levels commonly used in the home and are stringently regulated to avoid the possibility of intense exposure. To date, there is no credible evidence implicating the ovens in birth defects or other diseases.

PHYSICAL LABOR AND PREGNANCY. There is some evidence that strenuous work may contribute to preterm delivery. Women whose jobs involve at least two of the following may be at increased risk: standing more than three hours a day; working at a machine that produces vibration; strenuous physical lifting; repetitive, tedious work; and exposure to loud noise or extremes of hot or cold temperatures. Experts speculate that strenuous work releases catecholamines (stress hormones), which may increase uterine contractions and perhaps decrease placental blood flow.

Physiological changes that occur as pregnancy advances may also increase the risk of injury to pregnant women. For example, the center of gravity shifts, making tasks that involve balance or vertical climbing more difficult and creating a greater possibility of falling. Respiratory demands differ in pregnancy and may alter a woman's sensitivity to airborne dust and other irritants. Prolonged standing can cause faintness or dizziness due to pregnancy-caused changes in blood flow and blood pressure.

Because individual capacities differ, it is difficult to establish criteria for limitations on lifting or physical stress. However, NIOSH has established general safety guidelines on lifting that can be extrapolated to recommendations for lifting during pregnancy.

Among the factors that determine how much weight can safely be held is the horizontal distance between the body's centerline (a straight line from your head down through your body) and the held object. With an object that is held 6 inches from the body, most individuals can safely lift 60 pounds. Holding an object 12 inches away, 30 pounds can usually be lifted without harm. At 24 inches, the safety factor is reduced to 15 pounds. These guidelines pertain to infrequent lifting. Frequent, repetitive lifting requires lighter loads to maintain safety.

Workloads easily handled before pregnancy can usually continue to be handled during early pregnancy. As her abdomen expands, however, a pregnant woman must of necessity hold objects further away from her body's centerline. Thus, under the NIOSH guidelines, it is reasonable to project that as pregnancy advances, the weight of loads lifted should be reduced.

If your job requires lifting or involves any of the factors mentioned here, discuss them with your physician and find out whether you should ask for a modification in your job. Sometimes simple modifications such as lighter lifting, footrests while sitting, or additional rest breaks are sufficient to assure safety during pregnancy. Job modifications and frequent cervical checks are especially important for women who already are at higher risk of preterm delivery due to, for example, an incompetent cervix or a prior history of preterm delivery.

SAFEGUARDING REPRODUCTIVE HEALTH

Although a mother or father's exposure to drugs or chemicals can have an impact on fertility and the developing child, most babies are born healthy despite such exposures.

If a man or woman has been exposed to a potential teratogen, to evaluate risk a physician will need to know the extent and length of the exposure(s), as well as at what point during the pregnancy it occurred. If the exposure happened prior to conception and the drug or chemical has completely passed out of the mother's system, the fetus would not suffer harm. If it occurred during the pregnancy, defining the degree of developmental risk is more difficult.

Prospective parents who believe they may have been exposed to drugs or chemicals that will damage their developing fetus are often desperate for information. Articles in popular journals or newspapers often give inaccurate information or skew their articles to make the risk of exposures seem worse than it actually is.

If you believe you have been exposed to a substance that may harm your pregnancy, the first step in getting information is to ask your physician/obstetrician for advice. If he or she cannot provide you with sufficient information, call a pregnancy hot line or contact the nearest major medical center or university with a medical school. Many of these offer counseling on teratogenicity or have occupational and environmental health clinics that provide evaluation and management of exposed workers and citizens (see also Appendix B).

No one can say for certain which baby will be born healthy and which may be affected by drugs or chemicals. The surest way to avoid harming the unborn child is to safeguard your reproductive health.

Before Conception

There is much that both men and women can do before conception occurs, such as the following:

- Limit alcohol intake to no more than one to two drinks per week (preferably none) if you are trying to start a family.
- Stop smoking. Smoking can cause fertility problems in women and may also damage sperm in men. If you are planning to start a family, it's best to quit. Local chapters of the American Heart Association and the American Lung Association can provide kits to help you stop smoking on your own or can steer you to a smoking cessation clinic (check the white pages of your telephone book). (See p. 731 for information on stopping smoking.)
- Cease taking all nonessential drugs as soon as you decide you want to start a family. If you cannot stop on your own, talk to your doctor about entering a treatment program for substance abuse.
- Consider preconception counseling.
- Identify and limit exposure to potentially harmful chemicals present in the workplace and home.
- Observe all the rules of good nutrition (see Chapter 22, "The ABCs of Staying Healthy").

Once Pregnant

Women can take the following steps to safeguard the developing fetus:

- Stop taking all unnecessary drugs (preferably before pregnancy begins). Do not use any medication prescribed before becoming pregnant without first consulting your obstetrician. Discuss with him or her *any* medications prescribed by *any* physician, dentist, or specialist. There may be alternative medications that are safer for your baby.
- Attempt to identify and limit exposure to potentially harmful chemicals. If work or hobbies, such as gardening or crafts, involve the use of chemicals, consult your obstetrician regarding their possible impact and whether further exposure should be limited.

- Observe all the rules of good nutrition (see Chapter 22, "The ABCs of Staying Healthy").
- Do not smoke.
- Do not consume alcohol.

To Minimize Reproductive Hazards in the Workplace

If you are pregnant or are planning to have a family, be aware that chemicals at your place of work may affect your pregnancy. As explained throughout this chapter, exposure to chemicals can lower the fertility of both men and women as well as impact on the infant's development both within the womb and following birth. Here are some suggestions:

- To learn what kind of chemicals you are exposed to on the job, ask your firm to provide Material Safety Data Sheets (MSDSs). These will provide information on the type of chemicals in your worksite and their known effects.
- If the MSDSs do not list reproductive effects— and they may not—research them out on your own. Bring the MSDSs to your physician and ask him or her if any of the chemicals pose a problem. If your physician is not able to provide such information, your regional poison control center or pregnancy hotline may be able to assist you, or find out if your nearest major medical center or university medical school has occupational health expertise available for you to consult (see Appendix B).
  Note: There are many materials not included under OSHA's Hazard Communication Standard Act, which regulates the use of these data sheets (see p. 359). Noncovered materials include hazardous wastes regulated by the EPA, tobacco and tobacco products, wood and wood products, manufactured items, and food. If

you work in an industry using these products, you will have to do additional detective work to find out the materials or ingredients used in the product being manufactured.

- If you do work with chemicals, find out what kind of protective clothing is recommended— gloves, masks, respirators, and so forth—and make sure you use it. For chemicals covered by OSHA's Hazard Communication Standard Act, the type of protective gear should be listed on MSDSs. However, be aware that sometimes the information in these sheets is general (i.e., wear rubber gloves) rather than specific (i.e., wear rubber gloves made of butyl rubber). Find out if your firm is following proper ventilation procedures. If your company does not provide this information, ask your union or your physician for guidance.
- Ask your community library or union to order medical books detailing reproductive effects of chemicals. Among the best are *Hazardous Materials Toxicology* by John B. Sullivan and Gary R. Krieger, published in 1992 by Williams & Wilkins; *Chemically Induced Birth Defects* by James L. Schardein, published in 1985 by Marcel Dekker; and *Maternal-Fetal Toxicology: A Clinician's Guide* edited by Gideon Koren, published in 1990 by Marcel Dekker.
- If you belong to a union, find out if they have a health safety committee that can help you identify risks and demand protection. If they do not have such a committee, discuss the issue with your representative and attend your union local's meetings to make sure that issues of this sort are raised and become part of the agenda.
- If you don't belong to a union that has a covering health safety policy, you can call your regional poison control center (see Appendix B) or your local health department.

CHAPTER 12

Of Special Concern: Infants and Children

D aily, it seems, we hear alarming reports of air and water pollution, toxic waste sites, and newly uncovered carcinogens that are said to threaten the well-being of our children. One day the news focuses on asbestos insulation hidden in the schools where our children spend most of their time. The next, we hear suspicions that our children's nourishing fruits and vegetables are laced with cancer-causing pesticide residues . . . that our homes are situated dangerously close to power lines emanating low-frequency electromagnetic fields . . . or that the drinking water, soil, and even the paint we used to decorate our homes contain dangerous amounts of lead.

We feel acutely responsible to protect our children from environmental threats, but at times we can't distinguish precisely what constitutes a real risk, particularly when the health effects of many environmental hazards are not yet well understood or reports about them seem contradictory.

In this chapter, we discuss why children might be more vulnerable to environmental hazards and attempt to help prioritize these potential threats to children. (See Chapter 11, "Reproductive Effects and Prenatal Exposures," for information on the impact of environmental hazards on the developing fetus.)

RATING THE RISKS TO CHILDREN

Although the specter of health threats from environmental hazards raises parental concern, not all potential hazards are equal. In fact, the specific risks to children posed by many agents are scientifically controversial, not well studied, or not well defined.

Reassuringly, most public health experts rate the risk to children's health from environmental agents as significantly low on the list of pos-

sible causes of disease or death—significantly lower than risks posed by childhood infections, automobile accidents, or accidents in the home.

However, because the risks of childhood exposures to environmental agents may possibly contribute to cancer, chronic illness, and intellectual deficits, it is important to scrutinize the sources of potential threats.

WHY CHILDREN CAN BE MORE VULNERABLE

Children may be more sensitive than adults to environmental toxins. There are several reasons for this sensitivity:

Infancy and childhood are unique periods in terms of physical growth and mental development. An infant gains weight more rapidly during the first four to six months after birth than at any time during the rest of his or her life. All organs of an infant's body participate in this rapid growth spurt. Thus, chemicals that accumulate in the body during infancy may, in some instances, be incorporated into body tissues in greater amounts than in later childhood, when growth is slower.

This is especially relevant to environmental agents believed to cause cancer. The evolution of a cancer typically begins when a carcinogen interacts with a cell's DNA. In an infant or child, cells grow and divide rapidly. If this rapid division follows exposure to a carcinogen capable of altering DNA, it is possible that this alteration, or mutation, will become a permanent feature of the cell's DNA and be passed on to each subsequently created cell (see Chapter 7, "Cancer," for details on carcinogenesis). Cancers can take a long time—decades, in most cases—to develop: A person exposed to a carcinogen in infancy or childhood may not actually develop a detectable cancer until mid- or late adulthood.

A child's weight is a source of vulnerability. The effects of most environmental toxins are dose dependent, that is, the greater the amount absorbed relative to body weight, the greater the risk of injury. Because of a child's greater intake of food, water, and air relative to body weight, small amounts of a substance such as a pesticide may produce toxic effects in a child, whereas the same dose may be relatively harmless to an adult.

A number of other biological factors also render children more sensitive to toxins. Many of the body's organs and systems are not structurally or functionally mature at birth. For example, in the gastrointestinal system, many of the enzymes in the intestines, liver, and kidneys that detoxify substances are not yet fully operative, which means that foreign chemicals can be retained in newborns for longer periods of time than in adults. Thus, a greater proportion of a chemical is likely to accumulate in the body of an infant compared to that of an older child or adult.

One of the organ systems most susceptible to age-related effects is the nervous system. This is because the nervous system continues to develop after birth; neurons, the cells that comprise the brain, increase in number until about age two. The blood–brain barrier (see p. 89), which blocks many chemicals from entering the brain, is also not yet fully developed at birth. Some researchers believe that lead's effects on intelligence are greater in children in part because the lack of a mature blood–brain barrier allows a higher concentration of lead to accumulate in the brain than when exposure occurs later in life.

Children also have a higher metabolic rate and, because they breathe more rapidly, a higher rate of intake of air per unit of body weight. This means that in the same time period, twice as much of any chemical per volume of air inhaled in the atmosphere will reach the lungs of a child as that of an adult. A child will therefore take in relatively more of the chemicals found in direct or passive cigarette smoke, for example, than will an adult.

What happens when a child is exposed to environmental chemicals? For some toxins, the cause-and-effect results of exposure are direct and immediate. A child who drinks a household cleaner or plays in soil heavily laced with a pesticide may become ill or even die from its acute effect on the central nervous system. However, exposure to even low doses of some toxins, such as lead, can damage a child's health in ways that are not easily detected or that may not be apparent for many years.

The damaging effects of lead on children, such as learning disabilities and anemia, have been well documented (see Lead information sheet, p. 392, as well as pp. 241 and 256). The specific effects of most other environmental toxins on children are less clearly understood, in part owing to the limited methods and number of cases that scientists have at their disposal to gather information on toxins and their effects.

Researchers use animals (most frequently laboratory mice and rats) to study the effects of environmental hazards. If an environmental toxin causes certain physical and functional changes in young rodents, suspicion is raised about similar consequences in young children. However, the quantities of such environmental toxins necessary to cause damage in a child cannot be determined precisely from studies in animal models. Nor can it be assumed that a toxin's effect in another species will be the same in humans because of biological differences between species. For example, parts of the central nervous system that take about ten days to develop in rats can take up to two to three years to develop in a human (see Chapter 2, "Illness and the Environment: Finding the Links").

How Children Are Exposed to Environmental Toxins

Like adults, children may be exposed to chemicals in the environment through what they eat, breathe, or touch. Exposure to chemicals can begin prior to conception, affect the developing fetus (see Chapter 11, "Reproductive Effects and Prenatal Exposures") and continue at birth through breast feeding. For example, chemicals such as nicotine and polychlorinated biphenyls (PCBs) can be found in a mother's milk if she has been exposed to them in her diet, work, or daily environment. (Cow's milk is also subject to contamination by the chemicals and antibiotics possibly found in animal feed.) Drugs, both legally prescribed and illicit, can also be passed through breast milk.

For the most part, chemicals that are easily metabolized and excreted from the body will be found in breast milk only following a recent exposure, as when a drug such as cocaine is taken. However, substances such as PCBs and lead and other heavy metals, which are stored by the body, may be present in breast milk as the result of chronic, long-term, low-dose exposure.

It is important to emphasize that the presence of a chemical or other substance in breast milk does not automatically mean that an infant will absorb the chemical at a level that will cause harm. For most infants, human breast milk is the ideal source of nutrition. Except in cases where high occupational exposure has occurred, the benefits of breast feeding greatly outweigh the risks of harm from environmental toxins.

After infancy, a child's diet expands along with the potential sources of exposure to environmental toxins. Compared to an adult's diet, a child's diet contains relatively greater amounts of fruits and vegetables, providing, relatively speaking, a greater exposure to pesticide residues or any other contaminants that may be present on produce.

Young children search out, touch, and taste the world around them. This oral exploring can bring them into direct contact with toxic hazards, for example, lead in paint chips or dust, chemicals in cleaning agents, or pesticides on floors.

Children's Susceptibility to Toxins

As with adults, the susceptibility to toxins varies from child to child. A number of factors are capable of modifying the effects of environmental toxins.

Nutrition is an important modifier. Deficiencies in vital nutrients can affect the ability to modify a toxin, because such deficiencies may enhance or impede absorption and retention of environmental chemicals. For example, an iron or calcium deficiency may increase a child's metabolic uptake of lead. A child's general state of health is an important modifier as well. Medications or special diets may alter the chemical balance of the intestines and, therefore, increase or decrease the absorption of chemicals (see Box 12.1).

Box 12.1 DIET, EXERCISE, AND CHILDREN'S HEALTH

Diet in infancy and childhood has a major influence on future adult health. What and how much a child eats will help lay the foundation for his or her health in later years.

Not long ago, a diet that led to illness was usually one deficient in one or several nutrients. Today, vitamin deficiency diseases have been largely prevented, but we face another type of dietary imbalance that can lead to disease: nutritional excesses, specifically excesses in fat and cholesterol. Although some fat and cholesterol are essential in the diet, a diet too rich in these substances has been linked to the development of coronary artery disease, this country's most serious and widespread health problem. However, the American Academy of Pediatrics cautions that parents should not go overboard in limiting fat in a child's diet. Children need 30 percent fat in their diets to grow properly; this is the lower limit for fat restriction.

The key to healthy eating is to offer your children foods with a moderate amount of unsaturated fat and to limit foods high in saturated fat and cholesterol. Suggestions for modifying a family's diet may be found in Chapter 9, "Heart and Circulatory Ailments," and Chapter 22, "The ABCs of Staying Healthy."

An adequate amount of exercise is also important to a child's health. The low fitness level of today's children underscores their current lack of exercise. Consider these statistics from the President's Council on Physical Fitness and Sports:

- Nearly one-third of all children in the United States are overweight.
- Fifty percent of all youngsters do not get enough exercise to develop healthy cardiovascular systems.
- Half of all girls and one-third of all boys between ages six and seventeen cannot run a mile in less than ten minutes.
- Forty percent of boys and 70 percent of girls can do only one push-up, 25 percent of kids can't do a single sit-up properly, and 70 percent cannot lift themselves into a chin-up.

Modern conveniences and television make it easy for youngsters to be underactive. All children—boys and girls, born athletes and not—need exercise. Here are some guidelines for making your child active:

- Serve as an example. A child whose parents are fit and active will want to be that way, too.
- Exercise with your child; your participation in the sport or fitness program will make it special.
- Encourage the development of fitness skills: skipping, running, tossing, and catching balls.
- Demonstrate correct movements in a sport or activity, because children learn by mimicry; they need to first see whatever it is they are trying to do.

(continued)

Box 12.1 DIET, EXERCISE, AND CHILDREN'S HEALTH (*continued*)

- Don't push a child into any sport that he or she resists. This can create a negative attitude toward all sports and activities.
- Encourage activities that a child can carry throughout life: gardening, walking, swimming, cycling, tennis, and dance classes are better over the long haul than contact sports such as wrestling, football, rugby, and soccer, which become harder and more dangerous to do as one gets older.
- Check with your pediatrician before letting your child embark on any sport. The doctor can advise you about the appropriateness and level of activity.

Also important is the interaction between environmental chemicals and the social and economic milieu in which a child lives, as well as hygienic practices. For example, family hygiene practices, such as hand washing before meals, may be a determinant of exposure resulting from hand-to-mouth activity in children.

LEADING AGENTS FOR CONCERN

Although there is a new flurry of concern with each new report of an environmental "incident," the challenge to the American public, regulatory agencies, and parents of children growing up in this world is to keep problems in perspective while working to eliminate them. There are a number of substances that parents should be especially concerned about.

Tobacco Smoke

The smoke from cigarettes, pipes, and cigars contains many different chemicals, some of which are as dangerous to youngsters as the air pollutants from automobiles and factories. Cigarette smoke is a major contributor to indoor pollution that threatens the health of children.

There are two types of smoke given off by cigarettes—*sidestream smoke*, the smoke given off by the burning end of a cigarette and the type that primarily affects nonsmokers, and *mainstream smoke*, the smoke inhaled and then exhaled by smokers. Nearly 85 percent of the smoke that fills a room is sidestream smoke, and it contains more highly concentrated amounts of tar, nicotine, ammonia, and carbon monoxide than mainstream smoke. Exposure to this secondhand, or passive, smoke is recognized by the EPA as contributing to bronchitis, pneumonia, and other ailments in children, and as a carcinogen.

The 1986 reports by the National Research Council (NRC) and the surgeon general both concluded that passive smoking adversely affects children's health. These reports, and the Committee on Environmental Hazards of the American Academy of Pediatrics, recommended that children not be exposed to cigarette smoke.

A number of studies have linked parents' smoking to health problems in children. Children who live with smokers are nearly twice as likely as those who live in smoke-free households to suffer colds, asthma, and other respiratory problems, including bronchitis. Children with asthma are likely to be more severely affected by their illness if they live in a smoking household. A 1991 report by the U.S. National Center for Health Statistics found that almost twice as many children who live with a smoking parent were in fair to poor health as compared with children who lived in nonsmoking households. According to a study jointly funded by the National Institute of Child Health and Human Development, the Centers for Disease Control and Prevention, and the Office of Maternal and Child Health, children of smokers suffer significantly more respiratory infections, including bronchitis and pneumonia, and chronic ear infections.

Data from the U.S. National Health Interview Survey suggests that children of smoking mothers spend about 20 percent more time sick in bed than other children. A 1988 study at McGill University in Montreal suggests that exposure to tobacco smoke early in life can create small airway abnormalities that may adversely affect pulmonary function for life. Thus, not only are children of smokers more likely to be sick with respiratory illnesses than children of nonsmokers, they are also more likely to develop respiratory problems.

There are other effects that passive cigarette smoking may have on children. The NRC and the surgeon general have concluded that in adults exposure to passive smoke increases a nonsmoker's risk of lung cancer, although the extent of risk is not clear. It is possible that future studies will document a link between parental smoking and lung cancer later in the life of the exposed child.

There is speculation that cigarette smoke also may cause other health effects. According to a multicenter study of healthy adolescents, passive smoking, like active smoking, may lead to alterations in blood lipid profiles, which are predictive of an increased risk of coronary heart disease. Cadmium, a heavy metal released into the air by cigarette smoke, has been implicated in renal disease.

To protect their children, parents should refrain from smoking in the house and never smoke in the car.

Besides being exposed to toxic fumes, children who live with smokers are also exposed to the subtle message that smoking cigarettes is acceptable behavior. An alarming number of smokers take up the habit as children: More than 52 percent start smoking by age 18, according to the U.S. Office of Smoking and Health. Although most states prohibit the sale of cigarettes to minors, the laws are not uniform and often not well enforced; also, cigarette vending machines are easily accessible to underage smokers. (The U.S. Department of Health and Human Services has recommended, thus far without success, that states and cities ban the machines.) Perhaps the best preventative step parents can take themselves is simply not to smoke and thus not encourage their children to start a practice linked to coronary heart disease, stroke, chronic obstructive pulmonary disease, and cancers of the lung, mouth, larynx, and esophagus. (See Chapter 6, "Respiratory Ailments," and Chapter 22, "The ABCs of Staying Healthy," for information on the health effects of smoking and guidelines for quitting.)

Lead

Public health officials have concluded that lead is the number one environmental threat to children in all economic strata. According to the Department of Health and Human Services, an estimated 15 percent of the nation's children are exposed to lead levels high enough to have an impact on learning ability, and some researchers speculate that the number of children at risk is actually much higher.

Research clearly demonstrates that lead—even in small doses—can slow development, negatively affect a child's intelligence level, and cause learning disabilities and behavioral problems. Children exposed to low levels of lead while in the womb have been found to have impaired intelligence, attention span, and auditory and language functions, as well as behavioral problems such as hyperactivity, in early childhood. Such children may be able to recover from, or at least compensate for, the effects of lead poisoning only if they do not continue to be exposed to lead and if they live in a nurturing environment that fosters learning. Children who continue to be exposed to lead after birth perform poorly on tests that measure cognitive function throughout the first five years of life (see Box 12.2).

In addition to lowered intelligence, epidemiologic studies have associated low-level lead exposure with a form of behavioral disorder known as attention deficit disorder. (In the majority of cases involving this disorder, however, the cause cannot be traced.) Children with this disorder find it difficult to concentrate; they are easily distracted, hyperactive, and find it hard to control their impulses. As a consequence, they tend to perform poorly in school.

Children absorb a substantially higher percentage of lead than adults, and this is one of the reasons that they are more affected by lead than adults are.

How Lead Affects a Child's Cognitive Functioning. Fifty years ago, little was known about the effects of lead on mental development and function. Today, however, researchers know that exposure to lead in childhood can affect a child's mental development with potentially long-lasting effects. Scientists do not yet know precisely how lead exerts its damaging effects. However, a number of promising studies have pointed to some intriguing possibilities.

The brain begins to develop in the first trimester of a woman's pregnancy, but its complex network of cells continues to develop even after birth. (See Chapter 5, "The Brain and Nervous System," for a discussion on how the brain works and Chapter 11, "Reproductive Effects and Prenatal Exposures," for the development of the fetus.) During the first two years of life, the brain can be thought of as "organizing" itself. Its cells, called neurons, develop extensions called dendrites and axons. It is these cells that, with the help of chemicals called neurotransmitters, convey information that is translated into thought, action, and emotion. Over a child's first twenty-four months of life, the density of these cells increases as the brain acquires the complexity that will serve it through life. Lead appears to interfere with the development of this network.

Box 12.2 LANDMARK STUDIES OF LEAD AND CHILDREN

Researchers of childhood lead exposure have projected that perhaps as many as 55 percent of children living in poor urban areas have blood lead levels high enough to cause learning problems. One 1979 investigation by Herbert Needleman of 270 lead-exposed children in Boston, considered a landmark study, helped to definitively establish the role that lead plays in learning disabilities. Children who had high levels of exposure to lead, as demonstrated by the lead content of their baby teeth, showed impaired intelligence, attention span, and auditory and language functions. An interesting aspect of this study was that the teachers of these children had independently rated them as poor performers; those children who were the lowest performers had the highest measured levels of lead.

In 1989, researchers checked up on 132 of the subjects, now young adults out of high school. The results were startling. Those who had high levels of lead as children had a lower class standing when compared to their nonexposed peers. They had difficulty with reading, were clumsier, and had poorer hand–eye coordination. These children also had a higher school drop-out rate. The results of the study imply that the effects of childhood lead exposure persist into adulthood.

How Children Are Exposed to Lead

Many experts contend that the primary route of exposure to lead occurs when chips of lead-based paint are eaten or when lead dust from paint that has blistered, flaked, or powdered off walls is inhaled or swallowed, which is more likely in children who live in houses built before 1977, when the sale of lead-based paint for residential use was banned. Although this ban has begun to limit the number of children exposed to lead in their home environment, the federal government has not effectively dealt with the issue of lead paint contamination in some 24 million homes painted before 1977.

Early formulations of paint contained concentrations of lead as high as 50 percent. Gradually, as the dangers of lead were realized, manufacturers began to lower the levels of lead in paint until all residential lead-containing paint was banned. As a rule, however, consumers should assume that the older the house, the more likely it is not only to have been painted with lead-based paint, but to have been painted with paint containing very high concentrations of lead.

Renovating an older house can greatly increase the danger of lead poisoning if not done professionally or with great caution. Removing old paint by burning, sanding, or scraping can fill the air and coat surfaces with very fine lead particles. The finer the particle, the more likely that it will be absorbed by the lung during respiration. It is also more difficult to remove these fine lead dust particles from the house, especially if the floor boards are splintered or pitted. Special vacuums are required for adequate decontamination. If renovations and the cleanup following the renovation are done improperly, the walls of a house may be free of lead paint, but its floors, carpeting, windowsills, and furniture may be full of lead dust, which may not be noticeable to the naked eye (see Chapter 22, "The ABCs of Staying Healthy").

Drinking water contaminated by lead pipes, solder, and brass fittings can also elevate blood lead levels, as can living by a factory that uses lead in its manufacturing process. (House dust, dirt, and garden soil in these areas have been found to have a very high lead content from airborne lead contamination.) Burning old painted wood can also lead to exposure. Children whose parents work in industries that use lead are also at higher risk for lead exposure, because their parents can bring home lead dust on their work clothes, shoes, hair, and skin.

Living by a heavily traveled highway also can increase exposure to lead. For many years, leaded gasoline was the major source of lead pollution in the air and soil. With the Environmental Protection Agency (EPA)-mandated phaseout of lead and lead additives from gasoline, this source is not as prevalent as it once was, but many truck fuels still do contain lead. Soil in heavily trafficked areas (such as cities) and areas by highways are often contaminated because large quantities of lead settled to the ground in past years (see Chapter 15, "Soil").

Testing Lead Levels in Blood. When a child eats or inhales lead, it enters the bloodstream and accumulates in different organs, including the liver, kidney, and central nervous system, where it causes the symptoms associated with lead poisoning. Because lead appears to concentrate wherever high levels of calcium are found, most of the lead that a child takes in will eventually concentrate in bone, where it is stored. If lead that has been stored in bone is mobilized into the bloodstream, it can be redistributed to other organs, starting a fresh cycle of damage.

To date there is no reliable way to test for the amount of lead in bone, although a new, noninvasive procedure using X-ray fluorescence is now under study and looks promising. Currently, tests for lead measure the amount found in blood.

• It is imperative that children be tested for lead poisoning. According to the Centers for Disease Control and Prevention, unless they live in areas where widespread screening has revealed no problem, all children should be

---

Box 12.3 MINIMIZING THE RISKS FROM LEAD IN THE HOME

If you are concerned about lead levels in your home; here are some guidelines to follow:

- Ask your local health department to check your house for lead or to direct you to sources for home testing kits.
- If tests show that you have a major hazard, do not attempt to remove it yourself. Hire a qualified contractor to remove the lead. Improper lead abatement makes matters much worse. To find a qualified contractor, contact your regional Environmental Protection Agency (see Appendix A) or your state health department.
- Children (and pregnant women) should leave the area until the removal and renovations are finished and cleaned up. If that is impossible, seal off the rooms where the renovations are taking place. During the renovation, remove or seal all furnishings in plastic, including wall-to-wall carpeting. Wet mopping, rather than vacuuming, also is a better way to remove lead dust. Do not use torches or sanders to remove lead-based paint.
- If you are buying a home, try to test for lead and, if necessary, have the lead reduced before moving in.
- Test drinking water: Levels of lead should not exceed 15 parts per billion. If the water contains too much lead, find out why: Check to see if the water is coming through lead-soldered pipes. You may be able to reduce the risk of exposure by running cold water for a few minutes before collecting for drinking or cooking. Teach children to do the same. (See Chapter 13, "Water," for information on testing water.)
- To minimize lead levels in soil, cover lead-contaminated soil with clean soil that has been seeded or sodded, or cover the soil with bark chips or sand.
- Cut back on imported or large-size canned foods and juices as a food source for children; some cans have lead-soldered seams.
- Do not serve food or drinks in amateur or imported pottery; they are likely to contain lead or glazes that contain lead. Don't store liquids in lead crystal; the lead may leach out.
- Be sure that your child's diet has adequate amounts of calcium, iron, and protein, all of which have been shown to diminish the effects of lead exposure in laboratory animals.

---

tested for lead poisoning at twelve months and again at twenty-four months. Even children who do not have overt symptoms of lead poisoning should be tested, because many of lead's effects are subtle. Early subtle symptoms of lead poisoning can include lethargy, fatigue, feelings of irritability, headaches, and sometimes abdominal pain. Behavioral changes, weakness, clumsiness, and a general feeling of sickness can also signal lead poisoning. Frequently, however, there are no overt symptoms that will tell a parent that a child has lead poisoning. Even a physician cannot tell simply by observing a child whether or not the child has lead poisoning.

If a family moves, children should be tested after several months in the new location to ensure that there is no lead exposure.

- If a child shows elevated levels of lead in the blood, immediate measures must be taken. Children should be removed from the source of exposure if it is known. The source must be traced in order to prevent recurring exposure of the child and to prevent other children from being exposed.
- If a child's blood test reveals a high level of lead (above 35 micrograms per deciliter or, in some instances, above 25 micrograms per deciliter), depending upon certain factors, chelation therapy may be considered. This procedure involves giving the child medication(s) that draws lead out of the bone and into the bloodstream and then saturating the child with fluids so that the chelating medication(s) and lead are excreted in the urine. Chelation therapy can have unpleasant side effects and must be properly monitored to avoid damage to the kidneys.

Chelation therapy will often remove enough lead so that the child is no longer acutely poisoned, but it cannot completely remove the lead from the child's body. Once a child's blood lead level has dropped, some damaged tissues may repair themselves with time. Other forms of damage, however, particularly those to the central nervous system (which can include a lower IQ), may be permanent and irreversible.

Because removal of lead from the body is such a serious and difficult procedure and because the effects of lead exposure are so damaging, the best treatment for lead exposure is preventing it in the first place.

Air Pollution

Although there are few studies that directly investigate the effects of outdoor air pollution on youngsters, we can expect that children respond to indoor and outdoor pollutants much in the same way as adults do.

For information on the specific health effects of air pollutants, federal standards, and guidelines on how to reduce exposure, see Chapter 6, "Respiratory Ailments," and Chapter 14, "Air."

Among the leading air pollutants being investigated for their effects on children are the following:

Ozone. Ground-level ozone, which is formed by the interaction of sunlight and nitrogen oxides and hydrocarbons emitted in great quantities in motor vehicle exhaust, irritates the lungs and may lead to permanent structural damage as well as increased susceptibility to infection. Ozone is an outdoor pollutant that is carried by wind, so it has the potential to pollute areas at quite a distance from the actual source of pollution.

Studies of children have shown that exposure to high concentrations of ozone in the atmosphere can affect pulmonary function. For example, a study of children attending summer camp in New Jersey showed that children exercising in the outdoors do experience some impairment of lung function, at least temporarily, during periods when ozone levels are elevated. The long-term effects of exposure to ozone on the lungs of children is still unclear, since appropriate studies have not yet been conducted.

Respirable particulate matter from wood stoves. Particulate matter, tiny solid or liquid particles made up of smoke, dust, dirt, soot, and condensed chemical and metallic fumes, can impair breathing. When wood stoves are used as a source of heat, the wood smoke releases respirable particulate matter (RPM) both into the indoor and outdoor air. RPM particles can be inhaled into the respiratory system if they are small enough to become airborne. The particles can remain in the lungs for months and can cause nose and throat irritation as well as respiratory infections such as bronchitis.

A study conducted in the small Oregon town of Klamath Falls illustrates the problem. During the 1990 heating season, pollution levels in this small community, in which many homes use wood stoves for heating, violated EPA clean air standards on forty-five days. A study of 406 children in the community showed lung function to be adversely affected in the areas of the town with the highest levels of wood-smoke pollution. Additionally, children living in homes with wood-stove heat showed greater declines in lung function than children in homes without wood-stove heat.

Harvard University is currently conducting a major study of the effects of air pollution on children, the six cities study of air pollution and health. To date, the study has found a strong association between concentrations of air pollution containing inhalable particles and chronic cough, bronchitis, and chest illness. It has also found that air pollution can adversely affect lung function, although these changes appear to be transitory and reversible.

Nitrogen Dioxide.

Nitrogen dioxide is released by automobile exhaust, in tobacco smoke, by gas stoves, and by gas-fired or kerosene space heaters. Dispersed in the outside air, the gas itself is not viewed as harmful. However, in high concentrations, typically found indoors or in industry, nitrogen dioxide can damage the lungs and has been associated with bronchitis, pneumonia, and other respiratory illnesses.

One potentially problematic source of nitrogen dioxide in indoor environments is gas stoves. Gas stoves release nitrogen dioxide into the air when used for cooking. The pilot light also creates this gas. When a gas stove is used to heat parts of the house during the winter, indoor levels of the gas can reach extremely high concentrations, exceeding federal clean air standards.

A number of studies have investigated whether or not the presence of a gas stove or gas-fueled source of heat impairs the respiratory health of children. The results have been so inconsistent that no definitive statements can be made regarding these risks. It is probable that the amount of nitrogen dioxide released into the average household by gas stoves is insufficient to cause harm. However, it seems prudent to advise parents who use gas for cooking to keep children out of the kitchen while hot meals are being prepared, not to use gas-fired or kerosene space heaters in a child's room, and not to use a gas oven to heat a house.

Asbestos.

Asbestos is a fibrous material that was commonly used in insulation, especially around heating pipes, and in concrete water pipes until the 1970s. Asbestos fibers are dangerous when released into the air and inhaled (see Chapter 6, "Respiratory Ailments"). With heavy occupational exposure, the fine asbestos fibers taken up by the lung have caused cancers of the lung and pleural membranes.

Widespread concern about the effects of asbestos on children was first raised in the 1970s after national publicity about a New Jersey school in which asbestos sprayed on a ceiling had begun to come off in flakes and chunks. Because the latency period (the time that elapses between exposure and the development of a cancer) is more than fifteen years, there is concern that children exposed to asbestos in schools may develop cancer in later life.

In 1984, the EPA required that all school districts regularly survey their buildings for asbestos; however, in 1990, the EPA also recommended that asbestos-containing material that is undamaged should be left in place and a program be put in place to continuously monitor that the asbestos remains in intact condition. The health risks posed by this material arise only when it is airborne. Improperly removing asbestos can be much riskier than leaving it in place, restricting access to it, and routinely monitoring it to ensure that it is intact.

Pesticides

Pesticide products are used to control pests—among them insects, weeds, fungi, and rodents—and include insecticides, herbicides, fungicides, rodenticides, and fumigants (see p. 607). Children can be harmed by these chemicals if pesticide containers are carelessly left within their reach or if they are allowed to eat or play in soil that has been treated with pesticides.

Fumigants used to exterminate household pests such as cockroaches or termites are particularly dangerous to children because, in their gas form, they readily penetrate the lungs. Children are most commonly exposed to these products by putting objects contaminated with poison residues in their mouths, but there are also some uncommon routes of fumigant poisoning. In California, one infant was hospitalized after his diapers were sprayed with a cockroach extermination product. The pesticide penetrated his skin, causing severe, life-threatening effects to his central nervous system. Children's skin is thinner than adults and poisons can readily pass into a child's system through dermal contact. A child's room, toys, clothing, or bedding should *never* be sprayed with fumigants.

For most children, exposure to pesticides is not a routine occurrence. However, children of farm workers are often exposed to pesticides on a daily basis and therefore are at great risk of developing both acute and chronic health problems as a result of pesticide exposure.

Box 12.4   PESTICIDE EXPOSURE AND CHILDREN OF FARM WORKERS

In the United States, the agricultural work force comprises an estimated 2 million hired farm workers and another 3 million farm owners. They labor under some of the worst working conditions in this country (see Chapter 21, "The Workplace"). One of the dangers faced by farm workers is exposure to pesticides; because the children of farm workers and farm owners either live adjacent to pesticide-laden fields or work in their fields alongside their parents, they, too, face risks from pesticides.

Pesticides must be registered with the EPA before being used in the United States. However, pesticide products can contain so-called inert substances that do not require registration or even testing for health effects. In some cases, the inert ingredients are more toxic than the pesticide itself.

Health problems related to pesticide exposure can include respiratory tract irritation and contact dermatitis. Toxic effects of pesticides on the nervous system can lead to behavioral changes; acute poisoning affecting the nervous system can lead to death. Frequently, pesticide-related illness is mistaken for flu or gastroenteritis. Little is known about the contribution of pesticides to long-term chronic health problems because no appropriate studies on these effects have been conducted.

In addition to the dangers of direct contact, there is the possibility that pesticide residues in food can also cause harm to children. In 1986, a public advocacy group, the National Resources Defense Council (NRDC), conducted a study to determine whether levels of pesticide residues in fruits and vegetables pose a health hazard to preschoolers different than that to adults. Their study implied that children were uniquely vulnerable for two reasons: First, the typical child consumes fruits and vegetables at a relatively higher rate than an adult, and with this increased intake comes greater relative exposure to pesticides present in food. Second, children may be more vulnerable to the effects of toxic chemicals, including pesticides. The NRDC study concluded that, relative to their weight, preschoolers *are* exposed to levels of pesticides that are unsafe, increasing their risks of cancer and neurologic impairment.

The NRDC study is controversial. Nevertheless, the EPA has commissioned a study by the National Academy of Sciences to examine the safety of legal levels of residues in food, which is due out in 1993. The diets of infants and toddlers have been monitored since 1974 by the Food and Drug Administration (FDA). The results of these studies, called market basket surveys, are published regularly. These monitoring programs show that, in general, fruits and vegetables grown in the United States have pesticide residues well within the tolerance levels set by the EPA. Although the NRDC argues that the FDA's levels are too low, that its sampling is too limited, and that the method of analysis is inadequate, the matter remains to be resolved.

It is clear that there are gaps in the scientific knowledge concerning the scope of the potential problem of pesticide residues in food as it relates to children and that further studies need to be done. However, fruits and vegetables are such an important component of a child's diet that they should not be limited because of fear of pesticide residues.

As outlined in Box 12.5, parents can take precautions to limit exposure to pesticide residues.

Electromagnetic Fields

Electric power systems, including power lines, wiring, and lighting in the home, produce electric and magnetic fields. Since the late 1960s, there has been considerable scientific controversy over the potential effects of these fields on health.

In 1979, a study conducted in Denver reported a two- to fourfold increase in childhood leukemias as a result of exposure to electromagnetic fields (EMFs) emitted by overhead power lines. The study was widely publicized and triggered widespread concern among parents (see p. 596 for details of the study). Critics of the study argued that it contained many design flaws, including failure to differentiate other elements that may have been associated with the increased cancer rate.

Since 1979, there have been few studies conducted to confirm or refute the correlation between leukemia and EMFs, and the results have been inconclusive.

However, a more clear-cut correlation between exposure to low-frequency electromagnetic fields and the incidence of leukemia was suggested by a case-control study of Swedish children, which was reported in late 1992. The study included all children with cancer and all adults with leukemia or brain tumors, who were diagnosed between 1960 and 1985, from among the nearly one-half million people living within 300 meters of any 220- and 400-kV power lines in Sweden. The researchers found an association with proximity to the power line magnetic fields and the incidence of childhood leukemia.

Does living by a power line confer an added danger on children? For the moment, pending further evidence, the general consensus in the United States is that fears about leukemia and power-line exposure are unwarranted by the available data. This is not to say, however, that future studies will fail to verify that EMF exposure causes an increase in the risk of leukemia. Abroad, in September 1992, the Swedish National Board for Industrial and Technical Development, NUTEK, announced a new policy, which assumes that there is a connection between exposure to power-frequency magnetic fields and cancer, in particular, as it pertains to children.

Further research is definitely needed to resolve this issue.

Accidents

A child is many times more likely to be harmed in an accident at home or in a motor vehicle than to suffer harm from asbestos, EMFs, or pesticide residues in food. Accidents kill more children under age five than all diseases combined. For example, this year an estimated 135,000 children under age five will accidentally ingest poison and thousands of others will suffer injuries related to household products.

The factors that affect the likelihood of an accident occurring include age, gender (boys

---

Box 12.5 PESTICIDE SAFETY

• Store pesticides away from children and pets (a locked cabinet in an area with ventilation is best). Keep the children and pets away from areas where you mix or apply pesticides.

• Never transfer pesticides to soft-drink bottles or other containers that children associate with something to eat or drink. Always properly refasten lids.

• Rinse fruits and vegetables thoroughly with water, scrubbing them with a brush. Peel them if possible. Although this surface cleaning will not remove pesticide residues taken up into the growing fruit or vegetable, it will remove most of the existing surface residues, not to mention any dirt.

• Cooking or baking foods reduces some (but not all) pesticides.

• If you are growing your own vegetables, find out how the land was used previously. Choose a site that had limited or no chemical applications and where drift or runoff from your neighbor's garden or lawn will not result in unintended pesticide residues on your produce.

• If you get water from a private well, test it for pesticide residues. (Municipal water systems are routinely tested for pesticide residues.) Be cautious about using pesticides and other chemicals on your property, and never use or mix a pesticide near your well head.

• Use pesticides only when absolutely necessary, and then use only limited amounts. When used indoors, provide adequate ventilation during and after application, and keep children out of the area. If you hire a pest control company, oversee its activities carefully.

• If you use an indoor bug "bomb," keep children away from the treated area until thoroughly ventilated (at least overnight), and thoroughly scrub any area where bug spray may have settled before allowing them to play there. The label instructions may state that it is safe to return to the house in several hours; this time period may be acceptable for adults, but it is not acceptable for children.

• Keep children away from chemically treated lawns until the pesticides have settled into the soil (a process that is helped by rain or your sprinkler).

• Take children indoors and close windows before applying pesticides on your lawn or garden.

• If you are applying professional-grade chemicals, have a licensed, reputable firm spread the chemicals, and keep your children in or away from the house while this is being done.

Do not accept bland reassurances by anyone applying pesticides either outside or inside your home as to their safety. They are potentially toxic and can injure children.

---

have more accidents than girls), the child's personality, and socioeconomic status (children from disadvantaged families have a higher rate of injury and more serious injuries than those from more well-to-do families).

Box 12.6 explains how to make the home environment as safe as possible. As for older children, it is important that they learn streetwise ways: how to cross the street safely, how to ride a bicycle, how to travel on public transportation.

Box 12.6   THE CHILD-SAFE HOME

Use the following checklist to identify and correct potential dangers in your home. Some of the precautions relate to environmental hazards; others are general safety tips. Don't depend on close supervision. It's impossible to watch a child every minute of the day.

General

- Install properly placed and functioning smoke alarms. Replace the batteries twice each year.
- Post your regional Poison Control Center number by the telephone in case of an emergency (see Appendix B). Also post your doctor's name and number; the phone number of the local hospital; and your family's name, address, and phone number (for the babysitter). Post these numbers by all the telephones in the house.
- Reset hot water heater settings to prevent inadvertent scalding by children using bathroom or kitchen water.
- Keep buckets and pails out of the reach of children; if they have lids, keep them tightly shut. Dozens of small children have fallen into pails and drowned.

Kitchen

- Keep detergents, cleaning products, lighter fluid, furniture polishes, and insecticides in a locked cabinet or on a high shelf out of childrens' reach. Each time you use a product, secure the lid and store the product immediately after use.
- Keep household cleaners and personal-care products in their original containers with the appropriate label explaining treatment in case of accidental poisoning.
- Always turn pot handles toward the back of the stove when cooking, so that a small child can't pull them over.
- Tie cords from coffee makers, toaster ovens, and other appliances, or fasten wires along the wall with tape or insulated staples.
- Install safety latches on kitchen cabinets and drawers, especially those containing knives and other dangerous utensils.

Bathroom

- Install a medicine cabinet with a lock, or move medicines, vitamins, and mouthwashes to a locked closet. Small children can climb onto the sink and open the cabinet.
- Keep all drugs—both prescription and over-the-counter—in child-resistant containers.
- Destroy old medications by pouring them down the drain or toilet. Don't discard medicines in the trash.
- Keep a 1-ounce bottle of syrup of ipecac in the medicine chest to induce vomiting in an emergency (it can be purchased at a pharmacy). Store the product with other medicines in a locked cabinet.

(continued)

Box 12.6   THE CHILD-SAFE HOME (*continued*)

- Never leave your child in the bathtub unattended, even for a minute. Hundreds of young children drown in tubs each year. When filling the tub, run the cold water first and last, so there's no risk of burns from overly hot water or a hot metal faucet.

Living Rooms, Dining Rooms, and Bedrooms

- Use edge and corner cushions on sharp table corners. Injuries from tables send 70,000 babies to emergency departments every year.
- Cover unused outlets with safety covers or locking switch plates.
- Tie up cords to lamps, stereos, telephones, and other plug-in objects so baby can't pull the items over.
- Securely lock windows; don't rely on a screen to keep the baby from falling out the window.
- Put stickers or decals on glass doors to prevent toddlers from running through the glass.
- Never leave a baby unattended on a waterbed; babies have suffocated in a stomach-down position on waterbeds.
- Keep cigarette lighters or matches away from children. About 200 children die each year in fires associated with lighters; most of the victims are less than five years old.

Garage

- Keep kerosene, antifreeze, paints, solvents, and other hazardous products in their original containers. Never store them in cups, soft-drink bottles, and other food containers.

Pools

- Empty wading pools when not in use.
- Have your child learn to swim as early as possible. Toddlers can learn floating methods for emergency situations before they learn to swim. Community groups, such as YMCAs, often offer water safety and swimming programs.
- Children (even those who have been taught to swim) should not play in pools unsupervised.
- Use arm flotation devices for toddlers, not flotation vests—the vests can actually cause a toddler to tip over in the water and drown.
- Install a child-proof fence around permanent backyard pools for your child's safety and that of neighborhood children. Alarms are available that sound when a heavy object falls in the pool.

Nursery

Many parents assume products designed for use by babies are safe, but about 57,000 babies suffer serious or fatal injuries from the use of baby products each year.

(*continued*)

Box 12.6 THE CHILD-SAFE HOME (*continued*)

Cribs

- Make sure slats, spindles, or crib rods are spaced no more than 2⅜ inches apart. Babies have been injured when widely spaced slats have allowed arms, legs, and torso to slip through, but not the head. No slats should be missing or cracked.
- The mattress should fit snugly: If you can fit more than two fingers between the edge of the mattress and the crib side, the mattress is too small. A baby can suffocate if its head or body becomes wedged between the mattress and the sides of the crib.
- Never use plastic wrapping or bags to cover the mattresses or pillows. The plastic film can cling to a child's face, causing suffocation.
- Make certain corner posts are no higher than ⅝ inch to prevent clothing and cords from becoming entangled.
- Make certain there are no cutouts in the headboards and footboards that risk head entrapment.
- Cribs made before 1978, and particularly those made before 1970, may be coated with paint or varnish containing dangerous amounts of lead. If you plan to use an older crib, refinish it using lead-free paint designed for use on baby products.
- Remove all toys strung across the crib when the baby can push up on hands and knees or has reached five months of age. These babies can pull themselves up to a hanging crib toy and fall over it or become entangled in it, but they can't disentangle themselves or support their weight.

Toys

- Buy toys with a child's age, interests, and skill level in mind. Keep toys with small parts away from small children who can swallow or choke on them.
- If a toy chest has a free-falling lid, remove the lid or replace the hinge with one that holds the lid open in any position. Children have been killed by lids dropping on their heads or necks. Avoid chests with latches that could entrap a child inside.

Strollers

- Use a stroller with a wide base to prevent tipping.
- Be sure the seat belt and crotch strap securely attach to the frame. Be sure the seat belt buckle is easy to fasten and unfasten.
- Test the brakes to be sure they securely lock the wheels.

Changing Tables

- Choose a table with drawers or shelves that are easily accessible without leaving the baby unattended. The baby can roll off the table if left alone for even a few seconds.

(*continued*)

Box 12.6 THE CHILD-SAFE HOME (*continued*)

High Chairs

• Choose a chair has both waist and crotch straps that work independent of the tray, and use them every time. Children have died after becoming stuck when they slid down between the tray and seat of a high chair.

Playpens

• Never leave a child in a mesh-sided playpen with one side in the down position. When the side is down, the mesh forms a loose pocket that leaves a gap between the edge of the floor board and the mesh side. A baby can fall or roll into this pocket and suffocate.
• Look for playpen mesh with a small weave (less than ¼-inch openings), with no tears, holes, or loose threads.
• Make certain wooden playpens have slats spaced no more than 2⅜ inches apart.

Baby Gates

• Accordion-style wooden baby gates made before 1985 may have wide V-shaped openings along the top edge and diamond-shaped openings along the sides that are large enough to entrap a child's head or neck. Choose a gate with a straight top edge or an accordion-style gate with V openings no more than 1½ inches in width to prevent head entrapment.
• Do not count on a gate at the top of stairs to deter your infant: Almost all gates can be dislodged or climbed.

Motor Vehicle Accidents. Motor vehicle accidents (MVAs) are a leading cause of death and injury among children. On average, more than 16,000 children are killed every year and over 200,000 injured as a result of MVAs. Most of the serious injuries children suffer in cars are the result of striking some part of the vehicle interior or of being ejected from the vehicle as the result of a crash. However, a car does not need to be in an accident in order for a child inside the car to be injured; children can be seriously injured by sudden stops or turns as well.

Among the most serious and debilitating injuries children suffer in MVAs are head and neck traumas. Many, if not most, of these injuries can be avoided if the child is properly restrained by a car safety seat or seat belt. For small children, a safety seat offers more pro-tection than a seat belt. Therefore, car seats should be used until a child no longer fits into one comfortably (generally up to the time the child weighs 40 pounds); after that the car's built-in seat belt system should be used. The best position for a child's car seat is the center seat in the rear. Infants should be positioned so that they face backward; this will help spread the impact of the crash across the back of the infant. Toddlers may be allowed to face forward. Some type of child-restraint device is required by law in all fifty states; contact your department of transportation for your state's laws.

It is important to make sure that the safety seat is properly positioned. The seat belt strap should fit snugly around the car seat and the car seat's straps should fit snugly to the child. Do not place the shoulder straps under the child's arms.

Children who are too big for safety seats should be restrained with a seat belt and shoulder harness. The lap belt should be positioned over the thighs, not over the child's abdomen. If the child is too small for the car's shoulder harness (that is, it goes across the child's face or neck), use a safety-designed booster seat (never use pillows or cushions). Never allow a child to stand unrestrained in the backseat or to sit on your lap with the belt around the both of you (in an accident, the child would absorb the greatest impact of the crash.)

SCHOOL BUS SAFETY. Fatal pedestrian accidents can occur when young children get on and off school buses. School-age children—as well as their younger brothers or sisters who may meet them at the bus stop—should be made aware of safety practices on and around school buses. Children should remain seated when aboard a bus, and they and their drivers should be aware of how to use emergency exits. Children should stay ten feet away from the curb while waiting at bus stops; when getting off the bus, they should *never* step into the road until the bus has pulled away from the curb. Often, car drivers will ignore the flashing emergency lights and pass a stopped bus; bus drivers may not notice small children crossing in front or to the sides of the bus—particularly if the child is stooping over to pick up something he or she dropped. Also, make sure your children do not have dangling scarves, mittens, or straps which can get caught in the closing bus doors. You may wish to check with your child's school about the possibility of having adult safety monitors on buses.

Pedestrian Injuries. Motor vehicles can kill and severely injure children who are playing or walking along roadsides; over 1,000 children are killed every year this way and 80,000 injured. Children are most frequently injured by cars when they run out into traffic or play by driveways.

Toddlers and preschoolers are at especially high risk to be injured in pedestrian automobile accidents. They frequently run out into the street after a toy, pet, or older child without regard to oncoming cars. Young children (up to about age seven or so) must be closely supervised if they play near streets and should be accompanied by an adult when crossing the street. Children over age seven should be taught street-crossing skills (how to look for traffic, wait for the light, and so forth) but should still not be allowed to cross streets with heavy traffic on their own. Help your child plot a safe route home from school or from friends' houses or playgrounds; for example, teach them to cross at the corners, not in the middle of the street.

Bicycle Injuries. When children are old enough to ride bikes, make sure they know road safety rules and wear properly fitted helmets. Most auto–bike accidents occur as a result of a young bicyclist entering a road without stopping, turning without warning, weaving into traffic, or riding against the traffic. If the child will be riding the bike at night, the bike should have safety reflectors and lights, and the child should wear light-colored clothing.

Burns. Ninety percent of all childhood burns are caused by house fires. The most common cause of house fires is a smoldering cigarette. Another common cause is a child's experiments with a pack of matches or cigarette lighter—another reason why, if you have children, you should consider giving up smoking.

Children, especially those between the ages of one and two, are likely to be injured by scalding, from tipping hard-to-reach pots and containers. (A child's skin is thinner than an adult's and will scald or burn more deeply, more quickly, and at lower temperatures.) Scalding also can occur if a child drinks liquids that are too hot.

Because of this, a child should never be allowed to play unattended in the kitchen while the stove is on, even for a moment. If you must have the child with you while cooking, keep him or her safely ensconced in a playpen. Erect safety barriers around cooking stoves, electric baseboard heaters, space heaters, fireplaces, wood stoves, or other sources of heat. (Even when unlit, these can present a danger; for example, a child may ingest soot from a fireplace.) Restrict a child's access to such appliances as electric coffee pots, corn poppers, toasters, frying pans, irons, and so forth.

Box 12.7 MICROWAVES AND CHILDREN

Perhaps the greatest risk involving children and cooking at home is the simplest: burning. All children, especially latch-key children, or those who often cook for themselves unsupervised, are vulnerable to numerous kitchen-based risks. The afterschool period from 3 to 6 in the evening (when parents are often at or en route from work) is an especially vulnerable time for accidents among young children. Touching and spilling hot foods are major safety risks when preparing, cooking, and serving foods. The ubiquitous microwave also poses a hazard: liquids, such as those containing oils, can become extraordinarily hot in a few moments. Indeed, the number of burns in children caused by microwaves has been rising in recent years, according to burn center reports.

Many of the burns children experience are not due to spills: The Shriners Burn Institute in Cincinnati, Ohio, has documented that popping a jelly donut directly from the freezer into the microwave for thirty seconds can cause the jelly inside to reach 217°F—above the boiling point of water and hot enough to burn a child's throat.

Common sense and caution are the watchwords for protecting your children in the kitchen. Consider keeping the microwave off-limits until a child is seven years old or at least until your child is old enough to read and understand directions and is able to lift something out of the microwave without precariously standing on a chair or counter (thus risking both falling and spilling hot food on themselves).

Poisons. The number of childhood poisoning fatalities has declined in recent years, due to such factors as increased parental awareness of poisonings, child-proof containers for poisons, and the increased availability of poison center hot lines. However, the actual number of poisonings has not decreased, and thus it remains a serious problem. Medicines (i.e., aspirin and fever and cold preparations), plants, pesticides, and household cleaning agents are among the common poisonous substances that children are likely to ingest. Careless storage of hazardous substances is a major contributor to poisoning accidents, particularly in toddlers and young children; for example, cosmetics left out on bathroom shelves or bedroom dressers are a major source of childhood poisonings.

Toxic materials must be kept stored in locked cabinets. They should be kept in their original containers (so that in the event a child is poisoned, the container and its label of contents can accompany the child to the hospital).

Choking and Suffocation. A child can choke when an object lodges in his or her throat or airway and blocks the movement of air in and out of the lungs. The most common objects are coins and disc batteries. Very young children may choke on food.

Foods that are dangerous for children are

those that are round or sized such that they can obstruct the airway. Hot dogs, grapes, round candies, and nuts are among the foods that can cause problems. Nonfood items include small balls, rattles, and small pieces broken off from toys. Balloons are especially dangerous.

Toys designed for young children must meet standards set by the Consumer Product Safety Commission, which bans toys with small detachable components for use by children under age three. However, parents with older children may not realize that toys built for children over age three may endanger their younger child.

Young children can also die from suffocation if their faces become wedged against a pillow or mattress. The safest sleeping position for an infant is on his or her back, not on the stomach. A child can be strangled within a crib if the railings are spaced more than 2⅜ inches apart or if there is fancy woodwork in the headboard that could entrap a child's head. There should be no room between the mattress and the side of the crib (if you can insert two fingers in this space, the mattress does not fit snugly enough). Anything that can become wrapped around a child's neck (crib toys on strings, pacifier cords, blankets, or clothes with long ribbons or fringe, etc.) can cause strangulation.

Falls. Falls are a serious problem for young children; they account for about one-third of all emergency department visits by children. Danger is related to height: The higher the fall, the more likely that the child will be seriously injured.

Although the most serious falls are from windows on high floors (windows should be equipped with guard rails), injuries to children also result from falling from high chairs, bunk beds, cribs, and other pieces of furniture. Children under six years old should not be allowed to sleep in the top level of a bunk bed. If using a bunk bed, make sure that the space between the mattress and the guard rail will not permit a child to slide out. If there is a space larger than 3.5 inches, attach another board to close the gap.

Falls down stairs are often not deadly, because each step breaks the child's fall.

Baby walkers are dangerous and should never be used. Infants become too mobile when using them and are prone to fall down stairs or pull objects over onto themselves. (A fall down a flight of stairs in a baby walker is more likely to cause death or serious brain injury, because the fall is not broken until the child reaches the bottom stair.) If you allow your child to move about in a walker, he or she must be supervised and strong guard rails should be installed at the top of any steps. Don't use an expandable guard rail with V-shaped slats—a child's head can become stuck between them.

PARENTAL ACTION

If you are concerned about the effect that a specific environmental agent may have on your child, the best action you can take is to become informed. Throughout this book we address many of the environmental risk issues that affect children. For additional information, consult your pediatrician, a poison control center, or the local library. Other organizations, such as the EPA in Washington, D.C., which distributes literature free of charge about environmental hazards, the local chapters of the National Research Defense Council, or the organizations listed in our appendices, can be valuable resources. To form a complete, balanced view, be sure to consult medical sources (journals and books) as well as popular literature.

Twenty Common Symptoms
of Exposure to
Toxic Environmental Agents

Symptom Charts

In the past, patients and physicians alike have been mystified by physical complaints caused by something "right under the patient's nose"—a household cleaner, a chemical used at work, or a plastic or fixative used in a home hobbyist workshop. We sometimes grow so accustomed to the products and practices that we encounter in daily life that we do not even question them as a source of illness or irritation.

We now examine twenty common symptoms of illness in terms of the possible environmental factors found in the home, in the workplace, or outdoors that can cause them.

We hope that these charts will alert you to the ways in which environmental agents can affect your health and make you aware of possibilities and issues that you can discuss with your physician.

Agents encountered in our environment, including the workplace, *can* cause these twenty symptoms and they are often overlooked or ignored. However, the symptoms listed here can also be due to many other factors, including common and relatively minor illnesses. The information contained here should not be interpreted as implying that a symptom is necessarily or most likely the result of an environmental toxin. Rather, the information should be used as an aid in suggesting, eliminating, and identifying possible causes for symptoms with no immediate explanation.

The charts should not be used for self-diagnosis or as a substitute for a doctor's treatment.

HOW TO USE THE CHARTS

The discussion of each symptom is presented in two parts: The first part includes a definition of the symptom and presents a general discussion of its physiological causes and the possible disorders with which it can be associated. The second part discusses possible environmental causes of a symptom using self-assessment questions. Answering "yes" to the questions may reveal possible agents that might be the cause of your symptoms as well as possible sources of exposure.

Consult the information sheets that follow the charts for more information on the agents, including where else they are found in the environment, other symptoms associated with exposure, and whether or not they are particularly harmful to children or cause cancer. (Those agents set in *italics* are not listed in the information sheets.)

Consult "The Twenty Common Symptoms and Exposures in the Workplace," p. 422, to find the possible link(s) between your occupation and the twenty symptoms described here.

SYMPTOMS OF A MEDICAL EMERGENCY

If you develop any of the symptoms listed below, seek immediate medical treatment. Do not stop to consult the charts!

The following list, developed by the American College of Emergency Physicians, identifies emergency symptoms that are life-threatening or strongly indicate a serious condition and require prompt attention.

Abdominal pain if it is accompanied by continuous vomiting.

Severe asthma attacks that do not respond to normal asthma medication.

Insect bites or stings if they cause severe swelling, a generalized rash, or difficulty breathing.

Any pain resulting from injury if it is too severe to allow weight bearing or normal movement. This may be a sign of fracture, even if there is no swelling or deformity.

Permanent teeth that are knocked out. Place the tooth in a cup of milk and bring to the dentist or an emergency department. The replacement must be made within two hours.

Burns if they involve significant blistering or charring or involve the palms of the hands, the soles of the feet, the face, or groin.

Colds if they last more than one week.

Cuts if they are deep, bleed heavily, cause loss of movement or function, or have separated edges.

Eye injuries: from chemicals, acids, alkalis, or solid objects. In the case of chemicals, acids, and alkali irritants, flush the eye with water for ten to fif-teen minutes, then see a physician immediately. In the case of solid objects, *do not rub* the eye or apply pressure; cover lightly with a gauze or cloth patch and see a physician.

Foreign bodies in the nose or ears.

Chest pain if there is uncomfortable pressure, fullness, or squeezing pain in the center of the chest lasting two minutes or more or pain that spreads to the neck, arms, shoulders, or back. These symptoms can indicate a heart attack.

A head injury if it causes loss of consciousness, vomiting, sleepiness, difficulty in arousing the victim, change in mental acuity, or headache unrelieved by over-the-counter pain relievers.

Rashes if they look like small bleeding spots beneath the skin, are accompanied by high fever or sleepiness, or occur inside the eye or mouth.

Seizures. Move harmful objects out of the way of the victim, roll onto left side to prevent choking if vomiting, start rescue breathing if breathing ceases or is obstructed.

Vomiting or diarrhea if it lasts over twenty-four hours (twelve hours in the case of an infant), or at any time when either is bloody.

CONCEPTION DIFFICULTIES

For human reproduction to be successful and produce healthy babies, a complex system of hormone production, sex cell production, and libido must function and be well timed. The delicate nature of this system is evidenced by the prevalence of infertility; in the United States, more than one in eight couples is labeled as infertile.

The cause for many disorders of reproduction remains unknown. Various factors may contribute to infertility. Infrequent intercourse will limit the chances that sperm will be present when an egg is released into the fallopian tubes. Many physiological disruptions can interfere with conception, the successful joining of sperm and egg and its implantation in the wall of the uterus. (See Chapter 11, "Reproductive Effects and Prenatal Exposures," for more information.)

Illnesses That Affect Fertility

Illnesses such as sexually transmitted diseases, diabetes, thyroid disorders, and tuberculosis; emotional problems; or even noise have been linked to infertility in the female. In males, both emotional and physical stress may alter hormonal cycles and the production of sperm. Among these physical factors are heat, which may be caused by hot baths, weather, or restrictive undergarments; light; illnesses such as mumps and liver and hormone disorders; and lack of adequate oxygen (hypoxia). Undescended testes (cryptorchidism) can increase the temperature of the testes and diminish sperm counts.

Medications That Affect Fertility

Many drugs may affect both the male and female reproductive capacity. Among those that affect female fertility are corticosteroids; diethylestilbestrol; androgens; estrogens; progestins; anti-cancer drugs, such as antineoplastic agents, alkylating agents, and antimetabolites; drugs affecting the central nervous system; and anesthetic gases.

Drugs that are spermatotoxins, damaging or stopping production of sperm in males, include amiodarone, an antiarrhythmic drug; analogs of cyclosporine, an immune suppressant medication; valproic acid, an antiepileptic drug; and cancer chemotherapeutic agents.

Environmental Agents That Affect Fertility

Some research has focused on the direct effects that toxins may have on the female. Recently, there has been increased awareness that toxins may affect exposed males.

If you are having difficulty conceiving and you answer "yes" to any of the following questions, you should be aware of the possibility of toxic exposure.

ENVIRONMENTAL CONSIDERATIONS IN CONCEPTION DIFFICULTIES

Questions to Ask About Your Surroundings and Activities	Toxic Possibilities If You Answered Yes*	What to Do
Do you live in an old house with flaking paint and old plumbing? Are you renovating an old house? Do you live in an inner city?	You may be exposed to lead by eating paint chips, inhaling dust, or drinking contaminated tap water. Renovating may expose you to lead in old paint and pipes. Lead is a known spermatotoxin.	Consult your doctor. Avoid further exposure.
Do you live in a mobile home? Do you spend a lot of time indoors where there are gas appliances, new carpeting, particle board, or foam insulation?	All of these are sources of exposure to formaldehyde.	Improve ventilation in your home. Inform your doctor of your potential exposure.
Do you live near a smelter or other hazardous waste site?	There may be high levels of lead, arsenic, or cadmium emitted in the air near these facilities.	If symptoms persist, inform your physician about your place of residence.
Have you placed any pesticide products in your home?	Some roach powders contain boric acid.	Discontinue application of this pesticide and inform your doctor of your possible exposure.
Do you drink well water?	Well water may be contaminated by arsenic from natural sources.	Have your drinking water tested. Inform your doctor of the possibility of toxic exposure.
Do you regularly drink alcoholic beverages?	Drinking alcohol (ethanol) is believed to lower a man's production of the hormone testosterone and therefore may contribute to infertility.	Stop or reduce your alcohol consumption. Consult your doctor or a counselor if necessary for help.
Do you drink home-distilled moonshine whiskey or wine? Do you eat from glazed pottery dishes or cook with leaden pots?	All these are possible sources of exposure to arsenic, as well as lead, which is a known spermatotoxin.	Consult your doctor. Replace dishes and cookware with lead-free kitchenware. Discontinue drinking homemade alcoholic beverages.
Have you eaten seafood, bread, or seed grain?	Ordinarily these foods are safe, but in the past, environmental disasters have affected these foodstuffs, and it could possibly occur again. Fish has been contaminated with methylmercury from industrial discharge. Methylmercury is used as a fungicide for seeds intended for planting, but, in the past, these seeds have been accidentally ingested.	Consult your doctor. Discontinue eating these foods until the problem is resolved.

(continued)

ENVIRONMENTAL CONSIDERATIONS IN CONCEPTION DIFFICULTIES (*continued*)

Questions to Ask About Your Surroundings and Activities	*Toxic Possibilities If You Answered Yes**	*What to Do*
Are you taking dietary supplements, homeopathic medicines, products sold in health food stores, herbal medicines, or folk remedies?	Some of these products have contained contaminants such as arsenic and lead, a known spermatotoxin.	Inform your doctor of these supplements. Discontinue using folk medicines, which may cause other symptoms.
Do you smoke cigarettes? Are you exposed to side-stream smoke?	Cigarette smoking can impair the fertility of both men and women. You are inhaling nicotine, polycylic aromatic hydrocarbons, and tobacco contaminants, such as cadmium and formaldehyde.	Seek help to quit or reduce smoking. Avoid people who are smoking.
Do you smoke marijuana?	Tetrahydrocannabinol, the psychoactive ingredient in marijuana, lowers testosterone levels, affects sperm size and shape, and disrupts the menstrual cycle in laboratory animals.	Quit smoking marijuana.
Do you use cocaine, crack, heroin, or other illicit drugs?	Cocaine may inhibit testosterone production and decrease sperm counts leading to infertility. Women using heroin and other opioids have a decreased sexual desire. Also, many of these substances are contaminated with toxins, such as arsenic and lead, a known spermatotoxin.	Seek help to discontinue your substance abuse. Continued use of illicitly prepared drugs puts you at risk of exposure to many toxins.
Do you intentionally sniff glue or adhesives either to get high or because you use it in a hobby?	Inhaled glue or adhesives may contain toluene.	Seek help to discontinue abusing this substance. Hobbyists should ensure proper ventilation.
Do you work in a darkroom?	You may be exposed to benzene, boric acid, cadmium, formaldehyde, and mercury.	Consult your doctor.
Do you paint, print, dye, or batik?	You may be exposed to arsenic, benzene, boric acid, carbon disulfide, ethylene glycol ethers (glycols), formaldehyde, lead, manganese, mercury, styrene, toluene and other solvents, and xylene.	Consult your doctor about the materials used in your hobby. Be alert to toxins in hobbyist materials. Read labels, clean up properly, and work in a well-ventilated area.

(continued)

ENVIRONMENTAL CONSIDERATIONS IN CONCEPTION DIFFICULTIES (continued)

Questions to Ask About Your Surroundings and Activities	Toxic Possibilities If You Answered Yes*	What to Do
Do you make pottery or glaze pots?	Your hobby may expose you to arsenic, boric acid, cadmium, formaldehyde, lead, manganese, and mercury.	Consult your doctor about the materials used in your hobby. Be alert to toxins in hobbyist materials. Read labels, clean up properly, and work in a well-ventilated area.
Do you blow glass or make stained glass or neon light?	Your hobby may expose you to arsenic, boric acid, lead, manganese, and mercury.	Consult your doctor about the materials used in your hobby. Be alert to toxins in hobbyist materials. Read labels, clean up properly, and work in a well-ventilated area.
Do you make jewelry, do metalwork, or solder?	You may be inadvertently exposed to arsenic, benzene, cadmium, formaldehyde, lead, manganese, and mercury in your craft materials.	Consult your doctor about the materials used in your hobby. Be alert to toxins in hobbyist materials. Read labels, clean up properly, and work in a well-ventilated area.
Do you use rubber cement or other adhesives in your projects?	You may be exposed to benzene and carbon disulfide in rubber cement.	Consult your doctor about the materials used in your hobby. Be alert to toxins in hobbyist materials. Read labels, clean up properly, and work in a well-ventilated area.
Do you make wax, plastics, or resin sculpture?	You may be exposed to benzene and styrene.	Consult your doctor about the materials used in your hobby. Be alert to toxins in hobbyist materials. Read labels, clean up properly, and work in a well-ventilated area.
Do you target shoot? Are you a gunsmith, hunter, or marksman?	Your hobby may expose you to mercury and, in poorly ventilated indoor ranges, to lead-containing fumes from gunfire.	Consult your doctor. Choose a well-ventilated range.
Do you garden?	If you mix or apply gardening chemicals, you may be exposed to arsenic, carbon disulfide, chlorinated hydrocarbon insecticides, formaldehyde, mercury, and nicotine.	Consult your doctor. Discontinue applying these chemicals.

(continued)

ENVIRONMENTAL CONSIDERATIONS IN CONCEPTION DIFFICULTIES (*continued*)

Questions to Ask About Your Surroundings and Activities	Toxic Possibilities If You Answered Yes*	What to Do
Do you work with wood or refinish furniture? Do you remove paint or varnish?	Some paints, varnishes, and their removers may contain benzene, carbon disulfide, ethylene glycol ethers (glycols), manganese, styrene, toluene and other solvents.	Consult your doctor. Be alert to toxins in hobbyist materials. Read labels, clean up properly, and work in a well-ventilated area.

* See information sheets for more information.

COUGH, WHEEZING, AND SHORTNESS OF BREATH

Cough

Coughing is the body's attempt to clear the airways of irritants such as excess mucus, dusts, or aspirated food. A chronic cough is a sign of chronic bronchitis, which can have many causes with smoking and air pollution being the most common. Coughing has myriad causes. Asthma, infections, tumors, and irritating airborne particles can trigger coughing. Nasal congestion, whether from allergies or infections, can cause coughing because of a postnasal drip. Whether the cough is dry, whether there is sputum, and what color the sputum is offer clues to what might be causing the cough.

A dry cough can be due to allergies, asthma, viral pneumonia, or atypical pneumonia, such as legionella or mycoplasma. Clear or white sputum suggests an absence of bacterial infection. Yellow or green sputum suggests bronchitis, pneumonia, or sinus infection.

In small children, coughing can be due to aspirating (inhaling) small objects.

Although most coughs are due to respiratory problems, heart disease can sometimes be the source. Lungs get congested when the heart has trouble pumping, causing someone to cough up clear or blood-tinged sputum. Some heart problems can also produce a dry cough.

Gastrointestinal disease may cause a cough; gastroesophageal reflex is a common cause of chronic cough unrelated to smoking.

Wheezing

Wheezing, a distinctive high-pitched sound, occurs when blocked airways disrupt air flow. Wheezing is most commonly caused by an asthmatic reaction, which can be triggered by specific external irritants, such as cigarette smoke or allergies to airborne agents (see Chapter 6, "Respiratory Ailments"). Certain food additives, such as monosodium glutamate, and medications, including aspirin and other nonsteroidal anti-inflammatory drugs, can also trigger wheezing. Wheezing can also be a symptom of emphysema. In rare instances, a tumor can cause localized wheezing in susceptible persons.

Shortness of Breath

Long-term exposure to many inhaled dusts can cause scarring and fibrosis of the lungs and result in progressive shortness of breath or a gradually worsening cough; this type of permanent damage due to dusts is called *pneumoconiosis*. Examples of such dusts include silica, to which sand blasters, miners, and stone workers are exposed, and asbestos, to which many miners, construction workers, and electricians were exposed; cadmium, to which welders can be exposed, also can cause fibrosis. Symptoms of pneumoconiosis can appear and worsen years after the exposure has stopped.

Cigarette smoking also causes lung scarring, which manifests as shortness of breath in emphysema and or chronic bronchitis. Cigarette smoking can also aggravate pneumoconiosis.

Inhaled agents can also damage the lungs by triggering an immune reaction that damages the lungs by causing acute or chronic inflammation. The process is known as *hypersensitivity pneumonitis* (see p. 128). This is what occurs when farmers react to moldy hay and grains (farmer's lung) or horseback riders react to moldy barn straw (horseback rider's lung). If exposure to the trigger continues, it can lead to permanent damage.

Injury to the pleura, the delicate membranes

lining the chest cavity, can also make breathing difficult. Pleurisy, in which the lining is inflamed because of infection, makes breathing difficult because of pain. Asbestos can cause stiffening and thickening of the normally supple pleura and lead to shortness of breath. Mesothelioma, a rare and serious cancer that grows from the pleura, is also linked to asbestos exposure and may be present as shortness of breath (see pp. 124–127).

Although most substances that damage or irritate the airways are inhaled, other routes of exposure can lead to chronic lung damage. Substances that are injected into the bloodstream or absorbed through the skin can have lung toxicity. Skin contact with the herbicide paraquat can damage the lungs and high-dose radiation can cause lung scarring.

Sudden, severe shortness of breath (rather than a gradual onset of symptoms) can be caused by a wide range of substances including noxious gases such as chlorine, ammonia, or oxides of nitrogen, an overwhelming allergic reaction, or a severe response to drugs, such as heroin. A heart attack can also cause such severe symptoms.

Some medications can lead to breathing difficulties. Salicytes (aspirin), nonsteroidal antiinflammatory drugs (such as ibuprofen), and beta-adrenergic blockers (a type of drug prescribed widely to treat hypertension) can trigger asthma. Another class of antihypertensive drugs, the angiotensin-converting enzyme (ACE) inhibitors, can cause a cough as a side effect.

The injection of any illegal drug made for oral use that contains talc or the use of any illicit drugs containing insoluble debris, as well as the use of certain intravenous cancer chemotherapy drugs, can cause lung damage.

Exposure to many environmental agents may result in cough, wheezing, or shortness of breath. If you notice these symptoms, and you answer "yes" to any of the following questions, you should be aware of the possibility of toxic exposure.

ENVIRONMENTAL CONSIDERATIONS IN COUGH AND BREATHING DIFFICULTIES

Questions to Ask About Your Surroundings and Activities	Toxic Possibilities If You Answered Yes*	What to Do
Do you smoke? Are you exposed to side-stream smoke?	Cigarette smoking is the major cause of chronic bronchitis. Passive smoking can also be a serious problem.	Quit smoking. Avoid people who are smoking. If not possible, make sure the room is well ventilated.
Do you use illicit drugs?	Marijuana and inhaled cocaine and heroin can cause shortness of breath and lung damage.	Seek help to discontinue your substance abuse.
Do you live in an area that suffers from air pollution?	Ozone, sulfur dioxide, oxides of nitrogen, carbon monoxide, and particulate matter cause these symptoms.	Avoid prolonged outdoor exposure, especially on hot days.
Do you have asthma or an asthmatic reaction?	Animal danders, pollen, and nuisance and irritant dusts can cause or worsen symptoms. Chemicals such as diisocyanates can also do this.	Avoid allergens. If you have asthma, get medications. See whether symptoms follow specific activities.

(continued)

ENVIRONMENTAL CONSIDERATIONS IN COUGH AND BREATHING DIFFICULTIES (*continued*)

Questions to Ask About Your Surroundings and Activities	Toxic Possibilities If You Answered Yes*	What to Do
What kind of ventilation is used in your home, office, or other area in which you spend a lot of time?	Bacteria, fungi, pollen, and other debris in air-cooling systems and humidifiers can cause lung problems. Heating can dry respiratory membranes.	Clean air-conditioning filters and humidifiers. When the heat is on in your house, use a humidifier.
Do your symptoms get worse after gardening?	Problems may be due to pollens, bacteria and fungi on hay, or allergic reactions to certain pesticides.	Limit contact if possible and consider using an appropriate respirator.
Are you a woodworker?	Fungi and fungal spores in wood dusts and natural allergens present in wood (such as western red cedar) can cause symptoms in woodworkers. Petroleum distillates cause coughing in painters and woodworkers. Sawdust irritates the lungs.	Limit contact, but if that's not possible, wear an appropriate respirator and ensure good ventilation.
Do you sculpt?	Sculptors are exposed to silica from many stones, including granite, slate, and sandstone.	Ensure good ventilation and use an appropriate respirator.
Do you make ceramics?	Many clays contain silica. They may also contain talc (nuisance dusts), which can be contaminated with asbestos. Glazes can also contain silica. The major hazards come from working with these products in their dry or powdered form.	Use appropriate respirators and ensure good ventilation. Use a wet mop to clean up or a special vacuum cleaner.

* See information sheets for more information.

DIARRHEA

Diarrhea is defined as an increase in a person's normal stool production, either the quantity or consistency of stool, or the frequency of bowel movements. What can be normal for one person might be considered diarrhea by another.

Diarrhea from Illnesses

- Inflammatory bowel disease is a group of chronic disorders in which the bowel becomes inflamed without a known cause. In one inflammatory bowel disorder, Crohn's disease, the diarrhea may alternate with constipation. In another, ulcerative colitis, the diarrhea is often bloody. Weight loss, fatigue, anemia, and persistent cramping can occur with both of these illnesses.
- Irritable bowel syndrome causes recurring symptoms that are similar to Crohn's disease— loose stool that alternates with constipation and can be accompanied by cramps. In this disorder, however, the colon is structurally normal and other problems, such as anemia, don't develop. Stress triggers the symptoms in many cases.
- An inability to digest certain foods can cause diarrhea. The most familiar example is lactose intolerance, in which milk products are poorly digested because of a deficiency in the enzyme lactase. Abdominal bloating and gas tend to accompany diarrhea in this disorder.
- Several metabolic disorders cause diarrhea. An overactive thyroid gland or underactive pancreas can cause diarrhea. People with long-standing diabetes often develop diarrhea.
- Diarrhea can be caused by a wide range of bacterial, viral, and parasitic infections. *Escherichia coli*, *Shigella ssp.*, *Giardia lambia*, Norwalk virus, and *Entamoeba histolytica* are common culprits. Diarrhea often starts suddenly in someone who is otherwise healthy. In developing countries, contaminated water is a major source of severe diarrheal disease.

Diarrhea from Medications

Many drugs cause diarrhea. Antibiotics, like ampicillin and clindamycin, can upset the normal bacteria in the digestive system, causing an overgrowth of those bacteria that trigger diarrhea. In severe cases, this can produce a type of colitis from the overgrowth of the bacterium *Clostridium difficile*, which produces a toxin. Overuse of antacids that contain magnesium, such as Milk of Magnesia, and of all types of laxatives can cause diarrhea.

Drug withdrawal can produce diarrhea. When heroin or alcohol abuse is stopped, diarrhea can become a severe complaint.

Diarrhea from Environmental Agents

- Foods can harbor other poisons that cause diarrhea. Some contaminated deep-sea fish, shellfish, plants such as pokeweed (*Phytolacca americana*), autumn crocus (*Colchicum autumnale*), mayapple (*Podophyllum peltatum*), rosary pea (*Abrus precatorius*), castor bean (*Ricinus communis*), and mushrooms can cause diarrhea (see pp. 617–620). Fruits and vegetables can be contaminated with organophosphate and carbamate pesticides that cause diarrhea. Outbreaks have been reported with vegetables and watermelons.
- Heavy metals, such as nickel, cadmium, copper, and zinc, can cause diarrhea. By storing very acidic fruits in metal-lined containers, these metals can contaminate food and drinks.

Arsenic and copper can contaminate well water.

- Artificial sweeteners that contain a nonabsorbed sugar (such as sorbitol) can cause diarrhea if consumed in sufficient amounts. These sweeteners can be found in various elixirs (such as theophylline) and chewing gum.

Some toxic substances in the environment can cause diarrhea. If you experience diarrhea and answer "yes" to any of the following questions, you should be aware of the possibility of a toxic exposure.

ENVIRONMENTAL CONSIDERATIONS IN DIARRHEA

Questions to Ask About Your Surroundings and Activities	Toxic Possibilities If You Answered Yes*	What to Do
Did you suddenly develop diarrhea? Can you relate it to a specific meal, like a picnic?	Food poisoning, due to bacterial infection or toxins that contaminate food is common, especially with food that has not been properly prepared or refrigerated.	Consult your doctor if diarrhea persists.
Are you taking any medications?	Antibiotics, laxatives, and magnesium-containing antacids are common drugs that cause diarrhea.	Discontinue taking the drug if possible. Drink clear liquids, such as apple juice or sodas, to keep up with fluid and sugar loss. Avoid milk, and orange and tomato juices. With prolonged and severe diarrhea, special preparations may be needed to keep up with the volume and electrolyte losses.
Have you recently stopped using heroin, morphine, or other opiate/opioid-related drugs?	Diarrhea is one sign of opiate withdrawal.	Consult your doctor for detoxification treatment.
Do certain foods repeatedly trigger diarrhea?	Milk and milk products cause diarrhea in people who are lactase deficient. Gluten-containing products can trigger diarrhea in people with the diseases celiac or tropical sprue.	Avoid these foods or consume them in small quantities. Enzyme substitutes, such as Lactaid, may help people with lactose intolerance.
Are you drinking punch or fruit juices that have been stored in metallic containers?	Cadmium, copper, and zinc can leech into acidic drinks and food.	Consult your doctor. Store drinks and foods in plastic or glass containers.
Do you have hobbies, like photography or pottery, that might expose you to heavy metals?	Antimony, arsenic, lead, and mercury are some of the metals that cause diarrhea.	Inform your doctor. Check product labels on supplies that you work with.

(continued)

ENVIRONMENTAL CONSIDERATIONS IN DIARRHEA (*continued*)

Questions to Ask About Your Surroundings and Activities	*Toxic Possibilities If You Answered Yes**	*What to Do*
Have you taken any unusual herbal teas?	Teas made from juniper berries, horsetail, dock root, aloe leaves, buckthorn bark, senna leaves, or shave grass can cause diarrhea.	Stop use of teas. Consult your doctor.
Have you eaten seafood?	Deep-sea fish and shellfish can contain toxins that cause diarrhea.	Consult your doctor. Discontinue eating these foods until the problem is resolved.
Are you taking iron supplements?	A high dose of iron can cause diarrhea.	Consult your doctor.

* See information sheets for more information.

Two symptoms involving a sense of physical disorientation are dizziness and vertigo. If you are experiencing dizziness, you may feel dazed, faint, giddy, lightheaded, or unsteady. Vertigo is defined as the sensation that you or your environment is moving, rotating, or spinning; you may experience dizziness after or in-between attacks of vertigo.

Dizziness

Emotional stress, prolonged lying down, a change in position, turning your head too quickly, or injury can cause you to feel dizzy or faint. Heat stress can also cause dizziness when blood flow to the skin increases and blood flow to the brain decreases.

Dizziness from Illness and Trauma. The following medical conditions may cause dizziness: blood loss, dehydration, hyperventilation, anemia, anxiety, depression, high blood pressure, diabetes, ear or eye disease, cardiovascular problems, seizures, epilepsy, or other neurological disorders.

A *stroke* in which the blood supply to the brain is blocked or a blood vessel bursts, or a transient ischemic attack, a temporary disruption of blood supply to the brain, can cause dizziness or fainting.

In people over fifty, cervical osteoarthritis is a common disorder affecting the spine in the neck region. Pressure on the nerves and blood vessels in this area may cause dizziness and fainting to occur.

Sometimes dizziness or fainting may be associated with urination, defecation, coughing, or swallowing.

Dizziness may be a symptom in persons who develop a subdural hematoma or hemorrhage in which blood leaks under the outermost covering of the brain. Some types of tumors also are associated with dizziness. A tumorous growth on the nerve to the ear (an acoustic neuroma) may also cause dizziness.

Herpes zoster, a viral infection, may affect the nerve to the ear and cause dizziness. People with temporomandibular joint neuralgia, a disorder of the jaw joint, complain of dizziness.

Dizziness from Medications. Certain drugs can cause dizziness. They include antianxiety drugs; aspirin and other nonsteroidal anti-inflammatory drugs; blood pressure medicines; diuretics; nitrates; phenothiazines; phenytoin (Dilantin); tricyclic antidepressants; antituberculosis drugs; aminoglycoside antibiotics, such as streptomycin, kanamycin, and neomycin; chloroquine; and quinine.

Vertigo

Vertigo can be caused by injury of the brainstem. Labyrinthitis is an infection of the fluid-filled chambers in the inner ear that control balance, leading to vertigo. The cause is usually viral and the abnormal sensations may last one to three weeks. People, mostly the middle-aged, with Meniere's disease feel vertiginous from an increase in fluid in these chambers. Chronic middle ear infections may also cause dizziness.

Up to a third of patients with multiple sclerosis have vertigo.

Both pilots and divers often experience vertigo. Their disorientation is due to conflicting sensory cues as to their spatial orientation.

If you experience dizziness or vertigo and you answer "yes" to any of the following questions, you should be aware of the possibility of toxic exposure.

ENVIRONMENTAL CONSIDERATIONS IN DIZZINESS/VERTIGO

Questions to Ask About Your Surroundings and Activities	*Toxic Possibilities If You Answered Yes**	*What to Do*
Do you live in an old house with flaking paint and old plumbing? Are you renovating an old home? Do you live in an inner city?	Children especially may be exposed to lead by eating paint chips, inhaling dust, or drinking contaminated tap water. Renovating may expose you to lead in old paint and pipes.	Consult your doctor. Avoid further exposure.
Do you live in a mobile home? Do you spend a lot of time indoors where there are gas appliances, new carpeting, particle board, or foam insulation?	All of these are sources of exposure to formaldehyde.	Improve ventilation in your home. If your symptoms persist, consult your doctor.
Do you live near a smelter or other hazardous waste site?	There may be high levels of arsenic emitted in the air near these facilities.	If symptoms persist, inform your doctor of your place of residence.
Do you heat your house with a wood stove?	Arsenic-treated wood burning in a wood stove may be a source of this toxin.	Improve ventilation or replace your wood with untreated wood.
Do you use special products to clean your walls, clothing, or rugs? Do you use common hardware store products, such as waterless handcleaner?	Trichloroethylene, other halogenated hydrocarbon solvents, irritant gases, petroleum distillates, and turpentine are found in some common household cleaning and hardware store products.	Inform your doctor of any household products you are using. Work only in well-ventilated areas.
Have you eaten meat, fish, poultry, or eggs that could possibly be contaminated?	In the past, polybrominated biphenyls have contaminated these foodstuffs when it was accidently added to feedstock.	Inform your doctor of the possibility of having eaten tainted foodstuffs.
Have you recently eaten tainted fruit, seed grain, or vegetables?	These foodstuffs may be sprayed with chlorinated hydrocarbon insecticides or pesticides. Some vegetables naturally contain nitrates.	Thoroughly wash all fruits and vegetables before eating; avoid those that seem to cause dizziness. Consult your doctor if symptoms persist.
Have you recently eaten smoked fish, bologna, salami, pepperoni, bacon, frankfurters, corned beef, canned ham, or sausages?	Nitrites and nitrates are used in these foods to impart a smoked flavor and pink color and to prevent botulism.	Avoid eating foods known to contain nitrite and nitrate compounds. Check ingredient lists carefully. If your symptoms persist, consult your doctor.

(continued)

ENVIRONMENTAL CONSIDERATIONS IN DIZZINESS/VERTIGO (*continued*)

Questions to Ask About Your Surroundings and Activities	Toxic Possibilities If You Answered Yes*	What to Do
Have you eaten seafood, bread, or seed grain?	Ordinarily, these foods are safe, but environmental contamination has affected these foods, and it could possibly occur again. Fish has been contaminated with methylmercury from industrial discharge. Methylmercury is used as a fungicide for seeds intended for planting, but, in the past, these seeds have been accidently ingested.	Consult your doctor. Discontinue eating these foods until the problem has been resolved.
Do you eat from glazed pottery dishes or cook with leaden pots?	You may be ingesting high levels of lead.	Replace dishes and cookware with lead-free kitchenware.
Do you drink well water?	Well water may be contaminated by arsenic or nitrites and nitrates from natural sources or from groundwater contaminated by pesticide runoff.	Have your drinking water tested (see Box 13.2, p. 521). If symptoms persist, inform your doctor of the possibility of toxic exposure.
Are you taking dietary supplements, homeopathic medicines, or products sold in health food stores? Do you take herbal or traditional folk medicines?	These products have been contaminated with arsenic, cyanide, and lead.	Inform your doctor about these supplements. Discontinue using folk medicines, which may cause other symptoms.
Are you using any cough medicines, tonics, mouthwashes, liquid vitamins, or other over-the-counter medications?	These preparations may contain ethanol.	Discontinue the use of these substances. If your symptoms persist, consult your doctor.
Have you recently drunk whiskey or other alcoholic beverages? Do you drink home-distilled moonshine whiskey or wine?	Drinking alcohol (ethanol) can cause dizziness. Methanol and ethylene glycol have been found in preparations of homemade whiskey in which ethanol should have been used. Arsenic and lead have also been found as contaminants in homemade whiskey and wine.	**Seek immediate medical help.** With methanol poisoning symptoms may be mild initially but could progress to blindness, coma, and/or death. Ethylene glycol can cause renal failure.
Are you a cancer patient taking Laetrile? Have you chewed and ingested the seeds from apples, peaches, pears, apricots, or plums? Do you eat cassava in large quantities?	Laetrile is an unapproved anti-cancer drug made from cyanide-containing apricot seeds. Cyanide is also found in the seeds of other fruits and in the cassava plant.	Consult your doctor. Discontinue ingesting these products.

(*continued*)

ENVIRONMENTAL CONSIDERATIONS IN DIZZINESS/VERTIGO (*continued*)

Questions to Ask About Your Surroundings and Activities	*Toxic Possibilities If You Answered Yes**	*What to Do*
Do you sniff glue, typewriter correction fluid, or other substances? Do you snort substances, especially those believed to be aphrodisiacs?	If you sniff glue, you may inhale toluene or other solvents. Trichloroethylene can be inhaled from typewriter correction fluid. Organic nitrites can cause dizziness.	Seek help to discontinue abusing these substances.
Do you use cocaine, crack, heroin, or other illicit drugs?	These substances may be contaminated with toxins, such as arsenic and lead.	Seek help to discontinue your substance abuse. Continued use of illicitly prepared drugs puts you at risk of exposure to many toxic substances.
Do you smoke? Are you exposed to side-stream smoke?	You are inhaling nicotine, polycyclic aromatic hydrocarbons, and tobacco contaminants, such as cyanide and formaldehyde.	Seek help to quit or reduce smoking. Avoid people who are smoking.
Have you sprayed your pet or rooms with a flea-killer spray?	Over-the-counter flea and tick products may contain pyrethins (pyrethrum, pyrethrins, and pyrethroids).	Discontinue the use of these products. Consult your doctor if your symptoms persist.
Do you garden?	If you mix or apply gardening chemicals, you may be exposed to arsenic, benzene, carbon disulfide, chlorinated hydrocarbon insecticides, cyanide, formaldehyde, nicotine, mercury, cholinesterase inhibitors, petroleum distillates, or organic tin.	Consult your doctor. Discontinue applying these pesticides, insecticides, or herbicides.
Do you paint, dye, batik, or print? Do you make plastics or wax sculpture? Do you use adhesives, rubber cement, or solvent-based markers or colored inks in your art projects?	You may be exposed to aniline, arsenic, benzene, carbon disulfide, carbon tetrachloride and other halogenated hydrocarbon solvents, formaldehyde, ketones, lead, methanol, petroleum distillates, styrene, organic tin, toluene, turpentine, or xylene.	Consult your doctor about the materials used in your hobby. Be alert to toxins in hobbyist materials. Read labels, clean up properly, and work in a well-ventilated area.
Do you make pottery, glaze ceramics, or do enameling?	Your craft materials may expose you to arsenic, formaldehyde, lead, and methanol.	Consult your doctor about the materials used in your hobby. Be alert to potential toxins in hobbyist materials. Read labels, clean up properly, and work in a well-ventilated area.

(continued)

ENVIRONMENTAL CONSIDERATIONS IN DIZZINESS/VERTIGO (*continued*)

Questions to Ask About Your Surroundings and Activities	Toxic Possibilities If You Answered Yes*	What to Do
Do you blow glass or make stained glass? Do you make neon light?	You may be inadvertently exposed to excess levels of lead, methanol, organic tin, or turpentine.	Consult your doctor about the materials used in your hobby. Be alert to toxins in hobbyist materials. Read labels, clean up properly, and work in a well-ventilated area.
Do you work in a darkroom?	Using darkroom chemicals may expose you to benzene, carbon monoxide (released from methylene chloride), cyanide, irritant chemicals such as formaldehyde and cresol (phenol and phenolic compounds), and trichloroethylene (a halogenated hydrocarbon).	Consult your doctor about the materials used in your hobby. Be alert to potential toxins in hobbyist materials. Work in a well-ventilated area. (See Chapter 20.)
Are you a gunsmith, hunter, or marksman? Do you target shoot?	You may be exposed to cyanide, lead, selenious acid, and petroleum distillates.	Avoid or minimize exposure. Choose a well-ventilated range. Consult your doctor if your symptoms persist.
Do you work with wood or refinish furniture?	You may be exposed to benzene, carbon disulfide, carbon monoxide from exposure to methylene chloride in paint strippers, methanol, petroleum distillates, styrene, toluene, and trichloroethylene, as well as other halogenated hydrocarbon solvents.	Consult your doctor about the materials used in your hobby. Be alert to potential toxins in hobbyist materials. Work in a well-ventilated area.
Do you use a computer with a video display terminal at your workplace or home?	Dizziness is one of the complaints from people using video display terminals.	Adjust the lighting in your workspace; check your posture and the placement of the video display terminal relative to your body; take frequent breaks. Consult your doctor if your symptoms persist.
Do you work on internal combustion engines?	You may be exposed to carbon monoxide.	Work only in a well-ventilated area. Consult your doctor if your symptoms persist.
Do you make jewelry, weld, solder, or do metalwork?	Your materials may expose you to arsenic, benzene, cyanide, formaldehyde, halogenated hydrocarbon solvents, lead, and methanol.	Be alert to potential toxins in hobbyist materials. Work in a well-ventilated area. Consult your doctor if your symptoms persist.

* See information sheets for more information.

FEVER AND CHILLS

The body's temperature is an indicator of general health. Normal temperature falls between 97.0 and 100.2°F, a range influenced by individual variations, the time of day, and, for women, the stage of menstrual cycle (there is a slight, transient rise in body temperature during ovulation and menstruation). When body temperature rises above this range, you have a fever. Fevers may be accompanied by chills and a sensation of cold, sometimes with shaking.

Fever from Illness

Fever is frequently an indication that the body is fighting off an infection caused by a virus, bacterium, fungus, or parasite. It can occur with self-limited infections, such as influenza or upper respiratory ailments; with infections requiring treatment, such as an infection of the urinary tract; with diseases such as pneumonia, meningitis, bacterial endocarditis, tuberculosis, and Rocky Mountain spotted fever; or with tropical infections, such as malaria, Chagas's disease, and leishmaniasis.

Connective tissue disease, such as juvenile rheumatoid arthritis and temporal arteritis, can present with fever. Fever is also a symptom of some tumors, notably lymphomas (although other symptoms usually are present as well), and metastatic carcinoma (a cancer that has spread from its original or primary site to another place in the body) arising in the lung, pancreas, or stomach.

Other less common causes of fever include vasculitis (an inflammation of the blood vessels) and the rare inherited disease familial Mediterranean fever.

Very high fevers are common in children in response to common ailments, such as middle ear or upper respiratory infections, influenza, roseola, and measles.

Fever is also associated with sunstroke or heat stroke, and the body's temperature can be elevated by strenuous exercise under certain circumstances.

Fever from Medications

Fever can result from some drugs or as an allergic reaction to drugs, such as certain antibiotics, nonsteroidal anti-inflammatory agents, salicylates (aspirin), atropine, antihistamines, tranquilizers, and antimalarial drugs. Fever is an exceedingly rare, yet treatable, side effect of certain anesthetic agents; this complication is termed malignant hyperthermia.

If you experience fever or chills and you answer "yes" to any of the following questions, you should be aware of the possibility of toxic exposure.

ENVIRONMENTAL CONSIDERATIONS IN FEVER AND CHILLS

Questions to Ask About Your Surroundings and Activities	Toxic Possibilities If You Answered Yes*	What to Do
Have you accidently eaten any poisonous plants?	Jimsonweed (*Datura stramonium*), English or deadly nightshade, and other plants containing atropine or related substances cause fever. Children are particularly susceptible to even low doses of atropine, which can be fatal.	**Seek immediate medical help. This may be a life-threatening situation.**
Are you taking any dietary supplements or using products sold in health food stores?	Using dimethyl sulfoxide (DMSO) to treat arthritis or sports injuries or to heal scars may cause chills without fever.	Inform your doctor of these supplements.
Do you use illicit drugs?	Some street drugs, such as amphetamines, cocaine, and LSD, can cause fever.	Seek help to discontinue your substance abuse. Continued use of illicitly prepared drugs puts you at risk of exposure to many toxins and infections.
Do you intentionally sniff glue or adhesives either to get high or because you use it to build models?	These substances contain harmful petroleum distillates.	Seek help to discontinue abusing these substances. Hobbyists should ensure proper ventilation.
Do you garden?	Some insecticides and herbicides used for pest control in gardens contain certain dinitro derivatives of phenol and cresol.	Discontinue application of these chemicals and consult your doctor.
Do you blow glass, make stained glass, make pottery, glaze ceramics, or do enameling?	You may be suffering from metal fume fever from exposure to fumes of such metal oxides as aluminum, antimony, arsenic, cadmium, cobalt, lead, magnesium, manganese, nickel, selenium, silver, thallium, tin, or zinc.	Consult your doctor about the materials used in your hobby. Be alert to toxins in hobbyist materials. Read labels, clean up properly, and work in a well-ventilated area.
Do you paint, dye, engrave, etch, or develop photographs?	These activities may expose you to certain dinitro derivatives of phenol and cresol or petroleum distillates.	Consult your doctor about the materials used in your hobby. Read labels, clean up properly, and work in a well-ventilated area.
Do you work with wood or refinish furniture?	Many common solvents and furniture polishes contain petroleum distillates.	Consult your doctor if you have symptoms. Work in a well-ventilated area.

(continued)

ENVIRONMENTAL CONSIDERATIONS IN FEVER AND CHILLS (*continued*)

Questions to Ask About Your Surroundings and Activities	Toxic Possibilities If You Answered Yes*	What to Do
Do you make jewelry or metal sculpture, weld, or solder?	You may be suffering from metal fume fever from exposure to fumes of such metal oxides as aluminum, antimony, arsenic, cadmium, cobalt, lead, magnesium, manganese, mercury, nickel, selenium, silver, thallium, tin, and zinc in your materials.	Consult your doctor about the materials used in your hobby. Be alert to toxins in hobbyist materials. Work in a well-ventilated area.
Are you a gunsmith, hunter, or marksman?	You may be exposed to petroleum distillates.	Consult your doctor if you have symptoms. Clean and polish your guns in a well-ventilated area to avoid inhalation.

* See information sheets for more information.

HAIR LOSS

Hair grows from birth and increases throughout life, although some thinning occurs naturally as we age. Any excessive loss of hair—either all over the head or in patches—should be investigated.

In men and women, the most common type of hair loss is androgenetic alopecia, or male pattern baldness, which mostly affects the top of the scalp. It can occur in anyone who has the genetic makeup and the required level of male hormones. Women also can experience temporary hair loss due to hormonal shifts several months after having a baby.

Hair Loss from Illness or Trauma

Thinning hair may follow a severe illness, physical stress such as surgery, or psychological stress. It may be a symptom of disease affecting the whole body, such as a hereditary or endocrine disorder or an autoimmune disease.

Patchy hair loss may be due to a bacterial, viral, fungal, or protozoan infection of the skin and scalp. Both benign and cancerous tumors can destroy hair follicles, leading to patchy hair loss.

Trauma to the hair follicle, such as braiding, straightening, frequent pulling or twisting, bleaching, dyeing, or permanent waving, will also cause hair to fall out. Smooth, relatively healthy-appearing areas on the scalp without hair can be caused by a relatively common disease, alopecia areata.

Malnutrition and other diseases that prevent the body from absorbing enough nutrients can cause hair loss. Iron-deficiency anemia may lead to hair loss.

Hair Loss from Medications

Some medications may cause hair loss as a side effect. Among these are anticoagulants, anticancer drugs, antithyroid drugs, blood pressure medicines, oral contraceptives, anti-inflammatory drugs, and lithium. Radiation therapy will also cause hair to fall out (this is usually temporary, although it can be permanent if the dose is high enough).

If you have excessive hair loss or bald patches and you answer "yes" to any of the following questions, you should be aware of the possibility of toxic exposure.

ENVIRONMENTAL CONSIDERATIONS IN HAIR LOSS

Questions to Ask About Your Surroundings and Activities	*Toxic Possibilities If You Answered Yes**	*What to Do*
Do you use an antifungal or antidandruff shampoo?	If you are using a medicated shampoo too often, you may be exposing yourself to excessive amounts of selenium.	Discontinue use of the shampoo and consult your doctor.
Are you taking dietary supplements, vitamins, homeopathic medicines, or health food products?	Some of these products might be contaminated with substances such as thallium, arsenic, or selenium. Long-term use of very high doses of vitamin A (25,000+ IU daily) may cause hair loss.	Consult your doctor.
Do you use cocaine, crack, heroin, or other illicit drugs?	Cocaine can cause hair loss. In addition, many of these substances are contaminated with toxins such as lead, arsenic, and strychnine.	Seek help to discontinue your substance abuse habit. Continued use of illicitly prepared drugs puts you at risk of exposure to many toxins.
Do you garden? Has your house been sprayed for pests? Have you placed any antipest products in your home or sprayed your pets for pests?	You may be exposed to pesticides containing thallium, arsenic, and possibly copper. In addition, some roach powders contain boric acid.	Discontinue the application of pesticides. Consult your doctor.
Do you clean guns or other metal objects?	If you use gun blue to clean guns or other metal objects, you may be exposed to selenious acid (a selenium compound).	Consult your doctor and mention your use of gun blue.

* See information sheets for more information.

HEADACHE

A headache is a pain in the head that ranges from mild to extremely severe. It is one of the most common medical complaints, each year affecting as many as 24 million Americans severely enough to cause them to miss work. Most headaches do not indicate a life-threatening condition. Headaches that merit immediate medical attention are ones that come on suddenly, are extremely severe, or change in characteristic pattern or severity of pain. There are many different causes for a headache and they are diagnosed according to their patterns of occurrence, severity, onset, and location of the pain.

Common Types of Headaches

Among the most common, nonthreatening types of headaches are the following:

- Muscle tension headaches are characterized as a constant bandlike pressure that seems worst at the end of the day and may last from hours to weeks. This type is very common and usually associated with physical and psychological stress.
- Vascular headaches, including migraine and cluster headaches, are generally more severe. Symptoms may stem from alterations in the blood flow in the brain as blood vessels contract and then dilate. Migraines are experienced as recurring, throbbing pain felt on one side in the front of the head; they are sometimes preceded by vision changes and may be accompanied by nausea and/or vomiting. Migraine attacks may be brought on by alcohol or stress and may last days. Cluster headaches are so named because of the pattern of having a series of vascular headaches for a period of weeks to months (a cluster), followed by years of no recurrence.
- Sinus headaches are usually characterized by facial pain and often accompanied by nasal stuffiness and discharge, although the pain may be only at the top of the head. These headaches may also be accompanied by fever. Pain increases when the head is lowered because this increases the pressure in the sinuses.
- Nonspecific febrile headaches are accompanied by muscle aches and pains, cough, and sore throat.
- Individuals over forty who complain of pain in the back of the head and neck that gets worse if they move their neck may have cervical arthritis, an inflammation in the neck vertebrae.

Headaches from Serious Illnesses

A number of more serious ailments can cause headaches; among them are the following:

- Meningitis is an inflammation of the covering of the brain and/or spinal cord accompanied with fever, headache, nausea and vomiting, and a stiff neck.
- Subarachnoid bleeding (under the covering of the brain) may be due to vascular abnormality, hypertension, or trauma, causing a very sudden, diffuse, and severe pain with the person sometimes losing consciousness, vomiting, or having a stiff neck.
- Trigeminal neuralgia is experienced as jabs of pain in the face if facial trigger points are touched.
- Temporal arteritis is an inflammation of the blood vessels at the sides of the head near the eyes. It usually occurs in people over fifty and is often accompanied by generalized, chronic

muscle aches and weakness and intermittent vision problems, which can lead to blindness.

- Malignant hypertension, a sudden, high increase in blood pressure, can cause headache and blurring of vision and lead to a stroke or heart attack.
- An abscess or tumor within the skull can cause a headache. (It sometimes has a pattern that is unlike the other types of headaches.)
- A chronic subdural hematoma, a condition in which blood slowly collects under the covering of the brain, causes headaches as well as episodes of confusion, changes in thought, and drowsiness that appear over time. (This condition is seen mainly in people who have sustained a head injury; particularly, in people who abuse alcohol; or people who are elderly.)

Headaches from Medications

Headaches may be caused by medications, including ergot, caffeine, corticosteroids, sedatives, decongestants containing phenylephrine and caffeine, atropine, birth control pills, nitrites or nitrates (amyl nitrite or nitroglycerin), hydralazine, indomethacin, calcium channel blockers, disulfiram (Antabuse), antiparasitic drugs, oral antidiabetic agents, certain anticancer drugs, some antibiotics, and some anesthetics.

Some drugs, when combined with another substance, can cause headaches. For example, taking either a monoamine oxidase inhibitor or a blood pressure (hypertension) medication and drinking alcohol can result in a headache. Other examples include taking amphetamines and eating tyramine-containing foods (such as cheeses and pickled herring), or taking a monoamine oxidase inhibitor and eating tyramine-containing foods.

Some toxic substances in our environment can also cause headaches. If you experience headaches and you answer "yes" to any of the following questions, you should be aware of the possibility of toxic exposure.

ENVIRONMENTAL CONSIDERATIONS IN HEADACHE

Questions to Ask About Your Surroundings and Activities	Toxic Possibilities If You Answered Yes*	What to Do
Are you taking dietary supplements, homeopathic medicines, vitamins, or products sold in health food stores? Do you take herbal or traditional folk medicines?	Historically some of these products contained contaminants, such as cyanide and lead. Long-term use of very high doses of vitamin A (25,000 + IU) and vitamin D (1,000–3,000 IU/kg) daily may also cause headaches. Large doses of nutmeg may cause headaches.	Inform your doctor of these supplements. Discontinue using folk medicines, which may cause other symptoms. Consult your doctor for persistent headaches.
Are you being treated for acne or osteoporosis?	Long-term use of very high doses of vitamin A (25,000 + IU) daily may cause headaches. Used to treat or prevent osteoporosis, vitamin D in high doses (1,000–3,000 IU/kg/day) may also cause headaches.	Consult your doctor.

(continued)

ENVIRONMENTAL CONSIDERATIONS IN HEADACHE (*continued*)

Questions to Ask About Your Surroundings and Activities	Toxic Possibilities If You Answered Yes*	What to Do
Are you a cancer patient taking Laetrile? Have you chewed and ingested the seeds from apples, peaches, pears, apricots, or plums? Do you eat cassava in large quantities?	Laetrile is an unapproved and ineffective anticancer drug made from cyanide-containing apricot seeds. Cyanide is also found in the seeds of other fruits and in the cassava plant.	Consult your doctor. Discontinue ingesting these products.
Have you eaten large quantities of fruits and vegetables?	If the fruits and vegetables you have eaten were sprayed with pesticides, you may be exposed to chlorinated hydrocarbon insecticides, carbamates, and organophosphates (see pesticides). Certain vegetables, such as broccoli, collards, cauliflower, and spinach contain high concentrations of nitrates.	Wash all fruits and vegetables thoroughly to remove any pesticide residue. Remove from your diet vegetables high in nitrates.
Have you eaten Chinese food, canned soups, potato chips, gourmet seasonings, dry-roasted nuts, processed meats, instant gravies, or TV dinners or used the flavor enhancer Accent?	Monosodium glutamate (MSG), a flavor enhancer used in these foods, may produce the Chinese restaurant syndrome in certain individuals. Among its symptoms are headache, muscle tightness, flushing, and sweating.	Avoid ingesting MSG. Check ingredients listed on packages of these foods, request MSG-free Chinese dishes, and make sure sauces on foods are MSG-free.
Have you eaten fish at a recent meal?	Fishborne food poisoning may be caused either by toxins or actual bacteria infecting any seafood you may have eaten. Headache is a common symptom for many types of fishborne poisoning.	Seek immediate medical help. In certain kinds of fishborne food poisoning, symptoms may progress within hours to death or can leave survivors with nerve damage.
Have you recently eaten smoked fishes, bologna, salami, pepperoni, bacon, frankfurters, corned beef, canned ham, or sausages?	Nitrites and nitrates are used in these foods to impart a smoked flavor or pink color or to prevent botulism. These compounds, however may cause migrainelike headaches in some people.	Avoid eating foods known to contain nitrate and nitrite compounds. Check ingredients listings carefully. If headaches persist, consult your doctor.
Have you recently eaten cheeses, canned figs, pickled herring, chopped liver, pods or broad beans, yeast, coffee, chi-	These foods all contain tyramine, a substance that acts on certain nerve endings. An increased incidence of headaches	Avoid eating foods known to contain high levels of tyramine. These foods are particularly dangerous to anyone taking a

(continued)

ENVIRONMENTAL CONSIDERATIONS IN HEADACHE (*continued*)

Questions to Ask About Your Surroundings and Activities	*Toxic Possibilities If You Answered Yes**	*What to Do*
anti wine, or alcoholic beverages, especially beer?	occurs in some individuals following ingestion of tyramine-containing foods.	monoamine oxidase inhibitor (check with your doctor). If headaches persist, consult your doctor.
Have you eaten chocolate recently?	Chocolate has been found to be the food most likely to trigger migraine headaches.	Avoid eating chocolate or chocolate-flavored foods. If headaches persist, consult your doctor.
Do you eat many foods that contain artificial colorings and flavorings?	Food, drug, and cosmetic (FD&C) dyes, such as eosin B (D&C Red No. 25), eosin Y (D&C Red No. 3), erythrocin B (FD&C Red No. 3), phyloxine B (D&C Red No. 8), tartrazine (FD&C Yellow No. 5), and rose bengal, are among the agents that may be linked to headaches.	Change your diet to exclude foods with additives. Check ingredients listings carefully. If headaches persist, consult your doctor.
Do you use oil of peppermint or licorice flavorings?	Exposure to some flavoring agents such as oil of peppermint and licorice can cause headache.	Avoid foods containing these products.
Have you been without food for 5 or more hours during the day or for thirteen hours overnight?	A study of 1,800 women with migraine headaches found that fasting was a precipitating factor for headache.	Make sure to eat regularly and avoid long periods without nourishment.
Do you drink well water?	Groundwater may contain high levels of nitrites and nitrates.	Have your water tested for contaminants and naturally occurring compounds, such as nitrites and nitrates.
Have you recently stopped drinking coffee or caffeinated soft drinks? Does your headache begin on the weekends away from your normal routine?	You may be suffering from withdrawal from caffeine. In a quarter of all heavy coffee drinkers, a throbbing headache appears within 18 to 24 hours after the last caffeine ingestion. Headaches may occur on weekends when coffee breaks are infrequent.	Try to reduce the amount of coffee that you drink at all times, so that you won't experience such a large swing in the levels of caffeine in your body.

(*continued*)

ENVIRONMENTAL CONSIDERATIONS IN HEADACHE (*continued*)

Questions to Ask About Your Surroundings and Activities	Toxic Possibilities If You Answered Yes*	What to Do
Do you use an antiseptic mouthwash and/or toothpaste?	Accidental ingestion of boric acid may occur when it is used as an antiseptic in mouthwash and toothpaste. Alcohol (ethanol) may be found in some mouthwashes and has been linked to headaches.	Discontinue using these products. If your headache persists, consult your doctor.
Have you recently drunk whiskey or other alcoholic beverages? Do you drink home-distilled moonshine whiskey or wine? Do you eat from glazed pottery dishes or cook with leaden pots?	Alcoholic (ethanol) beverages and alcohol-containing cough preparations, tonics, and nonprescription drugs may produce headaches in certain people. Methanol has been found in homemade whiskey in place of ethanol. Lead has been found as a contaminant in homemade whiskey and wine, as well as glazes and pots.	Avoid drinking alcohol-containing preparations. **If methanol poisoning has occurred, seek immediate medical help!** Symptoms may be mild initially but could progress to blindness, coma, and/or death. To avoid further exposure to lead, replace dishes and cookware with lead-free kitchenware and do not drink homemade spirits.
Do you use cocaine, crack, heroin, marijuana, or other illicit drugs? Do you inhale amyl nitrite, butyl nitrite, or similar substances?	Cocaine can cause headaches. Many of these substances are contaminated with toxins such as lead. Smoking marijuana can produce the feeling of heaviness and pressure in the head in some individuals. Organonitrites (nitrites and nitrates) can cause headache.	Seek help to discontinue your substance abuse. Continued use of illicitly prepared drugs puts you at risk for exposure to many toxins.
Do you intentionally sniff glue, adhesives, or typewriter correction fluid to get high?	If you sniff glue, you may inhale toluene and other solvents, which in addition to causing intoxication can cause headache. Trichloroethylene, a halogenated hydrocarbon solvent, can be inhaled from typewriter correction fluid.	Seek help to discontinue your substance abuse.
Do you smoke? Are you exposed to side-stream smoke? Have you recently stopped smoking?	You are inhaling nicotine and tobacco contaminants, such as cadmium, formaldehyde, and cyanide, and absorbing these substances into your body. After quitting smoking, many people complain of headaches that are caused by nicotine withdrawal.	Quit or reduce smoking to reduce your exposure to these toxins. Seek help in quitting smoking from your doctor. Avoid people who are smoking.

(*continued*)

ENVIRONMENTAL CONSIDERATIONS IN HEADACHE (*continued*)

Questions to Ask About Your Surroundings and Activities	*Toxic Possibilities If You Answered Yes**	*What to Do*
Do you live in a high-pollutant urban area?	Headache is among the symptoms described in nonspecific air pollution syndrome. The existence of this syndrome has yet to be scientifically proven but refers to symptoms, such as headache, anxiety, backache, and fatigue, which affects healthy people when the air pollution level rises.	Consult your physician.
Do you live near a smelter, iron or steel production facility, fossil fuel-burning plant, or a municipal waste incinerator?	Living near a smelter or other airborne-toxin-emitting facility increases the likelihood of exposure to cadmium and other noxious fumes.	If your headaches persist, inform your doctor about your proximity to these facilities.
Do you live in an old house with flaking paint and old plumbing? Do you live in an inner city? Are you renovating an old home?	Children especially may be exposed to lead by eating paint chips, inhaling dust, or drinking contaminated tap water. Renovation may expose you to lead in old paint and pipes.	Avoid further exposure. Consult your doctor if headache persists.
Do you live in a mobile home? Do you spend a lot of time indoors where there are gas appliances, new carpeting, particle board, or foam insulation?	All of these are potential sources of exposure to formaldehyde. Improve the ventilation in your home.	If your headaches continue, consult your doctor.
Do you use special products to clean your walls, clothing, or rugs? Have you recently used any hardware store products such as degreasers, dewaxers, or other cleaners?	Irritant gases may be released from certain household cleaning products containing ammonia and chlorine. Trichloroethylene, other halogenated hydrocarbon solvents, and petroleum distillates are found in some common household cleaning products and hardware store products.	Work only in well-ventilated areas. Discontinue using any household products that seem to cause your symptoms. Consult your doctor if your headaches continue.
Has your house been sprayed for pests? Have you placed any antipest products in your home? Have you sprayed your pets for pests?	If you mix or apply pesticides or insecticides, you may be exposed to boric acid in roach powders, chlorinated hydrocarbon insecticides, or cholinesterase inhibitors.	Discontinue the use of these products. Consult your doctor if your headache persists.

(*continued*)

ENVIRONMENTAL CONSIDERATIONS IN HEADACHE (*continued*)

Questions to Ask About Your Surroundings and Activities	Toxic Possibilities If You Answered Yes*	What to Do
Does your discomfort grow worse during the day at work and disappear or diminish after you leave your workplace?	Your headache may be part of the sick building syndrome. Poorly designed or malfunctioning fluorescent lighting may also be one cause of headache.	Speak to your supervisor and see if others have similar complaints. Discuss your symptoms with an occupational health nurse at your workplace.
Do you make pottery, glaze ceramics, make neon lights, or do enameling?	Craft materials may expose you to antimony, boric acid, cadmium, chromium, copper, lead, manganese, mercury, and nickel. During the firing process to harden pottery, formaldehyde may be released from the clay.	Consult your doctor about the materials used in your hobby. Be alert to toxins in hobbyist materials. Read labels, clean up properly, and work in a well-ventilated area.
Do you paint?	You may be exposed to aniline, antimony, arsenic, benzene, boric acid, cadmium, carbon disulfide, chromium, copper, glycols, halogenated hydrocarbon solvents, lead, manganese, mercury, methanol, nickel, petroleum distillates, styrene, toluene, and turpentine.	Be alert to toxins in hobbyist materials. Read labels carefully, clean up properly, and work in a well-ventilated area. If your headaches persist, consult your doctor about the materials used in your hobby.
Do you dye, print, batik, etch, engrave, or do lithography?	Your craft materials may expose you to aniline in dyes and inks; antimony, benzene, boric acid, carbon tetrachloride, and formaldehyde in batik; copper; dinitro derivatives of phenol and cresol; glycols; manganese; methanol; nickel; petroleum distillates; styrene; organic tin; toluene; turpentine; and xylene. When overheated, batik wax may release formaldehyde.	Be alert to toxins in hobbyist materials. Read labels carefully, clean up properly, and work in a well-ventilated area. If your headaches persist, consult your doctor about the materials used in your hobby.
Do you silk-screen?	Your hobby may expose you to formaldehyde, petroleum distillates, styrene, toluene and other solvents, and xylene.	Be alert to toxins in hobbyist materials. Read labels carefully, clean up properly, and work in a well-ventilated area. If your headaches persist, consult your doctor about the materials used in your hobby.

(continued)

ENVIRONMENTAL CONSIDERATIONS IN HEADACHE (*continued*)

Questions to Ask About Your Surroundings and Activities	*Toxic Possibilities If You Answered Yes**	*What to Do*
Do you make plastics, resin, or wax sculptures?	You may be exposed to antimony oxide, which is added to plastics as a fire retardant; benzene; carbon tetrachloride; glycols; halogenated hydrocarbon solvents; petroleum distillates; and styrene.	Be alert to toxins in hobbyist materials. Read labels carefully, clean up properly, and work in a well-ventilated area. If your headaches persist, consult your doctor about the materials used in your hobby.
Do you work in a darkroom?	Using darkroom chemicals may expose you to benzene, boric acid, cadmium, carbon monoxide (which is metabolized in the blood from methylene chloride), chromium, cresol, cyanide, dinitro derivatives of phenol and cresol, fluorides, formaldehyde, mercury, and trichloroethylene.	Be alert to toxins in hobbyist materials. Read labels carefully, clean up properly, and work in a well-ventilated area. If your headaches persist, consult your doctor about the materials used in your hobby.
Do you work with or refinish furniture?	Woodworkers, varnish workers, paint removers, and refinishers may be exposed to aniline, benzene, glycol ethers, trichloroethylene and other halogenated hydrocarbon solvents, methanol, noise from power tools, petroleum distillates, styrene, and toluene. Paint stripping may expose you to methylene chloride, which is metabolized to carbon monoxide in the body.	Be alert to toxins in hobbyist materials. Read labels carefully, clean up properly, and work in a well-ventilated area. If your headaches persist, consult your doctor about the materials used in your hobby.
Do you blow glass or make stained glass?	You may be exposed to fumes containing antimony, boric acid, cadmium, copper, lead, manganese, methanol, nickel, organic tin, and turpentine.	Be alert to toxins in hobbyist materials. Read labels carefully, clean up properly, and work in a well-ventilated area. If your headaches persist, consult your doctor about the materials used in your hobby.

(*continued*)

ENVIRONMENTAL CONSIDERATIONS IN HEADACHE (*continued*)

Questions to Ask About Your Surroundings and Activities	Toxic Possibilities If You Answered Yes*	What to Do
Do you make jewelry or metal sculpture, solder, or weld?	You could be exposed to benzene, cadmium, chromium, copper, cyanide, formaldehyde-containing resins used in making molds for metal casting, halogenated hydrocarbon solvents, lead, manganese, mercury, methanol, nickel, and noise from power tools.	Be alert to toxins in hobbyist materials. Read labels carefully, clean up properly, and work in a well-ventilated area. If your headaches persist, consult your doctor about the materials used in your hobby.
Are you a gunsmith, hunter, or marksman? Do you target shoot or supervise target shooters?	You may be exposed to mercury and petroleum distillates. In poorly ventilated indoor shooting ranges, you may be exposed to lead-containing fumes from gunfire. Loud noise may also cause headache.	Avoid or minimize exposure. Choose a well-ventilated range and wear protective ear coverings. Consult your doctor if your headaches persist.
Do you listen to loud music, wear stereo headphones, or go to loud music concerts? Do you use power tools?	Some leisure-time activities may expose you to loud noise, which can cause headaches.	Be aware of the sound level while involved with your hobbies. Lower the volume of your music; wear protective hearing gear. Consult your doctor if your headaches persist.
Do you use leaf blowers or lawn mowers? Do you ride in or work on motorcycles, trucks, cars, snowmobiles, motorboats, or race cars?	These activities may expose you to noise as well as to carbon monoxide, both of which may cause a headache.	Be aware of the sound level involved in these activities. Wear protective hearing gear and work only in well-ventilated areas.
Do you garden?	If you mix or apply garden chemicals, you may be exposed to boric acid in roach powders, carbon disulfide, chlorinated hydrocarbon insecticides, cyanide, dinitro derivatives of phenol and cresol, fluorides, mercury nicotine, nitrites and nitrates, pesticides, petroleum distillates, and organotin compounds.	Discontinue applying these chemicals. Consult your doctor if your headaches persist.

(continued)

ENVIRONMENTAL CONSIDERATIONS IN HEADACHE (*continued*)

Questions to Ask About Your Surroundings and Activities	*Toxic Possibilities If You Answered Yes**	*What to Do*
Do you use a computer with a video display terminal (VDT) at your workplace or home?	Headache is one of the most common complaints from workers using VDTs.	Adjust the lighting in your workplace. Check your posture and the placement of the VDT relative to your body. Use an antiglare screen when possible. Take frequent breaks and try to control "job stress," which may be a factor in VDT-generated headache. Consult your doctor if your headaches persist.

* See information sheets for more information.

Changes in hearing can take many forms and have various causes. Some people suffer from tinnitus, in which they hear ringing, pulsing, buzzing, or roaring sounds; others experience muffling or complete deafness in one or both ears. The loss of hearing can be sudden or can occur gradually over a lifetime.

The ear is the hearing organ and transmits sound to the brain for interpretation. Sound travels from the external pinna, the outer ear on the side of the head, through the auditory canal, eardrum, and bones of the middle ear to the nerve connections of the inner ear. Sound is converted to electrical impulses and travels along nerves to the brain. Any blockage or disturbance of this pathway may affect hearing.

Some lessening of the ability to hear is associated with increasing age, although it is not clear whether this is "natural" or the result of cumulative trauma to the ear due to excessive, prolonged exposure to noise. (See Chapter 18, "Noise," for more information.)

Common Causes of Hearing Changes

- Infections, such as a cold, flu, sinus infection, runny nose, sore throat, or allergies such as hay fever, can reduce hearing or cause ringing in the ears by blocking the eustachian tube, which runs from the middle ear to the back of the nose (see Figure 18.1, p. 632).
- The passage of sound can be blocked if wax builds up in the ear canal; if a foreign body, such as an insect or bead, gets lodged in the auditory canal; or due to an infection or a tumor somewhere in the ear.
- A perforated eardrum, whether from infection or trauma, may also cause a decrease in hearing.
- Trauma to the ear or the head, such as a blow

to the head, a loud explosion, or the changes in pressure throughout the auditory canal and sinus passages that occur during air travel or when scuba diving, can damage parts of the hearing mechanism.

Numerous other medical problems can affect hearing. A physician should rule out such problems as nerve, blood vessel, or other tumors; arteriosclerosis; genetic diseases; and brain or nerve disorders. Hearing loss may also be a part of Meniere's disease, which affects the ear's function of balance. Otosclerosis, an abnormal growth that immobilizes one of the bones in the ear, can lead to hearing loss.

Hearing Changes from Medications

Hearing disturbances can be a side-effect of some medications, including certain blood pressure medicines, antimalarial drugs, fever and pain medications (i.e., high doses of aspirin), antibiotics, and caffeine.

Nonprescription medications, such as herbal medicines and substances used in folk medicines, are sometimes contaminated with other substances, such as lead, caffeine, and salicylates, which can affect hearing.

Illicitly prepared drugs, such as cocaine, crack, and heroin, are themselves toxic to the ear or they may be contaminated with toxins that affect hearing, such as lead and arsenic.

Hearing Changes from Environmental Agents

By far, the most prevalent and significant cause of hearing loss is noise-induced hearing loss caused by exposure to excessive levels of environmental or industrial noise. Such hearing loss accounts for a significant number of occupational disabilities (see p. 637).

In addition, studies with animals indicate that exposure to certain environmental chemicals and toxic substances can cause hearing loss or can exacerbate the vulnerability of the ear to damage induced by excessive noise (see Table 18.1, p. 635–636).

If you notice ringing or buzzing in your ears or a diminished ability to hear and you answer "yes" to any of the following questions, you should be aware of the possibility of toxic exposure.

ENVIRONMENTAL CONSIDERATIONS IN HEARING CHANGES

Questions to Ask About Your Surroundings and Activities	Toxic Possibilities If You Answered Yes*	What to Do
Do you live in an inner city or in an old house with flaking paint and old plumbing? Are you renovating an old home?	Children especially may be exposed to lead by eating paint chips, inhaling dust, or drinking contaminated tap water. Renovating may expose you to lead in old paint and pipes.	Consult your doctor. Avoid further exposure.
Do you drink home-distilled moonshine whiskey or wine? Do you eat from glazed pottery dishes or cook with leaden pots?	These are possible sources of exposure to lead.	Consult your doctor. Replace dishes and cookware with lead-free kitchenware. Discontinue drinking homemade spirits.
Do you take herbal medicines or folk remedies?	Nonprescription medications are sometimes contaminated with other substances, for example, lead.	Consult your doctor. Discontinue using folk medicines, which may cause other symptoms.
Do you use cocaine, crack, heroin, or other illicit drugs?	These substances are toxic. In addition, many of these substances are contaminated with toxins such as lead and arsenic.	Seek help to discontinue your substance abuse. Continued use of illicitly prepared drugs puts you at risk of exposure to many toxins.
Do you listen to loud music, wear stereo headphones, or go to loud music concerts? Do you ride or work on snowmobiles, motorcycles, motorboats, or race cars? Do you use power tools?	Some leisure-time activities may expose you to loud noise with the potential to damage your hearing. This noise typically does not cause pain and you may initially be unaware of its effect.	Prevention is the key to preserving your hearing. Lower the volume of your music; wear protective hearing gear to prevent any further damage to your hearing.
Do you target shoot or supervise target shooters?	Repeated loud bursts of noise may damage unprotected ears. In poorly ventilated indoor ranges, you may be exposed to lead-containing fumes from gunfire.	See your doctor for a hearing evaluation. To prevent further damage, wear protective ear coverings. If you shoot indoors, choose a well-ventilated range.

(continued)

ENVIRONMENTAL CONSIDERATIONS IN HEARING CHANGES (*continued*)

Questions to Ask About Your Surroundings and Activities	Toxic Possibilities If You Answered Yes*	What to Do
Do you garden?	If you mix or apply pesticides, you may be exposed to nicotine, arsenic, mercury, organic tin, or carbon disulfide.	Consult your doctor. Discontinue applying pesticides or insecticides.
Do you paint, print, dye, sculpt, solder, or make stained glass or ceramics?	You may inadvertently be exposed to lead; organic tin; or the solvents xylene, styrene, or toluene.	Consult your doctor about the materials used in your hobby. Be alert to toxins in hobbyist materials. Read labels, clean up properly, and work in a well-ventilated area.

* See information sheets for more information.

IRRITATION OR DRYNESS OF EYES, EARS, NOSE, THROAT, OR SINUSES

One of the most important functions of the nose is to filter the air of particles and expel them either through a sneeze or in mucus, which traps the particles. If the nose is excessively dry or irritated from environmental substances, it may not be able to perform that function.

Anything in the air that inflames or dries the mucous membranes that cover the nose, sinuses, mouth, and throat can cause discomfort. Some things will cause only mild irritation, whereas others (like cadmium) can be progressive and can ultimately lead to much more serious consequences.

Conditions that cause marked dehydration, such as excessive sweating, diarrhea, or uncontrolled diabetes, can dry the mucous membranes. Surfaces that are normally lubricated by moist surfaces now start to rub against each other without this protective barrier. Very dry eyes can lead to corneal ulceration, and a dry mouth will promote tooth decay.

Irritation and Dryness from Illness or Injury

- Bacterial and viral infections, as well as exposure to certain chemicals, can cause inflammation of the nose, sinuses (sinusitis), mouth (gingivitis, or gum inflammation), throat (sore throat), and eyes (conjunctivitis, or pink eye).
- Allergic reactions triggered by pollens, animal dander, certain chemicals, or other allergens cause inflammation of the mucus membranes. Allergic reactions are characterized by itchy eyes, sore throat, and itchy, flowing nose. Although the eyes may be red and runny and produce a whitish, mucousy, thready discharge, unlike inflammation due to infection, there is no yellow or puslike discharge.
- Foreign objects, such as dirt or an eyelash, often cause eye irritation. Foreign bodies can injure the eye, causing an abrasion of the cornea, the transparent part of the surface that overlies the pupil and iris. If this occurs, the eye may feel irritated even after the foreign body has been removed. A corneal abrasion, which is exceedingly painful, can be diagnosed by examining the eye with a special dye and a blue light and/or a slit lamp.
- Certain hormonal changes may cause nose, mouth, and throat dryness or irritation. Oral contraceptives may cause nose membranes to swell and run and the throat to become dry and irritated. Thyroid hormone may cause membranes to become dry and the tongue to increase in size. The hormonal changes that accompany pregnancy may cause the mucous membranes of the nose to swell and cause blockage and postnasal drip.
- Unusual diseases can cause eye irritation. Sjogren's syndrome, an autoimmune disease that tends to strike middle-aged women, causes dry eyes and mouth because of inflammation in the tear ducts and salivary glands. Reiter's syndrome, which mainly affects young men, causes conjunctivitis along with arthritis and urethritis.

Irritation and Dryness from Medication

- Medications, including antihistamines, antidepressants, and drugs used to treat high blood pressure, can dry the mouth.
- Drugs snorted into the nose, such as cocaine,

will cause drying of the nasal membranes and may cause a hole to form in the septum, the structure that divides the nose in half.

• Radiation treatment of the mouth for cancers can cause dryness and irritation.

Irritation and Dryness from Environmental Agents

• Environmental agents dispersed as aerosols, fumes, dusts, or gases (such as ozone) can cause irritation. Fumes of metal oxides can cause irritation accompanied by general flulike symptoms, a condition known as metal fume fever. Cadmium fumes can cause such severe irritation that a person may develop symptoms such as severe shortness of breath due to lack of oxygen caused by fluid accumulation in the lungs (pulmonary edema).

• Cigarette or marijuana smoking may dry the mouth and the throat; the hot smoke may also affect the ability of the vocal cords, which produce speech, to function at their peak.

If you experience irritation or dryness of your eyes, ears, nose, throat, or sinuses and you answer "yes" to any of the following questions, you should be aware of the possibility of toxic exposure.

ENVIRONMENTAL CONSIDERATIONS IN IRRITATION OR DRYNESS OF THE EYES, EARS, NOSE, THROAT, OR SINUSES

Questions to Ask About Your Surroundings and Activities	Toxic Possibilities If You Answered Yes*	What to Do
Do you smoke cigarettes? Are you exposed to side-stream smoke?	Smoke can irritate the eyes, nose, and throat.	Quit smoking. Avoid people who are smoking.
Do you live in an area of high industrial pollutants?	Irritant gases, including sulfur dioxide, nitrogen oxides, and ozone, can cause these symptoms.	Avoid prolonged outdoor exposure when air quality is poor.
Do you work in a tightly sealed building?	Cigarette smoke, chemicals, and dusts contribute to sick building syndrome. Ozone produced by photocopiers, as well as low humidity, can also cause symptoms.	If it's not possible to open windows, check with the department in charge of overseeing the air-conditioning and heating systems.
Do you use illicit drugs?	Snorting cocaine can cause a perforation of the membrane that divides the nose. Smoking heroin and marijuana can also irritate the eyes, nose, and throat.	Seek help to discontinue your substance abuse. Continued use of illicitly prepared drugs puts you at risk of exposure to many toxins.
Do you take medications?	High blood pressure medications and antihistamines can cause dryness of the mouth.	Consult your doctor.

(continued)

ENVIRONMENTAL CONSIDERATIONS IN IRRITATION OR DRYNESS OF THE EYES, EARS, NOSE, THROAT, OR SINUSES (*continued*)

Questions to Ask About Your Surroundings and Activities	*Toxic Possibilities If You Answered Yes**	*What to Do*
Do you drink well water?	Phenol has been found in well water and is known to cause sore throats.	Have your water tested.
Do you make ceramics?	Clay contains silica and nuisance dusts (including talc). Glazes can contain metals like antimony, manganese, and chromium, whose oxides can cause irritation as well as metal fume fever when the metal is heated.	Work in a well-ventilated area. Use an appropriate respirator.
Do you sculpt?	Nuisance dusts and silica can irritate the eyes, nose, and throat.	Work in a well-ventilated area. Use an appropriate respirator.
Do you garden?	Pesticides and pollens can irritate the nose and throat. Overexposure to the ultraviolet rays of the sun can irritate the eyes.	Wear protective eye glasses. Use pesticides as directed on windless days.
Do you spend a lot of time in the sun?	Ultraviolet radiation can damage eyes, causing a gritty feeling.	Wear protective sunglasses and avoid looking directly at the sun.

* See information sheets for more information.

MEMORY LOSS, CONCENTRATION CHANGES, AND CONFUSION

A lapse in memory, occasional confusion, or a lack of concentration may occur in anyone and is often simply thought of as absentmindedness. With normal aging, you also may begin to experience loss of memory for recent events. However, sudden or severe confusion, memory loss, or lack of concentration may signal an underlying medical problem.

Physiological Causes of Memory Loss and Confusion

A recent head injury could cause these symptoms, often when there is damage to the brain or bleeding inside the skull. A stroke in which a blocked or burst vessel prevents blood from reaching the brain and causes death of brain tissue, or a temporary cutoff of blood to the brain, a transient ischemia attack, can also create confusion or forgetfulness.

People with heart and lung disorders and diabetes may also experience these symptoms. Any physical stress such as a recent illness, fever, childbirth, surgery, or neurological disease can precipitate confusion and memory lapse or lack of concentration.

Psychological Causes of Memory Loss and Confusion

Mental stress, perhaps from a change in jobs, home, or in a relationship, may disrupt normal thought in an individual. A person may appear confused, forgetful, or distracted. An exaggerated reaction to a situation can also disrupt memory and normal thought patterns.

Psychotic individuals, those with severe mental disorders associated with distorted percep-tions, illogical thinking, and an inability to respond to or recognize reality, may appear confused and unable to remember or concentrate.

Dementia, or long-term loss of memory and intellectual function, may occur in the elderly or at any age in those with presenile dementia, neurosyphilis, Huntington's chorea, subdural hematoma, or a brain tumor. Almost half the incidence of dementia is caused by Alzheimer's disease, while another 30 to 40 percent is due to multiple strokes.

A deficiency in vitamins, such as B_{12}, or minerals, such as iron or zinc, in an elderly person may also be at the root of a state of confusion, lack of concentration, or memory loss.

Medications That Cause Memory Loss and Confusion

Almost any medication has, at some point, been reported to cause disruption in memory or concentration or cause confusion. Among the more likely types of drugs that can cause these symptoms as side effects are adrenal corticosteroids, amphetamines, antidepressants, antihistamines, atropine, barbiturates, beta-adrenergic blockers, bromides, clonidine, hypoglycemic agents (insulin and oral agents) used to treat diabetes, tranquilizers, sleeping pills (such as benzodiazepines, digitalis and lithium), and overly high doses of salicylates (aspirin).

Environmental Agents That Cause Memory Loss and Confusion

These symptoms may also be caused by some toxic substances in our environment. For example, ordinarily bread and seed grains are quite safe to eat, but there have been incidents in which these foodstuffs were contaminated with toxins. In a 1971 incident in Iraq, seed grains treated with a methylmercury-containing fungicide and intended for planting, were accidently used in bread, causing over 6,500 poisonings. Fish have been found contaminated with methylmercury from industrial discharges, notably in the Minamata Bay area of Japan, where mercury contamination of the bay in the 1950s caused widespread poisoning among local residents (see Box 1.2, p. 25).

If you experience sudden or disruptive memory loss, lack of concentration, or confusion and you answer "yes" to any of the following questions, you should be aware of the possibility of toxic exposure.

ENVIRONMENTAL CONSIDERATIONS IN MEMORY LOSS, CONCENTRATION CHANGES, AND CONFUSION

Questions to Ask About Your Surroundings and Activities	*Toxic Possibilities If You Answered Yes**	*What to Do*
Are you a habitual drinker? Do you drink to quiet your nerves or on the job? Have you recently been drinking whiskey?	Frequently drinking too much alcohol (ethanol) may cause loss of memory and confusion. Alcoholics also sometimes suffer blackouts or total losses of memory for a specific period. In some cases, methanol has been found in preparations of whiskey where ethanol was expected to have been used.	Seek help to cut down on your consumption of alcohol. Seek immediate medical attention in cases of methanol poisoning even if symptoms initially appear mild, as they can become quite severe.
Do you drink home-distilled moonshine whiskey or wine? Do you eat from glazed pottery dishes or cook with leaden pots?	All these are possible sources of exposure to lead (see also the entry above on methanol). In using lead-glazed pottery, imports and ceramics with chipped or worn protective glazes are especially risky.	Consult your doctor. Replace dishes and cookware with lead-free kitchenware. Discontinue drinking homemade spirits.
Have you eaten any wild mushrooms or any gathered by amateur mushroom collectors?	Ingesting certain types of wild mushrooms can cause mental confusion or disorientation in addition to other symptoms.	**Seek immediate medical help.**
Do you take herbal medicines or folk remedies? Are you taking dietary supplements, homeopathic medicines, or products from a health food store?	Historically some of these products contained contaminants, such as arsenic, cyanide, lead, or thallium. Ingestion of a toxic dose of many of these may cause disorientation.	Consult your doctor. Discontinue using folk medicines, which may cause other symptoms.

(continued)

ENVIRONMENTAL CONSIDERATIONS IN MEMORY LOSS, CONCENTRATION CHANGES, AND CONFUSION (*continued*)

Questions to Ask About Your Surroundings and Activities	Toxic Possibilities If You Answered Yes*	What to Do
Are you a cancer patient taking Laetrile? Have you chewed and ingested the seeds from apples, peaches, pears, apricots, or plums? Do you eat cassava in large quantities?	Laetrile is an unapproved anti-cancer drug made from cyanide-containing apricot seeds. Cyanide is also found in the seeds of other fruits and in the cassava plant.	Consult your doctor. Discontinue your ingestion of these products.
Are you a kidney dialysis patient?	Because of your impaired kidney function, you may be affected by aluminum in antacids taken with therapy as well as in the fluid used in the machine.	Inform your doctor of your symptoms and explore with him/her any aluminum connection.
Do you smoke? Are you exposed to side-stream smoke? Have you recently quit smoking?	You are inhaling nicotine and tobacco contaminants, such as cyanide, and absorbing these substances into your body. Also, while stopping smoking, the withdrawal from nicotine can cause impaired memory and concentration.	Seek help to quit or reduce smoking and for help in dealing with the effects of withdrawal. Avoid people who are smoking.
Do you take hallucinogens, such as LSD, mescaline, or PCP (phencyclidine) or smoke marijuana?	These drugs of abuse are associated with symptoms of confusion, lack of concentration, and memory lapse.	Seek help to discontinue your substance abuse. Continuing to use these substances may aggravate these symptoms.
Do you use cocaine, crack, heroin, or other illicit drugs?	Many of these substances are contaminated with toxins, such as lead and arsenic. Cocaine itself can cause confusion, memory problems, and lack of concentration.	Seek help to discontinue your substance abuse. Continued use of illicitly prepared drugs may expose you to many toxins.
Do you intentionally sniff glue or adhesives, typewriter correction fluid, or gasoline to get high?	Habitual glue sniffers who inhale toluene may show long-term effects similar to those in people exposed through work; these include short-term memory impairment and inability to concentrate. Trichloroethylene, a halogenated hydrocarbon solvent, is found in typewriter correction fluid, a substance sometimes inhaled for its intoxicating affect.	Seek help to discontinue your substance abuse. Long-term exposure to these chemicals can cause serious health problems.

(continued)

ENVIRONMENTAL CONSIDERATIONS IN MEMORY LOSS, CONCENTRATION CHANGES, AND CONFUSION (*continued*)

Questions to Ask About Your Surroundings and Activities	*Toxic Possibilities If You Answered Yes**	*What to Do*
Do you live in an inner city or an old house with flaking paint and old plumbing? Are you renovating an old home?	Children especially may be exposed to lead by eating paint chips, inhaling dust, or drinking contaminated tap water. Renovating may expose you to lead from old paint and pipes.	Consult your doctor. Avoid further exposure.
Do you work or live in cold conditions: outdoors, in chilled rooms, or in an inadequately heated room?	If you develop hypothermia, a cold-related disorder, as the temperature drops, it can impair your memory and affect your reasoning abilities and motor functions.	Dress to avoid the effects of cold temperatures and seek to improve your work conditions.
Do you use special cleaning products, especially for your walls, clothing, or rugs; degreasers, dewaxers; polishes; or waterless hand cleaners?	Various halogenated hydrocarbon solvents, including trichloroethylene, and petroleum distillates are found in some common hardware and household cleaning products.	Inform your doctor and tell him/her of any household products you are using. Work only in well-ventilated areas.
Have you stored clothing in mothballs or flakes?	Inhalation of high concentrations of naphthalene in mothballs may cause mental confusion.	Use this product only in well-ventilated areas.
Do you paint, print, photoetch, dye, or do lithography?	Some substances in hobbyist materials, such as arsenic, halogenated hydrocarbon solvents, lead, mercury, methanol, petroleum distillates, styrene, thallium, organic tin, toluene, and xylene, are toxic.	Consult your doctor about the materials used in your hobby. Be alert to potential toxins in hobbyist materials. Read labels, clean up properly, and work in a well-ventilated area.
Do you silk-screen or batik?	These activities may expose you to carbon tetrachloride, a halogenated hydrocarbon solvent; petroleum distillates; styrene; toluene and other solvents; and xylene.	Consult your doctor about the materials used in your hobby. Be alert to potential toxins in hobbyist materials. Read labels, clean up properly, and work in a well-ventilated area.
Do you make pottery or glaze ceramics?	These activities expose you to arsenic, carbon monoxide, lead, and mercury.	Consult your doctor about the materials used in your hobby. Be alert to potential toxins in hobbyist materials. Read labels, clean up properly, and work in a well-ventilated area.

(continued)

ENVIRONMENTAL CONSIDERATIONS IN MEMORY LOSS, CONCENTRATION CHANGES, AND CONFUSION (*continued*)

Questions to Ask About Your Surroundings and Activities	Toxic Possibilities If You Answered Yes*	What to Do
Do you work in a darkroom?	Using darkroom chemicals may expose you to methylene chloride, which directly affects your central nervous system and is metabolized to carbon monoxide in the body. You may also be exposed to cresol, cyanide, mercury, and trichloroethylene, a halogenated hydrocarbon solvent.	Consult your doctor about the materials used in your hobby. Be alert to toxins in hobbyist materials. Read labels, clean up properly, and work in a well-ventilated area.
Do you blow glass, make stained glass or jewelry, make neon lights, or do enameling?	These activities may expose you to arsenic, cyanide, lead, mercury, methanol, thallium, and organic tin.	Consult your doctor about the materials used in your hobby. Be alert to potential toxins in hobbyist materials. Read labels, clean up properly, and work in a well-ventilated area.
Do you do woodworking, furniture refinishing, paint stripping, or furniture polishing?	These activities can expose you to methanol, petroleum distillates, styrene, toluene, trichloroethylene, and other halogenated hydrocarbon solvents. Paint stripping may expose you to toluene and methylene chloride, which is metabolized to carbon monoxide in the body.	Consult your doctor about the materials used in your hobby. Be alert to potential toxins in hobbyist materials. Read labels, clean up properly, and work in a well-ventilated area.
Do you do metalwork, solder, or weld?	You may be exposed to arsenic, cyanide, halogenated hydrocarbon solvents, lead, and mercury.	Consult your doctor about the materials used in your hobby. Be alert to toxins in your hobbyist materials. Read labels, clean up properly, and work in a well-ventilated area.
Do you make plastics or wax sculptures?	You may be exposed to styrene, carbon tetrachloride, and petroleum distillates.	Consult your doctor about the materials used in your hobby. Be alert to toxins in hobbyist materials. Read labels, clean up properly, and work in a well-ventilated area.

(continued)

ENVIRONMENTAL CONSIDERATIONS IN MEMORY LOSS, CONCENTRATION CHANGES, AND CONFUSION (*continued*)

Questions to Ask About Your Surroundings and Activities	Toxic Possibilities If You Answered Yes*	What to Do
Are you a hunter, gunsmith, or marksman?	These activities may expose you to cyanide, lead, mercury, methanol, and petroleum distillates. In poorly ventilated indoor ranges, you may be exposed to lead-containing fumes from gunfire.	Avoid or minimize further exposure. If you shoot indoors, choose a well-ventilated range. If your symptoms persist, consult your doctor.
Do you garden? Has your house been sprayed for pests? Have you placed any antipest products in your home? Have you sprayed your pet(s) for pests?	In your quest against insect or rodent infestation, fungi, and weeds and also in fertilizing, you may be exposed to arsenic, carbon disulfide, chlorinated hydrocarbon insecticides, cyanide, mercury, nicotine, pesticides, petroleum distillates, thallium, and organic tin.	Consult your doctor. Discontinue applying pesticides.

* See information sheets for more information.

NAIL ABNORMALITIES

Nail disorders are usually not serious threats to health, but they may indicate the presence of other diseases or environmental exposures. Nails may be affected by trauma, infections, general state of health, drugs, or chemicals in the environment. Nail abnormalities manifest themselves in numerous ways: Nails may be stained or discolored (e.g., leukonychia is a white discoloration, white transverse bands are called Mees lines, and blue-black discoloration is common from trauma); they may hurt; the area around the nail may become inflamed (paronychia); the nail may separate from the underlying finger (onycholysis); or they may be brittle, deformed, easily destroyed, thinned, softened, pitted, thickened, form growths, or shed.

Common Nail Problems

Nail problems are numerous and some are quite common. Many of us have experienced an ingrown toenail (the nail grows into the flesh at the sides of the toe and causes pain) or any of the variety of bacterial, fungal, and viral infections that cause athlete's foot, ringworm, or warts. Other such microorganisms can cause nail discoloration, destruction, or paronychia.

Nail problems can be caused by trauma, for example, from ill-fitting shoes that constantly press against and irritate the nail, or from exposure to vibration on the job, for example, pneumatic drill users may develop nail thickening, brittleness, splitting, and discoloration. Trauma can cause the nail to separate from the nailbed, discoloration (blue-black discoloration under the nail from hemorrhage), or nail pain. Workers particularly prone to nail trauma include shoemakers, florists, weavers, butchers, packers, potters, rope makers and users, keypunch operators, as well as dancers and sports enthusiasts.

Medical Causes of Nail Abnormalities

Changes in the nails are sometimes seen if other body systems are diseased. When anemia is present, the nail may appear pale; people with chronic liver disease sometimes have white nails. People with chronic lung and heart disease can have nail clubbing (a bulbous finger deformity where the nail grows as a mound shape). People with thyroid disease, chronic renal failure, or diabetes may also find abnormalities appearing in the nails. Local infections in the vicinity of the nail bed also may disturb the growing nail.

Nail Abnormalities from Medications

Drugs mainly cause color changes but may also cause pain or even shedding of the nails. Antibiotics, anticancer drugs, antimalarial drugs, retinoids, and dapsone (used for treating, among other things, leprosy) are the main types of drugs that affect nails.

Nail Abnormalities from Environmental Agents

Toxic substances in our environment can also cause abnormalities in the nails. The way in which these substances affect the nails varies. External discoloring agents discolor the nails when they come into direct contact with the nails, such as dinitrobenzene and the chromates, whereas internal discoloring agents, such as silver, cause discoloration after being taken into the body.

Solvents, hydrofluoric acid, and formaldehyde act as irritants and corrosives, causing more immediate damage to the nails. Other agents can cause an allergic reaction, usually in the nail bed, for example, formaldehyde, nickel, or cosmetics.

Exposure to some environmental agents may be detected by their affect on the nails, for ex-ample, the appearance of Mees lines from exposure to the heavy metals arsenic and thallium.

If you notice any nail abnormalities that persist and you answer "yes" to any of the following questions, you should be aware of the possibility of toxic exposure.

ENVIRONMENTAL CONSIDERATIONS IN NAIL ABNORMALITIES

Questions to Ask About Your Surroundings and Activities	Toxic Possibilities If You Answered Yes*	What to Do
Do you take herbal medicines or folk remedies? Are you taking dietary supplements, homeopathic medicines, vitamins, or products from a health food store?	Nonprescription medications may be contaminated with arsenic or thallium. Long-term use of very high doses of vitamin A may cause brittle nails.	Inform your doctor of your self-medication.
Do you use cocaine, crack, heroin, or other illicit drugs?	These substances are toxic. In addition, many of these substances may be contaminated with toxins, such as arsenic.	Seek help to discontinue your substance abuse. Use of illicitly prepared drugs puts you at risk for exposure to many toxins.
Do you smoke?	Handling tobacco (presumably the nicotine content) can cause yellow to brown nail staining.	Quit or reduce smoking to limit your contact with this staining agent.
Are your hands constantly immersed in water? Do you frequently wash clothes or dishes?	Constant water immersion can contribute to the development of paronychia.	Avoid water contact with your hands. Use rubber gloves when you immerse your hands. To absorb sweat and keep hands dry, wear thin cotton gloves under rubber gloves.
Do you wear sculptured artificial nails or nail polish or hardener?	Acrylics in sculptured nails, nail polish remover, and formaldehyde in nail hardener may cause damage. Using nail polish may cause yellow-brown discoloration of the nails.	Discontinue applying these products.
Do your hands frequently have contact with oils and other chemicals at work?	Solvents, alkalis, acids, and motor oils can soften and damage your nails.	Avoid further contact by wearing barrier creams or gloves while on the job.

(continued)

ENVIRONMENTAL CONSIDERATIONS IN NAIL ABNORMALITIES (*CONTINUED*)

Questions to Ask About Your Surroundings and Activities	Toxic Possibilities If You Answered Yes*	What to Do
Do you garden?	Certain plants and bulbs contain potential allergens that may damage the nail. You may also be exposed to chemicals found in pesticides: arsenic, dinobuton and dinitro-*o*-cresol, paraquat and diquat, solvents, and turpentine.	Consult your doctor. Discontinue applying pesticides. Protect your hands from contact with plants and bulbs.
Do you dye, paint, sculpt, make stained glass, work in a darkroom, solder, weld, or make ceramics?	You may be exposed to acrylics, aniline, arsenic, chromium salts, dinitrobenzene, dinitro-*o*-cresol, hydrofluoric acid, formaldehyde, silver, thallium, and turpentine.	Consult your doctor about the materials used in your hobby. Be alert to toxins in hobbyist materials. Read labels, clean up properly, and work in a well-ventilated area.
Do you make jewelry or weld with silver solder?	You may be inadvertently exposed to acids, arsenic, or thallium.	Consult your doctor about the materials used in your hobby. Be alert to toxins in hobbyist materials. Read labels, clean up properly, and work in a well-ventilated area.

* See information sheets for more information.

NAUSEA

Nausea is a queasy feeling or an urge to vomit. It can be caused by anything from what is colloquially called a stomach virus to food poisoning or, in very rare cases, a brain tumor. A person's age, general health, and associated symptoms help sort out the cause.

Common Causes of Nausea

There are a number of common causes of nausea. These include gastritis (inflammation or irritation of the stomach, often associated with vomiting), enteritis (inflammation or irritation of the intestines, often associated with diarrhea), or gastroenteritis (inflammation of both, often associated with vomiting and diarrhea). Bacteria, viruses, parasites, and chemical irritants such as alcohol can bother the gastrointestinal tract. Food poisoning, overeating, and too much drinking are very common explanations for feeling nauseated. Nausea may be an early symptom of botulism, which occurs after the ingestion of improperly canned food. Other associated symptoms of botulism include visual disturbances and difficulty with speech and swallowing.

Anxiety, that feeling of "butterflies" in the stomach, is another common cause of nausea. Motion sickness, whether in a car or airplane, and noxious odors can cause nausea, as well.

Nausea from Illnesses

A range of abdominal disorders can trigger nausea. Stomach inflammation and ulcers, gall bladder disease (cholecystitis), liver inflammation (hepatitis), appendicitis, and intestinal obstruction can cause nausea. Kidney stones, pancreatitis, pelvic inflammatory disease, and twisted ovaries or testicles can also cause nausea. Depending on the underlying disorder, nausea can be the prelude to more severe symptoms, such as vomiting or extreme pain, or nausea can be the main symptom.

Hepatitis, an inflammation of the liver, merits special mention in discussing possible environmental causes of nausea. Because the liver metabolizes many chemicals found in the blood, thereby concentrating many toxins, it is particularly vulnerable to the effects of exposure. Hepatitis may be caused by viruses, drugs (including therapeutic doses of isoniazid and acetaminophen), alcohol, or chemicals, such as arsenic, carbon tetrachloride, dimethylformamide, and benzene. Other environmental factors—including poisonous mushrooms, pesticides, and excessive doses of vitamin A—can also injure the liver.

Hormones can cause nausea. Morning sickness of pregnancy is related to a surge in estrogens. Endocrine disturbances, such as diabetic crisis, also cause nausea.

Neurological problems can also make people sick to their stomachs. Migraine sufferers often suffer nausea with their headaches. People with an inflammation of the inner ear, a disorder known as labyrinthitis, also complain of nausea, but often with ringing in their ears or associated dizziness. Brain tumors, which may raise pressure inside the head, can cause nausea, but often there are other symptoms, such as severe headache or specific neurological problems such as diminished vision. Meningitis, strokes, and head injuries can also cause nausea.

Heart attacks, especially those involving the inferior wall of the heart, can cause nausea and vomiting. Chest pain, sweating, or shortness of breath may accompany the nausea in this case.

Nausea from Medications

Numerous drugs can cause nausea. Sometimes the nausea is a side effect that must be tolerated; other times nausea is an important warning of impending danger. For example, the antibiotics erythromycin and tetracycline often make people nauseated. Many cancer chemotherapy drugs cause nausea as a side effect but, frequently, this must be tolerated. On the other hand, excessive doses of a well-known heart drug, digitalis, are dangerous, and nausea is a warning symptom in this instance. Theophylline (an asthma medication) and opiates, such as codeine or morphine, can also cause nausea.

Nausea from Environmental Agents

Plants, such as mayapple (*Podophyllum peltatum*) or pokeweed berries (*Phytolacca americana* or *Phytolacca decandra*), as well as common plants, such as those of the Arum family (including philodendrum, dieffenbachia, and elephant ear) can trigger nausea.

Toxins that may cause brain swelling, such as excessive doses of vitamin A and carbon monoxide, readily cause nausea, although carbon monoxide can also cause nausea in the absence of brain swelling. Cocaine and amphetamines can cause bleeding in the brain, triggering nausea.

If you experience nausea and you answer "yes" to any of the following questions, you should be aware of the possibility of toxic exposure.

ENVIRONMENTAL CONSIDERATIONS IN NAUSEA

Questions to Ask About Your Surroundings and Activities	Toxic Possibilities If You Answered Yes*	What to Do
Did nausea start suddenly after a specific meal? Did someone else develop the same symptoms?	Food poisoning is common, often caused by bacteria, such as *Salmonella ssp.*, *Staphylococcus aureus*, *Campylobacter jejuni*, *Clostridium botulinum*, and *Bacillus cereus* type I.	Consult your doctor if symptoms persist.
Did you eat any plants, mushrooms, or herbs that might be poisonous?	Poisonous mushrooms can be hard to identify, even by an experienced mycologist. Common plants, such as philodendron and dieffenbachia, can be toxic. High doses of certain herbs, like caraway and cardamom, cause nausea. Mayapple and pokeweed can also cause nausea.	Consult your doctor.
Are you taking medications or vitamins?	High doses of vitamins A or D can cause nausea. Antibiotics are another common cause.	If not medically necessary, stop high doses of the vitamins. Consult your doctor regarding antibiotics or other medications.

(*continued*)

ENVIRONMENTAL CONSIDERATIONS IN NAUSEA (*continued*)

Questions to Ask About Your Surroundings and Activities	*Toxic Possibilities If You Answered Yes**	*What to Do*
Do you drink alcohol?	Alcohol can cause nausea in numerous ways: by irritating the stomach; injuring the liver, which results in hepatitis; and increasing toxic metabolites.	Stop or reduce your alcohol consumption. Consult your doctor or a counselor if necessary for help.
Are you drinking alcohol and taking medications at the same time?	Certain medications cause nausea and vomiting if mixed with alcohol. Antidepressants that are monoamine oxidase inhibitors can trigger a violent reaction if consumed with red wine or foods with a high tyramine content. Disulfiram (Antabuse), designed to maintain sobriety, as well as some antibiotics and antidiabetic drugs cause a severe reaction if alcohol is consumed, either in the obvious form of a drink or in less obvious forms, such as medicines or foods that contain alcohol.	Consult your doctor about whether it is safe to drink while taking a prescribed medication.
Is there a possibility that you are pregnant?	The rise in hormones causes nausea, mainly in early pregnancy.	Sweet or salty foods may help.
Do you work with wood?	You may be exposed to arsenic, benzene, boric acid, carbon tetrachloride, fluorides, formaldehyde, and phenol.	Work in a well-ventilated area. Follow instructions on labels about correct use of product. Inform your doctor of your activities.
Do you make jewelry?	You may be exposed to benzene, cadmium, inorganic mercury, and selenium.	Ensure adequate ventilation

* See information sheets for more information.

NUMBNESS AND WEAKNESS IN THE ARMS AND LEGS

Nearly everyone has experienced numbness or weakness in the arms and legs from sitting in one position too long or upon waking. We may have pressed on a nerve, stretched it, or temporarily cut off the blood supply. This feeling is usually relieved by moving around.

Numbness and Weakness from Trauma and Illness

Trauma and exposure to cold or heat can also have this effect. An individual who hyperventilates, breathing too rapidly and too deeply, may also experience some numbness and weakness of the limbs.

Certain medical conditions also may cause numbness and weakness in the arms or legs. Neck stiffness may signal cervical osteoarthritis in which pressure on the nerves and blood vessels in the neck region causes numbness and weakness in the arms. Raynaud's syndrome occurs in people whose blood vessels overreact to low temperatures. Carpal tunnel syndrome traps and pinches nerves in the wrist, causing numbness and weakness in the hands. Parvovirus B19, which causes fifth disease (erythema infectiosum), a mild communicable disease with a rash in children, has recently been reported to cause numbness and tingling in the fingers and toes of adults who are affected.

A person may experience numbness and weakness if the blood supply to the brain is disrupted by a bleeding or blocked artery (stroke) or temporarily by a narrowing of the arteries (transient ischemic attack). Diseases of the nervous system in which the covering of the nerves is damaged (demyelinating disease) may cause numbness and weakness of the limbs.

Long-term, irreversible numbness may be felt in those suffering from diabetes, alcohol abuse, chronic kidney disease, pernicious anemia, central nervous system damage from a tumor, syphilis, or nerve compression.

Numbness and Weakness from Medications

Some drugs, such as isoniazid (used to treat tuberculosis) and nitrofurantoin (an antibiotic used to treat urinary tract infections), may have numbness and weakness of the limbs as a side effect.

Numbness and Weakness from Activities

Divers may experience this sensation from improper decompression. Computer operators and assembly line workers may be affected because of repetitive motion (overuse syndromes).

If you experience numbness or weakness in your arms or legs and you answer "yes" to any of the following questions, you should be aware of the possibility of toxic exposure.

ENVIRONMENTAL CONSIDERATIONS IN NUMBNESS AND WEAKNESS IN THE ARMS AND LEGS

Questions to Ask About Your Surroundings and Activities	*Toxic Possibilities If You Answered Yes**	*What to Do*
Are you taking dietary supplements, homeopathic medicines, or products sold in health food stores? Do you take herbal or traditional folk medicines?	Historically, some of these products contained contaminants, such as arsenic and lead.	Inform your doctor of these supplements.
Have you recently eaten tainted fruit, seed grain, or vegetables?	These foodstuffs may be sprayed with chlorinated hydrocarbon insecticides or pesticides.	Thoroughly wash all fruits and vegetables before eating. Consult your doctor if symptoms persist.
Have you recently eaten mussels, clams, oysters, or other shellfish?	From May to October, shellfish may become poisonous from eating certain microscopic marine animals that produce a neurotoxin capable of causing numbness of the extremities.	**Seek immediate medical help: This is a medical emergency.**
Have you eaten any seafood, bread, or seed grain?	Ordinarily these foods are safe, but in the past environmental disasters have affected these foodstuffs and could possibly occur again. Fish has been contaminated with methylmercury from industrial discharge. Methylmercury is used as a fungicide for seeds intended for planting, but, in the past, these have been accidently ingested.	Consult your doctor. Discontinue eating these foods.
Have you eaten any home-canned foods? Have you eaten any previously cooked foods left at room temperature for a long time? Have you eaten canned olives, mushrooms, asparagus, tomatoes, beets, fish, peppers, or onions that may have gone bad?	Botulinum toxin is produced in these types of foods by *Clostridium botulinum* organisms. This toxin is the most potent poison known and affects the nerves. Persons affected by botulism may feel weakness in the limbs.	**Seek immediate medical help: This is a medical emergency.**
Have you eaten any unidentified wild plants?	Eating poison hemlock (*Conium*) and dog parsley (*Aethusa*) can cause gradually increasing weakness.	**Seek immediate medical help. This poisoning may be fatal.**

(*continued*)

ENVIRONMENTAL CONSIDERATIONS IN NUMBNESS AND WEAKNESS IN THE ARMS AND LEGS (continued)

Questions to Ask About Your Surroundings and Activities	Toxic Possibilities If You Answered Yes*	What to Do
Do you drink well water?	Well water may be contaminated by arsenic from natural or agricultural sources.	Have your drinking water tested. If symptoms persist, inform your doctor of the possibility of toxic exposure.
Do you drink home-distilled moonshine whiskey or wine? Are you a habitual drinker of alcoholic beverages?	Arsenic and lead have been found as contaminants in home-made whiskey and wine. Numbness may be a result of chronic ethanol (drinking alcohol) consumption.	Discontinue drinking home-made alcoholic beverages. Consult your doctor about your drinking habits.
Do you use cocaine, crack, heroin, or other illicit drugs?	Many of these substances are contaminated with toxins, such as arsenic or lead.	Seek help to discontinue your substance abuse. Continued use of illicitly prepared drugs puts you at risk of exposure to many toxins.
Are you habitually using any cough medicines, tonics, mouthwashes, liquid vitamins, or other over-the-counter medications?	These preparations may contain ethanol, which can cause numbness and weakness of the limbs.	Discontinue your use of these substances. If your symptoms persist, consult your doctor.
Do you live near a smelter or other hazardous waste site?	There may be high levels of arsenic or fluorides emitted in the air near these facilities.	If your symptoms persist, inform your doctor of your place of potential exposure.
Do you live in an inner city or an old house with flaking paint and old plumbing? Are you renovating an old home?	Children especially may be exposed to lead by eating paint chips, inhaling dust, or drinking contaminated tap water. Renovating may expose you to lead in old paint and pipes.	Consult your doctor. Avoid further exposure.
Has your house been sprayed for pests? Have you placed any antipest products in your home?	If you mix or apply insecticides, you may be exposed to chlorinated hydrocarbon insecticides.	Discontinue use of this product. Consult your doctor if symptoms persist.
Have you been treated for body lice?	Benzene hexachloride (lindane), a chlorinated hydrocarbon insecticide, is found in Kwell shampoo and sprays for body lice.	Discontinue your treatment. Consult your doctor if symptoms persist.
Do you use special products to clean your walls, clothing, or rugs? Do you use common hardware store products, such as waterless handcleaner?	Halogenated hydrocarbon solvents and petroleum distillates are found in some common household cleaning and hardware store products.	Inform your doctor of any household products you are using. Work only in well-ventilated areas.

(continued)

ENVIRONMENTAL CONSIDERATIONS IN NUMBNESS AND WEAKNESS IN THE ARMS AND LEGS (*continued*)

Questions to Ask About Your Surroundings and Activities	*Toxic Possibilities If You Answered Yes**	*What to Do*
Do you garden?	If you mix or apply pesticides or insecticides, you may be exposed to arsenic, carbon disulfide, chlorinated hydrocarbon insecticides, halogenated hydrocarbon solvents, organic mercury, pesticides, petroleum distillates, thallium, or organic tin.	Consult your doctor. Discontinue applying pesticides or insecticides.
Do you paint, print, batik, or dye? Do you use rubber cement or other adhesives in your projects? Do you do wax sculpture?	You may be exposed to arsenic, carbon disulfide, carbon tetrachloride and other halogenated hydrocarbon solvents, lead, manganese, petroleum distillates, styrene, thallium, or organic tin.	Consult your doctor about the materials used in your hobby. Be alert to toxins in hobbyist materials. Read labels, clean up properly, and work in a well-ventilated area.
Do you blow glass or make stained glass?	You may be exposed to arsenic, lead, manganese, or organic tin.	Consult your doctor about the material used in your hobby. Be alert to toxins in hobbyist materials. Read labels, clean up properly, and work in a well-ventilated area.
Do you make pottery, glaze ceramics, or do enameling?	You may be exposed to arsenic, lead, or manganese.	Consult your doctor about the materials used in your hobby. Be alert to toxins in hobbyist materials. Read labels, clean up properly, and work in a well-ventilated area.
Do you work in a darkroom?	Using darkroom chemicals may expose you to methylene chloride, a halogenated hydrocarbon solvent, which is metabolized to carbon monoxide.	Consult your doctor about the materials used in your hobby. Be alert to toxins in hobbyist materials. Read labels, clean up properly, and work in a well-ventilated area.
Do you work with wood or refinish furniture?	You may be exposed to carbon disulfide, halogenated hydrocarbon solvents, manganese, petroleum distillates, and styrene. Paint strippers may be exposed to methylene chloride, a halogenated hydrocarbon solvent, which is metabolized to carbon monoxide.	Consult your doctor about the materials used in your hobby. Be alert to toxins in hobbyist materials. Read labels, clean up properly, and work in a well-ventilated area.

(*continued*)

ENVIRONMENTAL CONSIDERATIONS IN NUMBNESS AND WEAKNESS IN THE ARMS AND LEGS (*continued*)

Questions to Ask About Your Surroundings and Activities	Toxic Possibilities If You Answered Yes*	What to Do
Are you a hunter, gunsmith, or marksman? Do you target shoot or supervise target shooters?	You may be exposed to lead, petroleum distillates, or selenium (see selenious acid).	Choose a well-ventilated shooting range. Consult your doctor if your symptoms persist.
Do you work on internal combustion engines?	You may be exposed to carbon monoxide.	Work only in a well-ventilated area. Consult your doctor if symptoms persist.
Do you make jewelry, weld, solder, or do metalwork?	You may be inadvertently exposed to arsenic, halogenated hydrocarbon solvents, lead, manganese, or thallium.	Consult your doctor about the materials used in your hobby. Be alert to toxins in hobbyist materials. Read labels, clean up properly, and work in a well-ventilated area.

* See information sheets for more information.

RASH

Rash is a nonspecific term that refers to areas of redness, inflammation, or blisters on the skin. In certain circumstances, almost anything can cause a rash—from contact with benign substances, such as excessive quantities of water or sun, to specific industrial toxins. Because large surface areas of skin are directly exposed to the outside world and its contaminants, the environment often plays a significant role in the development of skin problems (see Chapter 4, "Skin Ailments").

Some Common Causes of Skin Rashes

- Infections can be caused by a fungus, such as ringworm (tinea corporis); a virus, such as herpes, chickenpox (varicella), measles, German measles (rubella), or shingles (herpes zoster); or a bacterium, such as staphylococcus, streptococcus, or impetigo.
- Infestations of the skin by parasites, such as scabies or lice (pediculus), may present as rashes. Bug bites, for example, from bedbugs, can appear as numerous itchy, slightly raised spots on the skin.
- Physical agents, such as cold, sun, heat, pressure, and water, may irritate the skin and cause rashes. Heat and humidity are responsible for prickly heat, a rash common in young children.
- Allergic reactions are a common cause of rash and include the appearance of hives (bright red, slightly raised patches, that blanch on pressure, are usually evanescent, and itchy). Hives may appear as a reaction to a particular food, medication, or temperature.

- Contact dermatitis accounts for 80 to 90 percent of all skin disease caused by occupational exposure. In these cases skin comes into direct contact with a substance and results in inflammation from either irritation or an allergic reaction.
- Some substances act as skin irritants, and direct contact may cause red patches with itching, burning, or pain. Long-term contact may lead to dry, scaly lesions.
- Other substances act as skin allergens, leading to skin lesions that can resemble those caused by irritants, although the reaction involves the sensitization of the immune system. There are thousands of allergens present in the home, work, and outdoor environment.

Rash from Medications

Many medications cause rash (drug rash) as a side effect, including salicylates (aspirin), nonsteroidal anti-inflammatory agents (ibuprofen), certain antibiotics (tetracycline, doxycycline, and sulfa-type antibiotics), barbiturates, phenytoin (Dilantin), bromide, and phenothiazines. Some topical first-aid medications, such as neomycin, thimerosal, and benzocaine, cause rash.

Some biocides and germicides, such as formaldehyde, parabens, quaternium-15, and kathon CG, a mixture of two isothiazolinones, can also lead to a rash.

Environmental exposures to many substances can also result in skin rash. If you notice a change in your skin and you answer "yes" to any of the following questions, you should be aware of the possibility of toxic exposure.

ENVIRONMENTAL CONSIDERATIONS IN A RASH

Questions to Ask About Your Surroundings and Activities	Toxic Possibilities If You Answered Yes*	What to Do
Have you recently been handling food or preparing meals? Have you eaten any food that consistently causes a skin rash?	Foods primarily cause hives (urticaria); less often, they cause allergic contact dermatitis (mango, gingko). The most common allergenic foods are dairy products, eggs, citrus fruits (particularly strawberries and pineapple), flour, grains, honey, menthol, nuts, meats, seafood, vanillin, and vegetables, such as carrots or asparagus.	Identify and avoid the offending agent.
Have you recently been walking outdoors, hiking, or gardening?	Contact with a variety of plants, including poison oak, poison ivy, and poison sumac, may cause a skin reaction.	Avoiding contact with these plants is important. Depending on the severity of the rash, treatment may include soaks, topical medications, lotions, or oral medication from your doctor.
Have you been cleaning, washing, polishing, or using a waterless handcleaner?	Common substances such as water, soaps, and detergents can cause rash. Waterless handcleaner and furniture polish contain petroleum distillates, which can affect the skin. Oven cleaners, spot removers, and furniture polishes often contain trichloroethane. If you are wearing rubber gloves, chemicals added to the rubber (e.g., accelerators and antioxidants) can cause a rash.	Protect your hands from contact with water and harsh chemicals by wearing rubber or vinyl gloves (although you may develop sensitivity to rubber gloves as well).
Are you wearing new shoes or clothing? Are you wearing clothing made from silk or wool?	Itching rashes are known to be caused by some textiles, such as silk and wool, and textile finishes that contain formaldehyde, formaldehyde resins, or dyes. The two most common causes of shoe dermatitis are the rubber accelerators added to the rubber and leather tanning agents (potassium dichromate). Allergic reactions also occur from phenolic resins used in footwear and clothing.	You may need to consult your doctor to attempt identifying the fabrics or items of clothing that cause the rash. Once they are identified, avoid them.

(continued)

ENVIRONMENTAL CONSIDERATIONS IN A RASH (*continued*)

Questions to Ask About Your Surroundings and Activities	Toxic Possibilities If You Answered Yes*	What to Do
Do you wear perfumes, colognes, or cosmetics? Do you use hairspray?	There are numerous substances in many cosmetics and colognes that may cause a skin rash, notably fragrances, hair dyes, preservatives (e.g., *p*-phenylenediamine), and stabilizers, as well as chromium, formaldehyde, and trichloroethane (in hairspray).	It is difficult to identify the precise cause of such skin problems; you may need to work with your doctor. Once identified, avoid further exposure. If the problem persists, consult your doctor.
Do you use hair preparations, such as cold wave lotion or permanent hair dyes?	The skin may be sensitized to thioglycolates in wave lotions or *p*-phenylenediamine, toluenediamines, and other aromatic amine compounds.	If you notice a rash consistently following a hair treatment, discontinue using this preparation. In some cases, switching to a different formulation may help.
Have you been renovating your home or upgrading your insulation?	Fiberglass can cause pinpoint lesions (small pinpricklike dots) with intense itching.	Keep your body covered and shower right after working with fiberglass to help reduce irritation.
Do you work in a darkroom?	A skin rash may be caused by contact with reducing and oxidizing agents, alkalis, solvents, color developers, chromate (chromium), cobalt, formaldehyde, mercury, *p*-phenylenediamine, and PBA-1 (persulfate bleach accelerator) found in photographic chemicals.	Be alert to potential skin irritants and allergens in photographic chemicals. Read labels, avoid skin contact, and clean up properly. Consult your doctor if your rash persists.
Do you make jewelry?	You may be exposed to fluxes, solvents, mercury, nickel, and enamels.	Be alert to potential skin irritants and allergens in hobbyist materials. Read labels and clean up properly. Consult your doctor if your rash persists.
Do you paint, ink, or dye?	You may be exposed to materials containing acrylics, chromate (chromium), cobalt, nickel, *p*-phenylenediamine in inks and dyes, petroleum distillates, solvents, and turpentine.	Be alert to potential skin irritants and allergens in hobbyist materials. Read labels and clean up properly. Consult your doctor if your rash persists.

(*continued*)

ENVIRONMENTAL CONSIDERATIONS IN A RASH (*continued*)

Questions to Ask About Your Surroundings and Activities	Toxic Possibilities If You Answered Yes*	What to Do
Do you silk-screen?	You may be exposed to solvents, soaps, and detergents; an abundance of water; chemicals added to rubber (antioxidants, accelerators); formaldehyde; and dyes.	Be alert to potential skin irritants and allergens in hobbyist materials. Read labels and clean up properly. Consult your doctor if your rash persists.
Do you make ceramics?	You risk exposure to cobalt in glazes, mercury, nickel, clay dust, wet clay, acids, and alkalis. Soaps and detergents used to clean up may also affect the skin.	Be alert to potential skin irritants and allergens in hobbyist materials. Read labels and clean up properly. Consult your doctor if your rash persists.
Do you refinish furniture or work with wood?	Woodworkers may be exposed to sawdust and other nuisance dusts, wood bleaches, shellacs, lacquers, varnishes, turpentine, and other solvents and certain woods, including cedar, ebony, mahogany, pine, fir, rosewood, satinwood, teak, and cocobolo. Even the soaps and detergents used to clean up may affect the skin.	Be alert to potential skin irritants and allergens in hobbyist materials. Read labels and clean up properly. Consult your doctor if your rash persists.
Do you garden?	You may be exposed to poison oak, poison ivy, and poison sumac; other irritating plants, such as chrysanthemums, ragweed, English ivy, primrose, tulips, hyacinths, garlic onions, sagebrush, feverfew, liverwort, lichens,and primrose; organomercurials (mercury); pesticides; formaldehyde; and halogenated hydrocarbon solvents.	Use garden chemicals with care, reading instructions and avoiding direct skin contact. Try to identify those plants that cause your rash and avoid them.

* See information sheets for more information.

SMELL DISTURBANCES

Disturbances of the sense of smell can take several forms. You can lose your sense of smell (anosmia) or have it decreased (hyposmia). It can become distorted (dysosmia) so that things smell foul (cacosmia) or so that you sense different smells without the presence of a stimulus (parosmia).

The ability to smell may become altered for a number of reasons. Odors must travel from the environment up the nasal cavity to reach the olfactory nerves, which then carry electrical impulses to the brain; this is where the interpretation of smell occurs. Any disruption in this path will affect the sense of smell. As we age, our sense of smell often diminishes. Elderly people complain about food losing its taste because sensing flavor depends on both smell and taste.

Common Causes of Altered Smell

The most common ailments that diminish the sense of smell by blocking the passages in the nose are colds, allergies, flu, sinus infections, or nasal polyps (small growths on the inside of the nose). Less frequently, overgrowth of the adenoids, a deviation in the septum dividing the two nasal passages, or a tumor will block the airflow and decrease the sense of smell.

A head injury affecting the front part of the nervous system or brain or a skull fracture can damage the sense of smell. Five to ten percent of all major head injury cases result in some dysfunction in the sense of smell.

Medical Disorders That Alter Smell

Many diseases of other body systems also affect the sense of smell, including infections, tumors, neurological problems, endocrine disorders, hereditary disease, cirrhosis of the liver, and kidney failure. Hallucinations of odor may be associated with certain psychological disorders.

Damage to nervous tissue in the brain by a stroke or by toxic chemicals may alter our sense of smell. Smell is distorted in some people who are born with certain errors in the way the body handles its various chemical reactions. A hereditary disease that results in a missing liver enzyme has been shown to cause a buildup of a substance responsible for a fish odor complaint.

Dietary deficiencies can affect the sense of smell, particularly deficiencies in vitamin A, vitamin B_{12}, or zinc.

Medications That Alter Smell

Smell may be altered as a side effect of a number of medications, dietary supplements, and nose drops, including some antibiotics, blood pressure medicines, anticoagulants, and antihistamines. Cancer chemotherapy and radiation treatment to the head may also damage nerve cells that carry smell sensation to the brain.

Environmental Agents That Alter Smell

Many substances in the environment can interact and interfere with the sense of smell. We can lose our sense of smell temporarily or permanently. When the ability to perceive an odor is temporarily lost but then returns in a few minutes after the cause is removed, this is called *smell adaptation*. When the ability to detect a particular chemical completely disappears, it is called *olfactory fatigue;* it can remain for a variable amount of time.

The way in which environmental substances affect our ability to smell varies. Some substances, such as hydrogen sulfide, block or alter the sites in the lining of the nose that pick up the stimulus for smell. Other substances, for example, chromium and formaldehyde, hinder the sense of smell by causing a general inflammation of the tissues in the nose. Certain substances, including lead, mercury, and trichloroethylene, may actually destroy nerve tissue and prevent the smell "message" from reaching the brain.

The brain may also act to modify our sense of smell by sending signals back to the nerves, which pick up smell messages. This theory may explain why we "adapt" to some odors: The more we are exposed to these odors, the less we notice them.

A relatively new class of chemicals called malodor counteractants are being added to our environment. These substances are used to neutralize an offensive odor. They prevent our perception of foul odors. Malodor counteractants are found in industrial cleaning agents, often used in hospitals, sewers, waste water treatment plants, industrial plants, and garbage landfills.

If you notice that your sense of smell is decreased, absent, or distorted and you answer "yes" to any of the following questions, you should be aware of the possibility of toxic exposure.

ENVIRONMENTAL CONSIDERATIONS IN SMELL DISTURBANCE

Questions to Ask About Your Surroundings and Activities	Toxic Possibilities If You Answered Yes*	What to Do
Do you smoke? Are you exposed to side-stream smoke?	You are inhaling nicotine and tobacco contaminants, such as cadmium, formaldehyde, and cyanide, and absorbing these substances into your body.	Quit or reduce smoking. Avoid people who are smoking.
Are you taking any dietary supplements or vitamins, or using products sold in health food stores?	Taking high doses of vitamin D or using dimethyl sulfoxide or cyanide-containing health food products may affect your sense of smell.	Consult your doctor. Discontinue using folk medicines, which may cause other symptoms.
Have you recently changed toothpastes?	Some toothpastes have been shown to affect the sense of smell.	Change brand or type of toothpaste.
Do you live in a mobile home? Do you spend a lot of time indoors where there are gas appliances, new carpeting, particle board, or foam insulation?	All of these are sources of exposure to formaldehyde, which can reduce your ability to smell.	Improve the ventilation in your home. If your smell disturbance continues, consult your doctor.
Do you use oil of peppermint?	Repeated exposure to oil of peppermint has been reported to decrease the ability to smell.	Avoid this product.

(continued)

ENVIRONMENTAL CONSIDERATIONS IN SMELL DISTURBANCE (*continued*)

Questions to Ask About Your Surroundings and Activities	*Toxic Possibilities If You Answered Yes**	*What to Do*
Do you paint; make ceramics, pottery, or jewelry; or do enameling or metalwork? Do you work in a darkroom?	You may be exposed to benzene and other petroleum distillates, cadmium, chromium, cyanide compounds, halogenated hydrocarbon solvents, mercury, nickel, nuisance dusts, and vanadium.	Consult your doctor about the materials used in your hobby. Be alert to potential toxins in hobbyist materials. Read labels, clean up properly, and work in a well-ventilated area.
Are you a gunsmith, hunter, or marksman?	These hobbies may expose you to benzene and other petroleum distillates, cyanide, mercury, and nickel.	Avoid further exposure. Consult your doctor if your problem continues.
Do you have a hobby or work in any occupation that generates nuisance dusts?	Your sense of smell may be affected by high concentrations of nuisance dusts.	Use respiratory protective gear in poorly ventilated workplaces. Consult your doctor if your problem persists.

* See information sheets for more information.

TREMOR

A tremor is a shaking or involuntary rhythmic or irregular movement of a part or parts of the body. A small amount of tremor is normal when attempting to maintain a posture or during movement. Abnormal tremors are usually more pronounced and are associated with many disorders.

Classifications

Tremors are classified as static (or resting), postural, and intention tremors.

Static tremors occur during rest and often disappear when the person begins to move; this is the type of tremor frequently seen in people with Parkinson's disease, or Parkinsonism.

Postural tremors occur either when trying to maintain a posture or throughout the movement of a limb. Included in this category are anxiety tremors, which are seen in depressed persons or those with psychiatric disease; tremor of fatigue, which occurs with exhaustion; and essential tremor, an inherited tremor, which can occur at any age and usually affects the upper limbs.

A number of ailments can cause postural tremors, including an overactive thyroid condition; liver dysfunction or failure; kidney failure; lung disorders and malabsorption syndromes (an inability to digest and/or absorb nutrients from the intestine); poisonings; acute illnesses, including infections; and as a result of lesions in certain parts of the brain.

Intention tremors occur when an arm or leg is moved toward a goal. This kind of movement is seen in people who have a disease affecting the cerebellum section of the brain (including multiple sclerosis) or who have taken too much anticonvulsant medication, such as phenytoin (Dilantin).

Neurological Causes of Tremor

Neurological problems, including stroke, and degenerative diseases of the brain, can cause tremors.

A rare cause of tremor that is found in infants four to eighteen months of age is *spasmus nutans*, a rhythmic nodding or rotatory tremor of the head occuring when the infants are sitting up. This problem usually disappears by two years of age.

Tremor from Medications

Many kinds of drugs can cause tremor as a side effect, including antipsychotic drugs, such as phenothiazines and haloperidol; antidepressive drugs, such as tricyclics and lithium; stimulants, such as amphetamines; epinephrine used to treat glaucoma; thyroid hormones; theophylline, an asthma medication; and phenytoin (Dilantin), an anticonvulsant.

Tremors caused by medication are usually fairly benign with the exception of tardive dyskinesia. Older people are more prone to develop tremor, and it takes longer for medication-related tremors to subside in them. Sedative–hypnotic drugs (including barbiturates, such as phenobarbital, and benzodiazepines, such as Valium and Librium) and antipsychotic drugs can also cause tremor during withdrawal.

A serious side effect of therapy with antipsychotic medications (phenothiazine and haloperidol) is *tardive dyskinesia*, a disorder causing involuntary and repetitive movements. It may occur months to years after therapy begins. Movements of the face and mouth, such as lip smacking, chewing, grimacing, and protrusion of the tongue, are most common. However, abnormal, repetitive movements of the limbs and body may also occur. Sedative-hypnotics may also cause tremor as an indication of over-use.

Tremor from Environmental Agents

Some toxic substances in our environment can also cause tremor. Ordinarily safe foods, such as fish, bread, and seed grains, have been affected by contaminants, such as methylmercury, in a few isolated incidents. In a 1971 incident in Iraq, seeds treated with fungicide containing methylmercury were intended to be planted but were mistakenly ingested, causing over 6,500 poisoning cases. In the Minamata Bay in Japan in the 1950s, fish were found contaminated by methylmercury from industrial discharge. Methylmercury attacks the nervous system, producing tremors as one of its effects.

If you have a tremor and you answer "yes" to any of the following questions, you should be aware of the possibility of toxic exposure.

ENVIRONMENTAL CONSIDERATIONS IN TREMOR

Questions to Ask About Your Surroundings and Activities	Toxic Possibilities If You Answered Yes*	What to Do
Do you live in an inner city or an old house with flaking paint and old plumbing? Are you renovating an old home?	Children especially may be exposed to lead by eating paint chips, inhaling dust, or drinking contaminated tap water, although tremor is not the most common or severe symptom of lead exposure. Renovating may expose you to lead in old paint and pipes.	Consult your doctor. Avoid further exposure.
Do you drink many cups of coffee, tea, or soft drinks? Have you taken over-the-counter diet pills, stimulants, cold or allergy medicines, or pain relievers?	These products all may contain caffeine or phenylpropanolamine, stimulants that, in large doses, can affect your central nervous system and cause tremors.	Eliminate sources of these stimulants in your diet and in any medications you use. Examine ingredient lists on baked goods, frozen dairy desserts, and gelatin puddings.
Do you drink home-distilled moonshine whiskey or wine? Do you eat from glazed pottery dishes or cook with leaden pots?	All these are possible sources of lead, although tremor is not the most common or severe symptom of lead exposure. Whiskey and wine also contain ethanol, which can cause tremor.	Consult your doctor. Replace dishes and cookware with lead-free kitchenware. Discontinue drinking homemade spirits.
Are you a regular drinker? Have you recently stopped drinking alcohol after a long period of regular drinking?	You may have a problem with chronic alcohol abuse, which can be associated with tremor. Tremulousness and delirium tremens are part of the withdrawal syndrome associated with alcoholism.	Seek help to end your abuse of alcohol. Sometimes medical attention is necessary to control the symptoms of withdrawal.

(continued)

ENVIRONMENTAL CONSIDERATIONS IN TREMOR (*continued*)

Questions to Ask About Your Surroundings and Activities	Toxic Possibilities If You Answered Yes*	What to Do
Have you stopped smoking in the past few weeks? Are you trying to give up smoking?	Tremulousness is part of temporary withdrawal.	Eat a balanced diet. Don't drink caffeine or eat sweets until withdrawal symptoms pass.
Do you take herbal medicines or folk remedies? Are you taking dietary supplements, homeopathic medicines, or products from a health food store?	Over-the-counter products sold as remedies (such as ginseng) may be contaminated with arsenic, lead, or thallium, as well as with other stimulants.	Consult your doctor. Discontinue using folk medicines, which may cause other symptoms.
Do you take cough medicine, tonics, liquid vitamins, or other over-the-counter drugs? Do you use mouthwash?	All of these products contain ethanol, which can be associated with tremor.	Discontinue the use of these products. Inform your doctor if your symptoms persist.
Do you use cocaine, crack, heroin, phencyclidine (PCP), amphetamines, marijuana, or other illegal drugs? Do you snort drugs from plastic or paper bags?	Using and abusing cocaine, PCP, amphetamines, and marijuana has caused tremors in some users. These substances may also be contaminated with toxins, such as arsenic or lead. Inhaling fluorocarbons from bags can be more than merely intoxicating. Tremor or even sudden death may occur.	Seek help to discontinue your substance abuse. Use of illegal drugs may expose you to many toxins.
Do you intentionally sniff glue or adhesives, or typewriter correction fluid to get high?	If you sniff glue or adhesives, you are inhaling toluene or other solvents, which in addition to causing intoxication can cause substance tremor. Trichloroethylene, a halogenated hydrocarbon solvent, can be inhaled from typewriter correction fluid.	Seek help to discontinue your substance abuse.
Do you use special products to clean your walls, clothing, or rugs? Have you accidently ingested a toilet bowl cleaner, disinfectant, metal cleaner, furniture polish, or a household bleach?	Trichloroethylene and other halogenated hydrocarbon solvents are found in some common household cleaning products.	**Seek immediate medical attention in cases of ingestion.** Otherwise inform your doctor of any household products you are using. Work only in well-ventilated areas.

(*continued*)

ENVIRONMENTAL CONSIDERATIONS IN TREMOR (*continued*)

Questions to Ask About Your Surroundings and Activities	*Toxic Possibilities If You Answered Yes**	*What to Do*
Do you garden? Has your house been sprayed for pests? Have you placed any antipest products in your home?	If you mix or apply insecticides, pesticides, or fertilizers, you may be exposed to arsenic, thallium, chlorinated hydrocarbons, mercury, nicotine, and vanadium.	Consult your doctor. Discontinue applying any of these products.
Do you make jewelry or weld with silver solder?	You may inadvertently be exposed to mercury, cadmium, or thallium.	Consult your doctor about the materials used in your hobby. Be alert to toxins in hobbyist materials. Read labels, clean up properly, and work only in a well-ventilated area.
Do you make ceramics?	You may be exposed to arsenic, lead, manganese, mercury, or vanadium.	Consult your doctor about the materials used in your hobby. Be alert to toxins in hobbyist materials. Read labels, clean up properly, and work only in a well-ventilated area.
Do you paint, print, dye, do lithography or enameling, blow glass, or make stained glass or neon lights? Are you using rubber cement or other adhesives in your art projects?	You may be exposed to arsenic, carbon disulfide, halogenated hydrocarbon solvents, lead (in stained-glass making and enameling), manganese, mercury, thallium, vanadium, or xylene. Some adhesives and inks contain ethanol.	Consult your doctor about the materials used in your hobby. Be alert to toxins in hobbyist materials. Read labels, clean up properly, and work in a well-ventilated area.
Do you work in a darkroom?	Using darkroom chemicals may potentially expose you to methylene chloride, which is rapidly metabolized to carbon monoxide in the body; trichloroethylene, mercury, and vanadium.	Consult your doctor about the materials used in your hobby. Be alert to toxins in hobbyist materials. Read labels, clean up properly, and work in a well-ventilated area.
Do you weld, solder, or do metalwork?	You may be exposed to arsenic, halogenated hydrocarbon solvents, lead, manganese, and mercury.	Consult your doctor about the materials used in your hobby. Be alert to toxins in hobbyist materials. Read labels, clean up properly, and work in a well-ventilated area.

(*continued*)

ENVIRONMENTAL CONSIDERATIONS IN TREMOR (*continued*)

Questions to Ask About Your Surroundings and Activities	Toxic Possibilities If You Answered Yes*	What to Do
Are you a gunsmith, hunter, or marksman? Do you target shoot?	You may be exposed to lead and mercury.	Avoid or minimize exposure. Choose a well-ventilated range. Consult your doctor if your symptoms persist.
Do you refinish furniture? Do you remove paint or varnish?	Some paints, varnishes, and paint and varnish removers may contain carbon disulfide, trichloroethylene, and other halogenated hydrocarbon solvents. Paint strippers may also be exposed to methylene chloride, which is rapidly metabolized to carbon monoxide in the body.	Consult your doctor about the materials used in your hobby. Be alert to toxins in hobbyist materials. Read labels, clean up properly, and work in a well-ventilated area.

* See information sheets for more information.

URINE COLOR CHANGES

Urine is so consistently yellow that a marked change in color can be alarming. Many things alter urine color, transforming its usual yellow hue into shades of red, orange, blue, green, or black.

Urine color depends largely on what is being filtered through the kidneys and how concentrated the urine is. Dehydration deepens the usual yellow color. Loss of the ability to concentrate urine, as happens in uncontrolled diabetes, can result in nearly colorless urine.

Urine Color Changes from Illness and Trauma

A bacterial or viral infection, such as cystitis (a bladder infection) or pyelonephritis (a kidney infection), can change the usual clear appearance of urine to a murky one. Infection with the bacteria *Pseudomonas aeruginosa* can cause a greenish hue. Blood in the urine turns it red, although small amounts (detectable only on laboratory exam) will not change its color. Blood can come from different areas within the urinary system. At the level of the kidney, it is usually due to the inflammatory process glomerulonephritis, a somewhat rare condition. Glomerulonephritis can also be caused by other diseases, including the autoimmune disease lupus and streptococcal skin infections, or, possibly, toxins such as carbon tetrachloride.

Bleeding can come from injury to the ureters, tubes that link the kidneys to the bladder. Most frequently this is due to the passing of kidney stones. Severe flank pain is often present. Bladder injury, from a bacterial infection or toxins, such as the chemotherapy drug cyclophosphamide (Cytoxan), or the illicit drug methaqualone (Quaaludes), can cause hemorrhagic cystitis, a severe inflammation of the bladder in which there is blood in the urine. Blood in the urine along with urinary frequency and urgency are the usual symptoms.

Hepatitis can turn the urine cola or amber colored because of the accumulation of bilirubin pigments (derived from the bile that is secreted by the liver). Viruses, drugs, and toxins that cause liver damage can indirectly change the color of urine.

Urine Color Changes from Medications

A large number of drugs can turn the urine a variety of colors. Rifampin, used to treat tuberculosis, and phenazopyridine (Pyridium), used to relieve the pain of cystitis, turn the urine bright orange; the antidepressant amytryptyline can turn urine blue-green. These color changes are harmless. In some instances, color changes can indicate toxicity, such as with the high blood pressure medication methyldopa, which can turn it black.

Some common over-the-counter drugs can cause harmless changes in urine color. Clorets (because of chlorophyll), Doan's Pills (because of methylene blue), and Listerine (because of thymol) can turn the urine blue or green.

Urine Color Changes from Environmental Agents

Urine often changes color because of substances being filtered within the body, such as pigments, by-products of drugs, or toxins. Toxins can either directly change the color of urine or cause such alteration indirectly by first injuring tissue that then releases pigmented substances that are filtered by the kidney. An example of this is when a toxin destroys red blood cells, which release hemoglobin pigments when the cells rupture; the urine's reddish cast comes from hemoglobin pigments released into the bloodstream, not from bleeding within the urinary system. Drugs, such as quinine, certain snake or spider bites, and chemicals, such as phenol and cresol, can also cause blood cells to burst.

Similarly, the breakdown of muscle cells releases myoglobin, a dark pigment that, when filtered by the kidneys, turns the urine dark red or burgundy colored. Such muscle breakdown can occur due to ingestion of alcohol and certain drugs, including phenothiazines and illicit drugs, such as phencyclidine (PCP) and cocaine, and as a result of a severe crush injury, an electrical injury, or grand mal seizures. Myoglobin can also be released after carbon monoxide, copper sulfate, or zinc phosphate poisoning.

Certain foods can change the urine's color as a harmless effect. For example, beets, rhubarb, and blackberries can turn it red.

If you experience changes in urine coloration and you answer "yes" to any of the following questions, you should be aware of the possibility of toxic exposure.

ENVIRONMENTAL CONSIDERATIONS IN URINE COLOR CHANGES

Questions to Ask About Your Surroundings and Activities	Possible Toxins If You Answered Yes*	What to Do
Have you eaten red vegetables or fruits?	Beets, rhubarb, and blackberries can turn urine red.	Don't worry; this isn't harmful.
Have you taken any medications?	Rifampin and phenazopyridine (Pyridium) turn urine bright orange. Many other medications turn urine blue, green, and black (see above).	Ask your physician if the medication could be the problem.
Are you using illicit drugs?	Methaqualone (Quaaludes) can cause hemorrhagic cystitis, turning urine red.	Seek help to discontinue your substance abuse. Use of illicit drugs may expose you to many toxins.
Do you drink a lot of alcohol?	Alcohol can change the color of urine by causing liver damage and releasing bilirubin pigments in the urine or by causing muscle breakdown and releasing myoglobin pigments. Alcohol can also interfere with the kidneys' ability to concentrate urine, thereby making it very light.	Stop or reduce your alcohol consumption. Consult your doctor or a counselor if necessary for help.

(continued)

ENVIRONMENTAL CONSIDERATIONS IN URINE COLOR CHANGES (*continued*)

Questions to Ask About Your Surroundings and Activities	*Possible Toxins If You Answered Yes**	*What to Do*
Have you had a significant physical injury, such as one sustained in sports or a severe car accident?	Myoglobin, the pigment released by crushed muscle fibers, will turn the urine burgundy. This is a serious problem because large amounts of myoglobin can cause kidney failure.	**Seek immediate medical attention (already likely because of the injury).**
Have you taken clothing in or out of storage?	If you inhaled or swallowed naphthalene-containing mothballs, this could cause brown or black urine.	Consult your doctor.

* See information sheets for more information.

PAIN ON URINATION, DIFFICULTY URINATING, OR DECREASED URINATION

In women, bladder infections caused by bacteria are the most likely cause of urinary problems that include frequency (urinating more often than usual), urgency (urinating without being able to wait comfortably), and pain. Use of a diaphragm can aggravate the problem, resulting in increased incidence of infection and pain. Sexually transmitted diseases, such as chlamydia or herpes, can cause similar symptoms. Postmenopausal women may experience urinary discomfort because of estrogen depletion.

In men, urinary discomfort is more commonly due to an infection of the urethra or of the prostate, rather than the bladder. Older men often suffer from urinary frequency and difficulty starting the stream because of enlargement of the prostate.

Difficulty urinating can also be due to diseases or toxins that change the bladder's normal muscle tone—either by increasing or by decreasing it.

Pain or Difficulty Urinating from Illnesses

Absence of any urine output, as distinct from severely decreased urine output, often suggests that there is something physically blocking the ureters or that the kidneys have failed entirely. Kidney stones composed of calcium oxalate or uric acid stones are a likely cause of blockage. Frequent consumption of rhubarb or very high doses of vitamin C can cause oxalic acid stones to form. The anti-inflammatory drug phenylbutazone causes uric acid stones, and fluorinated anesthetics like halothane, cause oxalic acid stones.

Severe blood loss, dehydration, or heart failure can significantly decrease blood flow to the kidneys, causing them to fail. Neurologic problems such as multiple sclerosis or spinal cord injuries can prevent the bladder from emptying normally.

Pain or Difficulty Urinating from Medications

Many medications including tricyclic antidepressants, such as amitriptyline (Elavil), and atropine, a drug that is used medically but is also, in rare cases, used to incapacitate robbery victims, can interfere with normal bladder-emptying function. Some antibiotics, including isoniazid, sulfonamides, and fluoroquinolones, as well as pain-killing drugs, such as morphine, codeine, and hydromorphone (Dilaudid) can cause urinary difficulties. Methaqualone (Quaaludes), an illegal drug, causes severe cystitis (bladder inflammation) with bleeding.

Pain or Difficulty Urinating from Environmental Agents

Foodborne neurotoxins can also impair bladder function. Botulism, usually from foods that have been improperly preserved at home, causes difficulty urinating.

Poisonous mushrooms, such as the *Amanita* species, can cause severe dehydration and loss of blood volume, resulting in kidney shutdown.

Toxins that severely damage the kidneys or reduce blood flow to the kidneys will markedly decrease urine output. Heavy metals (like platinum) and drugs (like the sulfonamides, anticonvulsants, and amphetamines) can damage the kidneys. Naphthalene, an ingredient of mothballs and turpentine, a widely used solvent, can also make urination painful. Other damaging agents include benzene and carbon tetrachloride.

If you experience pain on urination, difficulty urinating, or decreased urination, and you answer "yes" to any of the following questions, you should be aware of the possibility of toxic exposure.

ENVIRONMENTAL CONSIDERATIONS IN PAIN ON URINATION, DIFFICULTY URINATING, OR DECREASED URINATION

Questions to Ask About Your Surroundings and Activities	Toxic Possibilities If You Answered Yes*	What to Do
Are you taking antibiotics?	Isoniazid, sulfonamides, and fluoquinolone antibiotics can cause urinary problems.	Consult your doctor.
Are you taking painkillers?	Morphine, hydromorphone (Dilaudid), and codeine can cause difficulty urinating.	If possible, decrease usage. Consult your doctor, because suddenly stopping may cause symptoms of withdrawal.
Do you use illicit drugs?	Methaqualone (Quaaludes) causes hemorrhagic cystitis. Phencyclidine (PCP, or angel dust) can cause kidney failure. LSD can cause urinary obstruction.	Consult your doctor. Seek help to discontinue your substance abuse. Use of illicitly prepared drugs may expose you to many toxins.
Have you stored clothing in mothballs or flakes?	Mothballs may contain naphthalene, which can make urination painful.	Avoid mothballs and deodorizers that contain naphthalene.
Do you inhale glue either to get high or because you use it to build models?	Toluene and other solvents have been linked to kidney problems that decrease urine output.	Seek help to discontinue your substance abuse. Ensure proper ventilation.
Do you make ceramics?	Glazes can contain heavy metals such as lead or chromium that can cause kidney damage and decreased urine output.	Consult your doctor about the materials used in your hobby. Ensure adequate ventilation and use an appropriate respirator.
Do you paint?	Solvents, such as toluene and turpentine, can damage the kidneys.	Consult your doctor about the materials used in your hobby. Ensure good ventilation.

* See information sheets for more information.

VISION CHANGES

Eyesight is an extremely important sense for gathering information and responding to the environment, and vision disturbances can have great impact upon your life. You can notice a change in vision from very benign conditions, such as the need for corrective lenses (glasses), or from life-threatening ones, such as bleeding, a blood vessel blockage, or a brain tumor. Any change in the ability to see merits a consultation with a doctor.

Complete loss of sight is a medical emergency; it may follow a recent head or eye injury that may have injured the eye, nerves, eye muscles, or parts of the brain that form the delicate visual system. Always wear eye protective gear when engaged in occupations, household chores, and hobbies that have potential eye hazards. Loss of vision is also a side effect of some medications, including certain antimalarial drugs.

Blurred or double vision is seen due to many causes, ranging from food poisoning (botulism), diabetes, thyroid ailments, alcohol (ethanol) intoxication; intoxication from inhaling halogenated hydrocarbons or other chemicals that can impair central nervous system functioning (such as toluene); or as a side effect of a number of medications, such as certain antibiotics, antidepressants, and heart medications. When evaluating the cause, a doctor will need to rule out neurological, blood pressure, glaucoma, and other possibilities.

Vision Changes from Illnesses or Injuries

A frequent cause of eye injuries is foreign body accidents, in which something enters the eye and scratches the cornea (the transparent surface that overlies the pupil and iris) or penetrates the eye. The extent of damage depends upon the type of object and its force upon entering.

Other vision changes often accompany aging, such as presbyopia (nearsightedness), cataracts (a clouding in the lens of the eye, which impairs vision), and macular degeneration (a deterioration of the retina that results in loss of vision not correctable with eyeglasses or contact lenses). Glaucoma, an elevation in the pressure inside the eye (intraocular), occasionally causes blurring of vision or pain; commonly, there are no initial symptoms until serious damage has occurred. Routine eye examinations for a pressure measurement are crucial to detect an elevation of intraocular pressure.

Eyesight can be affected by eye infections caused by bacteria, fungus, or viruses; these require medical treatment. One common condition, conjunctivitis, or pink eye, manifests as gritty, burning, tearing red eyes and may be due to either an infection, allergies, or chemical exposure.

Migraine headaches (severe recurrent headaches) can be associated with seeing flashing lights or floating spots. Other visual disturbances include nightblindness, caused by an inadequate amount of vitamin A in the diet or by some medications, and nutritional amblyopia, or poor vision, which occurs in chronic alcohol abusers who are deficient in B vitamin.

Vision Changes from Environmental Agents

The most common cause of serious toxic eye injury is contact with corrosive substances, their vapors, or fumes; such substances include alkalis, acids, solvents, detergents, and other chemicals. Regardless of the substance, immediate and copious washing of the eye is recommended when damage is due to contact with a dangerous substance.

If you notice a change in your ability to see and you answer "yes" to any of the following questions, you should be aware of the possibility of toxic exposure.

ENVIRONMENTAL CONSIDERATIONS IN VISION CHANGES

Question to Ask About Your Surroundings and Activities	*Toxic Possibilities If You Answered Yes**	*What to Do*
Are you taking dietary supplements, homeopathic medicines, vitamins, or products sold in health food stores? Do you take herbal or traditional folk medicines?	Historically some of these products contained contaminants, such as lead, thallium, cyanide, and arsenic. Long-term use of very high doses of vitamin A (25,000+ IU) and vitamin D daily may affect your vision.	Consult your doctor. Discontinue using folk medicines, which may cause other symptoms.
Are you being treated for acne or osteoporosis?	High doses of vitamin A for acne treatment can cause blurred or double vision. Used to treat or prevent osteoporosis, vitamin D in high doses may cause cataracts or exophthalmos (an eye alignment deviation).	Consult your doctor.
Do you drink home-distilled moonshine whiskey or wine?	Methanol has been found in preparations of whiskey where ethanol (drinking alcohol) should have been used. Lead has also been found as a contaminant in homemade whiskey and wine.	**Seek immediate medical help.** Initially symptoms may be mild but could progress to blindness, coma, and/or death.
Do you intentionally sniff glue or adhesives, typewriter correction fluid, or other substances?	If you sniff glue or adhesives, you are inhaling toluene or other solvents, which in addition to causing intoxication can cause blurring of vision. Trichloroethylene can be inhaled from typewriter correction fluid.	Seek help to discontinue your substance abuse.
Do you use cocaine, crack, heroin, or other illicit drugs?	These substances are contaminated with toxins, such as lead and arsenic.	Seek help to discontinue your substance abuse. Continued use of illicit drugs may expose you to many toxins.

(continued)

ENVIRONMENTAL CONSIDERATIONS IN VISION CHANGES (*continued*)

Question to Ask About Your Surroundings and Activities	Toxic Possibilities If You Answered Yes*	What to Do
Do you smoke?	Smokers inhale nicotine and tobacco contaminants, such as cyanide. Tobacco amblyopia, a rare partial loss of vision, is caused by cyanide in cigarette smoke or a nutritional deficit associated with smoking.	Seek help to quit or reduce smoking.
Are you a cancer patient taking Laetrile? Have you chewed and ingested the seeds from apples, peaches, pears, apricots, and plums? Do you eat cassava in large quantities?	Laetrile is an unapproved anti-cancer drug made from cyanide-containing apricot seeds. Cyanide is also found in the seeds of other fruits and in the cassava plant.	Consult your doctor. Discontinue ingesting these products.
Have you eaten seafood, bread, or seed grain?	Ordinarily these foods are safe, but in the past environmental disasters have affected these foodstuffs, and it could possibly occur again. Fish has been contaminated with methylmercury from industrial discharge. Methylmercury is used as a fungicide for seeds intended for planting, but, in the past, they have been accidently ingested.	Consult your doctor. Discontinue eating these foods until the problem is resolved.
Do you eat from glazed earthenware dishes, live in an old house with flaking paint and old plumbing, or live in an inner city?	Children especially may be exposed to lead by eating paint chips, inhaling dust, or drinking contaminated tap water. Lead has been associated with visual impairment, blindness, and permanent brain damage.	**Seek immediate medical help.**
Have you eaten any home-canned foods? Have you eaten any previously cooked foods left at room temperature for a long time? Have you eaten canned olives, mushrooms, asparagus, tomatoes, beets, fish, peppers, or onions that may have gone bad?	Botulinum toxin is produced in these types of foods by *Clostridium botulinum* organisms. This toxin is the most potent poison known and affects the nerves.	**Seek immediate medical help. This is a medical emergency.**

(*continued*)

ENVIRONMENTAL CONSIDERATIONS IN VISION CHANGES (*continued*)

Question to Ask About Your Surroundings and Activities	*Toxic Possibilities If You Answered Yes**	*What to Do*
Do you use a computer with a video display terminal at your workplace or home?	If you use a video display terminal you may experience eyestrain and blurred vision. However, there is no evidence that video display terminals cause permanent or temporary eye damage.	Work shorter hours. Take a short break often and eliminate any glare.
Do you paint; dye; print; make stained glass, jewelry, or ceramics; target shoot; or refinish or work with wood?	You may be exposed to methanol, lead, phenols, carbon disulfide, toluene, xylene, and halogenated hydrocarbon solvents including carbon tetrachloride. Paint strippers may be exposed to methylene chloride, which is metabolized to carbon monoxide in the body.	Consult your doctor about the materials used in your hobby. Be alert to potential toxins in hobbyist materials. Read labels, clean up properly, and work in a well-ventilated area.

* See information sheets for more information.

WEAKNESS (GENERALIZED), FEELING "UNDER THE WEATHER," OR DEPRESSION

A sense of weakness, being "under the weather," or depression can lead you to feel vaguely ill without being able to point to a specific cause. Although minor mood swings are common, they become a cause for concern if the low feelings persist or worsen.

Weakness and Depression from Illness or Stress

Sometimes stress; major life events, such as a divorce or death (reactive depression); an unhealthy life-style; or overactivity may weaken you and cause you to feel overwhelmed. Depression is more common at certain times of life, such as at adolescence, after giving birth, at midlife, menopause, or upon retirement. Increased susceptiblity to bouts of depression may have no apparent cause.

Poor physical conditioning or an inadequate amount of sleep may make you feel "blue."

An infectious illness such as influenza or mononucleosis may be followed by a period of depression. Other medical conditions that may make you feel weak or "under the weather" include infectious illnesses, anemia, cardiorespiratory illness, a malignancy, and nutritional deficiency.

Myasthenia gravis is a chronic progressive disease that causes muscular weakness. The face and throat are usually affected first but the weakness spreads further.

Chronic fatigue syndrome is a recently named complex of symptoms, including fatigue and depression, which can be incapacitating. The cause(s) and diagnosis are still unclear.

Premenstrual syndrome (PMS) is a condition of irritability that has been cited as sometimes occuring in the days before a woman has her menstrual period. PMS encompasses feelings of mild unhappiness to severe depression. Many women notice mild changes associated with their menstrual cycles, but a doctor's advice should be sought if the mood changes begin to disrupt the daily routine.

Weakness and Depression from Prescribed Drugs

Drugs may have side effects that may cause you to have vague feelings of being ill. Among those known to cause weakness and low feelings are birth control pills, tranquilizers and antidepressants, barbiturates or other sedative-hypnotics, antihistamines, atropine or related drugs, analgesics, salicylates, antipsychotics such as chlorpromazine, hypoglycemic drugs, digitalis, thiazide diuretics, methyldopa, corticosteroids, reserpine, thyroid drugs, amphetamines, and beta-adenergic blocking agents. Consult your doctor if you notice these feelings while being treated with any of these medications.

You must be especially vigilant if taking several medications prescribed by different doctors for different conditions. Your pharmacist can help you assemble a list of your medications and their possible interactions for you to discuss with your doctors.

Weakness from Substance Abuse

Recreationally used tranquilizers, benzodiazepines, barbiturates or other hypnotics, and amphetamines can cause weakness.

Alcohol has a depressant effect on the nervous system, and excessive drinking can cause feelings of being "worn out," tired, and listless. Alcohol is a major contributor to the absence from work and illness. (Prolonged heavy drinking also causes permanent damage to the liver and nervous system.)

If you experience weakness, depression, or a feeling of being under the weather and you answer "yes" to any of the following questions, you should be aware of the possibility of toxic exposure.

ENVIRONMENTAL CONSIDERATIONS IN WEAKNESS (GENERALIZED), FEELING "UNDER THE WEATHER," OR DEPRESSION

Questions to Ask About Your Surroundings and Activities	Toxic Possibilities If You Answered Yes*	What to Do
Do you live in an inner city or an old house with flaking paint and old plumbing? Are you renovating an old home?	Children especially may be exposed to lead by eating paint chips, inhaling dust, or drinking contaminated tap water. Renovating may expose you to lead in old paint and pipes.	Consult your doctor. Avoid further exposure. Collect a water sample for chemical analysis if you suspect contamination.
Have you eaten any home-canned foods? Have you eaten any previously cooked foods left at room temperature for a long time? Have you eaten canned olives, mushrooms, asparagus, tomatoes, beets, uneviscerated fish, peppers, or onions that may have gone bad?	Botulinum toxin is produced in these types of foods by *Clostridium botulinum* organisms. This toxin is the most potent poison known and affects the nerves.	**Seek immediate medical help. This is a medical emergency.**
Have you eaten seafood, bread, or seed grain?	Ordinarily these foods are safe, but in the past environmental disasters have affected these foodstuffs, and it could possibly occur again. Fish has been contaminated with methylmercury from industrial discharge. Methylmercury is used as a fungicide for seeds intended for planting, but, in the past, they have been accidently ingested.	Consult your doctor. Discontinue eating these foods until the problem is resolved.
Have you eaten contaminated meat, milk, or eggs?	When polybrominated biphenyls were accidently added to livestock feed in Michigan, consumers of these products showed signs of weakness and depression.	Consult your doctor. Discontinue eating these foods until the problem is resolved.

(continued)

ENVIRONMENTAL CONSIDERATIONS IN WEAKNESS (GENERALIZED), FEELING "UNDER THE WEATHER," OR DEPRESSION (*continued*)

Questions to Ask About Your Surroundings and Activities	Toxic Possibilities If You Answered Yes*	What to Do
Have you recently eaten smoked fish, bologna, salami, pepperoni, bacon, frankfurters, corned beef, canned ham, or sausages?	Nitrites and nitrates are used in these foods to impart a smoked flavor or pink color or to prevent botulism. Nitrites have been associated with lethargy and weakness.	Avoid eating foods known to contain nitrite compounds. Check ingredient lists carefully. If your symptoms persist, consult your doctor.
Do you drink well water?	Well water may contain high levels of nitrites and nitrates.	Have your well water tested for nitrites and nitrates.
Are you taking any dietary supplements or using products sold in health food stores?	Long-term use of very high doses of vitamin A (25,000+ IU) and vitamin D may cause weakness. Historically, some products sold in health food stores contained contaminants such as arsenic, cyanide, lead, and thallium.	Consult your doctor. Discontinue using folk medicines, which may cause other symptoms.
Do you take herbal medicines or folk remedies?	Nonprescription medications are sometimes contaminated with other substances, for example, lead.	Consult your doctor. Discontinue using folk medicines, which may cause other symptoms.
Do you drink home-distilled moonshine whiskey or wine? Do you eat from glazed pottery dishes or cook with leaden pots?	All these are possible sources of exposure to lead.	Consult your doctor. Replace dishes and cookware with lead-free kitchenware. Discontinue drinking homemade spirits.
Have you had too much alcohol?	The hangover that follows excessive alcohol (ethanol) consumption may be associated with weakness or feeling under the weather.	Limit your intake of alcoholic beverages. Seek help to curb your drinking.
Do you smoke? Are you exposed to side-stream smoke?	You are inhaling nicotine and tobacco contaminants, such as cadmium and cyanide, and absorbing these substances into your body.	Seek help to quit or reduce smoking. Avoid people who are smoking.
Have you recently quit smoking?	Depression has been associated with nicotine withdrawal.	Seek counseling help if you find yourself becoming depressed when quitting smoking. Consult your doctor about nicotine replacement therapy to assist your withdrawal.

(*continued*)

ENVIRONMENTAL CONSIDERATIONS IN WEAKNESS (GENERALIZED), FEELING "UNDER THE WEATHER," OR DEPRESSION (*continued*)

Questions to Ask About Your Surroundings and Activities	*Toxic Possibilities If You Answered Yes**	*What to Do*
Do you use cocaine, crack, heroin, or other illicit drugs? Do you inhale amyl nitrite, butyl nitrite, or similar substances?	Many of these substances are contaminated with toxins, such as arsenic and lead. Using organic nitrites (nitrites and nitrates) can cause weakness.	Seek help to discontinue your substance abuse. Continued use of illicit drugs puts you at risk of exposure to many toxins.
Are you a cancer patient taking Laetrile? Have you chewed and ingested the seeds from apples, peaches, pears, apricots, or plums? Do you eat cassava in large quantities?	Laetrile is an unapproved anti-cancer drug made from cyanide-containing apricot seeds. Cyanide is also found in the seeds of other fruits and in the cassava plant.	Consult your doctor. Discontinue ingesting these products.
Are you being treated for acne or osteoporosis?	Long-term high doses of vitamin A for acne treatment can cause weakness. Used to treat or prevent osteoporosis, vitamin D in high doses may also cause weakness.	Consult your doctor.
Has your house been sprayed for pests? Have you placed any antipest products in your home?	If you mix or apply pesticides or insecticides, you may be exposed to boric acid in roach powders, chlorinated hydrocarbon insecticides and organophosphates (carbamates).	Discontinue the application of pesticides. Consult your doctor.
Do you sniff glue or typewriter correction fluid to get high?	If you sniff glue, you may inhale toluene and other solvents. Trichloroethylene can be inhaled from typewriter correction fluid.	Seek help to discontinue your substance abuse.
Have you been treated for body lice?	Benzene hexachloride (lindane), a chlorinated hydrocarbon insecticide, is found in Kwell shampoo and sprays for body lice.	Discontinue the use of this product. Consult your doctor if your symptoms persist.
Do you use a dust product to control fleas on your pet?	Carbamate dusts (pesticides) are used for flea control on pets.	Discontinue the use of this product. Keep pets away from furniture, where family members may come into contact with the chemicals. If weakness persists, consult your doctor.

(*continued*)

ENVIRONMENTAL CONSIDERATIONS IN WEAKNESS (GENERALIZED), FEELING "UNDER THE WEATHER," OR DEPRESSION (*continued*)

Questions to Ask About Your Surroundings and Activities	Toxic Possibilities If You Answered Yes*	What to Do
Do you use special products to clean your walls, clothing, or rugs? Have you recently used any hardware store products, such as degreasers, dewaxers, or other cleaners?	Trichloroethylene, other halogenated hydrocarbon solvents, and petroleum distillates are found in some common hardware store and household cleaning products.	Work only in well-ventilated areas. Consult your doctor if your symptoms persist.
Do you garden?	You may be exposed to benzene, carbon disulfide, chlorinated hydrocarbon insecticides, copper, cyanide, dinitro derivatives of phenol and cresol, mercury, nitrites, pesticides (organophosphate and carbamate agents), petroleum distillates, thallium, tin, and other hazardous chemical components.	Discontinue applying these chemicals. Consult your doctor if your symptoms persist.
Do you blow glass or make stained glass or neon lights?	You may be exposed to fumes containing antimony, arsenic, lead, magnesium, manganese, mercury, nickel, selenium, or tin.	Consult your doctor about the materials used in your hobby. Be alert to toxins in hobbyist materials. Read labels, clean up properly, and work in a well-ventilated area.
Do you make pottery, glaze ceramics, or do enameling?	You may be exposed to fumes of aluminum, antimony, arsenic, cadmium, cobalt, copper, lead, magnesium, manganese, mercury, nickel, selenium, tin, or zinc while firing pottery. Potters may also be exposed to boric acid and boron compounds.	Consult your doctor about the materials used in your hobby. Be alert to potential toxins in hobbyist materials. Read labels, clean up properly, and work in a well-ventilated area.
Do you make jewelry, weld, solder, or do metalwork?	You may be exposed to the fumes of aluminum, antimony, arsenic, cadmium, copper, magnesium, manganese, mercury, nickel, selenium, thallium, tin, or zinc and to benzene, cyanide, halogenated hydrocarbon solvents, and lead. If you use tools for grinding, drilling, and polishing, you may be exposed to cobalt.	Consult your doctor about the materials used in your hobby. Be alert to potential toxins in hobbyist materials. Read labels, clean up properly, and work in a well-ventilated area.

(*continued*)

ENVIRONMENTAL CONSIDERATIONS IN WEAKNESS (GENERALIZED), FEELING "UNDER THE WEATHER," OR DEPRESSION (*continued*)

Questions to Ask About Your Surroundings and Activities	Toxic Possibilities If You Answered Yes*	What to Do
Do you paint, dye, silk-screen, print, or use colored inks or markers?	You may be inadvertently exposed to aniline, benzene, boric acid and boron compounds, carbon disulfide, carbon tetrachloride and other halogenated hydrocarbon solvents, dinitro derivatives of phenol and cresol, lead, mercury, petroleum distillates, styrene, thallium, tin, toluene, xylene, or zinc.	Consult your doctor about the materials used in your hobby. Be alert to potential toxins in hobbyist materials. Read labels, clean up properly, and work in a well-ventilated area.
Do you use rubber cement or other adhesives in your art projects?	You may be exposed to benzene, carbon disulfide, halogenated hydrocarbon solvents, or xylene in various adhesives.	Consult your doctor about the materials used in your hobby. Be alert to toxins in hobbyist materials. Read labels, clean up properly, and work in a well-ventilated area.
Do you work in a darkroom?	Using darkroom chemicals may expose you to benzene, boric acid and boron compounds, methylene chloride (which is metabolized to carbon monoxide), cresol, cyanide, dinitro derivatives of phenol and cresol, mercury, and trichloroethylene.	Consult your doctor about the materials used in your hobby. Be alert to potential toxins in hobbyist materials. Read labels, clean up properly, and work in a well-ventilated area.
Do you use leaf blowers or lawn mowers, ride or work on motorcycles, snowmobiles, trucks, or cars? Do you work on internal combustion engines?	These activities may expose you to carbon monoxide and petroleum distillates.	Work in well-ventilated areas. Consult your doctor if you continue to feel weak or under the weather.
Do you make plastics, resin, or wax sculpture?	You may be exposed to benzene, carbon tetrachloride and other halogenated hydrocarbon solvents, petroleum distillates, and styrene.	Consult your doctor about the materials used in your hobby. Be alert to potential toxins in hobbyist materials. Read labels, clean up properly, and work in a well-ventilated area.
Are you a gunsmith, hunter, or marksman? Do you target shoot?	You may be exposed to mercury and petroleum distillates and lead-containing fumes from gunfire at shooting ranges.	Avoid or minimize exposure. If you shoot indoors, choose a well-ventilated range. Consult your doctor if your symptoms continue.

(*continued*)

ENVIRONMENTAL CONSIDERATIONS IN WEAKNESS (GENERALIZED), FEELING "UNDER THE WEATHER," OR DEPRESSION (continued)

Questions to Ask About Your Surroundings and Activities	Toxic Possibilities If You Answered Yes*	What to Do
Do you work with wood or refinish furniture?	Paint strippers and finishes may expose you to benzene, carbon disulfide, methylene chloride (which is metabolized to carbon monoxide in the body), other halogenated hydrocarbon solvents including trichloroethylene, petroleum distillates, styrene, and toluene.	Consult your doctor about the materials used in your hobby. Be alert to potential toxins in hobbyist materials. Read labels, clean up properly, and work in a well-ventilated area.

* See information sheets for more information.

Information Sheets

These information sheets provide further details about many of the common environmental toxins referred to throughout the book and in the Symptom Charts (pp. 275–358). Arranged alphabetically, the information sheets profile numerous chemical hazards and include some notable biological hazards, such as botulism, as well as physical hazards, such as ionizing radiation, lasers, and noise.

HOW TO READ THE INFORMATION SHEETS

A brief physical description of the environmental agent (or class of agents) is found in the opening paragraph, along with common synonyms or alternative names.

Sources of Exposure lists the major types of industries or activities through which exposure is likely to occur.

Routes of Exposure lists the means by which an agent can enter the body. There are four major pathways of entry: absorption through contact with the skin and/or mucous membranes; ingestion, the advertent or inadvertent eating or drinking of the agent; injection; and inhalation of fumes, of evaporated vapors of a gas, of respirable solid dust particles, or of liquids dispersed as aerosols or mists. (Many solid substances gain entry through inhalation when, for example, they are heated and the solid is transformed into a fume or gas, or when the solid is ground and forms a respirable dust.)

Symptoms of Exposure describes the *acute* symptoms (those that arise immediately after exposure to the agent, or that are caused after one exposure to a toxic level of the agent) as well as *long-term* or *chronic* symptoms (those that emerge over time, or that are caused by the cumulative effect of prolonged exposure to a toxic agent at lower than immediately toxic levels).

Alerts highlight special concerns regarding the ability of an agent to harm developing fetuses or women and men in their reproductive capacity (Pregnancy and Reproductive Alert), to harm children (Child Alert), or to cause cancer (Cancer Alert).

OSHA/NIOSH Standards cite federal regulations and/or recommendations of the levels of exposure to a potentially hazardous agent that are considered within an acceptable range for the workplace (permissible exposure limits, or PELs). The federal PEL standards are expressed either as a time-weight average (TWA) over an eight-hour day and/or short-term exposure limit (STEL). The TWA is intended to protect the majority of workers exposed at that level for an eight-hour day, five days a week for a work lifetime of forty years. The STEL is a level over a short period of time (typically, fifteen minutes) above which it would be dangerous to be exposed to the agent. Of course, some agents are so toxic that any exposure for even shorter periods would be dangerous, and are so noted.

The federal standards are set by the Occupational Safety and Health Administration (OSHA), the federal agency responsible for enforcing exposure standards as well as the standards regarding hazard communication for employees. OSHA bases its regulations upon the recommendations made by the National Institute for Occupational Safety and Health (NIOSH), the federal agency responsible for research in safety and health. It helps to keep in mind the difference in the intent between these standards; both OSHA standards and NIOSH recommendations are listed here if they differ.

In some cases, there isn't a federal standard and/or NIOSH recommendation; in these instances, we have supplied the recommendations of the American Conference of Governmental Industrial Hygienists (ACGIH), and the levels are expressed as threshold limit values (TLV); TLV refers to airborne concentrations of chemical substances to which a majority of workers may be exposed over an eight-hour workday, for forty-hour workweeks for a working lifetime without adverse effect and are generally time-weighted averages calculated over an eight-hour period.

Exposure to concentrations less than those listed may produce ill effects in some people as there is a wide range in individual susceptibility to these substances.

The OSHA Hazard Communication Standard mandates that workers who are exposed to toxic substances on the job are to be provided with information about the nature of these hazards and training about protective measures needed for job safety. Many states have "right-to-know" legislation which mandates that employers make even more specific information available to their workers.

For a listing of OSHA and NIOSH standards, we recommend readers to the *NIOSH Pocket Guide to Chemical Hazards*, last published in 1990 by the U.S. Department of Health and Human Services and periodically updated (available for sale as DHHS (NIOSH) publication No. 90-117 by the Superintendent of Documents, U.S. Government Printing Office, Washington, D.C. 20402 .)

Abbreviations and Acronyms Found in the Information Sheets

ACGIH	American Conference of Governmental Industrial Hygienists
TLV	threshold limit value (time-weighted average over eight-hour period)
PEL	permissible exposure limit (TWA concentrations that must not be exceeded during any eight-hour work shift of a forty-hour workweek)
STEL	short-term exposure limit (unless otherwise noted, a fifteen-minute TWA exposure that should not be exceeded at any time during the workday)
TWA	time weighted average concentrations (usually over an eight-hour day but up to a ten-hour workday during a forty-hour workweek)
EPA	Environmental Protection Agency
FDA	Food and Drug Administration
cm^3	cubic centimeter (volume)
fibers/cm^3	fibers per cubic centimeter
g	gram (= 1,000 mg)
L	liter (= 1,000 mL)
m^3	cubic meter (volume)

(continued)

m	meter (= 100 cm)
mg	milligram
mg/m^3	milligram of a substance per cubic meter of air (at 68°F and 1 atmosphere pressure)
mL	milliliter
J/cm^2	joules per square centimeter (measure of work expended or energy per square centimeter)
mW/cm^2	milliwatt per square centimeter
mppcf	millions of particles of a particular cubic foot of air (measure of vapor)
ppm	parts of a substance (vapor of gas) per million parts of air

INFORMATION SHEETS

Acetates

Acetates are a group of organic compounds used as solvents and in the manufacture of a variety of consumer products. They include butyl acetate, ethyl acetate, and propylene glycol monomethyl ether acetate (PGMEA) among others.

SOURCES OF EXPOSURE: Workers may be exposed to acetates if they use them as solvents for cellulose, resins, oils, and fats or in manufacturing paints, enamels, varnishes, lacquers, photographic film, drugs, furniture polish, and other products.

ROUTES OF EXPOSURE: Inhalation and ingestion.

SYMPTOMS OF EXPOSURE: Exposure to acetates will irritate the eyes, nose, and skin. In high concentrations, they may also cause headache, drowsiness, and unconsciousness.

Long-term, or chronic, exposure to butyl acetate, ethyl acetate, and PGMEA may damage the lining of the nose and cause loss of the sense of smell. Some acetates may cause liver and kidney damage.

OSHA/NIOSH STANDARDS: The federal standards (PELs) are methyl acetate, 200 ppm (610 mg/m^3) with a STEL of 250 ppm (760 mg/m^3); ethyl acetate, 400 ppm (1,400 mg/m^3); *n*-propyl acetate, 200 ppm (840 mg/m^3) with a STEL of 250 ppm (1,050 mg/m^3); isopropyl acetate, 250 ppm (950 mg/m^3) with a STEL of 310 ppm (1,185 mg/m^3); *n*-butyl acetate, 150 ppm (710 mg/m^3) with a STEL of 200 ppm (950 mg/m^3); isoamyl acetate, 100 ppm (525 mg/m^3); *n*-amyl acetate, 100 ppm (525 mg/m^3); *sec*-amyl acetate, 125 ppm (650 mg/m^3); *sec*-butyl acetate, 200 ppm (950 mg/m^3); and *tert*-butyl acetate, 200 ppm (950 mg/m^3).

Acrylics

Acrylics are a class of compounds related to acrylic and methacrylic acid. They are liquids with a strong odor and are easily joined together (polymerized). Acrylics are widely used in manufacturing and include acrylic acid; methyl, ethyl, and butyl acrylate; methacrylic acid; and methyl, ethyl, butyl, and isobutyl methacrylate.

SOURCES OF EXPOSURE: Acrylics are used in the manufacture of paints and lacquers; as solvents; and as an adhesive for paper, leather, and textiles. Dentists use acrylics to fill teeth and make bridges; orthopedic surgeons, as bone cement; and manicurists, to make sculptured nails. Plexiglass, artificial eyes, and contact lenses are made from acrylics, as are some floor coverings.

ROUTES OF EXPOSURE: Ingestion, skin absorption, and inhalation.

SYMPTOMS OF EXPOSURE: Contact with acrylics may cause irritation of the skin, eyes, and nose; slower and weaker heartbeat; kidney degeneration; and impairment of brain function. Allergic reactions causing skin inflammation with tingling and burning sensations (paresthesias) and tenderness of the limbs have been reported.

Long-term, or chronic, exposure can result in allergic contact reactions and damage to the nerves in the limbs. Contact with the nails can cause paronychia (inflammation of the skin around the nail), nail discoloration, onycholysis (separation of the nail from the underlying finger), and thinning and splitting of the nails.

OSHA/NIOSH STANDARDS: The OSHA standard (PELs) for acrylic acid is a TWA of 10 ppm (30 mg/m^3); methyl acrylate, 10 ppm (35 mg/m^3); ethyl acrylate, 5 ppm (20 mg/m^3); butyl acrylate, 10 ppm (55 mg/m^3); methacrylic acid, 20 ppm (70 mg/m^3); and methyl methacrylate, 100 ppm (410 mg/m^3).

Aluminum

Aluminum is a soft, lightweight, silver-white metal. Its many compounds have various industrial uses.

SOURCES OF EXPOSURE: Aluminum is found in the ores of cryolite and bauxite. The most dangerous exposures occur in the smelting and refining processes. Patients on kidney dialysis are also at risk for aluminum toxicity (from the dialysis fluid).

The salts of aluminum are used as astringents, deodorants, and antiseptics. Aluminum and its alloys are used in building ships, cars, and aircraft and making jewelry. Its compounds are also used in paints, china, pottery, and rubber products and in processing petroleum.

Aluminum may be ingested from processed foods, for example, pickles, antacids, and buffered aspirin, but is generally cleared by the kidneys.

Hobbyists who make jewelry and ceramics and metalwork (aluminum may be used for metal casting and sandblasting) may be at risk for toxic exposure.

ROUTES OF EXPOSURE: Ingestion (antacids), injection (intravenous dialysis fluid), or inhalation.

SYMPTOMS OF EXPOSURE: Inhalation of aluminum oxide fumes released if aluminum is heated may cause metal fume fever, a flulike illness whose symptoms include metallic taste in the mouth; eye, nose, and throat irritation; cough; difficulty breathing; fatigue; headache; fever; chills; sweating; nausea; vomiting; muscle aches; and weakness. Those exposed often recover in one to two days if not reexposed. At some point during continuous exposure to aluminum oxide fumes, tolerance develops (the fumes no longer cause symptoms). However, over the weekend or after a period without exposure, the tolerance is lost, and "Monday morning fever" may occur.

Ingestion of aluminum salts may cause burning of the mouth and throat, vomiting, watery or bloody diarrhea, painful spasm of the anal sphincter, blood in the urine, diminished urine output, jaundice, collapse, and convulsions. Skin, eye, nose, mouth, and throat irritations occur from exposure to aluminum salts.

Particles of aluminum may damage the cornea of the eye.

Long-term, or chronic, exposure to aluminum-containing skin solutions may cause red, bumpy rashes.

Patients with end-stage renal disease whose kidneys are failing may become poisoned from aluminum-containing dialysis fluid or, less commonly, by long-term ingestion of antacids, which contain aluminum. This "dialysis dementia," possibly due to aluminum poisoning, may affect brain function causing personality changes, difficulty in speaking, incoordination, memory loss, tremor, muscle twitching or spasm, dementia, and seizures. It may also cause weakness, shortness of breath, and softening and bending of the bones with pain.

CANCER ALERT: A higher incidence of lung and bladder cancer have been reported in aluminum-exposed workers.

OSHA/NIOSH STANDARDS: The OSHA standard (PELs) for total aluminum dust is a TWA of 15 mg/m³; respiratory fractions, 5 mg/m³; pyro powders, 5 mg/m³; welding fumes, 5 mg/m³; soluble salts, 2 mg/m³; and alkyls, 2 mg/m³.

Aniline

Aniline is a clear, colorless, oily liquid. It has a distinctive odor.

SOURCES OF EXPOSURE: Aniline is used widely in the manufacture of a variety of everyday products such as dyes, paints, varnishes, shoe polishes, inks, rubber, and drugs.

Hobbyists who paint, dye, print, or refinish furniture may be exposed to aniline.

ROUTES OF EXPOSURE: Skin absorption of liquid and vapor, inhalation of vapors, and ingestion.

SYMPTOMS OF EXPOSURE: Aniline irritates the eyes. Depending upon the amount of exposure, it can cause a range of effects from headache, respiratory abnormalities, weakness, dizziness, irritability, drowsiness, confusion, lethargy, and stupor to convulsions, coma, cyanosis (blue skin discoloration), and even death. Jaundice (yellow skin discoloration) and pain on urination can be delayed effects.

Aniline poisoning can produce a blue-violet discoloration of the nails.

Long-term, or chronic, exposure may cause weight loss, weakness, and irritability.

CANCER ALERT: Aniline dye workers have shown an increased rate of bladder cancers.

CHILD ALERT: Infants have died from absorption of aniline from cloth-marking ink stenciled on diapers. After washing, the inked diapers are safe.

OSHA/NIOSH STANDARDS: The federal standard (PEL) is 2 ppm (19 mg/m³).

Antimony

Antimony is a soft, silver-white metal. It forms many compounds, such as antimony trioxide, antimony trisulfide, and antimony trichloride and pentachloride. Stibine, a very toxic gas, is produced when acid interacts with metals containing antimony.

SOURCES OF EXPOSURE: Antimony is found naturally in several ores. Mining, refining, and smelting may expose workers to antimony. It is used in industry to make alloys (including pewter), abrasives, ant paste, battery components, paints, pigments and lacquers, flameproofing compounds, glass, pottery, enamels, glazes, drugs, matches, fireworks, and explosives. Antimony is also used in dyeing, blueing steel, and coloring other metals.

Antimony compounds have been used to treat certain tropical diseases.

Hobbyists should be aware of potential exposure to antimony while making ceramics and glazing, soldering, making glass, dyeing, and painting.

ROUTES OF EXPOSURE: Inhalation, ingestion, and skin absorption.

SYMPTOMS OF EXPOSURE: Inhalation of metal oxide fumes released if antimony is heated may cause metal fume fever, a flulike illness whose symptoms include a metallic taste in the mouth; eye, nose, and throat irritation; cough; difficulty breathing; fatigue; headache; fever; chills; sweating; nausea; vomiting; muscle aches; and weakness. Those exposed often recover in one to two days if not reexposed. At some point during continuous exposure to fumes, tolerance develops (the fumes no longer cause symptoms). However, over the weekend or after a period without exposure, the tolerance is lost, and "Monday morning fever" may occur.

Ingestion may cause irritation of the mouth, nose, and stomach; nausea, vomiting; severe bloody diarrhea; difficulty breathing; coma; and sometimes death. The kidney and liver may also be affected.

Inhalation of stibine causes headache, nausea, vomiting, weakness, jaundice (yellow skin discoloration), and anemia, whose symptoms include fatigue, pallor, shortness of breath, palpitations, headache, dizziness, and fainting.

Long-term, or chronic, exposure to fumes and dust may cause an itching skin rash known as antimony spots, bleeding gums, itching irritation of the eyes, laryngitis, headache, weight loss, and anemia. Miners may get a pneumonia caused by silica contamination of the dust.

Chronic ingestion may lead to dry throat, nausea, headache, sleeplessness, loss of appetite, and dizziness. The liver and kidney become affected later on.

CANCER ALERT: Antimony is a suspected lung carcinogen.

CHILD ALERT: Young children could be poisoned by ingesting ant paste.

PREGNANCY AND REPRODUCTIVE ALERT: A Russian study has reported miscarriages and premature births in antimony-exposed women. Menstrual cycle disorders have been reported in antimony-exposed women.

OSHA/NIOSH STANDARDS: OSHA and NIOSH recommend a TWA of 0.5 mg/m^3.

Arsenic

Arsenic is a steel-gray metal that forms several poisonous compounds. Among them is arsine gas, which may be released when acids react with metals. Arsenic is found naturally in the earth's crust in ores of copper, lead, and zinc.

SOURCES OF EXPOSURE: Arsenic can be found as a contaminant in soil, food, shellfish (although organic arsenic in shellfish is nontoxic), tobacco, coal dust, well water, and air near smelting plants as well as in the air when arsenic-treated wood is burned in wood stoves.

Arsenic is a component of numerous insecticides, weed killers, rodenticides, fungicides, some paints, wallpaper, and some medicines. Moonshine whiskey may also be contaminated with arsenic.

Hobbyists who make ceramics, blow glass, weld, print, dye, paint, and garden may be at risk for exposure to arsenic.

Illicitly prepared drugs, such as cocaine or heroin, may be contaminated with arsenic.

ROUTES OF EXPOSURE: Ingestion, inhalation of vapors, skin contact by injection.

SYMPTOMS OF EXPOSURE: Ingestion of a toxic dose of arsenic can cause abdominal pain, nausea, vomiting, watery or bloody diarrhea, restlessness, headache, dizziness, memory loss, chills, convulsions, tremors, paralysis, and heart irregularities.

Inhalation of arsenic dusts can cause breathing difficulties, restlessness, cyanosis (blue-gray skin discoloration), and cough.

Inhalation of arsenic oxide fumes may cause metal fume fever, a flulike illness whose symptoms include a metallic taste; eye, nose, and throat irritation; cough; difficulty breathing; fatigue; fever; chills; sweating; nausea; vomiting; muscle aches; and weakness. Those exposed often recover in one to two days if not reexposed. During continuous exposure to these fumes, tolerance develops (the fumes no longer cause symptoms). However, over the weekend or after a period without exposure, the tolerance is lost, and "Monday morning fever" may occur.

Exposure to arsine gas may initially cause headache, malaise, weakness, shortness of breath, nausea, and vomiting. The classical symptoms include stomach pain, dark urine, and jaundice (yellow skin discoloration).

Long-term, or chronic, exposure to arsenic may lead to nausea, vomiting, diarrhea, changes in skin color (darkening) and texture, hair loss, Mees' lines (horizontal white bands on the nails), shedding of the nails, longitudinal brown bands on the nails, and diffuse brown nails (discoloration of nails as either bands or the whole nail). Other more serious symptoms include memory loss, alterations in mental functions, numbness and loss of sensation in the limbs, muscle weakness, incoordination, hearing loss, and visual impairment.

CANCER ALERT: Arsenic and its related compounds can cause cancers of the lungs, liver, skin, and perhaps other body systems.

CHILD ALERT: Children can be poisoned by coming into contact with arsenic-containing insecticides (especially ant pastes, pesticides, or rodenticides) and then sucking on their unwashed hands. Another potential route of exposure is eating large quantities of sprayed fruits and vegetables that have been treated with arsenic-containing compounds and not washed adequately. Children may be exposed to arsenic through skin contact or ingestion through mouthing and play activities on wooden playground equipment treated with copper arsenate.

PREGNANCY AND REPRODUCTIVE ALERT: Arsenic's ability to cause chromosomal damage may affect fertility.

OSHA/NIOSH STANDARDS: The OSHA standard (PEL) is a TWA of 0.010 mg/m^3. NIOSH considers arsenic an occupational carcinogen and recommends a ceiling limit of 0.002 mg/m^3.

Asbestos

Asbestos is a generic term for several fibrous, mineral silicates, including chrysotile, amosite, anthophyllite, and crocidolite. This fibrous mineral was widely used, particularly from the 1930s through the 1960s, in construction because of its flexibility, strength, and ability to insulate. Although it was recognized as a health hazard by the Romans more than 2,000 years ago, the EPA did not begin to regulate the use of asbestos until 1974. In 1989, the EPA ordered a phaseout of nearly all industrial uses of asbestos; however, this order was overturned by an appeals court in 1991. (See pp. 124–127 for description and background.)

SOURCES OF EXPOSURE: Workers who mine asbestos are obviously exposed. Many people who work with asbestos-containing products such as brake pads, tiles, and insulation on steam pipes, furnaces, and electric wire are also at risk for exposure. People can be indirectly exposed by living near an asbestos plant or by living with someone who returns home with asbestos on his or her clothes.

ROUTE OF EXPOSURE: Inhalation.

SYMPTOMS OF EXPOSURE: The effects of asbestos are delayed. A relatively brief period of exposure, such as six months, can result in symptoms that usually do not appear until at least twenty years after exposure. The longer the exposure, however, the more likely symptoms will occur.

Because asbestos causes extensive scarring (fibrosis) of the lung, the main symptom of long-term exposure is shortness of breath; however, cough and sputum production are also common.

CANCER ALERT: Asbestos causes cancer, particularly lung cancer and mesothelioma, a rare cancer of the membrane lining the chest or abdominal wall. Exposure to asbestos has also been shown to cause cancers of the mouth, pharynx, larynx, esophagus, stomach, intestines, rectum, and kidney (see p. 147).

Smoking greatly increases the likelihood of lung cancer in people exposed to asbestos. One study found that asbestos-exposed smokers have ten times the death rate from lung cancer as exposed nonsmokers. Kidney cancer and gastrointestinal cancers also have been associated with asbestos.

OSHA/NIOSH STANDARDS: The OSHA standard (PEL) for fibers greater than 0.005 mm in length is a TWA of 2 million fibers/m³ per cubic centimeter of air. Employers must institute worker surveillance and protection measures at a TWA of 0.1 fiber/cm³. NIOSH considers asbestos to be a carcinogen and recommends reducing exposure to the lowest possible concentration. For fibers greater than 0.005 mm, NIOSH recommends a REL of 100,000 fibers/m³ in a 400-L air sample.

Benzene

Benzene is a clear, colorless liquid that evaporates easily. It is a known carcinogen widely used in industry for chemical production and as a solvent.

SOURCES OF EXPOSURE: Benzene is a widely used industrial solvent and a pollutant of air, soil, and water. Gasoline is composed of 1 to 2 percent benzene. Benzene can be a component in paint, ink, adhesives, paint removers, and degreasers.

Hobbyists who paint, print, sculpt in wax, work with wood, refinish furniture, make jewelry, and garden may be at risk for exposure to benzene.

ROUTES OF EXPOSURE: Primarily inhalation, but ingestion and skin contact as well.

SYMPTOMS OF EXPOSURE: Mild exposure from inhalation or ingestion of benzene causes dizziness, weakness, euphoria, headache, nausea, vomiting, tightness in the chest, and staggering. More intense exposure causes blurring of vision, tremors, shallow and rapid breathing, violent excitement, delirium, unconsciousness, and convulsions. Poisoning with massive amounts of benzene can lead to coma. Exposure may be fatal.

The following symptoms may continue for weeks after exposure: insomnia, agitation, headache, drowsiness, nausea, and loss of appetite.

Skin contact with benzene causes irritation, scaling, and cracking.

Long-term, or chronic, exposure from inhalation of benzene begins with headache, loss of appetite, drowsiness, nervousness, and pale skin. A skin rash (petechiae) and abnormal bleeding may also occur. Exposure could lead to death from blood abnormalities, such as aplastic anemia and acute myelocytic and monocytic leukemia.

Benzene's ability to cause chromosomal damage may affect fertility.

CANCER ALERT: Workers chronically exposed to benzene have a higher incidence of leukemia, aplastic anemia, and lymphoma.

PREGNANCY ALERT: Persistent low-level exposure to benzene may affect the unborn child.

OSHA/NIOSH STANDARDS: The OSHA standard (PEL) is a TWA of 1 ppm with a STEL of 5 ppm. NIOSH considers benzene to be an occupational carcinogen and recommends limiting exposure to the lowest feasible concentration with a STEL of 1 ppm (3.2 mg/m³) for sixty minutes.

Boric Acid and Boron Compounds

Boric acid is a white crystalline powder. Among other compounds containing boron (a brownish-black powder found in minerals) are borax (sodium borate), sodium perborate, boron trifluoride, and boron oxide. The boron hydrides include pentaborane, a colorless liquid with a sweet odor; decaborane, a white crystalline solid with a strong, chocolate color; and diborane, a colorless gas with an unpleasant odor.

SOURCES OF EXPOSURE: Boric acid is used as a pesticide against cockroaches; to fireproof textiles; to weatherproof wood; as a preservative;

and to manufacture glass, cosmetics, cements, leather, carpets, and artificial gems.

Accidental ingestion of boric acid may occur when it is used as an antiseptic in mouthwash and toothpaste. It is also found in soap and, in extremely low, nontoxic concentrations in contact lens solution. Excessive use on surgical wounds, burns, and ulcers has caused toxicity.

Boron is used in metal processing and in nuclear reactors. Borax is a cleaning and bleaching agent. Other boron compounds are used to soften water and are found in algicides, fertilizers, fumigants, and herbicides.

Pentaborane, decaborane, and diborane are used as rocket fuels, industrial catalysts, and in the synthesis of carborane polymers and the manufacture of semiconductors.

Hobbyists involved with pottery, enameling, glazes, printing, dyeing, painting, and photography may risk exposure to boric acid.

ROUTES OF EXPOSURE: Ingestion, inhalation, and absorption through broken skin, mucous membranes, and body cavities.

SYMPTOMS OF EXPOSURE: After ingestion of boric acid or borates occurs, a progression of vomiting and diarrhea with mucus and/or blood, skin reddening and blistering, weakness, lethargy, muscle twitching, tremors, headache, restlessness, convulsions, high fever, abnormalities in urine output, coma, and death may occur.

Boron oxide dust irritates the nose, mouth, and throat.

Decaborane and pentaborane potently affect the central nervous system and cause excitability, headaches, muscle twitching, convulsions, dizziness, loss of the ability to concentrate, incoordination, and sleepiness.

Diborane irritates the mucous membranes of the respiratory tract. Exposure symptoms are similar to metal fume fever: difficulty breathing, cough, chills, fever, chest pain, nausea, and drowsiness. Headache, dizziness, fatigue, and weakness may occur.

Long-term, or chronic, exposure to boric acid, borates, and inorganic related compounds causes loss of appetite, weight loss, vomiting, diarrhea, skin rash, hair loss, convulsions, and anemia.

Chronic exposure to diborane can lead to wheezing, shortness of breath, dry cough, and hyperventilation.

CHILD ALERT: Infants and young children may be affected when a boric acid preparation is used to treat diaper rash. Because children often play on the floor where roach powder containing boric acid is laid down, cases of poisoning have occurred.

REPRODUCTIVE ALERT: Boric acid has been shown to be a spermatotoxin and may cause difficulty in conceiving.

OSHA/NIOSH STANDARDS: The federal standard (PEL) for boron trifluoride is 1 ppm (3 mg/m^3) as a ceiling; boron oxide, 10 mg/m^3; diborane, 0.1 ppm (0.1 mg/m^3); pentaborane, 0.005 ppm (0.01 mg/m^3), STEL, 0.015 ppm (0.03 mg/m^3); decaborane, 0.05 ppm (0.03 mg/m^3), STEL, 0.15 ppm (0.9 mg/m^3). NIOSH does not have a recommendation for a boron trifluoride ceiling limit because there is no reliable short-term monitoring method.

Botulism

Botulinus toxin produced by the *Clostridium botulinum* bacillus causes botulism, one type of food poisoning. This toxin is the most poisonous substance known.

SOURCES OF EXPOSURE: The organism or its spores or toxin can be found in underprocessed, nonacid canned foods. The foods most often associated with botulism are meats, fish, vegetables, olives, and fruits. Home-canned foods are particularly susceptible.

Spores of *C. botulinum* are found in the soil and air.

ROUTE OF EXPOSURE: Ingestion (contaminated food).

SYMPTOMS OF EXPOSURE: The major symptoms are vomiting, double vision, and paralysis.

Within eight hours to eight days after eating contaminated foods, nausea, vomiting, and sometimes diarrhea, stomach pain, and bloating occur. This progresses to dry or sore mouth and throat, fatigue, lid drooping, difficulty speaking and swallowing, blurred or double vision, weakness, constipation, breathing difficulty, inability to urinate, and paralysis of the muscles controlling breathing and muscles of the limbs. About half of those severely poisoned die.

Most symptoms disappear in three to four weeks, except for weakness, which can last for more than a year.

CHILD ALERT: Botulism can occur in infants who are fed contaminated honey, fresh fruits, vegetables, or almost any other food if it has been mishandled.

Cadmium

Cadmium is a bluish silver-white metal that is easily worked and can be polished. It is widely used in industry.

SOURCES OF EXPOSURE: Cadmium is present in soil, water, air, and food. Food is the most likely source of exposure for those not exposed via their occupations. Food may be contaminated from its cadmium-containing vessels, such as cadmium-glazed pots and pans, or from vending machines dispensing liquids and soldered with cadmium-containing materials. Electroplated ice trays are also a source of exposure.

Air pollution affects those living near zinc and lead smelters and other cadmium-emitting plants. Other sources of cadmium exposure are waste incineration, fossil-fuel burning, sewage sludge, and phosphate fertilizers. Smokers are exposed to cadmium contained in tobacco.

Cadmium is found in antiseborrheic (dandruff and oily discharge) medications, antiseptics, and pesticides.

Hobbyists working in poorly ventilated work-spaces may be exposed to toxic levels of cadmium dust and fumes. Among those at risk are jewelry makers using cadmium–silver solder, ceramics makers, glass makers, welders, photographers, metal sculptors, and painters (cadmium is a frequent component in various paint pigments).

ROUTES OF EXPOSURE: Ingestion and inhalation. During the course of exposure, cadmium accumulates in the body.

SYMPTOMS OF EXPOSURE: After ingesting a toxic dose of cadmium, chills, nausea, vomiting, diarrhea, headache, muscle ache, stomach pain, and salivation may follow.

Inhalation of cadmium fumes causes symptoms of metal fume fever, a flulike illness whose symptoms can include fever; chills; sweating; headache; nausea; vomiting; difficulty breathing; chest pain; a metallic taste in the mouth; eye, nose, and throat irritation; cough; headache and weakness. Those exposed often recover in one to two days. At some point during continuous exposure to cadmium fumes, tolerance can develop (the fumes no longer cause symptoms). However, over the weekend or after a period without exposure, the tolerance is lost, and "Monday morning fever" may occur. Cadmium exposure may also cause decreased urine output, fever, and sometimes fatal lung edema (the lungs fill with fluid).

Long-term, or chronic, exposure to cadmium through inhalation causes loss of the sense of smell, runny nose, cough, shortness of breath, weight loss, fatigue, irritability, yellow rings on the teeth, kidney damage, and bone pain.

CANCER ALERT: Cadmium is regarded as a potential workplace carcinogen by NIOSH for lung cancer. A link with cancer of the prostate is more controversial.

REPRODUCTIVE ALERT: Cadmium's potential to cause chromosomal damage may affect fertility.

CHILD ALERT: Children may be exposed to cadmium if they are allowed to use arts and crafts materials designed for adult use. Cadmium is a frequent component in various paint pigments. They may inhale pigment dusts or ingest paints through poor painting techniques, such as pointing the brush with the lips or by putting their paint-splashed fingers in their mouths. Children should always use arts and crafts materials specifically labeled for their age group.

PREGNANCY ALERT: Women exposed to cadmium while pregnant more frequently deliver babies of low birth weight.

OSHA/NIOSH STANDARDS: The OSHA standard (PEL) for cadmium fume is a TWA of 0.1 mg/m^3 with a ceiling of 0.3 mg/m^3; and cadmium dust, 0.2 mg/m^3 with a ceiling of 0.6 mg/m^3. NIOSH treats cadmium dust and fumes as occupational carcinogens, and recommends reducing exposure to the lowest feasible level.

Caffeine

Caffeine is a widely consumed, naturally occurring substance found in coffee and tea. Americans consume about 15 million pounds of caffeine in coffee each year, and another 2 million pounds is added to foods.

SOURCES OF EXPOSURE: Caffeine is found naturally in coffee beans, tea leaves, kola nuts, cocoa trees, and ilex plants. It is used to formulate cola, some noncola soft drinks, cocoa, and chocolates. As a flavoring agent, it is added to pastries and desserts.

A cup of brewed coffee has 75 to 155 mg of caffeine; instant coffee, 86 to 99 mg; tea, 60 to 75 mg; and decaffeinated coffee, 2 to 4 mg. About a quarter to a third of all Americans take in more than 500 to 600 mg (three to five cups of coffee or tea) each day.

Caffeine is also found in over-the-counter preparations (i.e., stimulants, diet pills, cold and allergy preparations, and pain relievers) and in some prescription medications.

ROUTE OF EXPOSURE: Ingestion.

SYMPTOMS OF EXPOSURE: Ingestion of large quantities can cause stomach irritation (heartburn), vomiting, and convulsions. Mood disturbances (i.e., anxiety, jitteriness, tremulousness, agitation, and irritability) may occur. High-caffeine consumers also report depression and sleep disturbances.

Seizures, cardiopulmonary arrest, and deaths have been reported from an oral dose of 5.3 g in a child. The adult lethal dose ranges from 5 to 10 g, which is approximately equivalent to 65 cups of coffee, 100 cups of tea, or 200 cola soft drinks.

Long-term, or chronic, exposure to caffeine may cause restlessness, stomach pain, headache, nausea, vomiting, fever, agitation, rapid and/or irregular heartbeat, hyperventilation, convulsions, and respiratory failure.

Withdrawal of caffeine can cause headache.

Carbon Dioxide

Carbon dioxide is a colorless, odorless gas found naturally in the air. When its concentration becomes too high, it acts as an asphyxiant, replacing life-sustaining oxygen in the air that is inhaled. Its solid form is utilized as dry ice.

SOURCES OF EXPOSURE: Carbon dioxide is a major air pollutant that has been steadily increasing each year in the environment. The burning of fossil fuels and global deforestation contribute to the buildup of carbon dioxide.

Carbon dioxide is released into the air by animals and from fermentation, volcanic activity, and combustion (burning). Sparkling mineral spring water contains carbon dioxide in solution. Dry ice is the solid form of carbon dioxide.

ROUTE OF EXPOSURE: Inhalation.

SYMPTOMS OF EXPOSURE: At lower concentrations, exposure to carbon dioxide causes shortness of breath and headache. At higher concentrations (10 percent), visual disturbances, tinnitus (ringing in the ears), tremor, and loss of consciousness may result.

Long-term, or chronic, exposure in animals to carbon dioxide at low concentrations causes degeneration in the lungs, liver, kidney, and brain.

OSHA/NIOSH STANDARDS: The OSHA standard (PEL) is a TWA of 10,000 ppm (18,000 mg/m³). NIOSH recommends a TWA of 5,000 ppm (9,000 mg/m³) with a ceiling of 30,000 ppm (54,000 mg/m³) for a ten-minute duration.

Carbon Disulfide

Carbon disulfide is a clear, colorless liquid with a sweet smell. Widely used in industry, carbon disulfide acts as an organic solvent for fats, resins, rubber, and other compounds.

SOURCES OF EXPOSURE: Carbon disulfide is a human-made product used in making rayon and rubber and as an insecticide, corrosion inhibitor, grease remover, disinfectant, and grain and soil fumigant. It is also a solvent in rubber cement and in paints, varnishes, and paint and varnish removers.

Minute amounts are found naturally in coal and crude oil.

Hobbyists who paint, varnish, garden, and use rubber cement may be inadvertently exposed to carbon disulfide.

ROUTES OF EXPOSURE: Inhalation, skin absorption, and accidental ingestion.

SYMPTOMS OF EXPOSURE: Inhaling a toxic dose of carbon disulfide causes difficulty in breathing, cough, restlessness, mouth and stomach irritation, nausea, vomiting, headache, blurred vision, lethargy, and mood changes. Symptoms may progress to agitation, delirium, hallucinations, mania, convulsions, and unconsciousness. Exposure can be fatal. In cases where victims have regained consciousness, they have experienced irritability, muscle spasm, vision problems, and disturbed behavior.

Skin contact causes reddening, burning, cracking, and peeling and may progress to a second-degree burn.

Ingestion causes headache, dark blue skin discoloration, slowed breathing, loss of consciousness, tremors, convulsions, and death.

Long-term, or chronic, exposure by inhalation or skin contact may cause odd sensations in the limbs, muscle weakness, irritability, loss of memory, blurred vision, loss of appetite, insomnia, depression, personality changes, partial blindness, hearing loss, dizziness, weakness, and tremor.

Hearing loss may result from long-term exposure to the combination of high levels of noise and carbon disulfide. Complete loss of the sense of smell or a decreased ability to smell has also been reported in workers repeatedly exposed to carbon disulfide.

Workers chronically exposed to carbon disulfide have been reported to have more coronary heart disease.

REPRODUCTIVE ALERT: Chronic exposure to carbon disulfide can cause lowered sperm counts, abnormal sperm, a higher incidence of miscarriage, and menstrual irregularities.

OSHA/NIOSH STANDARDS: The OSHA standard (PEL) is a TWA of 4 ppm (12 mg/m³), and a STEL of 12 ppm (36 mg/m³). NIOSH recommends 1 ppm (3 mg/m³) TWA with a STEL of 10 ppm (30 mg/m³).

Carbon Monoxide

Carbon monoxide is a colorless, odorless gas. In the United States, it is the leading cause of deaths by poisoning.

SOURCES OF EXPOSURE: The exhaust from car engines is a major source of carbon monoxide in our environment. Carbon monoxide is emitted from any flame or combustion device, such as kerosene heaters or stoves. Fire victims are often affected by carbon monoxide. Burning natural gas or petroleum fuels emits carbon monoxide.

The smoke from cigarettes, pipes, and cigars is another common source. Smokers have a significantly higher blood level of carbon monoxide. Inhaling side-stream smoke also raises the blood level.

Workers in environments with high carbon monoxide levels are at risk of exposure. The paint stripper methylene chloride is also a source of exposure because it is metabolized to carbon monoxide. Hobbyists who use methylene chloride to strip paint or varnish in small home workshops and photo film processors are particularly at risk.

ROUTES OF EXPOSURE: Inhalation (carbon monoxide) and skin absorption (methylene chloride).

SYMPTOMS OF EXPOSURE: Inhaling a toxic dose of carbon monoxide causes headache, lethargy, irritability, increased breathing rate, chest pain, confusion, impaired judgment, shortness of breath, nausea, and fainting.

Exposure to higher concentrations may lead to hyperactivity, bizarre behavior, and convulsions and may be fatal.

Long-term, or chronic, exposure may lead to poor memory and mental deterioration and has been linked with hearing loss.

Delayed effects, occurring two to four weeks after significant exposure, may include visual loss, dementia, retardation, memory loss, lack of coordination in speech, personality changes, loss of bladder control, and difficulties in gait.

PREGNANCY ALERT: The developing fetus is very vulnerable to carbon monoxide poisoning. Smoking mothers more frequently deliver low-birth-weight babies.

OSHA/NIOSH STANDARDS: The federal standard (PEL) is a TWA of 35 ppm (40 mg/m^3) with a 200-ppm (229 mg/m^3) ceiling.

Carbon Tetrachloride

Carbon tetrachloride (tetrachloromethane and perchloromethane) is a clear, colorless liquid with a smell similar to ether. A suspected carcinogen, in industry it is being gradually replaced by less toxic solvents. Carbon tetrachloride is chemically classified as a halogenated hydrocarbon compound.

SOURCES OF EXPOSURE: The FDA has banned the use of carbon tetrachloride in most products. Exposure is limited to those who work in certain industries.

Hobbyists working with wax sculpture and batik, where carbon tetrachloride is used to remove wax, may be exposed.

ROUTES OF EXPOSURE: Inhalation, ingestion, and absorption through the skin.

SYMPTOMS OF EXPOSURE: Initially, exposure from inhalation, ingestion, or skin absorption may cause stomach pain; nausea; vomiting; dizziness; headache; lightheadedness; eye, nose, and throat irritation; blurred vision; incoordination; and confusion, which may progress to unconsciousness. A symptom-free period may follow lasting from one day to two weeks.

Later, symptoms of liver or kidney damage may develop: nausea; vomiting; jaundice (yellow skin discoloration) with a swollen, tender liver; decreased urine; swelling of the limbs (edema); and fluid retention with a sudden weight increase. Fever, diarrhea, unconsciousness, irregular pulse, and even death may occur.

The main findings after exposure to a toxic dose are coma, infrequent urination, and yellow skin discoloration.

Long-term, or chronic, exposure by inhalation or skin absorption of low doses may produce the same symptoms as mentioned above. Other vague symptoms may also indicate poisoning: fatigue; loss of appetite; vomiting; stomach discomfort; weakness; nausea; blurred vision; memory loss; burning, pricking or tingling sensations; and tremors.

CANCER ALERT: Carbon tetrachloride is a suspected carcinogen. Chronic exposure to carbon tetrachloride may play a role in the development of liver cancer. Repeated skin contact causes inflammation and may lead to skin cancer.

OSHA/NIOSH Standards: The OSHA standard (PEL) is a TWA of 2 ppm (12.6 mg/m³). NIOSH considers carbon tetrachloride to be an occupational carcinogen and recommends a 2-ppm (12.6 mg/m³) ceiling in a 45-liter sample for sixty minutes.

Chloroprene

Chloroprene is a colorless liquid with a pungent odor, chemically classified as a halogenated hydrocarbon compound. It is used in producing synthetic rubbers, such as neoprene and duprene, and polychloroprene latex.

Sources of Exposure: According to NIOSH, about 2,500 workers could potentially be exposed to chloroprene in their workplaces in the United States.

Routes of Exposure: Inhalation of vapors and skin absorption.

Symptoms of Exposure: Chloroprene causes hair loss, skin and eye irritation, sore throat, inflammation of the gums, and tooth enamel erosion.

Long-term, or chronic, exposure may damage the lungs, nervous system, liver, kidneys, spleen, and heart.

Cancer Alert: An increase in lung cancer among exposed workers has been reported. Some evidence has also linked chloroprene with cancers of the skin and liver. However, NIOSH has not made recommendations on these possibilities because of insufficient data.

Reproductive Alert: An increase in miscarriages has been reported in wives of male chloroprene workers.

OSHA/NIOSH Standards: The OSHA standard (PEL) is a TWA of 25 ppm (90 mg/m³).

NIOSH recommends a STEL of 1 ppm (3.6 mg/m³).

Chromium

Chromium is a hard silver metal used for its resistance to corrosion and for its bright, reflective finish. As an essential trace element, it is needed in small amounts by the body for insulin binding. Chromium-containing compounds include the chromates, chromic acid, and the chromium oxides. Some chromium compounds, such as chrome oxide, are suspected carcinogens.

Sources of Exposure: Chromium is found naturally in our diet, specifically in brewer's yeast, meats, fish, fruits, and vegetables. The most dangerous exposure to chromium is industrial. Chromium is used in chemical synthesis, steel-making, electroplating, leather-tanning, and as a radiator and plumbing antirust agent.

Hobbyists using chromium-containing substances for painting (e.g., chrome green, zinc yellow, strontium yellow and chrome yellow pigments), glazing ceramics (e.g., lead chromate, zinc chromate, and iron chromate), dying, etching, engraving, metalwork and welding (metal dusts and fumes), enameling, and photographic developing should avoid skin contact and only work in well-ventilated areas.

Routes of Exposure: Inhalation, ingestion, and skin absorption.

Symptoms of Exposure: If ingested, chromium will cause dizziness, intense thirst, stomachache, vomiting, bleeding disorders, shock, and urine abnormalities. Death may follow.

Inhaling chromium dusts or mists causes coughing, wheezing, chest pain while breathing, fever, headache, shortness of breath, and loss of weight. Inhalation of chromium oxide fumes causes symptoms of metal fume fever, a flulike illness whose symptoms can include fever; chills; sweating; headache, nausea; vomiting; difficulty breathing; chest pain; eye, nose, and throat irritation; cough; a metallic taste in the mouth; headache; and weakness. Those exposed often recover in one to two days if not reexposed. At some point during continuous exposure to chromium oxide fumes, tolerance develops (the fumes no longer cause symptoms). However, over the weekend or after a period without exposure, the tolerance is lost, and "Monday morning fever" may occur.

Skin contact will irritate and corrode the skin and cause yellowing of the nails. Exposure from skin contact causes allergic contact dermatitis.

Long-term, or chronic, exposure may cause skin ulcers. Inhalation of chromium fumes may cause nasal ulcers; bleeding; growths and a foul discharge from the nose; loss of the sense of smell; irritated, red, and runny eyes; bronchitis; asthma; and perhaps vomiting, nausea, and loss of appetite from liver damage.

CANCER ALERT: Exposure to certain chromium compounds is associated with a higher incidence of lung cancer.

CHILD ALERT: Chromium is excreted in breast milk.

Some hobbyist materials, such as paints and glazes, contain chromium compounds. To avoid exposure to these potentially dangerous materials, make sure that children use nontoxic arts and crafts supplies designed for their age group.

OSHA/NIOSH STANDARDS: OSHA standards for chromic acid and chromates (as CrO_3) are a PEL ceiling of 0.1 mg/m^3; a TWA for chromium (II) and chromium compounds (including chromic oxide, chromic sulfate, chromic chloride, chromic potassium sulfate, and chromite ore) of 0.5 mg Cr/m^3. A TWA of 0.05 mg Cr/VI is the standard for certain water-insoluble compounds designated as confirmed human carcinogens, including zinc chromate, calcium chromate, lead chromate, barium chromate, strontium chromate, and sintered chromium trioxide. NIOSH considers all chromium compounds, including chromic acid, to be potential occupational carcinogens.

Cobalt

Cobalt is a silver-gray, hard, brittle, and magnetic metal. It is found in several minerals in low concentrations. Cobalt is also found in trace amounts in the body. It combines with oxygen, sulfur, and arsenic to form many cobalt-containing compounds.

SOURCES OF EXPOSURE: Cobalt is used in alloys with several other metals that are used in electrical, automotive, and aircraft industries. It is used in magnets and grinding and polishing tools. Radioactive cobalt is used in treating cancer.

Hobbyists can be exposed to cobalt in enamels, glazes when heated (cobalt oxide is a glaze ingredient), paints and inks (e.g., cobalt violet, cobalt green, cobalt yellow, and cerulean blue), dyes, and photographic chemicals; in making glass and pottery; and if they use tools for grinding, drilling, or polishing.

ROUTES OF EXPOSURE: Inhalation and ingestion.

SYMPTOMS OF EXPOSURE: Contact with cobalt can irritate the eyes and skin. Inhalation of cobalt dusts causes irritation of the nose and throat and an asthmalike disorder with coughing, malaise, and wheezing. Excessive inhalation or ingestion of cobalt may cause vomiting, diarrhea, a sensation of heat, nerve deafness, and convulsions.

Inhalation of cobalt oxide fumes may cause metal fume fever, a flulike illness whose symptoms include a metallic taste in the mouth; eye, nose, and throat irritation; cough; difficulty breathing; fatigue; fever; headache; chills; sweating; nausea; vomiting; muscle aches; and weakness. Those exposed often recover in one to two days, unless reexposed. At some point during continuous exposure to cobalt oxide fumes, tolerance develops (the fumes no longer cause symptoms). However, over the weekend or after a period without exposure, the tolerance is lost, and "Monday morning fever" may occur.

Long-term, or chronic, exposure to cobalt in beer (increases the head or foam) has affected the heart muscle (cardiomyopathy). Cobalt can affect the lungs, causing asthma or pulmonary fibrosis after exposure to the fine dust of tungsten carbide and cobalt ("hard metal"). Chronic exposure can also cause allergic contact dermatitis.

CHILD ALERT: A report of a child who ingested a large quantity of magnets showed blood, thyroid, and heart disorders attributed to cobalt and iron toxicity.

OSHA/NIOSH STANDARDS: The OSHA standard (PEL) is a TWA of 0.05 mg/m^3.

Copper

Copper is a red-brown metal found naturally in the earth's crust and in the body. Used widely in industry, copper has the ability to conduct electricity and heat well. Its compounds have many applications.

SOURCES OF EXPOSURE: Copper may be found as a contaminant in food, especially shellfish, liver, mushrooms, nuts, and chocolate, and in water from copper piping. Beverages dispensed through copper or brass pipes in vending machines and food or drink stored in copper or brass containers may contain a high copper concentration.

Copper sulfate is used in astringents, deodorants, and antiseptics. Kidney dialysis patients and burn victims may be exposed to copper during the course of their treatment.

Copper is a component of certain insecticides, fungicides (Bordeaux mixture), and algicides. Copper is also a component of certain intrauterine devices.

Hobbyists who paint, make ceramics (copper carbonate is used as a glaze ingredient), work with metal (copper fumes arise in casting and copper nitrate is used as a metal colorant), make

stained glass (copper sulfate is used as a patina on lead came), blow glass (copper nitrate is used to stain glass), and dye (copper sulfate is used as a mordant) may risk exposure to copper.

ROUTES OF EXPOSURE: Ingestion; inhalation of copper-containing sprays, dust, or fumes; skin absorption (e.g., extensive application of copper salts to areas of burned skin, and particles in the eye).

SYMPTOMS OF EXPOSURE: Ingesting a toxic dose of copper may cause a metallic taste in the mouth, a burning mouth and throat, nausea, retching, green-blue-colored vomit, burning stomach pain, and the urge to defecate without results. Watery or bloody diarrhea may occur, although it is less common. Lethargy, red-colored urine or decreased urination, skin bronzing, collapse, convulsions, and coma may follow in severe poisonings.

Inhalation of large doses of copper dust or fumes may cause a sore throat and cough, eye irritation, swelling of the eyelids, sinus irritation, nausea, stomach pain, and diarrhea. Symptoms of metal fume fever also occur: muscle aches; headache; nausea; vomiting; fever; chills; eye, nose, and throat irritation; cough; weakness; and fatigue. Those exposed often recover in one to two days if not reexposed. At some point during continuous exposure to fumes, tolerance develops (the fumes no longer cause symptoms). However, over the weekend or after a period without exposure, the tolerance is lost, and "Monday morning fever" may occur.

Long-term, or chronic, exposure from copper-containing skin solutions may cause red, bumpy lesions on the skin and even green-blue discoloration.

CANCER ALERT: Continued inhalation of copper-containing sprays is linked with an increase in lung cancer among exposed workers.

OSHA/NIOSH STANDARDS: The federal standard (PEL) for copper fume, dusts, and mists is 0.1 mg/m^3.

Cyanide

Cyanide is a rapidly acting lethal poison. It exists as a gas and liquid and combines to form a variety of other compounds, many of which are also toxic, some of which are solid (such as salts).

SOURCES OF EXPOSURE: Many common plants contain cyanide compounds in their seeds (apple, peach, pear, and plum), leaves, bark, or roots (cassava). The burning of cigarettes releases hydrogen cyanide, which may affect smokers and others exposed to side-stream smoke.

Certain medications and products sold in health food stores may cause cyanide toxicity. Laetrile, an unapproved and ineffective anticancer drug, and nitroprusside, a drug given intravenously for severe high blood pressure, produce cyanide in the body.

Cyanide-containing compounds that are used in industry include acrylonitrile in the production of synthetic rubber; cyanamide as a fertilizer; cyanide salts in metal cleaning, hardening, and refining; and cyanogen chloride and hydrogen cyanide in chemical synthesis.

The burning of plastic furniture and natural fibers, such as wool and silk, in house fires releases cyanide.

Hobbyists who may be exposed include jewelry makers (cyanide salts are used in electroplating gold and silver), gardeners, photographers, solderers, metalworkers (cyanide salts are used in electroplating, electroforming, and coloring metals), and gunsmiths.

ROUTES OF EXPOSURE: Inhalation, ingestion, and skin absorption.

SYMPTOMS OF EXPOSURE: Ingestion or inhalation of large doses of cyanide or cyanide compounds causes unconsciousness, convulsions, and death within fifteen minutes. Smaller doses of cyanide compounds may cause dizziness, rapid breathing, vomiting, diarrhea, weakness, flushing, headache, drowsiness, rapid pulse, and unconsciousness. Death may occur depending upon the compound and its dose.

Skin contact with a solution of cyanide salts may cause itching, discoloration, and corrosion.

Long-term, or chronic, exposure to cyanide from eating cassava is associated with causing a type of neuropathy. Chronic exposure from tobacco smoking is associated with "tobacco amblyopia," a partial loss of vision.

Repeated inhalation of low doses of hydrogen cyanide and cyanide salts causes dizziness, weakness, headache, changes in taste and smell, breathing difficulty, hoarseness, eye and nose irritation, loss of appetite, weight loss, tremor, and mental deterioration.

CHILD ALERT: Eating seeds of apple, cherry, peach, apricot, plum, and pear may poison small children. The fatal dose ranges from five to twenty-five seeds if the seed capsule is chewed and broken. Accidental poisonings in children from Laetrile have been reported.

OSHA/NIOSH STANDARDS: The OSHA standard (PEL) for hydrogen cyanide is a STEL of 4.7 ppm (5 mg/m^3); and cyanides is 5 mg/m^3. For cyanides, NIOSH recommends a 4.7-ppm (5 mg/m^3) ceiling for 10 minutes.

Dibromochloropropane

Dibromochloropropane (DBCP) is a liquid previously used as a fumigant and to kill roundworms. It has been withdrawn from the marketplace because it can cause sterility in men. It is classified chemically as a halogenated hydrocarbon.

SOURCES OF EXPOSURE: DBCP was used as a fumigant on citrus, grape, peach, pineapple, soy bean, tomato, banana, and other perennial crops. Workers in factories producing this pesticide were also exposed.

ROUTES OF EXPOSURE: Inhalation and ingestion.

SYMPTOMS OF EXPOSURE: DBCP is a mild irritant. It is toxic to the liver and kidney.

Cancer Alert: NIOSH considers DBCP an occupational carcinogen.

Reproductive Alert: DBCP is a spermatotoxin. Long-term, or chronic, exposure to DBCP in males decreases sperm counts and contributed to infertility and sterility.

OSHA/NIOSH Standards: The OSHA standard (PEL) is a TWA of 0.001 ppm. NIOSH considers dibromochloropropane to be an occupational carcinogen and recommends reducing exposure to lowest levels feasible.

Diisocyanate(s)

The diisocyanates, used in polyurethanes, are combined with other molecules to reduce their volatility and therefore air contamination. These more stable diisocyanate combinations include toluene diisocyanate (TDI), the most common; hexamethylene diisocyanate (HDI); diphenylmethane diisocyanate (MDI); and isophorone diisocyanate.

Sources of Exposure: Polyurethanes are used in paints, rubbers, adhesives, and textile finishes and as insulation, cushioning material, molds, and coatings.

Hobbyists making plastics sculpture may be exposed to diisocyanates used to make polyurethane.

Route of Exposure: Inhalation.

Symptoms of Exposure: The main toxicity comes from exposure to the aerosolized diisocyanate. Eye, nose, and throat irritation are usually the first symptoms to occur. Dry cough, shortness of breath, and wheezing can follow. Occupational asthma has occurred and can be severe.

Long-term exposure can cause permanent loss of lung function.

Cancer Alert: NIOSH considers toluene diisocyanate (TDI) an occupational carcinogen.

OSHA/NIOSH Standards: The OSHA standard (PEL) for TDI is a TWA of 0.005 ppm (0.04 mg/m^3) with a STEL of 0.02 ppm (0.15 mg/m^3); and MDI, a ceiling of 0.02 ppm (0.2 mg/m^3). NIOSH considers TDI an occupational carcinogen and recommends a TWA for TDI of 0.005 ppm (0.04 mg/m^3) with a STEL of 0.02 ppm (0.15 mg/m^3); MDI, 0.05 mg with a ceiling of 0.2 mg for ten minutes; and HDI, 0.035 mg with a ceiling of 0.14 mg for ten minutes.

Dimethylformamide

Dimethylformamide (DMF) is a colorless liquid with a fishy odor widely used as an industrial solvent. Sometimes called the universal organic solvent, DMF has powerful solvent properties for many organic compounds and a slow rate of evaporation.

Sources of Exposure: Mainly used for the production of polyurethanes and acrylic fibers, DMF is also used to manufacture pesticides, pharmaceuticals, dyes, petroleum products, and other chemicals.

Routes of Exposure: Skin (primarily) absorption, inhalation, and ingestion. Skin contact can occur by wearing contaminated shoes and clothing.

Symptoms of Exposure: Symptoms include nausea, vomiting, abdominal pain, dizziness, headaches, loss of appetite, and intolerance to alcohol. The reaction to alcohol can mimic that seen in people taking the drug disulfiram—flushing and palpitations. DMF primarily injures the liver, causing a chemical hepatitis.

It is not known whether long-term exposure to DMF causes chronic liver disease.

OSHA/NIOSH Standards: The federal standard (PEL) is 10 ppm (30 mg/m^3).

Dimethyl Sulfoxide

Dimethyl sulfoxide (DMSO) is a clear, colorless liquid that acts as a solvent for many substances. Used as an industrial solvent for many years,

DMSO also has the ability to penetrate the skin and carry other chemicals along with it into the bloodstream. Although some people have proclaimed DMSO to be a wonder drug, its safety and efficacy are controversial.

SOURCES OF EXPOSURE: DMSO, a by-product of paper manufacturing, is used in industry as a solvent. It is also sold as a remedy for arthritis and sports injuries and to treat scars and scleroderma (a fibrous thickening of the skin). Intravenous DMSO has been used experimentally in animals to treat head injuries, spinal-cord trauma, and brain swelling (cerebral edema). In medical laboratories, DMSO is used to preserve platelets.

ROUTES OF EXPOSURE: Skin absorption, ingestion, and intravenous infusion.

SYMPTOMS OF EXPOSURE: DMSO can cause nausea, vomiting, stomach cramps, chills, chest pains, drowsiness, and transient garlic odor of the breath. It may cause visual disturbances and convulsions.

Kidney, liver, and red blood cell damage may result from large doses given intravenously.

Long-term, or chronic, exposure to DMSO causes dermatitis, an irritation resulting from repeated, direct contact with the skin. The skin becomes red and sore and itches. DMSO has been ranked in the top ten most potentially irritating solvents.

OSHA/NIOSH STANDARDS: Not applicable.

Dinitro Derivatives of Phenol and Cresol

Dinitro derivatives of phenol and cresol are a group of chemicals used as insecticides and herbicides. They include *dinitrophenol* (DNP); dinitro-*o*-cresol (DNOC), a yellow, odorless solid; and *dinobuton* among others.

SOURCES OF EXPOSURE: These dinitro derivatives are used as insecticides and herbicides and

also in explosives, dyes, photographic chemicals, and wood preservatives.

Hobbyists at risk include gardeners, dyers, and photographers.

ROUTES OF EXPOSURE: Inhalation, skin absorption, and ingestion.

SYMPTOMS OF EXPOSURE: Skin contact causes skin irritation, and ingestion causes oral irritation. The key symptom of poisoning is high fever. Other symptoms are weakness, malaise, headache, prostration, thirst, nausea, vomiting, blurred vision, excessive sweating, rapid heartbeat, apprehension, and breathing difficulty. Later symptoms may progress to black and blue skin discoloration, delirium, tremors, convulsions, infrequent urination, blood in the urine, yellow skin discoloration, coma, and sometimes death.

Long-term, or chronic, exposure to dinitro derivatives by agricultural workers has not caused any symptoms. DNOC and dinobuton have caused yellow discoloration of the nails.

OSHA/NIOSH STANDARDS: The federal standard (PEL) for DNOC is 0.2 mg/m^3; for DNP, none, but a guideline of 0.2 mg/m^3 is useful.

Dinitrobenzene

Dinitrobenzene is a liquid organic nitro (nitrogen- and oxygen-containing) compound.

SOURCES OF EXPOSURE: Dinitrobenzene is used in the manufacture of celluloid, dyes, explosives, and floor polishes and in certain chemical processes.

ROUTES OF EXPOSURE: Inhalation, skin absorption, and ingestion.

SYMPTOMS OF EXPOSURE: Exposure to a toxic dose may cause headache, irritability, dizziness, weakness, nausea, vomiting, difficulty breathing, palpitations, drowsiness, and unconsciousness. Death may occur.

Ingestion causes a bitter almond taste, irritation of the mouth and throat, and thirst. There may be diminished vision, hearing loss, and ringing in the ears.

Long-term, or chronic, exposure may cause anemia, with symptoms ranging from fatigue, pallor, shortness of breath, and palpitations to headache, dizziness, fainting, ringing in the ears, irritability, difficulty sleeping or concentrating, sensitivity to cold, loss of appetite, indigestion, nausea, bowel movement irregularity, abnormal menstruation, and loss of libido or impotence. A yellowish discoloration of the skin, eyes, nails, and hair may occur.

OSHA/NIOSH Standards: The federal standard (PEL) is 1 mg/m^3.

Dinitrophenol

See **Dinitro Derivatives of Phenol and Cresol.**

Dinitrotoluene

See **Trinitrotoluene and Dinitrotoluene.**

Dioxin

Dioxins are a group of chemicals belonging to the chlorinated hydrocarbon insecticides. Of the seventy-five various members of the group, 2, 3, 7, 8-tetrachlorodibenzo-*p*-dioxin (TCDD) is the most toxic and most studied. TCDD is colorless and odorless as a solid. Dioxin is no longer manufactured for commercial use in the United States but still occurs as a by-product contaminant in the manufacture of other chemicals.

Sources of Exposure: The food chain is the major route of human exposure, especially fish, meat, and dairy products. Food accounts for 98 percent of total adult exposure. See Box 13.8, p. 538 for information on bioaccumulation of dioxin.

Small amounts of dioxins are produced naturally in volcanoes and by forest fires, but major environmental disasters such as the spraying of Agent Orange in Vietnam, contamination at Love Canal in Niagara Falls, New York, and the explosion of the chemical plant in Seveso, Italy, have exposed thousands to potentially dangerous levels of this toxin.

Routes of Exposure: Inhalation and skin absorption.

Symptoms of Exposure: Exposure to TCDD may cause burning of the eyes, nose, and throat; headache; dizziness; loss of appetite; nausea; and vomiting. The face may become itchy and red and swell after a day or two. Bumps, pimples, and cysts may develop on the face, forearms, neck, shoulders, and body within several weeks. Chloracne (blackheads with small yellow cysts) may appear after a month, along with muscle aches and weakness, liver enlargement, insomnia, irritability, and loss of sexual desire. Memory impairment, bouts of anger, and other emotional disorders have also been reported.

Cancer Alert: The EPA and NIOSH consider TCDD to be a probable human carcinogen and a cancer promoter when exposure occurs with certain other agents. Agricultural workers using dioxin-containing pesticides have been found to have increased incidences of non-Hodgkin's lymphoma and soft-tissue sarcoma.

Child Alert: Ingesting contaminated soil and the frequency of hand-to-mouth activity puts children at risk for exposure.

Pregnancy Alert: Because dioxins can cross the placenta and accumulate in breast milk, fetuses and nursing infants whose mothers were exposed may also be at risk.

OSHA/NIOSH Standards: OSHA has not set a permissible exposure limit for dioxin. NIOSH recommends that workplace exposure be reduced to the lowest feasible level because of probable carcinogenicity.

Epoxy Resins

Epoxy resins are synthetic plastics made by linking epoxy monomers together with the aid of epoxy hardeners, or curing agents. Most commerical epoxy resins are formed by the reaction of epichlorohydrin and bisphenol A or diglycidyl ethers (DGE).

Epoxy resins are strong, have adhesive properties, and are resistant to chemicals and electricity. NIOSH recommends that "epichlorohydrin be handled in the workplace as if it were a human carcinogen."

SOURCES OF EXPOSURE: Epoxy resins are used in industrial paints, coatings, adhesives, and laminates.

ROUTES OF EXPOSURE: Inhalation and skin absorption.

SYMPTOMS OF EXPOSURE: Epoxy resins do not have any harmful effects except when heated, releasing irritating vapors. Inhalation of these vapors may cause difficulty in breathing.

Epoxy monomers and hardeners can irritate the skin and can also cause allergic skin rashes with redness, hives, itching, blistering, swelling, and pain. Accidental ingestion of epoxy hardeners can irritate the lining of the gastrointestinal tract. Inhalation of vapors of hardeners can cause asthma.

Epichlorohydrin irritates the eyes, skin, and nose. It causes blistering and deep-seated skin pain. Inhalation can cause nausea, vomiting, stomach discomfort, difficulty breathing, headache, cough, and blue skin discoloration. Bisphenol A may cause a skin reaction after exposure to light. DGE also may cause irritation and sensitization of the skin.

Long-term, or chronic, exposure to epichlorohydrin in animal models has produced lung, kidney, and liver injury.

CANCER ALERT: NIOSH considers epichlorohydrin and DGE occupational carcinogens.

REPRODUCTIVE ALERT: In rats epichlorohydrin acted as a spermatotoxin causing infertility. DGE in animals may damage cells in the testes and blood.

OSHA/NIOSH STANDARDS: The OSHA standard (PEL) for epichlorohydrin is a TWA of 2 ppm (8 mg/m^3); and for DGE, a TWA of 0.1 ppm (0.5 mg/m^3). NIOSH recommends reducing exposure to epichlorohydrin to lowest feasible concentration and considers both epichlorohydrin and DGE occupational carcinogens.

Ethanol

Ethanol (grain alcohol, spirit of wine, cologne spirit, ethyl alcohol, ethyl hydroxide, and ethyl hydrate) is a colorless, volatile, flammable liquid. Beer, wine, and cocktails contain ethanol, or drinking alcohol. Social drinking is a very common practice, but ethanol is a drug, and excessive consumption may cause damage to both the body and mind. Ethanol is also used commercially as a solvent, antifreeze, and fuel.

SOURCES OF EXPOSURE: Ethanol is found in alcoholic beverages, cough medicines, tonics, mouthwashes, liquid vitamins, and over-the-counter drugs. It is used as an antiseptic and as a solvent or processing agent to make pharmaceuticals, plastics, lacquers, polishes, plasticizers, perfumes, cosmetics, rubber accelerators, explosives, synthetic resins, nitrocellulose, adhesives, inks, and preservatives. Ethanol is also used in chemical synthesis.

ROUTES OF EXPOSURE: Ingestion, inhalation, and skin absorption.

SYMPTOMS OF EXPOSURE: Mild to moderate ingestion of alcohol may cause an initial relaxation, flushing of the skin, inebriation, loss of inhibitions, increased urination, incoordination, and visual impairment. In large doses, ethanol may markedly impair memory, concentration, judgment, and coordination and cause slurred speech, loss of balance, and blurred vision. Alcohol intake can also cause impotence in men. Excessive intake may cause loss of consciousness and may even be fatal.

The hangover, or common abstinence syndrome, may be associated with tremor, agitation, sleep disturbances, hyperexcitability, nausea, vomiting, weakness, headache, flushed faces, red eyes, and excessive sweating.

Inhalation of ethanol may cause eye and nose irritation, headache, drowsiness, tremors, and fatigue.

Long-term, or chronic, exposure to ethanol may lead to weight loss; nutritional deficiencies; cirrhosis of the liver with fluid retention, swelling, and jaundice; cardiomyopathy, a damaging of the muscle tissue of the heart; chronic gastritis, an inflammation of the lining of the stomach and intestine with diarrhea; destruction of the pancreas; pain or loss of sense or ability to move the extremities; and mental deterioration with memory loss, tremor, and impaired judgment.

Alcohol withdrawal may occur in those habitual drinkers when they abstain from alcohol. The symptoms include fear, sleeplessness, tremors, restlessness with hallucinations, quickened heartbeat, convulsions, and delirium tremens, its more serious form, in some. Those who chronically abuse alcohol may have flushed, veiny faces; husky voices; shaky hands; and bruises.

CHILD ALERT: Children are especially susceptible to the effects of alcohol because it is rapidly absorbed from the lining of the gastrointestinal tract and lungs.

PREGNANCY ALERT: Pregnant women who habitually drink alcohol may put their unborn children at risk for lowered birth weight and intrauterine growth retardation (IUGR) as well as fetal alcohol syndrome, a cluster of irreversible physical and mental defects (see p. 234).

REPRODUCTIVE ALERT: Ethanol intake may lower testosterone production and contribute to infertility.

OSHA/NIOSH STANDARDS: The federal standard (PEL) for airborne exposure is 1,000 ppm ($1,900$ mg/m^3).

Ethylenediamine

Ethylenediamine is a colorless, clear, thick liquid. It is a very alkaline substance with an odor similar to ammonia. It is one of the most potent sensitizers of the skin.

SOURCES OF EXPOSURE: Ethylenediamine is used as a stabilizer in some cosmetics, perfumes, and topical medications. It is used as a solvent and found in synthetic waxes, fungicides, and insecticides. Ethylenediamine is used in the curing process of epoxy resins and polyurethanes.

ROUTES OF EXPOSURE: Inhalation and skin absorption.

SOURCES OF EXPOSURE: Ethylenediamine vapor can irritate the eyes, skin, and respiratory tract. It may be linked to occupational asthma.

OSHA/NIOSH STANDARDS: The federal standard (PEL) is 10 ppm (25 mg/m^3).

Ethylene Oxide

Ethylene oxide is a colorless gas with a sweet odor. It is among the top twenty-five chemicals produced in the United States. In certain circumstances, ethylene oxide may be an explosion hazard.

SOURCES OF EXPOSURE: Ethylene oxide is used in laboratories for producing organic chemicals and plastics. Foodstuff, books, leather, soil, paper, and textiles are fumigated with ethylene oxide. Up to 100,000 workers in hospital central supply departments may be at risk for exposure because it is used to sterilize dental and surgical instruments.

ROUTE OF EXPOSURE: Inhalation.

SYMPTOMS OF EXPOSURE: Solutions of ethylene oxide may cause skin irritation, blisters, burns, allergic inflammation of the skin, and frostbite. High vapor concentrations may irritate the eyes, nose, throat, and lungs and cause headache, nausea, vomiting, diarrhea, fluid to accumulate in the lungs, difficulty breathing, drowsiness, and unconsciousness. Delayed effects include weakness, incoordination, and heart electrical abnormalities.

Long-term, or chronic, exposure may cause nerve damage affecting coordination and recent memory.

CANCER ALERT: Studies of ethylene oxide workers have found an excess rate of deaths from leukemia.

PREGNANCY ALERT: One study has shown a higher rate of spontaneous abortion among pregnant sterilizing staff in hospitals in Finland.

REPRODUCTIVE ALERT: Ethylene oxide can increase the frequency of mutation in humans and may potentially affect the sex cells leading to difficulty conceiving.

OSHA/NIOSH STANDARDS: The OSHA standard (PEL) is a TWA of 1 ppm (1.8 mg/m^3). NIOSH considers ethylene oxide an occupational carcinogen and recommends a TWA of less than 0.1 ppm (0.18 mg/m^3) and a ceiling of 5 ppm (9 mg/m^3) for a ten-minute duration.

Fluorides

Fluorides are compounds containing the element fluorine. Most are gases at room temperature; sulfur pentafluoride is a liquid.

SOURCES OF EXPOSURE: Fluorides are widely used in industry to produce chemical compounds, as a catalyst and wood preservative, to clean metals, in smelting, in pesticides, and in many other processes.

People living near manufacturing areas can be exposed to low levels of fluorides continually or to large amounts in cases of industrial accidents (neighborhood fluorosis).

Oral fluoride supplements, fluoridated water, and fluoride-containing toothpastes are used to prevent tooth decay and have not caused adverse effects at such low dosages.

ROUTES OF EXPOSURE: Inhalation and ingestion.

SYMPTOMS OF EXPOSURE: Inhalation of fluorine derivatives may cause immediate irritation of the skin, eyes, nose, mouth, and lungs; coughing; choking; and chills and then after one to two days, fever, coughing, difficulty breathing, and blue skin discoloration from lack of oxygen. Between 10 and 30 days later, the symptoms may disappear. Other fluorides may cause sleepiness, convulsions, and difficulty breathing.

Ingesting neutral fluorides may cause salivation, nausea, vomiting, diarrhea, and stomach pain that may progress to weakness, tremors, breathing difficulties, wrist and foot spasms, convulsions, coma, and sometimes death.

Long-term, or chronic, exposure to low concentrations in the air may cause nosebleeds and sinus trouble. Inhaling or ingesting more than 6 mg of fluorine daily in industrial dusts, insecticide, or excessive amounts of fluoride in the water causes fluorosis: weight-loss, brittle bones, weakness, fatigue, malaise, joint stiffness, severe headaches, nausea, vomiting, diarrhea, and discoloration of the teeth.

OSHA/NIOSH STANDARDS: The federal standard (PEL) for inorganic fluorides is a TWA of 2.5 mg/m^3. The exposure limit for fluorine is 1 ppm; fluoride salts, 2.5 mg/m^3; boron trifluoride, 1 ppm; bromine pentafluoride, 0.1 ppm; carbonyl fluoride, 2 ppm; chlorine trifluoride, 0.1 ppm; nitrogen trifluoride, 10 ppm; oxygen difluoride, 0.05 ppm; perchloryl fluoride, 3 ppm; selenium hexafluoride, 0.05 ppm; sulfur hexafluoride, 1,000 ppm; sulfur pentafluoride, 0.01 ppm; sulfur tetrafluoride, 0.1 ppm; sulfuryl fluoride, 5 ppm; and tellurium hexafluoride, 0.02 ppm.

Fluorocarbons

Fluorocarbons are colorless, mostly nonflammable gases, although a few are liquids. Depending upon their chemical structure, they are classified as fluoroalkanes and fluoroalkenes. Fluorocarbons include such products as Freons. The use of fluorocarbon propellants has been limited because of their association with the breakdown of the protective ozone layer of the atmosphere (see p. 29).

SOURCES OF EXPOSURE: Fluorocarbons are used as refrigerants, aerosol propellants, and anesthetics and in fire extinguishers, foam blowing agents, dry cleaning, and degreasing electronic equipment.

ROUTE OF EXPOSURE: Inhalation.

SYMPTOMS OF EXPOSURE: Under most working conditions, fluorocarbons have a low level of toxicity. Inhalation of fluorocarbons can cause irritation of the nose and mouth, light-headedness, dizziness, altered consciousness, irregular heartbeat, tremor, incoordination, and even sudden death.

Long-term, or chronic, exposure to fluoroalkenes has been associated with liver and kidney damage.

CHILD ALERT: Fluorocarbons have been abused because of their effect on the central nervous system. Inhaling certain propellants from paper or plastic bags can cause light-headedness and altered consciousness but also sudden death.

OSHA/NIOSH STANDARDS: Federal standards (PEL) for some widely used fluorocarbons are bromotrifluoromethane, 1,000 ppm (6,100 mg/ m³); dibromodifluoromethane, 100 ppm (860 mg/m³); dichlorodifluoromethane, 1,000 ppm (4,950 mg/m³); dichloromonofluoromethane, 1,000 ppm, (4,200 mg/m³); dichlorotetrafluoroethane, 1,000 ppm (7,000 mg/m³); fluorotrichloromethane, 1,000 ppm (5,600 mg/m³); tetrachlorodifluoroethane, 500 ppm (4,170 mg/ m³); and trichlorotrifluoroethane, 1,000 ppm (7,600 mg/m³).

Fluorocarbon Polymers

Fluorocarbons polymers or fluoroplastics are produced by linking together fluorocarbons (see above), and include such products as the nonstick surface polytetrafluoroethylene (Teflon and Silverstone) and fluorinated polyethylene propylene.

SOURCES OF EXPOSURE: Fluorocarbon polymers are used to create nonstick surfaces for cookware, utensils, and bandages and in electrical insulation and components, gaskets and valves, sealants, corrosion-resistant linings, exterior finishes, low-temperature lubricants, and lightweight synthetic clothing.

ROUTE OF EXPOSURE: Inhalation.

SYMPTOMS OF EXPOSURE: Exposure to hightemperature breakdown products of fluorocarbon polymers may cause polymer fume fever, a flulike illness with chills, fever, malaise, weakness, numbness and tingling in the arms and fingers, throat pain, difficulty in breathing, and joint and muscle aches, which lasts only one to two days.

OSHA/NIOSH STANDARDS: There is no OSHA standard. NIOSH recommends good work practices, engineering controls, and medical management.

Food, Drug, and Cosmetic Dyes

Food, drug, and cosmetic (FD&C) dyes are artificial coloring agents. These ingredients may be found in drug formulations, foods, and cosmetic preparations to enhance or give color to these products. They include eosin B (D&C red No. 25), eosin Y (D&C red No. 3), erythrocin B (FD&C red No. 3), Phyloxine B (D&C No. 8), tartrazine (FD&C yellow No. 5), amaranth (FD&C yellow No. 2), enythrosine (FD&C No. 3), and rose bengal. The FDA sets a safety level for these additives, meaning that there is no evidence of harm to the general population by use of these substances. However, individuals may react to a particular dye even though most others do not.

SOURCES OF EXPOSURE: Food, drug, and cosmetic dyes are found in many products including lipsticks, nail polishes, soft drinks, powdered drinks, candy, ice cream and other desserts, mouthwashes, toothpastes, antihistamines, antiasthma drugs, tooth powders, and vaginal douches.

ROUTE OF EXPOSURE: Ingestion.

SYMPTOMS OF EXPOSURE: Headache and gastrointestinal, respiratory, skeletal, dermatologic, and other neurological symptoms have been linked to ingestion of foods containing these dyes.

Ingestion of FD&C yellow No. 5 may cause an allergic reaction with symptoms ranging from hives and a mild runny nose to swelling of the skin, mucous membranes, internal organs, and brain; asthma; and anaphylaxis. Persons sensitive to aspirin may also react to tartrazine. Amaranth (FD&C yellow No. 2) may cause generalized itching, hives, and swelling of the skin, mucous membranes, internal organs, and brain. Sunset yellow (FD&C yellow No. 6) may cause purpura (allergic skin hemorrhages). Ponceau (FD&C No. 4) may cause heaviness in the chest. Erythrosine (FD&C No. 3) may interfere with the thyroid gland functioning.

Long-term, or chronic, exposure to certain FD&C dyes may cause cancer in laboratory animals and may be banned by the FDA in the future. These include FD&C red No. 3, FD&C red No. 8, FD&C red No. 9, FD&C red No. 19, FD&C red No. 37, and FD&C orange No. 17.

CHILD ALERT: A controversial claim states that certain artificial food additives may contribute to hyperactivity and other behavioral disturbances in children.

Formaldehyde

Formaldehyde (formalin, methyl aldehyde, and methylene oxide) is a colorless gas with an irritating, pungent odor widely used in industry. It has many commercial and medical applications.

SOURCES OF EXPOSURE: Formaldehyde is used medically as a disinfectant, antiseptic, deodorant, tissue preservative, and embalming agent. In industry, it is used in urea-foam insulation, paint pigment, fertilizer, paper, foundry, leather tanning, and plastic molding manufacturing. Formaldehyde also is used to treat textiles for wrinkle resistance.

The skin may come into contact with formaldehyde in cosmetics, paper, plastics, and medications.

Formaldehyde is an environmental pollutant found outdoors in smoke and smog and is released indoors, especially in mobile homes, from particle board, gas appliances, and carpeting.

Hobbyists who work in a darkroom (formaldehyde is in hardeners, stabilizers, and in color-processing systems), batik (wax when overheated may decompose to release formaldehyde), or make pottery (formaldehyde may be released from clay during the firing process) may be at risk for toxic exposure. Also at risk are metalworkers (formaldehyde-containing resins are used during mold making for metal casting) and woodworkers (formaldehyde is found in resin glues, fiberboard, and plywood).

ROUTES OF EXPOSURE: Ingestion and inhalation.

SYMPTOMS OF EXPOSURE: Ingestion of a toxic dose of formaldehyde is followed by stomach pain, vomiting, diarrhea, collapse, loss of consciousness, and death.

Inhalation of formaldehyde at low doses causes burning of the eyes, nose, and mouth and tearing of the eyes. It significantly reduces the sense of smell. Asthma and dermatitis may appear in some individuals. Higher doses may cause nausea, dizziness, cough, chest pain, shortness of breath, and wheezing.

Skin contact with formaldehyde may cause an allergic, red, itching skin condition. This is occasionally seen on eyelid skin as a result of contact with formaldehyde-containing nail polish.

Long-term, or chronic, exposure to low levels of formaldehyde in mobile homes has caused symptoms of sick-building syndrome, characterized by irritation of the eyes, nose, mouth, and throat; chronic colds or cough; chronic headaches; memory lapse; and drowsiness (see Box 14.7, p. 557).

Direct contact with formaldehyde can stain, soften, and eventually damage the nails.

REPRODUCTIVE ALERT: Some evidence of effects upon reproductive system (menstrual disorders, inflammation of the reproductive tract, sterility, and low birth weight in newborns were found in exposed garment workers).

CANCER ALERT: Chronic exposure may increase the risk of cancer (particularly nasal cancer and possibly lung cancer), although data from human studies are controversial.

OSHA/NIOSH STANDARDS: The federal standard (PEL) is a TWA of 1 ppm with a STEL of 2 ppm. NIOSH considers formaldehyde an occupational carcinogen and recommends minimizing workplace exposure levels and limiting exposure to the lowest feasible level.

Glutaraldehyde

Glutaraldehyde is a new disinfectant that has been used instead of formaldehyde. It comes as a solution of varying strengths, ranging from a 2 to 50 percent solution.

SOURCES OF EXPOSURE: In the medical setting, it is especially useful for sterilizing equipment without the need to heat the equipment.

ROUTES OF EXPOSURE: Skin contact, inhalation, and ingestion.

SYMPTOMS OF EXPOSURE: Skin contact with glutaraldehyde causes contact dermatitis. Inhalation of glutaraldehyde causes irritation of the eyes, throat, and lungs. Cough, chest tightness, headache, and asthmalike symptoms have also been reported.

PREGNANCY ALERT: Exposure to glutaraldehyde has been linked to fetal damage in mice and DNA damage in chickens and hamsters.

OSHA/NIOSH STANDARDS: The federal exposure limit (PEL) is 0.2 ppm.

Glycols and Derivatives

Glycols are a group of chemicals related to alcohols. They are used widely as solvents and antifreeze compounds. Some commonly used glycols are ethylene glycol and propylene glycol. An important subgroup of glycols are glycol ether compounds, which include ethylene glycol monomethyl ether (2-methoxyethanol), ethylene glycol monomethyl ether acetate, ethylene glycol monobutyl ether, ethylene glycol monoethyl ether (2-ethoxyethanol), ethylene glycol monoethyl ether acetate, diethylene glycol, and diethylene glycol monoethyl ether.

SOURCES OF EXPOSURE: Glycols are used as solvents for resins, lacquers, varnishes, gum, perfume, inks, paints, varnishes, and dyes. They are also found in cleaning products, liquid soaps, cosmetics, and hydraulic fluids. They are used in chemical synthesis. Propylene glycol is a constituent of injectable drugs, such as vitamins, antihistamines, and barbiturates.

Hobbyists who paint, print, dye, sculpt in resin, and refinish furniture may be exposed inadvertently to glycols in their materials.

ROUTES OF EXPOSURE: Inhalation, skin absorption, and ingestion.

SYMPTOMS OF EXPOSURE: Glycols and glycol ethers are eye, nose, and throat irritants.

Ingesting a large dose of ethylene glycol or diethylene glycol can cause initial intoxication followed by vomiting, cyanosis (blue skin discoloration) of peripheral extremities, headache, rapid heart rate, rapid breathing, difficulty in breathing, muscle tenderness, stupor, lack of urination, unconsciousness, and convulsions. Death may occur in adults from a dose of 100 g of ethylene glycol; for diethylene glycol, 15–100 g may be fatal. A much smaller dose may be fatal to a child.

Exposure to ethylene glycol ethers may cause sleepiness, difficulty breathing, and severe kidney and liver damage.

Long-term, or chronic, exposure from inhalation of ethylene glycol may cause loss of appetite, decreased urine output, unconsciousness, and jerky eye movements. Symptoms of chronic exposure to ethylene glycol ethers and derivatives include fatigue, lethargy, headache, nausea, loss of appetite, and tremor.

PREGNANCY ALERT: Animal studies have linked ethylene glycol monoethyl ether, ethylene glycol monomethyl ether, and their acetates to birth defects and miscarriages.

REPRODUCTIVE ALERT: Ethylene glycol ethers may interfere with the production of human sperm and cause difficulty conceiving.

OSHA/NIOSH STANDARDS: There is no OSHA standard for ethylene glycol. The American Conference of Governmental Industrial Hygienists (ACGIH) set a threshold limit value (TLV) of 10 mg/m^3 for particulate ethylene glycol and 100 ppm (260 mg/m^3) for the vapor. The OSHA standard for glycol ethers for a TWA are: 2-methoxyethanol, 25 ppm (80 mg/m^3); ethylene glycol monomethyl ether acetate, 25 ppm (120 mg/m^3); 2-ethoxyethanol, 200 ppm (740 mg/m^3); ethylene glycol monoethyl ether acetate, 100 ppm (540 mg/m^3); and ethylene glycol monobutyl ether, 50 ppm (240 mg/m^3). NIOSH recommends reducing exposure to glycol ethers to the lowest feasible level.

Grain Dust

Grain dust is produced whenever stores of grain are moved. The dust is composed of grain fragments; other plant material; fungi; bacteria; mold spores; toxins from mold and bacteria; rodent, bird, and insect debris and fecal excreta; silica from the soil; and chemicals, such as fungicides, herbicides, pesticides, and fumigants.

SOURCES OF EXPOSURE: Grain dust arises from stores of wheat, barley, rye, oats, corn, legumes (e.g., soybeans), and oil seeds, such as rape.

High concentrations of grain dust in the air may explode if ignited and, thus, present a fire hazard. Accidental poisonings from herbicides, fungicides, fertilizers, fumigants, and pesticides are also a risk.

ROUTE OF EXPOSURE: Inhalation.

SYMPTOMS OF EXPOSURE: Inhalation of grain dust may cause cough, shortness of breath, wheezing, and asthma and could lead to pneumonia.

Long-term, or chronic, exposure to grain dust can cause irritation of the throat, eyes, skin, and lungs; runny nose (rhinitis); and bronchitis with cough, phlegm production, and difficulty breathing. Grain fever is a flulike illness that produces fever, chills, headache, malaise, muscle aches, and sometimes cough and chest tightness.

OSHA/NIOSH STANDARDS: OSHA regulations for general industry contain requirements for the general aspects of occupational safety in grain elevators and feed mills, for example, dust control and protective equipment. The ACGIH has recommended a TLV for grain dust of 10 mg/m^3 for total dust and 5 mg/m^3 for respirable dust. NIOSH has made various recommendations for the control of combustible dusts, for machine guarding, and for personal protective equipment.

Halogenated Hydrocarbon Solvents

Halogenated hydrocarbons are chemically related compounds used as solvents. They include carbon tetrachloride (see information sheet), methyl chloride, trichloroethylene (see information sheet), 1,1,1-trichloroethane, tetrachloroethylene, dichloromethane (methylene chloride; see information sheet), tetrachloroethanes, ethylene dichloride, and ethylene chlorohydrin.

Sources of Exposure: Because of their ability to dissolve other substances, halogenated hydrocarbons are used in many hardware and household products as degreasers, dewaxers, and other cleaners. They are also used as propellants, fumigants, insecticides, refrigerants, and solvents and in chemical synthesis.

Routes of Exposure: Inhalation, skin absorption, and ingestion.

Symptoms of Exposure: Exposure to halogenated solvents may cause a range of effects on the skin, stomach and intestines, lungs, nervous system, kidneys, liver, and blood. These effects include stomach pain, nausea, vomiting, diarrhea, irritation of the eyes and nose, breathing difficulty, weakness, tingling and numbness, muscle twitching, drowsiness, dizziness, confusion, hyperactivity, fainting, slowed breathing, irregular pulse, skin discoloration, decreased urine output, coma, and death.

Skin contact with halogenated solvents can cause redness, itching, inflammation, and burns.

Long-term, or chronic, exposure to halogenated hydrocarbon solvents produces fatigue, loss of appetite, nausea, occasional vomiting, stomachache, weakness, weight loss, blurred vision, visual impairment, loss or decrease in the sense of smell, wheezing, yellow skin discoloration, memory loss, numbness and tingling in the limbs, joint pain, tremors, skin inflammation, confusion, hallucinations, sleepiness, and fainting.

Cancer Alert: Some of the halogenated hydrocarbon solvents are suspected carcinogens.

OSHA/NIOSH Standards: The OSHA standard (PEL) for carbon tetrachloride is a TWA of 2 ppm (12.6 mg/m^3); dichloroethylene, 200 ppm; methyl chloride, 50 ppm (105 mg/m^3) with a STEL of 100 ppm (210 mg/m^3); methylene chloride, 500 ppm (1,740 mg/m^3) with a ceiling of 1,000 ppm and maximum peaks of 2,000 ppm for a five-minute duration in a two-hour period; tetrachloroethylene, 25 ppm (170 mg/m^3); 1,1,2-trichloroethane, 10 ppm (45 mg/m^3); tetrachloroethane, 1 ppm (7 mg/m^3) for skin; trichloroethylene, 50 ppm (270 mg/m^3) with a STEL of 200 ppm.

NIOSH considers the following occupational carcinogens: carbon tetrachloride; methyl chloride; tetrachloroethylene; 1,1,2-trichloroethane; tetrachloroethane; and trichloroethylene.

NIOSH recommends for carbon tetrachloride a STEL of 2 ppm (12.6 mg/m^3) for a 60-minute period; for methyl chloride and methylene chloride reducing concentrations to lowest feasible levels; for tetrachloroethylene, 1 ppm (7 mg/m^3) for skin; for 1,1,2-trichloroethane, 10 ppm (45 mg/m^3); for tetrachloroethane, 1 ppm (7 mg/m^3) for skin; for trichloroethylene, 25 ppm.

Hemlock

Poison hemlock (*Conium maculatum*), water hemlock (*Cicuta maculata* and other *Cicuta* species), and dog parsley (*Aesthusa cynapium*) are poisonous members of the parsley family. Water hemlock contains the most deadly of these poisons.

Sources of Exposure: Poison hemlock grows as a weed alongside roads and ditches and in many open areas around the United States. Water hemlock grows throughout the United States around streams and marshes.

ROUTE OF EXPOSURE: Ingestion.

SYMPTOMS OF EXPOSURE: Ingestion of the *Cicuta* species may cause stomach pain; nausea; vomiting, perhaps with blood; sweating; diarrhea; convulsions; and cyanosis (blue skin discoloration) and lead to a cessation of breathing or heart attack. Ingestion of the less toxic *Conium* or *Aethusa* species may cause nausea, vomiting, salivation, fever, and increasing muscle weakness until breathing stops.

CHILD ALERT: Children may be at particular risk because of their likelihood of eating wild plants.

Hydrazine and Related Compounds

Hydrazine is a clear, colorless liquid, which is widely used, as are its related compounds, methylhydrazine, 1,1-dimethylhydrazine, 1,2-dimethylhydrazine, and phenylhydrazine.

SOURCES OF EXPOSURE: Hydrazines are used in the manufacture of many chemicals and in detergents, plasticizers, pharmaceuticals, insecticides, and herbicides. Some hydrazines are also used as rocket propellants.

ROUTES OF EXPOSURE: Inhalation and skin absorption.

SYMPTOMS OF EXPOSURE: Direct contact of hydrazine solution with the eye may cause permanent damage. Exposure to hydrazine vapor can cause temporary blindness lasting 24 hours. Other hydrazines may cause mild temporary eye problems. Exposure to hydrazine irritates the skin, mouth, nose, throat, and eyes and causes dizziness, nausea, vomiting, weakness, excited behavior, and convulsions. Hydrazine is toxic to the liver and kidneys.

Long-term, or chronic, exposure to hydrazines may cause kidney and liver damage. Symp-

toms of liver damage include malaise, lethargy, nausea, vomiting, itching, pain in the right upper stomach area, loss of appetite, dark urine, and light-colored loose stools. Symptoms of kidney damage include nausea, vomiting, decreased mental activity, itching, hiccups, muscle twitching, fatigue, loss of appetite, malaise, weakness, light-headedness, and a pale or yellow skin discoloration.

Repeated exposure to hydrazine can decrease or lead to loss of the sense of smell. The hands of workers repeatedly exposed to hydrazine hydrate may develop contact dermatitis.

CANCER ALERT: Hydrazine is a suspected skin carcinogen. In animals, hydrazines have caused lung and liver cancers.

OSHA/NIOSH STANDARDS: The OSHA standard (PEL) for a TWA for hydrazine is 0.1 ppm (0.1 mg/m^3); 1,1-dimethylhydrazine, 0.5 ppm (1.0 mg/m^3); phenylhydrazine, 5 ppm (22 mg/m^3); and methylhydrazine, a 0.2-ppm (0.35 mg/m^3) ceiling. NIOSH considers the following hydrazine compounds occupational carcinogens and recommends ceiling values: hydrazine, 0.03 ppm (0.04 mg/m^3); 1,1-dimethylhydrazine, 0.06 ppm (0.15 mg/m^3); phenylhydrazine, 0.14 ppm (0.6 mg/m^3) in a two-hour period; and methylhydrazine, 0.04 ppm (0.08 mg/m^3) in a two-hour period.

Hydrofluoric Acid

Hydrofluoric acid (HF) is a corrosive acid with many applications in industry and in household products.

SOURCES OF EXPOSURE: HF is used widely in industry to prepare high-octane gasoline, to refine petroleum, to clean metal casings, to make drugs and germicides, to frost and etch glass, and in leather tanning. It is used to manufacture dyes and plastics. HF is also found in antirust products.

Hobbyists who glaze pottery and develop photographs may be exposed to HF.

ROUTES OF EXPOSURE: Ingestion and inhalation.

SYMPTOMS OF EXPOSURE: Ingestion of HF may cause severe pain and difficulty swallowing; drooling; vomiting, perhaps with blood; stomach pain; and black tarry stools.

Inhalation may cause irritation of the respiratory tract with coughing and difficulty breathing. Rapid breathing, air hunger, difficulty breathing, and cyanosis (blue skin discoloration) may result from its affect on the larynx at the entrance to the respiratory system.

Skin contact with HF can cause severe, painful burns depending upon the acid concentration. Death has been reported from limited skin contact (2.5 percent of the body surface area, which is equivalent to the sole of the foot) and by inhalation.

Long-term, or chronic, exposure to HF may cause nail pain and longitudinal brown bands in the nails.

CHILD ALERT: Most ingestions of household materials containing HF occur in small children between the ages of one and four years of age.

OSHA/NIOSH STANDARDS: The federal standard (PEL) is 3 ppm with a STEL of 6 ppm.

Hydrogen Sulfide

Hydrogen sulfide is a colorless gas released when sulfur compounds decompose. There is an odor of rotten eggs at low concentrations.

SOURCES OF EXPOSURE: Hydrogen sulfide is found naturally below ground in caves or coal mines, in volcanoes, and in the soil. It is released from decaying fish, sewage, manure, and septic tanks. Occupational exposure may occur from the manufacture of paper, viscose rayon, silk, rubber, and petroleum; damp mines; hot sulfur springs; leather tanning; roofing asphalt tanks; the burning of wool, hair, food, and hides; metal refining; and production of heavy water for nuclear reactors.

ROUTE OF EXPOSURE: Inhalation.

SYMPTOMS OF EXPOSURE: Exposure to a high concentration of hydrogen sulfide gas is a leading cause of sudden death in the workplace. After inhaling hydrogen sulfide, the eyes become painfully irritated, halos are seen around lights, and blurred vision, headache, insomnia, nausea, vomiting, weakness, sore throat, cough, dizziness, loss of the sense of smell, drowsiness, and difficulty breathing may occur. At very high concentrations, coma, slow breathing, and death may ensue.

Long-term, or chronic, exposure to hydrogen sulfide gas causes headache, weakness, low blood pressure, nausea, loss of appetite, weight loss, unsteadiness, eye irritation, and cough.

OSHA/NIOSH STANDARDS: The OSHA standard (PEL) is a TWA of 10 ppm (14 mg/m^3) with a STEL of 15 ppm (21 mg/m^3). NIOSH recommends a ceiling of 10 ppm (15 mg/m^3) for a ten-minute period.

Chlorinated Hydrocarbon Insecticides

The chlorinated hydrocarbon insecticides are commercial, synthetic chemicals used to control the insect population. They may persist in the environment and in organisms from weeks to years after being applied. A classic example is dichlorodiphenyltrichloroethane (DDT), which is now banned in most countries.

The four chemical types include benzene hexachloride; DDT and its related compounds; the cyclodienes and related compounds (aldrin, chlordane, endosulfan, dieldrin, endrin, chlordecone [kepone], heptachlor, mirex, and isobenzan); and toxaphene and its related compounds.

SOURCES OF EXPOSURE: Fruits, seed grain, or vegetables sprayed with these insecticides may cause poisonings. Milk and meat may contain dichlorodiphenyl-dichloroethylene (DDE), the breakdown product of DDT. Benzene hexachloride (lindane) is used as an agricultural and residential insecticide and is also found in Kwell shampoo and sprays for body lice. Chlordane was used for residential subterranean termite control.

Hobbyists who garden are at risk.

ROUTES OF EXPOSURE: Ingestion, inhalation, and skin absorption.

SYMPTOMS OF EXPOSURE: In general these insecticides act as central nervous system stimulants. Symptoms vary with each type of insecticide, but, except for DDT, severe poisonings initially may cause seizures within the first five to six hours after ingestion, failure to breathe, and, in some cases, death.

Ingestion of 5 g or more of dry DDT may cause nausea, severe vomiting, headache, dizziness, and gradual weakness and numbness of the limbs. Ingestion of more than 20 g can cause twitching of the eyelids, tremors, muscle spasms; agitation and confusion may occur before or separate from the seizures.

In mild poisonings, chlorinated hydrocarbon insecticides may cause dizziness, nausea, stomach pain, and vomiting.

Ingestion or massive skin exposure to benzene hexachloride can cause vomiting and diarrhea and, later, convulsions. Mild exposure can cause dizziness, headache, nausea, tremors, and muscle weakness.

Long-term, or chronic, exposure may cause loss of weight and appetite. Chronic exposure to eldrin may also cause temporary deafness and disorientation. Chronic exposure to DDT may cause malaise; headache; dizziness; tingling sensation of the tongue, face, and lips; apprehension; tremor, and confusion. Chronic exposure to chloredecone causes permanent neurologic damage.

Chloredecone (kepone) is a suspected spermatotoxin that may cause difficulty conceiving. Other agents suspected of affecting the male reproductive system are benzene hexachlorides (lindane), DDT, methoxychlor, aldrin, chlordane, and dieldrin.

CANCER ALERT: Some of these chemicals have been found to be carcinogenic in laboratory animal studies.

OSHA/NIOSH STANDARDS: The OSHA standard (PEL) for aldrin/dieldrin is a TWA of 0.25 mg/m^3; DDT, 1 mg/m^3; kepone, none; and methoxychlor, 10 mg/m^3. NIOSH considers aldrin/dieldrin an occupational carcinogen and recommends the lowest reliably detectable level and 0.15 mg/m^3 TWA by the NIOSH-validated method; DDT, the lowest possible reliably detectable level and 0.5 mg/m^3 TWA by the NIOSH-validated method; and kepone, 1 mg/m^3 TWA.

Iron

Iron is a silver-gray metal. It forms many compounds including hematite (an iron ore), magnetic iron oxide, the very toxic iron pentacarbonyl, and various iron salts.

SOURCES OF EXPOSURE: Toxicity from iron exposure is associated more with ingestion of iron-containing products by children than with work-related exposure. Iron salts are found in vitamin supplements. Workers are generally affected by inhalation of iron oxide fumes.

ROUTES OF EXPOSURE: Ingestion, inhalation, and intravenous feeding.

SYMPTOMS OF EXPOSURE: Ingestion of a toxic dose of iron may initially cause nausea, stomach pain, vomiting, and diarrhea and, in severe cases, lethargy, restlessness, disorientation, coma, pallor, and rapid heartbeat. Vomiting may cease, followed 12 to 24 hours later by life-threatening symptoms: vomiting blood, dark stools, lethargy, coma, convulsions, cyanosis (blue skin discoloration) of peripheral extremities, difficulty breathing, low blood pressure, and increased heart rate.

Inhalation of iron oxide fumes causes metal fume fever, a flulike illness whose symptoms are a metallic taste in the mouth; eye, nose, and throat irritation; cough; difficulty breathing; fatigue; fever; chills; sweating; nausea; vomiting; muscle aches; and weakness. Those exposed often recover in one to two days. At some point during continuous exposure to iron oxide fumes, tolerance develops (the fumes no longer cause symptoms). However, over the weekend, or after a period without exposure, the tolerance is lost, and "Monday morning fever" may occur.

Exposure to iron-containing dusts and fumes can cause irritation and inflammation of the eyes.

Long-term, or chronic, exposure to iron oxide by inhalation causes siderosis, a benign lung condition, in which iron gets deposited in the lungs. Cough, wheezing, and shortness of breath may develop, although most workers do not develop any symptoms.

Long-term iron exposure may damage the liver and pancreas.

CHILD ALERT: Iron tablets are among the most common agents accidently ingested by children.

OSHA/NIOSH STANDARDS: The federal standard (PEL) for iron oxide fumes is a TWA of 10 mg/m³. No other iron compounds are regulated. NIOSH recommends a TWA of 5 mg/m³.

Irritant Gases

Irritant gases are a group of diverse gases that produce a similar type of injury: They all cause an inflammation of the lining of the respiratory tract. The extent of injury depends on the concentration and type of gas. Ammonia, chlorine, sulfuric acid mist, sulfur dioxide, and nitrogen oxides are the common irritant gases. More esoteric irritants include phosphorus oxychloride, acrolein, and phosgene.

SOURCES OF EXPOSURE: Ammonia is used primarily in the manufacture of fertilizer. It is also used in the manufacture of other chemicals and pharmaceuticals, synthetic fibers, dyes, plastics, and refrigerants, and in petroleum refining, mirror silvering, glue making, and leather tanning.

Chlorine is used in household bleaches; water purification; bleaching cloth and paper; chemical processes; pharmaceutical manufacturing; making solvents for dry cleaning, paint thinners, and degreasing agents; refrigerants; cosmetics; and plastics and resin manufacturing. Storage and transport accidents account for many exposures.

Sulfur dioxide and nitrogen oxides are found as air pollutants.

ROUTES OF EXPOSURE: Inhalation and ingestion.

SYMPTOMS OF EXPOSURE: Respiratory irritation is the major symptom of exposure to these gases. Inhaling irritant gases causes coughing, choking, hoarseness, throat and chest pain, difficulty in swallowing and speaking, difficulty breathing, headache, nausea, vomiting, and weakness. Eye irritation, tearing, and a runny nose may also be present. After six to eight hours, chest tightness, air hunger, dizziness, frothing at the mouth, and blue skin discoloration may occur. Death may follow.

A single exposure to certain respiratory irritants may cause permanent loss of the sense of smell.

Inhalation of high concentrations of ammonia causes restlessness, chest tightness, frothing at the mouth, blue skin discoloration, and a rapid heart rate.

Inhalation of sulfur dioxide may cause coughing, choking, headache, dizziness, and weakness. Chest tightness, difficulty breathing, frothing at the mouth, and cyanosis (blue skin discoloration) may follow.

Long-term, or chronic, exposure to irritant gas fumes may cause chronic cough, bronchial pneumonia, and stomach upsets.

Sulfur dioxide in air pollution has been shown to aggravate chronic heart and lung diseases including asthma and coronary artery disease. Long-term exposure to sulfur dioxide may cause breathing difficulties, cough, and sputum production.

Prolonged exposure to chlorine gas may produce corrosion of the teeth.

CHILD ALERT: High sulfur dioxide levels in the air have been shown to adversely affect children. Increased rates of respiratory tract infections have been seen in children when these levels were raised (see p. 118).

OSHA/NIOSH STANDARDS: The OSHA standard (PEL) for ammonia is a STEL of 35 ppm (27 mg/m³); chlorine, a 1-ppm (3 mg/m³) ceiling; sulfuric acid, 1 mg/m³; sulfur dioxide, 5 ppm (10 mg/m³); nitrogen dioxide, 5 ppm (9 mg/m³); nitrogen oxide, 25 ppm (30 mg/m³); phosphorus oxychloride, 0.1 ppm (0.6 mg/m³); acrolein, 0.1 ppm (0.25 mg/m³); and phosgene, 0.1 ppm (0.4 mg/m³).

NIOSH recommends for ammonia a 35-ppm (27 mg/m³) ceiling for 15 minutes; chlorine, a 1-ppm (3 mg/m³) ceiling for 15 minutes; sulfuric acid, 1 mg/m³; sulfur dioxide, 5 ppm (10 mg/m³); nitrogen dioxide, 1 ppm (1.8 mg/m³); nitrogen oxide, 25 ppm (30 mg/m³); and phosgene, 0.1 ppm (0.4 mg/m³) with a 0.2-ppm (0.8 mg/m³) ceiling for 15 minutes.

The ACGIH recommends a TLV for phosphorus oxychloride of 0.1 ppm (0.6 mg/m³).

Ketones

The ketone family is a group of chemicals with a similar structure. They are widely used as solvents in industry and common household products, and as chemical intermediates used in the production of other chemicals. They include acetone, diacetone, methyl ethyl ketone, methyl *n*-propyl ketone, methyl *n*-butyl ketone (MBK or MNBK), and methyl isobutyl ketone.

SOURCES OF EXPOSURE: Ketones are used as solvents and chemical intermediates; in paint, lacquer, varnish, plastics, rubber cement, dyes, celluloid, photography chemicals, rubber, inks, paper, textiles, pharmaceuticals, and cosmetics (e.g., nail polish remover); and in manufacturing explosives.

Hobbyists who use inks, dyes, paint and varnish removers, lacquers, metal-cleaning compounds, epoxy resins, and dewaxers may be exposed to ketones.

ROUTES OF EXPOSURE: Inhalation, accidental ingestion, and skin absorption.

SYMPTOMS OF EXPOSURE: In high concentrations, ketones may cause eye, nose, and throat irritation; headache; nausea; light-headedness; vomiting; dizziness; incoordination; and unconsciousness.

Long-term, or chronic, exposure can cause a dry, scaly skin inflammation. Exposure to MBK may affect the nervous system and produce numbness in the hands and feet and weakness of the forearms, legs, head, and feet. Recovery may take up to several years.

OSHA/NIOSH STANDARDS: The OSHA standard (PEL) for a TWA for acetone is 750 ppm (1800 mg/m³); diacetone, 50 ppm (240 mg/m³); methyl ethyl ketone, 200 ppm (590 mg/m³); methyl *n*-propyl ketone, 200 ppm (700 mg/m³); MBK, 100 ppm (410 mg/m³); and methyl isobutyl ketone, 100 ppm (410 mg/m³). NIOSH recommends a TWA for acetone of 250 ppm (590 mg/m³); diacetone, 50 ppm (240 mg/m³); methyl ethyl ketone, 200 ppm (590 mg/m³); methyl *n*-propyl ketone, 150 ppm (530 mg/m³); MBK, 1 ppm (4 mg/m³); and methyl isobutyl ketone, 50 ppm (200 mg/m³).

Laser Light

Laser light is a narrow focused beam of high-intensity energy.

SOURCES OF EXPOSURE: Lasers are used in industry in welding/cutting and metalworking. One million workers are directly involved with laser applications such as craftspeople, operators of lasers, and laser service personnel. Lasers are used to treat diseases in many fields including dermatology and ophthalmology.

Routes of Exposure: Absorption of laser energy (primarily through the eye).

Symptoms of Exposure: Exposure to laser light may decrease vision due to severe damage to the cornea or retina of the eye.

Lead

Lead is a blue or silver-gray, soft metal found in ores, seawater, soil, and as various minerals. The amount of lead in the environment has steadily increased, making it one of the top environmental pollutants. It is especially hazardous to children (see pp. 256–260).

Sources of Exposure: Lead is found in the air from various sources, notably car exhaust fumes, as well as from smelters; firing ranges; and the burning of lead-based-painted wood, newspapers, magazines, and battery casings. It is found in the soil and house dust (from old, flaking lead-containing paint).

Adults are most commonly exposed to toxic levels of lead through inhalation of lead-containing dust in the workplace. Family members can be exposed to lead on work clothes and shoes brought into the home.

Exposure to lead can occur when it leaches into food after being cooked or served in unfired or improperly fired pottery or leaden pots. Lead can leach into liquids, particularly home-distilled moonshine whiskey and wine stored in pottery. Lead piping and lead-lined tanks, common in older plumbing systems, are responsible for lead leaching into tap water.

Some herbal medicines, including traditional folk medicines, and cosmetics have been contaminated with lead.

Illicitly prepared drugs, such as cocaine, amphetamines, or heroin, may be contaminated with lead.

Hobbyists at high risk for lead exposure include those that target shoot, make stained glass and ceramics, solder, do car or boat repair, or do home remodeling.

Routes of Exposure: Inhalation; ingestion; injection; absorption through the skin; and via bullets retained in joints, lungs, or the abdomen. In children, lead toxicity is most often due to ingestion.

Symptoms of Exposure: If a toxic dose of lead is ingested or, more rarely, injected, a metallic taste in the mouth, stomach pain, vomiting, behavioral changes, diarrhea, and black stools will occur. This may progress to further symptoms, including decreased urine output, collapse, and coma.

Inhalation of lead oxide fumes causes metal fume fever, a flulike illness with symptoms including a metallic taste in the mouth; eye, nose, and throat irritation; cough; difficulty breathing; fatigue; fever; chills; sweating; headache; nausea; vomiting; muscle aches; and weakness. Those exposed often recover in one to two days. At some point during continuous exposure to the fumes, tolerance develops (the fumes no longer cause symptoms). However, over the weekend or after a period without exposure, the tolerance is lost, and "Monday morning fever" may occur.

Symptoms of lead poisoning from sniffing leaded gasoline initially include insomnia with nightmares, nausea, vomiting, irritability, anxiety, and restlessness. Continued exposure leads to tremor, spasmodic involuntary movement of the arms and/or legs and face muscles, confusion, mania, and seizures.

Long-term, or chronic, exposure from ingestion, skin absorption, or inhalation may manifest as loss of appetite, weight loss, constipation, apathy or irritability, occasional vomiting, fatigue, dizziness, headache, weakness, a sweet metallic taste in the mouth, insomnia, visual impairment, bluish (lead) gumline, and stomach discomfort. In children, chronic exposure manifests as loss of newly acquired skills and behavioral disorders. Visual impairment from inflammation of the optic nerve and even blindness has been reported in children.

Lead poisoning may cause nail pain, white

spots or patches on the nails, or even shedding of the nails.

More advanced symptoms include intermittent vomiting; irritability; nervousness; weakening of memory and the ability to concentrate; numbness in the legs; incoordination; pains in the arms, legs, and joints; sharp, recurrent stomach pains (lead colic); difficulty in moving the foot or wrist (wrist or foot drop); hearing loss; kidney disease; menstrual irregularities; and miscarriage.

Severe symptoms are persistent vomiting, incoordination, stupor, lethargy, tremor, delirium, convulsions, and coma. Death may occur.

CHILD ALERT: Lead poisoning is a major environmental hazard to children, particularly those from ages six months to five years. Children are very vulnerable to lead toxicity because they absorb more lead than adults and are less able to excrete it. Classically, lead poisoning occurs in young, malnourished children living in deteriorating urban housing.

The hands, clothing, toys, and play areas of children may be contaminated with lead-containing paint chips and dust. Children become poisoned with lead by inadvertent hand-to-mouth activities. They also may eat lead-containing paint and plaster chips and crawl on floors with contaminated dust and dirt. Other sources of lead exposure include food, polluted air, lead-glazed pottery, toys, topsoil near smelter dumps or freeways, and folk remedies. Children may also be exposed to lead through the contaminated clothes of parents who come into contact with lead in the workplace.

Nursing babies may be exposed to lead through breast milk containing high levels of the substance.

Sniffing leaded gasoline or "huffing" will cause symptoms in children.

Some hobbyist materials, such as paint pigments, glazes, and stained glass kits, also contain lead. Always use crafts materials designed specifically for children and look for nontoxic labeling.

PREGNANCY AND REPRODUCTIVE ALERTS: Lead is associated with miscarriages, an increased risk of birth defects, and impaired growth and development of the developing fetus and infant. Lead-exposed men may have abnormal sperm and low sperm counts, which are linked to reduced fertility.

OSHA/NIOSH STANDARDS: The OSHA standard (PEL) is a TWA of 0.050 mg/m^3. NIOSH recommends a TWA of less than 0.100 mg/m^3. The air level should be maintained so that the blood lead levels in workers remain less than or equal to 0.060 mg/100 g whole blood.

Magnesium

Magnesium is a light silvery-white metal. It is an essential component of the body's chemical reactions. Magnesium is found naturally in ores, in asbestos, talc, seawater, and salt deposits.

SOURCES OF EXPOSURE: Most toxicity results from ingesting large doses of magnesium sulfate. Magnesium sulfate is used medically to stimulate bowel action and to treat toxemia, a disorder of pregnancy. However exposure in the workplace can result from inhalation of magnesium-containing fumes.

Hobbyists who make ceramics and glass, weld, and paint may risk exposure to magnesium.

ROUTES OF EXPOSURE: Inhalation, ingestion, injection, and rectal administration.

SYMPTOMS OF EXPOSURE: Inhalation of magnesium oxide fumes causes metal fume fever, a flulike illness whose symptoms include a metallic taste in the mouth; eye, nose, and throat irritation; cough; difficulty breathing; fatigue; fever; chills; sweating; nausea; vomiting; muscle aches; and weakness. Those exposed often recover in one to two days. At some point during continuous exposure to the fumes, tolerance develops (the fumes no longer cause symptoms).

However, over the weekend or after a period without exposure, the tolerance is lost, and "Monday morning fever" may occur.

Magnesium oxides and fumes are mild eye, nose, and skin irritants.

Ingestion of large doses of magnesium sulfate causes stomach pain, vomiting, watery or bloody diarrhea, and collapse. Injection or rectal administration of magnesium sulfate can cause flushing, restlessness, thirst, slowed breathing, paralysis, coma, and death.

Long-term, or chronic, exposure by ingestion of magnesium-containing antacids can cause kidney failure.

OSHA/NIOSH Standards: The federal standard (PEL) for magnesium oxide fume is 10 mg/m^3. NIOSH states there is insufficient documentation to justify the OSHA standard.

Manganese

Manganese is a red-gray or silver soft metal found naturally in the earth's crust.

Sources of Exposure: Manganese is used widely in industry to make steel and other alloys, paint, varnish, ceramics, glass, inks, dyes, matches, and fireworks. Manganese is used as an antiknock agent in gasoline. Exposure may occur during the mining, refining, or smelting of this metal.

Hobbyists who make ceramics and glass, or who paint, varnish, print, dye, and weld risk exposure to manganese.

Routes of Exposure: Inhalation, skin absorption, and ingestion.

Symptoms of Exposure: Inhalation of manganese oxide fumes causes metal fume fever, a flu-like illness whose symptoms are a metallic taste in the mouth; eye, nose, and throat irritation; cough; difficulty breathing; fatigue; fever; chills; sweating; nausea; vomiting; muscle aches; and

weakness. Those exposed often recover in one to two days. At some point during continuous exposure to manganese oxide fumes, tolerance develops (the fumes no longer cause symptoms). However, over the weekend or after a period without exposure, the tolerance is lost, and "Monday morning fever" may occur.

Inhaling manganese dust may cause irritation of the nose and throat, cough, difficulty breathing, pneumonia, headache, and itching.

Ingestion, inhalation, or skin absorption of a toxic dose of manganese cyclopentadienyl tricarbonyls (antiknock gasoline additives) causes swelling, bleeding, nerve and kidney damage, hyperactivity, convulsions, and coma.

Long-term, or chronic, exposure from inhalation of manganese dust and fumes can begin with apathy, loss of appetite, drowsiness, headache, spasms, weakness of the legs, irritability, and joint pain. "Manganese madness" may follow with confusion, bizarre behavior, uncontrolled emotions, hallucinations, impotence, poor libido, sleep disturbances, and slurred speech. Numbness of the limbs, skin inflammation, enlargement of the liver, tremors, muscle cramps, difficulty walking, and a fixed facial expression may also occur. Miners of manganese have developed Parkinson's disease–like symptoms.

Chronic exposure to manganese cyclopentadienyl tricarbonyls (antiknock gasoline additives) may cause insomnia, disturbing dreams, emotional instability, hyperactivity, convulsions, and psychosis.

OSHA/NIOSH Standards: The federal standard (PEL) is a ceiling of 5 mg/m^3. NIOSH recommends a TWA of 1 mg/m^3 and a STEL of 3 mg/m^3.

Mercury

Elementary mercury is a silver liquid, but mercury also exists in inorganic (salts) and organic compounds. Elemental and inorganic mercury compounds are widely used as material for, or as part of the manufacturing process of, scientific instruments, electrical equipment, disk batteries, felt, dental amalgams, disinfectants, and caustic soda.

SOURCES OF EXPOSURE: Exposure from organic mercury compounds is generally from environmental sources, such as atmospheric contamination from mining, refining, or smelting, or from contamination of the marine environment from industrial effluent. The burning of fossil fuels, such as coal, also adds mercury to the air. Foods, especially seafood or grains treated with the fungicide methylmercury, can contain organic mercury compounds. Until recently, mercury was found in many latex house paints and at potentially toxic levels in freshly painted rooms.

Medical equipment and dental care have also been sources of exposure to mercury and its various compounds.

Hobbyists who make jewelry and ceramics, paint, work in a darkroom, and do metalwork may risk exposure to mercury.

ROUTES OF EXPOSURE: Ingestion, inhalation of vapors or dusts, injection of organic mercury, and skin absorption.

SYMPTOMS OF EXPOSURE: After ingestion of mercury salts, a metallic taste in the mouth, thirst, severe stomach pain, vomiting, and bloody diarrhea appear; urine output may diminish or stop; and death may follow.

Inhaling high concentrations of mercury vapor leads to shortness of breath, cough, fever, nausea, vomiting, diarrhea, inflammation of the lining of the mouth, salivation, and a metallic taste in the mouth. This may progress to severe difficulty breathing and kidney failure.

Inhaling toxic doses of organic mercurials causes a metallic taste in the mouth, dizziness, clumsiness, slurred speech, diarrhea, and convulsions, which may be fatal. Exposure to organic methylmercury causes difficulty speaking, incoordination, narrowing of the field of vision and sometimes blindness, and behavioral changes.

Inhalation of mercury oxide fumes causes symptoms of metal fume fever, a flulike illness whose symptoms can include fever; chills; sweating; headache; nausea; vomiting; difficulty breathing; chest pain; eye, nose, and throat irritation; cough; a metallic taste in the mouth; headache; and weakness. Those exposed often recover in one to two days if not reexposed. At some point during continuous exposure to the fumes, tolerance develops (the fumes no longer cause symptoms). However, over the weekend or after a period without exposure, the tolerance is lost, and "Monday morning fever" may occur.

Mercury is a skin irritant and can cause allergic skin rashes.

Long-term, or chronic, exposure by ingestion or injection of elemental or organic mercury or ingestion of mercury salts may cause itching or weeping skin reactions, inflammation of the lining of the mouth, salivation, diarrhea, anemia, liver damage, and kidney failure with the cessation of urine.

Chronic inhalation of mercury vapor or dusts or organic vapor or skin absorption may lead to tremors, salivation, inflammation of the lining of the mouth, loose teeth, pain and numbness in the limbs, diarrhea, anxiety, headache, weight loss, loss of appetite, hearing defects, loss of concentration, memory defects, mental depression, insomnia, irritability, instability, hallucinations, and mental deterioration.

Changes in the sense of smell have also been reported with inhalation of elemental mercury vapors.

CHILD ALERT: Pink disease (acrodynia) is an allergic reaction to mercury in infants and children. Its symptoms include restlessness, irritability, redness, swelling, coldness, irritation and burning of the hands and feet, inflammation of the mouth, loose teeth, hair and nail loss in severe cases, and, infrequently, death. Teething powders, lotions, ointments, and diaper rinses had previously contained mercury compounds.

Inhalation of high concentrations of mercury vapor is often fatal in children as well as adults.

PREGNANCY ALERT: Exposure to methylmercury has been linked with birth defects as well as neurological damage in the offspring of women exposed during pregnancy. (See Box 1.2, p. 25 for information on Minamata disease.)

OSHA/NIOSH STANDARDS: The federal standard (PEL) for inorganic mercury is a TWA of 0.05 mg/m^3; the standard for organic mercury is a TWA of 0.01 mg/m^3.

Methanol

Methanol (methyl or wood alcohol) is a colorless, volatile liquid that is distilled from wood. It is available in different concentrations in many everyday products, such as windshield washer fluid and Sterno canned heat.

SOURCES OF EXPOSURE: Methanol is used as a dry gas; an antifreeze; a paint remover; a gasoline additive; a solvent in shellac, varnish, paints, stains, duplicating fluids, cements, dyes, and inks; and in chemical synthesis (especially in making formaldehyde), and in denatured alcohol.

Methanol-contaminated whiskey has caused epidemics of methanol toxicity, including deaths.

ROUTES OF EXPOSURE: Ingestion, inhalation, and skin absorption.

SYMPTOMS OF EXPOSURE: Exposure by inhalation, skin absorption, or ingestion of a mildly toxic dose of methanol causes fatigue, headache, nausea, and then a temporary blurred vision, which may be permanent in some cases. A moderately toxic dose will cause severe headache, dizziness, lethargy, confusion, stomach pain, nausea, vomiting, and slowed breathing and heart rate. Temporary or permanent blindness

may occur after two to six days. In severe poisoning, symptoms may progress to rapid breathing, coma, and death.

Long-term, or chronic, exposure to inhaled methanol may at first be recognized as blurred vision and may progress to complete blindness.

Skin contact may cause paronychia (inflammation adjacent to the nail) and even nail loss.

OSHA/NIOSH STANDARDS: The federal standard (PEL) is a TWA of 200 ppm (260 mg/m^3) with a STEL of 250 ppm (325 mg/m^3).

Methyl Bromide, Methyl Chloride, and Methyl Iodide

Methyl bromide, methyl chloride, and methyl iodide are all colorless gases. Chemically they are classified as halogenated hydrocarbon compounds. They are very toxic, damaging almost all types of cells in the body.

SOURCES OF EXPOSURE: These gases are used in chemical synthesis; as insect fumigants for soil, grains, fruits, and warehouses; and as rodenticides. Flour, cereals, rice, grain, seed dates, and nuts are preserved with methyl bromide.

ROUTES OF EXPOSURE: Inhalation and skin absorption.

SYMPTOMS OF EXPOSURE: Inhalation or skin absorption of a mildly toxic dose of these gases causes irritation of the eyes, nose, and mouth; headache; nausea; vomiting; blurred vision; slurred speech; dizziness; malaise; euphoria; weakness or paralysis; difficulty breathing; drowsiness; confusion; and hyperactivity. Tremor, incoordination, muscle twitching, disturbed behavior and emotion including depression, and decreased or no urine output may be seen after exposure.

Exposure to high doses of these gases causes breathing difficulty, convulsions, and coma. Death may ensue.

Irritation and blistering result from skin contact.

Long-term, or chronic, exposure to these gases causes blurred vision; a decrease in the ability to smell; numbness of the limbs; incoordination; muscle pain; behavioral changes including depression, irritability, and insomnia; short-term memory loss; confusion; speech disturbances; hallucinations; sleepiness; fainting; seizures; and difficulty breathing.

Chronic low-dose skin exposure to methyl bromide causes drying, scaling, and itching.

CANCER ALERT: Methyl bromide, methyl chloride, and methyl iodide are considered by NIOSH to be occupational carcinogens. Methyl iodide is a suspected skin carcinogen.

OSHA/NIOSH STANDARDS: The federal standard (PEL) for methyl bromide is a TWA of 5-ppm (20 mg/m^3) ceiling; methyl chloride, 50 ppm (105 mg/m^3) with a STEL of 100 ppm (210 mg/m^3); and for methyl iodide, 2 ppm (10 mg/m^3). NIOSH considers all three substances occupational carcinogens and recommends reducing exposure to the lowest feasible concentration.

Methylene Chloride

Methylene chloride (dichloromethane, methylene dichloride, and methylene bichloride) is a colorless liquid with a pleasant odor. It is chemically classified as a halogenated hydrocarbon solvent. Methylene chloride is metabolized in the body to form carbon monoxide, which may contribute to ischemia and heart attacks.

SOURCES OF EXPOSURE: Methylene chloride is used in industry to extract substances at low temperatures; as a solvent for fat, oil, wax, and esters; and as a paint remover and degreaser.

Residents who live near methylene chloride production and use facilities or near hazardous waste sites that store methylene chloride have an increased risk of exposure.

Hobbyists who do woodworking (methylene chloride is in paint strippers); work in a dark-room; and use adhesives, aerosols, and paint thinners may be at risk for exposure.

ROUTES OF EXPOSURE: Inhalation and skin absorption.

SYMPTOMS OF EXPOSURE: At levels below 500 ppm, exposure may cause euphoria, sluggishness, light-headedness, irritability, sleepiness, and dizziness. Exposure to higher concentrations may produce headache; impaired concentration and coordination; loss of balance; eye, nose, and throat irritation; nausea; flushing; confusion; slurred speech; heart pain; and difficulty breathing. Exposure may lead rapidly to unconsciousness.

Long-term, or chronic, exposure may cause headache, dizziness, nausea, memory loss, tingling in the hands and feet, fatigue, and unconsciousness.

CANCER ALERT: The EPA considers methylene chloride a probable human carcinogen. NIOSH considers it an occupational carcinogen. Some studies indicate an association with increased incidences of liver, pancreatic, and biliary tract cancer.

PREGNANCY ALERT: Methylene chloride can cross the placenta and may be found in breast milk. Although it is unclear whether methylene chloride has direct effects on the developing fetus, increased carbon monoxide (a breakdown product of methylene chloride) may have adverse effects on the fetus (see Carbon Monoxide information sheet).

OSHA/NIOSH STANDARDS: The OSHA standard (PEL) is a TWA of 500 ppm with a ceiling of 1,000 ppm (2,000 ppm maximum in any two-hour period). NIOSH considers methylene chloride an occupational carcinogen and recommends reducing exposure to the lowest feasible concentration.

Microwaves

Microwaves are a form of electromagnetic energy (see Chapter 16, "Radiant Energy").

SOURCES OF EXPOSURE: In the home, microwave ovens are a potential source of exposure. Applications of microwave technology in industry are rapidly expanding.

ROUTE OF EXPOSURE: Microwave energy is directly absorbed by the body.

SYMPTOMS OF EXPOSURE: Only the effects caused by heating of the tissues, which includes thyroid damage, have been well studied. Other reported symptoms include headache, sleepiness and insomnia, fatigue, irritability, dullness, sweating, breathing difficulty, chest pain, irregular heartbeat, and other heart problems.

Long-term, or chronic, exposure to microwaves may be associated with decreased vision due to cataract formation, nail abnormalities including transverse ridging and onycholysis (separation of nail from the underlying finger), changes in menstrual patterns and other reproductive system changes, loss of memory, decreased sexual ability, emotional instability, and the symptoms mentioned above.

PREGNANCY AND REPRODUCTIVE ALERTS: Several animal studies report low birth weight, birth defects, stillbirths, and abnormal behavior in newborns. Occupational studies have found associations with retarded fetal development, congenital effects in newborns, decreased milk production in nursing mothers, and an increase in miscarriages in women working with microwaves.

Naphthalene

Naphthalene is a solid white substance with a "mothball" odor. Although some old-fashioned household deodorizers and mothballs may still contain naphthalene, most preparations now use the less toxic p-dichlorobenzene.

SOURCES OF EXPOSURE: Naphthalene may be used in some mothballs and in the manufacture of resin, dyes, tanning agents, lampblack, smokeless powder, and other compounds.

ROUTES OF EXPOSURE: Ingestion and inhalation.

SYMPTOMS OF EXPOSURE: Ingestion of naphthalene can cause nausea, vomiting, diarrhea, urinary difficulties or dark urine, and jaundice. Excitement, coma, and convulsions may also occur in severe poisonings.

Inhalation of high concentrations of naphthalene can cause eye irritation, headache, mental confusion, excitement, malaise, profuse sweating, vomiting, stomach pain, and visual disturbances. Jaundice, dark urine, and kidney failure may occur later.

Long-term, or chronic, exposure to naphthalene vapor may cause cataracts. Itching, redness, scaling, weeping, and crusting of the skin may result from continual handling of naphthalene.

CHILD ALERT: Naphthalene may be present in the household as an ingredient in some mothballs and deodorizers. Ingestion of approximately 2 g of naphthalene can be lethal to young children under age six.

OSHA/NIOSH STANDARDS: The federal standard (PEL) is 10 ppm (50 mg/m^3) with a STEL of 15 ppm (75 mg/m^3).

Nickel

Nickel is a silver-white magnetic metal found naturally in ores in the earth's crust. It has many industrial uses as a pure metal, an alloy, and nickel compounds. Nickel carbonyl is found in many chemical reactions and processes.

SOURCES OF EXPOSURE: Nickel is found as a contaminant in the air principally from the combustion of fossil fuels, such as petroleum and coal. Air, soil, and water may be polluted with nickel where it is mined, smelted, or refined.

Minute amounts of nickel are found in numerous food products including tea, cocoa, baking soda, and ground nuts. Using stainless-steel cooking utensils adds nickel to foods as does using fats and oils hydrogenated with nickel catalysts.

Nickel is found in costume jewelry, which may cause a skin reaction or contact allergic dermatitis. Dental alloys, some surgical implants, and fluid used in dialysis machines may contain nickel.

Hobbyists who make ceramics (nickel is used in colorants), jewelry, or who green glass, enamel (some enamels contain nickel), dye, print, paint, varnish, or do metalwork (nickel fumes may be released during metal casting and oxyacetylene welding) risk exposure to nickel.

ROUTES OF EXPOSURE: Inhalation of dusts, aerosols, and airborne compounds (major route of occupational exposure); accidental ingestion of nickel compounds or contaminated drinking water; injection of soluble nickel salts from contaminated intravenous fluid; and by leaching out of soluble nickel salts from catheters that remain inside the body. Skin contact with nickel may result in a reaction, but little nickel is absorbed by this route.

SYMPTOMS OF EXPOSURE: In nickel-sensitive individuals, intravenous infusion of nickel-containing solutions can cause allergic reactions and even anaphylaxis, a life-threatening allergic reaction.

Metallic nickel is nontoxic. However, if nickel salts are ingested, they may irritate the stomach, causing nausea, vomiting, gastrointestinal distress, and diarrhea. Other reported symptoms include giddiness, lassitude, headache, cough, and shortness of breath.

Inhalation of nickel oxide fumes causes metal fume fever, a flulike illness whose symptoms may include a metallic taste in the mouth; eye, nose, and throat irritation; cough; difficulty breathing; fatigue; fever; headache; chills; sweating; nausea; vomiting; muscle aches; and weakness. Those exposed often recover in one to two days. At some point during continuous exposure to nickel oxide fumes, tolerance develops (the fumes no longer cause symptoms). However, over the weekend or after a period without exposure, the tolerance is lost, and "Monday morning fever" may occur.

Inhalation of nickel carbonyl may cause nausea, vertigo, headache, shortness of breath, and chest pain; hours or days later chest tightness, central chest pain, dry cough, rapid breathing, and profound weakness occur, which can be fatal.

Long-term, or chronic, exposure via inhalation of dusts and aerosols is associated with irritation of the lining of the nose, loss of the sense of smell, asthma, lung irritation, and bronchitis.

CANCER ALERT: An increased incidence of cancer of the lung and nasal passages has been associated with nickel carbonyl exposure.

CHILD ALERT: The death of a young child who ingested a nickel compound from a chemistry hobby set has been reported.

PREGNANCY ALERT: Although nickel carbonyl has been demonstrated to be a potent teratogen in rats, studies of Welsh women employed during the two world wars show no teratogenic effects. However, the possibility of nickel exposure affecting a fetus remains.

OSHA/NIOSH STANDARDS: The OSHA standard (PEL) for soluble compounds of inorganic nickel is a TWA of 0.1 mg/m^3, and 1.0 mg/m^3 for insoluble compounds; and nickel carbonyl, a TWA of 0.001 ppm (0.007 mg/m^3). NIOSH considers all these substances to be occupational carcinogens, and recommends for inorganic nickel compounds a TWA of 0.015 mg/m^3 and nickel carbonyl, 0.001 ppm (0.007 mg/m^3).

Nicotine

Nicotine is a colorless, bitter-tasting liquid that evaporates easily. Found naturally in the leaves of the tobacco plant, nicotine is the main active component in cigarettes and cigars.

SOURCES OF EXPOSURE: Nicotine is found in all forms of tobacco, chewing tobacco, snuff, and tobacco substitutes, such as nicotine gum, and in many insecticide mixtures.

ROUTES OF EXPOSURE: Inhalation (primarily), skin absorption, and ingestion.

SYMPTOMS OF EXPOSURE: Exposure to a small dose of nicotine may cause rapid breathing, nausea, vomiting, dizziness, headache, diarrhea, rapid heartbeat, sweating, and salivation. A period of weakness is then followed by recovery. In addition to the above symptoms, a large toxic dose of nicotine may cause burning of the mouth, throat, and stomach; confusion; agitation; disturbed hearing and vision; restlessness; incoordination; prostration; convulsions; slowed breathing; coma; and even death.

Long-term, or chronic, exposure to small amounts of nicotine-containing pesticides has no reported effects. Tobacco smoking is associated with increased incidence of coronary heart disease and cancer of the mouth, bladder, and respiratory tract.

Withdrawal from smoking is associated with several physical symptoms, primarily from nicotine withdrawal: slowed heartbeat, lowered blood pressure, sweating, and rapid breathing. Other symptoms include a craving for cigarettes, anxiety, nervousness, irritability, impaired memory and concentration, depression, hostility, headaches, muscle cramps, stomach and bowel problems, increased appetite, weight gain, and insomnia.

REPRODUCTIVE ALERT: Nicotine is believed to be toxic to sperm, and because it collects in cervical mucus, it may affect fertility.

CHILD ALERT: Children may be poisoned if they eat cigarettes, snuff, or nicotine gum. They may also be exposed through side-stream smoke, inhaling the smoke from another person's cigarette. Infants exposed to environments with high concentrations of tobacco smoke have a higher incidence of pneumonia and bronchitis.

OSHA/NIOSH STANDARDS: The federal standard (PEL) is a TWA of 0.5 mg/m^3.

Nitrites and Nitrates

Nitrites and nitrates, chemical groups that include many compounds, have numerous diverse uses.

SOURCES OF EXPOSURE: Nitrites and nitrates are used in fertilizers and, as by-products of this use, are found as unwanted contaminants in well water. Nitrite is used in pickling and salting processes to preserve the pink color of meat; nitrate and nitrite compounds are also used as preservatives of meats and fish, including smoked fishes, bologna, salami, pepperoni, bacon frankfurters, corned beef, canned ham, and sausages. Nitrates and nitrites may be found in heart and blood pressure medications (they are used medically to dilate the blood vessels in the heart, to lower blood pressure, and as burn preparations). Nitroglycerin and ethylene glycol nitrite are used to make dynamite.

Nitrates are found naturally in vegetables, such as spinach, beets, radishes, eggplant, celery, cauliflower, broccoli, lettuce, collards, and turnips. Preserved meats and fish also contain nitrate and nitrite compounds. These include smoked fishes, bologna, salami, pepperoni, bacon, frankfurters ("hot dog headaches"), corned beef, canned ham, and sausages.

Hobbyists who garden and use nitrite- or nitrate-containing fertilizers may be at risk.

Organic nitrites (amyl, butyl, isobutyl, and isoamyl nitrites) historically have been abused as putative sexual aids.

ROUTES OF EXPOSURE: Ingestion, injection, inhalation, and skin and mucous membrane absorption.

SYMPTOMS OF EXPOSURE: Acute exposure to nitrites and nitrates may cause headaches, flushing, vomiting, dizziness, collapse, lowered blood pressure, blue skin discoloration, convulsions, coma, and difficulty breathing and cessation.

Long-term, or chronic, exposure may cause the symptoms listed above. Repeated exposure of nitroglycerin workers creates a tolerance in which the substance no longer causes adverse effects, such as headaches. However, the tolerance disappears rapidly and so poisoning may occur with a previously tolerated amount. Cessation of long-term exposure to nitrates can cause heart attack.

CANCER ALERT: Nitrosamines, formed from the interaction of nitrates and nitrites with amines, are suspected carcinogens in humans. These nitrosoamines are found in surface water from fertilizer contamination, pesticides, industrial cutting fluids, plastics and plasticizers, and toiletries.

CHILD ALERT: Infants are particularly susceptible to nitrate/nitrite toxicity. They may be seriously affected by the presence of more than 10 ppm of nitrogen as nitrate in well water. The hemoglobin in their blood may be altered to form methemoglobin and oxygen transfer to the tissues can be severely decreased.

OSHA/NIOSH STANDARDS: The OSHA standard (PEL) for nitroglycerin is a ceiling of 2 mg/m^3; and ethylene glycol dinitrate, a ceiling of 1 mg/m^3. NIOSH recommends for nitroglycerin and ethylene glycol dinitrate a ceiling limit of 0.1 mg/m^3.

Nitrogen

Nitrogen is a colorless, odorless gas that is a natural component of air. It is used to dilute oxygen in compressed air. Although not toxic itself, it can act as an asphyxiant if it decreases the amount of oxygen in the air inhaled.

SOURCES OF EXPOSURE: Nitrogen is found in the air and in compressed air.

ROUTE OF EXPOSURE: Inhalation.

SYMPTOMS OF EXPOSURE: Nitrogen bubbles in the body cause decompression sickness, or the bends, in divers, miners, and other compressed-air workers who surface too quickly. Symptoms range from skin itch, joint and muscle pain, vertigo, and difficulty breathing to blindness, paralysis, shock, and death.

Long-term, or chronic, exposure to nitrogen can cause damage to the heart and brain if the periods when the body lacks oxygen are prolonged.

Nuisance Dusts

Nuisance dusts, a term that refers to diverse dusts, both organic and inorganic, are generated in many workplaces and cause various types of occupational lung disease. Among the many inorganic dusts are chalk, potash, and iron oxide. Organic nuisance dusts can come from woodworking.

SOURCES OF EXPOSURE: Any workplace contaminated with dust from grinding, milling, or other processes is a hazard.

Hobbyists, particularly sculptors and potters, may be inadvertently exposed to dusts in contaminated workspaces.

ROUTE OF EXPOSURE: Inhalation.

SYMPTOMS OF EXPOSURE: Depending upon the type and concentration of the dusts in the environment, the reaction to dust may result in inflammation of the breathing tubes. The symptoms may include runny nose, sore throat, cough with or without mucus (bronchitis), difficulty breathing, chest tightness, and wheezing.

Long-term, or chronic, exposure to nuisance dusts can result in a range of symptoms from hyposmia (a decreased sense of smell) from chronic irritation of the lining membranes of the nose, to chronic bronchitis, asthma, or emphysema, associated with cough, wheezing, and difficulty breathing.

OSHA/NIOSH STANDARDS: The ACGIH recommends the TLVs for tin oxide and Portland cement of 10 mg/m^3; nonasbestiform talc, 2 mg/m^3.

Oil of Peppermint

Oil of peppermint, a flavoring agent, contains menthol and terpenes, a class of hydrocarbons.

SOURCES OF EXPOSURE: Many consumer products contain oil of peppermint as a flavoring.

ROUTES OF EXPOSURE: Inhalation and ingestion.

SYMPTOMS OF EXPOSURE: Exposure to oil of peppermint may cause heartbeat irregularities; swelling of the tongue, lips, and lining of the mouth; hives; flushing; and headache.

Long-term, or chronic, exposure to oil of peppermint has caused decreased or complete loss of the ability to smell in exposed workers.

Oxalic Acid

Oxalic acid is a corrosive acid that is a colorless liquid when in solution.

SOURCES OF EXPOSURE: Oxalic acid is widely used in manufacturing many common products such as inks, dyes, and bleaches. Household products containing oxalic acid include toilet bowl cleaners, disinfectants, metal cleaners, furniture polish, antirust products, and bleaches.

Hobbyists involved with ceramics, photography (oxalic acid is found in some toners), dyeing (oxalic acid is used as a mordant to fix dye to the fabric), bleaching, printing, lithography, drawing with ink, paint removing, varnishing, and wood or metal cleaning may be exposed through their craft materials.

ROUTES OF EXPOSURE: Inhalation and ingestion.

SYMPTOMS OF EXPOSURE: Direct contact with the skin causes corrosion and ulceration, localized pain, blue skin discoloration, and gangrene. Ingesting oxalic acid may cause irritation and corrosion of the mouth, esophagus, and stomach accompanied with pain and vomiting. Tremors, convulsions, shock, and collapse may follow. The kidneys may be damaged. Death may result after ingesting between 5 and 15 g of oxalic acid.

Long-term, or chronic, exposure to mist or dust may cause inflammation of the nose and throat and poisoning as described above.

OSHA/NIOSH STANDARDS: The federal standard (PEL) is a TWA of 1 mg/m^3 with a STEL of 2 mg/m^3.

Ozone

Ozone (O_3) is a blue gas with a pungent smell that is produced by ultraviolet light acting on molecular oxygen. Increased ozone levels on the ground cause respiratory problems and are a major component of smog (see p. 552). Destruction of the ozone layer in the upper portion of the stratosphere (possibly due to chlorofluorocarbons) renders us more vulnerable to the harmful effects of ultraviolet light (see p. 29).

SOURCES OF EXPOSURE: Ozone is created from a reaction between the ultraviolet rays of sunlight and oxidants such as nitrogen oxides or automobile exhaust, adding to air pollution in industrialized settings. It is produced by electric arc welding and photocopiers. Increased exposure also occurs while traveling at high altitudes.

ROUTES OF EXPOSURE: Inhalation and direct exposure of the eyes.

SYMPTOMS OF EXPOSURE: Ozone may cause irritation of the mucous membranes of the eyes and respiratory tract, including the nose, throat, and lungs. Ozone can cause cough, fatigue, headache, chest pain, and severe shortness of breath. It may also cause severe respiratory distress in which the lungs fill with fluid.

Long-term, or chronic, exposure can cause chronic eye and lung irritation.

OSHA/NIOSH STANDARDS: The OSHA standard is a TWA of 0.1 ppm (0.2 mg/m^3) with a

STEL of 0.3 ppm (0.6 mg/m³). NIOSH recommends a STEL ceiling of 0.1 ppm (0.2 mg/m³).

para-Phenylenediamine

para-Phenylenediamine is an organic dye, which is a strong skin sensitizer.

SOURCES OF EXPOSURE: para-Phenylenediamine is used as a preservative in cosmetics and topical medications. It is also found in inks, dyes, permanent hair dyes, and rubber.

ROUTE OF EXPOSURE: Skin contact.

SYMPTOMS OF EXPOSURE: Skin contact with para-phenylenediamine can cause an allergic contact skin reaction with itching, burning, or pain and a rash with pink to red skin patches. Significant exposure can cause yellow skin discoloration.

Long-term, or chronic, exposure may cause chronic dermatitis (dry, scaly patches on the skin with itching).

Paraquat and Diquat

Paraquat and diquat are water-soluble herbicides. They are classified as bipyridylium quaternary ammonium compounds based upon their chemical structure. Even though they are very toxic when first applied, they are inactivated by contact with the soil and rapidly decomposed by sunlight, quickly eliminating (in days) their toxic risk.

Accidental or intentional ingestion produces serious damage. From 33 to 50 percent of those who accidently ingest paraquat will die. The fatal dose of paraquat may be as little as 4 mg/kg; for diquat, 30 mg/kg.

SOURCES OF EXPOSURE: In 1978 when paraquat was sprayed on marijuana in Mexico, this herbicide was brought to general attention, but its presence in marijuana has not caused symptoms in this country due to the small quantities and decomposition associated with burning. Paraquat is also sprayed on cotton plants to dry the leaves during harvesting. Diquat is used mostly for aquatic weed control.

ROUTES OF EXPOSURE: Ingestion, skin absorption, and inhalation.

SYMPTOMS OF EXPOSURE: A primary target of paraquat toxicity is the lung. Inhalation and ingestion of paraquat can cause an oxidant-mediated lung injury that results in respiratory distress syndrome and acute lung injury and fibrosis; the only known therapy is lung transplantation. Skin contact with paraquat causes irritation and ulceration of the skin, nails, eyes, and lining of the nose.

Paraquat ingestion causes burning in the mouth and throat, nausea, cough, difficulty breathing, headache, vomiting, stomach pain, and diarrhea. By the fifth day, the victim may be coughing up blood, have little urine output, and ulceration of the tongue, esophagus, and stomach. Yellow or blue skin discoloration, fever, fast heart rate, and difficulty breathing may develop within a few hours. Ingestion of paraquat is frequently fatal.

Diquat ingestion causes stomach cramps, vomiting, and diarrhea and may progress to sparse urine output, irregular heartbeat, difficulty breathing, coma, and convulsions and can even cause death.

Long-term, or chronic, exposure to paraquat has caused nosebleeding; nose, mouth, and throat irritation; cough; headache; eye and skin irritation; and damaged fingernails. White or brown bands, ridging, softening, or thickening may develop in the nails, or there may be permanent nail loss.

Prolonged skin contact with diquat has caused transverse white or brown bands, a softening or thickening to develop in the nails, and permanent nail loss.

Paraquat is chemically similar to 1-methyl-4-phenyl-1,2,3,6-tetrahydropyridine (MPTP), which is known to cause Parkinsonism, a disease of the nervous system that causes tremors and rigidity of the muscles (see p. 105).

OSHA/NIOSH Standards: The OSHA standard (PEL) for the respirable dust of paraquat is 0.1 mg/m³; and diquat, 0.5 mg/m³.

Pesticides (Cholinesterase Inhibitors)

Cholinesterase-inhibiting pesticides are a group of pesticides used to control soft-bodied insects in agriculture. It is composed of two groups: the *organophosphate* insecticides, such as diazinon, malathion, and parathion, and the *carbamates*, one of which is carbaryl. They are grouped together because they act on the body in a similar way.

Sources of Exposure: Pesticides are found as contaminants in the air, water, and soil. Dusts, concentrates, and wettable powders are available to the public for use in home gardens. Commonly available formulations contain from 1 to 95 percent pure material. Tetraethyl pyrophosphate (TEPP) and malathion concentrates are available to the public, placing hobbyists who garden at risk for exposure.

Carbamate dusts are used both to control fleas on dogs and cats and in typhus and plague control programs.

Organophosphates are responsible for four out of five systemic poisonings from agricultural chemicals in California. Another potential source of exposure to pesticides is their residue on and in contaminated food and beverage products.

Routes of Exposure: Skin absorption, inhalation, and ingestion.

Symptoms of Exposure: The key findings of exposure to a toxic dose of these pesticides are disturbances of vision, difficulty breathing, and stomach problems. Reaction to a mild poisoning consists of loss of appetite, headache, dizziness, weakness, anxiety, stomachache, tremors of the tongue and eyelids, and visual problems.

A moderately toxic dose causes nausea, salivation, tearing, stomach cramps, vomiting, sweating, slow pulse or elevated pulse, and muscle twitchings.

Severe poisoning causes diarrhea with loss of bowel control, breathing difficulty, possibly cyanosis (blue skin discoloration) due to blockage of breathing by secretions, convulsions, and coma. Exposure can be fatal.

Delayed effects have appeared several days to weeks after poisoning and include calf pain, weakness, unsteadiness, and paralysis of the fingers, hands, and forearms.

Long-term, or chronic, exposure to low doses may produce severe symptoms since effects may last up to six weeks and become cumulative. Persistent muscle weakness may result from exposure to some of these pesticides.

Child Alert: Children may be poisoned by eating large quantities of sprayed fruits and vegetables that have not been adequately washed or from being exposed to lawns that have recently been treated with these pesticides.

OSHA/NIOSH Standards: The OSHA standard (PEL) for parathion is a TWA of 0.1 mg/m³; malathion, 10 mg/m³; and carbaryl, 5 mg/m³. OSHA has no standard for methyl parathion. NIOSH recommends for parathion a TWA of 0.05 mg/m³; methyl parathion, 0.2 mg/m³; malathion, 10 mg/m³; and carbaryl, 5 mg/m³.

Petroleum Distillates

Petroleum distillates are liquids obtained by refining crude oil. Chemically, they are branched-chain or straight-chain hydrocarbons. They are very widely used in almost all industries. They include petroleum ether (benzine), petroleum naphtha, rubber solvent naphtha, Stoddard solvent, varnish maker's and painter's naphtha, gasoline, kerosene, mineral seal oil, diesel oil, fuel oil, and *n*-hexane.

Sources of Exposure: Petroleum distillates are used as heating, cooling, and jet fuels and solvents. They are found in many household products, such as furniture polish, paint thinner, and lighter fluid. Petroleum distillates are found in waterless hand cleaners.

Pesticides, camphor, metals, or halogenated compounds may be dissolved in petroleum distillates.

Hobbyists involved with painting (petroleum distillates are used as paint thinners), printing (petroleum distillates are used in silk screen poster inks), wax sculpture, furniture finishing, woodworking, gardening, guns, hunting, and shooting may be at risk for exposure to petroleum distillates.

ROUTES OF EXPOSURE: Ingestion and inhalation.

SYMPTOMS OF EXPOSURE: The main findings in petroleum distillates exposure are lung irritation and nervous system effects.

After inhaling or ingesting petroleum distillates, headache, nausea, vomiting, difficulty breathing, and coughing possibly with bloody mucus may occur. Fever and cough may indicate pneumonia. Severe inhalation exposure may lead to very rapid, noisy breathing, cyanosis (blue skin discoloration) from lack of oxygen, coma, convulsions, and sometimes death. Weakness, dizziness, confusion, slow and shallow breathing, unconsciousness, and convulsions may follow ingestion of large amounts of petroleum distillates.

Skin contact causes irritation.

Long-term, or chronic, exposure from inhalation of petroleum distillates may cause dizziness, weakness, weight loss, nervousness and pain, and tingling and/or numbness in the limbs.

Workers exposed to benzene have reported a decreased or complete loss of their ability to smell. *n*-Hexane, a fraction of naphtha, may cause peripheral neuropathy.

CHILD ALERT: Ingestion by children of common household products that contain petroleum distillates is very common. Calls to a poison control center typically report ingestion of gasoline, lacquer thinner (benzene, Stoddard solvent, naphthas), furniture polish (mineral seal oil), kerosene, and charcoal lighter fluid.

Half of the hospital admissions for hydrocarbon poisonings are for children under three years of age. The most common type of hydrocarbon exposure is ingestion of petroleum distillates.

Teenagers may be involved in sniffing petroleum distillates.

OSHA/NIOSH STANDARDS: The OSHA standard (PEL) for petroleum naphtha is a TWA of 400 ppm (1,600 mg/m^3); gasoline, 300 ppm; mineral oil mist, 5 mg/m^3; rubber solvent naphtha, 400 ppm; Stoddard solvent, 100 ppm; and *n*-hexane, 50 ppm. There is no federal standard for kerosene vapor in workroom air. NIOSH recommends a TWA of 350 mg/m^3 for petroleum naphtha with a ceiling of 1,800 mg/m^3.

Phenol and Phenolic Compounds

Phenol (carbolic acid) is a white crystalline powder that is also available as a solution in water. Among its many derivatives are the creosotes (wood tar or coal tar); cresol; and the antioxidants, 2, 6-di-*tert*-butyl-*p*-cresol or butylated hydroxytoluene (DBPD, BHT), 4,4'-thio-bis(6-*tert*-butyl-*m*-cresol) and pentachlorophenol and related chlorinated phenols.

SOURCES OF EXPOSURE: Phenolic compounds have been used as antiseptics, disinfectants, caustic agents, germicides, fungicides, insecticides, topical anesthetics, antioxidants, wood preservatives, and herbicides. Phenol has been found as a contaminant in well water.

Hobbyists at risk are photographers (cresol).

ROUTES OF EXPOSURE: Ingestion, skin absorption, and inhalation.

SYMPTOMS OF EXPOSURE: After skin contact with all but the most dilute solutions of phenol or its derivatives, the skin blanches or turns red and may begin to slough off. Eye contact causes severe damage and may lead to blindness.

Other symptoms from either ingestion or skin absorption include profuse sweating, intense thirst, nausea, vomiting, diarrhea, loss of appetite, blue skin discoloration, hyperactivity, stupor, deep and rapid breathing, stomach pain, muscle pain, rapid and weak pulse, convulsions, coma, and difficulty breathing. If death does not occur immediately, the skin may yellow, urine may darken (from a product of phenol metabolism), and/or urine output may decrease.

Inhalation or skin absorption of cresol may cause muscle weakness, headache, dizziness, dimness of vision, ringing in the ears (phenol effect also), reduction in or loss of the sense of smell, rapid breathing, mental confusion, coma, and death.

Long-term, or chronic, exposure may cause the above symptoms. Chronic exposure to phenol-contaminated well water has caused sore throat, diarrhea, and dark urine.

Prolonged contact with cresol will discolor the skin and may cause liver and kidney damage. Chronic exposure to beta-naphthol may cause bladder tumors, anemia, and clouding of the lens of the eye.

CANCER ALERT: Trichlorophenols and 2,4-dimethyl phenol may be carcinogens or may be contaminated with carcinogens, such as dioxins.

OSHA/NIOSH STANDARDS: The OSHA standard (PEL) for phenol is a TWA of 5 ppm (19 mg/m^3); cresol, 5 ppm (22 mg/m^3); BHT and 4,4'-thio-bis(6-*tert*-butyl-*m*-cresol, 10 mg/m^3; and coal-tar products, 0.2 mg/m^3. There is no OSHA standard for creosote. NIOSH recommends for phenol a TWA of 5.2 ppm (20 mg/m^3) with a ceiling of 15.6 ppm (60 mg/m^3) for a fifteen-minute duration; cresol, 2.3 ppm (10 mg/m^3); and coal-tar products, 0.1 mg/m^3.

Phenolic Resins

Phenolic resins are a group of plastics manufactured by reacting phenol with an aldehyde, usually formaldehyde. Those most commonly used commercially include phenolformaldehyde, melamine formaldehyde, resorcinol formaldehyde, *p-tert*-butylphenol formaldehyde, furfuryl formaldehyde, and cardolite.

SOURCES OF EXPOSURE: Phenolic resins are used to make foam and synthetic leathers, for examples, used in footwear and clothing. Cured or hardened resin is used for automobile, electrical, and appliance parts.

ROUTES OF EXPOSURE: Direct skin contact and inhalation.

SYMPTOMS OF EXPOSURE: Skin contact with phenolic resins may cause irritation or allergic contact dermatitis with dryness, chapping, redness, and possibly blistering. Vitiligo (white patches in the skin caused by the loss of pigment) has also been reported.

Inhalation of dust, fumes, or particles has been associated with irritation of the eyes, nose, and throat; cough; rash; and phlegm production.

Long-term, or chronic, exposure to inhaled phenolic resin fumes has been associated with difficulty breathing (airway obstruction).

Phosphorus and Its Compounds

Yellow phosphorus is a yellow or colorless waxy substance. It ignites in air to form white fumes and green light. Red phosphorus is a red, granular, nonvolatile, insoluble, and almost unabsorbable substance. Phosphine is a colorless gas with a nauseating odor. Some other commonly found phosphorus-containing compounds are phosphoric acid, phosphorus chlorides and sulfides, and metal phosphides. Phosphides include zinc, aluminum, and calcium phosphide.

SOURCES OF EXPOSURE: Yellow phosphorus is found in rodent and insect poisons, fireworks, and fertilizers. Phosphorus sesquifluoride, a nontoxic substance, is now found on the heads of safety matches. Phosphides are used in rat poisons, which on contact with water may release phosphine. Phosphine may also be released when water or acid reacts with metal phosphides present in metal ores.

ROUTES OF EXPOSURE: Ingestion and inhalation. For phosphorus, direct skin contact can cause burns.

SYMPTOMS OF EXPOSURE: Ingestion of yellow phosphorus may cause nausea; vomiting; diarrhea; irregular heartbeats; and garlic odor of the breath, vomitus, and stools. Within one to two days, coma and death may occur or there may be a day or two of improvement. Symptoms may return and worsen. Death may occur up to three weeks after poisoning. In adults very small doses of yellow phosphorus can be fatal.

Inhaling phosphorus can cause the same symptoms as acute phosphorus ingestion. Inhaling phosphine or phosphides causes nausea, vomiting, fatigue, cough, yellow skin discoloration, tingling or burning sensations, incoordination, tremor, blurred vision, difficulty breathing, irregular heartbeats, convulsions, collapse, coma, and sometimes death.

Skin contact with phosphorus may cause severe burns.

Long-term, or chronic, exposure to yellow phosphorus, phosphine, or phosphides can cause toothache, followed by swelling and destruction of the jaw, or "phossy jaw." Weakness, weight loss, loss of appetite, and fractures may also occur. Inhalation of fumes may cause cough, bronchitis, and pneumonia.

CHILD ALERT: Yellow phosphorus has often been mixed with molasses or peanut butter, spread on bread, and put out as bait for rodents and roaches. Poisonings have occurred when children have mistakenly eaten this bait.

OSHA/NIOSH STANDARDS: The federal standard (PEL) for yellow phosphorus is 0.1 mg/m^3; phosphoric acid, 1.0 mg/m^3; phosphorus trichloride, 0.2 ppm (1.5 mg/m^3) with a STEL of 0.5 ppm (3 mg/m^3); phosphorus pentachloride, 1.0 mg/m^3; and phosphorus pentasulfide, 1.0 mg/m^3; for phosphine is a TWA of 0.3 ppm (0.4 mg/m^3) with a STEL of 1 ppm (1 mg/m^3).

Poison Ivy/Oak/Sumac

Poison ivy (*Rhus radicans*), poison oak (*Rhus toxicodendron*, *Rhus diversiloba*), and poison sumac (*Rhus vernix*) are related plants of the *Rhus* species. These plants have a milky sap containing urushiol, a toxin that causes severe skin reaction in about half of the people who are exposed to it (see p. 163).

SOURCES OF EXPOSURE: Poison ivy grows throughout the United States except in California and Nevada. Poison oak is found on the Pacific Coast and in an area bounded by New Jersey, northern Florida, and Texas. Poison sumac grows mainly in the South and East, from Texas to New Jersey.

ROUTES OF EXPOSURE: Direct contact, ingestion, and inhalation of smoke from burning plants.

SYMPTOMS OF EXPOSURE: A pattern of lines form on the skin causing itching, swelling, bumps, blisters, crusts, and oozing in twelve hours to one week after exposure. Limb swelling, swelling of the larynx or pharynx, decreased urination, weakness, malaise, and fever may also occur.

Long-term, or chronic, exposure may increase the intensity of the symptoms.

CHILD ALERT: Infants do not readily react to poison ivy or oak, but by the age of three, children are highly susceptible. They are often exposed during their play in wooded areas. They should be taught to identify these plants and avoid them.

Polybrominated Biphenyls

Polybrominated biphenyls (PBBs) are chemically classified as aromatic hydrocarbons (having rings of carbon and hydrogen atoms) that contain bromine molecules. These compounds were used in the manufacture of heat-resistant plastics, but PBBs are no longer manufactured in the United States. If ingested, they are stored in the body fat and are only slowly excreted.

SOURCES OF EXPOSURE: As a fine powder, PBBs are added to plastics as a flame retardant. Accidental exposure to PBBs occurred in Michigan in 1973 when PBBs were added to animal feedstock and the contaminated cattle, chickens, sheep, and swine were then consumed.

ROUTE OF EXPOSURE: Ingestion.

SYMPTOMS OF EXPOSURE: Long-term, or chronic, exposure to PBB-contaminated meat, milk, and eggs has been reported to cause acne, dry skin, skin darkening, nail discoloration, prolonged healing of cuts, nausea, fatigue, headache, blurred vision, dizziness, depression, nervousness, sleepiness, weakness, loss of balance, joint pain, insomnia, and back and leg pain. PBBs may also interfere with the immune system, cause liver damage, and adversely affect the sensory nerves.

CANCER ALERT: Animals exposed to PBBs have developed liver tumors.

REPRODUCTIVE ALERT: PBBs are reported to affect both the female and male reproductive capacity and may cause difficulty conceiving.

OSHA/NIOSH STANDARDS: No standards have been established.

Polychlorinated Biphenyls

Polychlorinated biphenyls (PCBs) are a group of 209 chemicals whose chemical structures consist of two fused rings of carbon and hydrogen with chlorine atoms attached. Usually found as mixtures of PCBs, these substances range from colorless to light brown oils, viscous liquids, and sticky semisolids. The EPA banned the production of PCBs in 1977 because of their carcinogenic potential.

SOURCES OF EXPOSURE: Because PCBs are chemically stable, they persist in toxic waste sites and are found in illegally dumped waste oil, transformer fluids, and old household appliances such as refrigerators. PCBs were used in transformers and capacitors in industrial and medical equipment and in fluorescent light fixtures.

PCBs are found in the soil, in sediment in rivers and bays, and in food sources such as fish and animal fat. In 1968 in Japan over 1,600 people exposed to PCBs through contaminated cooking oil developed rice oil disease, or *yusho* (see p. 534 and Figure 17.1, pp. 600–601 for more information).

ROUTES OF EXPOSURE: Inhalation and skin absorption.

SYMPTOMS OF EXPOSURE: Exposure to PCBs may cause chloracne (the development of blackheads with small yellow cysts) and enlargement of the liver.

Long-term, or chronic, exposure may cause weight loss, loss of appetite, nausea, vomiting, yellow skin discoloration, stomach pain, headache, dizziness, and swelling of the limbs.

CANCER ALERT: The EPA considers PCBs to be probable human carcinogens based upon animal studies showing increased incidence of cancers of the liver, pituitary gland, and gastrointestinal tract; leukemia; and lymphoma.

CHILD ALERT: PCBs accumulate in breast milk and may affect nursing infants who cannot effectively excrete this toxin.

PREGNANCY AND REPRODUCTIVE ALERTS: Fetuses and newborns are very sensitive to PCBs because they lack the liver enzyme necessary to breakdown and excrete PCBs. PCBs may possibly cause developmental and toxic effects on the human fetus.

PCBs interfere with conceiving because of their ability to prevent the implantation of the fertilized egg in the womb in laboratory animals.

OSHA/NIOSH Standards: The federal standard (PEL) is a TWA airborne concentration of 1 mg/m^3 for PCBs containing 42 percent chlorine; and PCBs containing 54 percent chlorine, 0.5 mg/m^3. NIOSH recommends a ten-hour TWA of 0.001 mg/m^3 based on the minimum reliable detectable concentration of PCBs. NIOSH also recommends that workplace exposure be reduced to the lowest feasible level because of PCBs' carcinogenic potential.

Polynuclear Aromatic Hydrocarbons

Polynuclear aromatic hydrocarbons (PAHs) (polynuclear aromatics and polycyclic organic matter) are composed of three or more fused rings of carbon and hydrogen atoms. They are solids at room temperature. Among the hundreds of such compounds are benzo[*a*]pyrene (B [*a*] P), benzo[*e*]pyrene, chrysene, and dibenz-[*a,b*]anthracene.

Sources of Exposure: According to one study, the smoke from one cigarette contains 10 to 50 ng B[*a*]P, 18 ng chrysene, 40 ng dibenz[*a,b*]anthracene, and 12 to 140 ng benz[*a*]anthracene. PAHs are also found in barbecued and smoked meats and fish, roasted peanuts and coffee, refined vegetable oil, wheat, rye, and lentils.

PAHs are found in the air from natural sources, such as forest fires and volcanoes, but mostly from human-made sources, such as burning coal, wood, petroleum products, and oil and from coke production, burning refuse, and car exhaust. Water, soil, and air may also be contaminated. People living near oil refineries and in cities with heavy traffic may be exposed to higher levels of PAHs.

Routes of Exposure: Inhalation and ingestion.

Symptoms of Exposure: No significant effects have been found with acute exposure.

Long-term, or chronic, exposure is associated with redness and burning of the skin, warts on areas exposed to the sun that may go on to become cancerous, irritation of the eyes with sensitivity to light, cough, bronchitis, and blood in the urine.

Cancer Alert: Epidemiologic studies of exposed workers have found increased incidences of cancers of the skin, lung, bladder, kidney, and gastrointestinal tract. Long-term exposure is associated with cancers of the lung, lip, pharynx, bladder, and kidney; lymphoma; and perhaps leukemia.

Pregnancy Alert: PAHs may affect the fetus. PAHs are excreted in breast milk and can affect nursing infants of mothers exposed to PAHs.

Reproductive Alert: Animal studies have shown that PAHs cross the placenta and destroy the functioning of the female's eggs, sometimes causing infertility.

OSHA/NIOSH Standards: OSHA standard (PEL) is a TWA for air in the workplace of 0.2 mg/m^3. NIOSH considers these substances to be occupational carcinogens and recommends that the workplace exposure limit be set at the lowest feasible concentration (which was 0.1 mg/m^3 when the recommendation was made).

Pyrethrum and Pyrethroids

Pyrethrum is an insecticidal dusting powder derived from the chrysanthemum and contains six active ingredients, the most active of which are pyrethrins I and II. Pyrethroids are synthetic pesticides that include allethrin, bioresmethrin, cypermethrin, permethrin, decamethrin, and fenvalerate. These synthetic agents are used in sprays as knockdown agents to kill flying insects.

Sources of Exposure: Many household insecticide sprays contain pyrethroids. Over 2,000 commercially available products contain pyrethrins, including over-the-counter flea and tick sprays.

ROUTES OF EXPOSURE: Inhalation and direct skin contact.

SYMPTOMS OF EXPOSURE: Except for many people who are allergic (see below), pyrethrum and pyrethroids are not particularly toxic, causing contact dermatitis, paleness, fast heartbeat, and sweating. Exposure to pyrethrins has caused tingling on the feet and hands, cough, shortness of breath, dizziness, vomiting, and diarrhea. Skin contact with pyrethroids may cause local burning, pricking, or tingling sensations that resolve in about a day; numbness on the face; dizziness; fatigue; and a fine rash.

Some individuals may be specifically allergic to the chrysanthemum (pyrethrum) family and may develop acute allergic symptoms, including swelling of the breathing passages, which may result in death if the person does not receive medical treatment.

Long-term, or chronic, exposure to pyrethrum may cause skin roughening, itching, and asthma especially in those who are sensitive to ragweed pollen.

OSHA/NIOSH STANDARDS: The federal standard (PEL) is a TWA of 5 mg/m^3 for pyrethrum.

Ionizing Radiation

Ionizing radiation is a form of energy that has the ability to change the structure of atoms when it interacts with matter. It includes X rays, gamma rays, alpha and beta particles, neutrons, and charged heavy nuclei (see Chapter 16, "Radiant Energy").

SOURCES OF EXPOSURE: Ionizing radiation is found naturally in the environment from the decay of radioactive elements and in cosmic rays from outer space. It is also produced artificially from X-ray machines, high-energy accelerators, and other devices. Some medical procedures expose us to ionizing radiation.

ROUTES OF EXPOSURE: External contact (radiation passes through body), inhalation of radioactive particles, direct skin contact with radioactive soils or dusts, and ingestion.

SYMPTOMS OF EXPOSURE: See Chapter 16, "Radiant Energy," for information on exposure to ionizing radiation.

OSHA/NIOSH STANDARDS: See Chapter 16, "Radiant Energy."

Rosin

Rosin (colophony) is a brittle material that becomes sticky when heated. It does not conduct heat or electricity and is noncorrosive. Wood rosin is distilled from the wood of pine trees, and gum rosin is obtained from the distillation of turpentine.

SOURCES OF EXPOSURE: Rosin is found in hot-melt glues and adhesive tapes and some cosmetics, particularly mascara. Rosin is also used as a flux in welding and for electrical soldering. Rosin is used on the bows of stringed instruments and on the stage surface to prevent slipping of performing artists.

Hobbyists who make stained glass, paint, solder, and weld are at risk for exposure to rosin flux fumes.

ROUTES OF EXPOSURE: Direct skin contact and inhalation.

SYMPTOMS OF EXPOSURE: Exposure to rosin may cause itching, burning, and a skin rash with pink to red patches or scaly plaques. Inhalation of rosin core solder fumes and dust can cause asthma.

Long-term, or chronic, exposure causes lesions that are dry and scaly, possibly with itching and crusty breaks in the skin, and asthma.

OSHA/NIOSH STANDARDS: The TLV adopted by the ACGIH for rosin core solder pyrolysis products is 0.1 mg/m^3.

Selenium

Selenium is a gray metal that exists naturally in the soil and in the body, where it plays a role in oxygen metabolism. Selenium may react with either acid and water or hydrogen gas to produce hydrogen selenide. Other selenium compounds include selenite salts, selenium dioxide, selenious acid, selenium oxide, selenium diethyldithiocarbamate, and selenium hexafluoride.

SOURCES OF EXPOSURE: Selenium is found naturally in the air, seawater, and minerals in the earth. As a pollutant, selenium is found in the air as selenium dioxide, a by-product of copper and nickel smelting and silver refining. Selenium may be found in low levels in wells and drinking water. It is used in some dietary supplements and as a nonapproved treatment for cystic fibrosis.

Selenium is widely used in the manufacture of electronic equipment, glass, ceramics, and pigment. It is used as an alloy with stainless steel, copper, and other steels; to vulcanize rubber; and in pesticide and fungicide preparations.

Hobbyists involved with stained glass making (selenium dioxide is used as a patina), glassblowing (selenium and selenium dioxide are used as colorants), jewelry making, ceramics, paints and pigments, dyes, and photography (selenium is used as a toner) may be exposed to selenium. Gun owners may be exposed to a very toxic form of selenium (selenious acid) when using gun blue to clean guns.

ROUTES OF EXPOSURE: Ingestion, inhalation of dust and vapor, and skin absorption of liquid.

SYMPTOMS OF EXPOSURE: Exposure to toxic doses of selenium and its compounds may cause irritation of the eyes, nose, throat, and skin; difficulty breathing; stomachache; diarrhea; and garlic odor of the breath.

Inhalation of selenium oxide fumes causes metal fume fever, a flulike illness whose symptoms are a metallic taste in the mouth; eye, nose, and throat irritation; cough; difficulty breathing; fatigue; fever; chills; sweating; nausea; vomiting; muscle aches; and weakness. Those exposed often recover in one to two days. At some point during continuous exposure to selenium oxide fumes, tolerance develops (the fumes no longer cause symptoms). However, over the weekend or after a period without exposure, the tolerance is lost, and "Monday morning fever" may occur.

Inhalation of hydrogen selenide causes irritation of the eyes, nose, mouth, and throat; coughing; sneezing; chest tightness; and difficulty breathing. Exposed workers have also reported a decreased or complete loss of their sense of smell.

Long-term, or chronic, exposure to selenium dioxide dust may cause "rose eyes," a puffy reddening of the eyelid, and perhaps also an inflammation of the eyes.

Chronic selenium exposure may cause white horizontal streaking on the nails, paronychia (inflammation of the skin around the nail), hair loss, irritability, fatigue, nausea, vomiting, garlic odor of the breath, and a metallic taste in the mouth. Other reported effects include muscle tenderness, tremor, light-headedness, and flushing.

PREGNANCY ALERT: Selenium can pass through the placenta and can be found in newborns.

OSHA/NIOSH STANDARDS: The federal standard (PEL) for selenium compounds (as Se) is 0.2 mg/m^3; selenium hexafluoride, 0.05 ppm (0.4 mg/m^3); and hydrogen selenide, 0.05 ppm (0.2 mg/m^3).

Silicon

Silicon exists either in its free form, known as *silica*, or combined with other minerals, or *silicate*. Free silica causes extensive pulmonary fibrosis, a permanent scarring of the lung tissue. Some silicates, such as asbestos, also cause lung damage. Although sand is almost pure silica, the grains are too big to inhale. It is the smaller dust particles that cause lung disease (see Chapter 6, "Respiratory Ailments").

Sources of Exposure: Stone such as quartz, granite, flint, chert, opal, chalcedony, and diatomite are major sources of exposure. Although sand poses no risk, sandblasting poses a large risk because the process converts the silica to particles small enough to be inhaled deep within the lung.

Hobbyists involved with plastics sculpture (many fillers contain free silica), metalworking (fine silica from sandblasting the surfaces), glass-blowing (silica in raw materials), stone sculpture (silica from stones), mold making (silica used as a separator), and ceramics (silica and silicates from clays and free silica in glazes) may be at risk for exposure to silicon. Potter's rot, grinder's consumption, and stone-mason's disease are other names for silicosis from inhalation of dust containing free silica.

Route of Exposure: Inhalation.

Symptoms of Exposure: After a relatively short period of exposure, such as nine months, a rapidly progressive, downhill course can ensue. Usually, however, symptoms result from long exposure.

Long-term, or chronic, exposure to silica may cause progressive, massive fibrosis or silicosis. The main symptom of this disease is shortness of breath and a progressive dry cough and wheezing. The disease is often complicated with infection, such as coexisting tuberculosis and sometimes complicated by autoimmune diseases. Unlike asbestos, silica has not been linked to cancer.

OSHA/NIOSH Standards: The federal standards (PELs) for crystalline silica in the form of breathable dust are: for cristobalite and tridymite a TWA of 0.5 mg/m^3; for quartz and tripoli, 0.1 mg/m^3. NIOSH considers these substances occupational carcinogens and recommends a TWA of 0.05 mg/m^3.

Silver

Silver is a shiny, white metal. Silver and its related compounds (silver salts) are used in medicine (e.g., silver nitrate, silver proteinates, and silver picrate), industry, and jewelry making.

Sources of Exposure: Silver is used industrially in metal and alloy working; in jewelry making; in electronics; in photographic film preparation; in the manufacture of mirrors, inks, and dyes; and as a chemical reagent in manufacturing. Silver compounds are used medicinally as antiseptics and local styptics. Newborns are treated with silver nitrate eyedrops to protect against gonococcal infection.

Hobbyists who make silver jewelry (silver is used in casting jewelry pieces) and ceramics (in applying metallic coatings) or work in a darkroom (silver nitrate is used as a hypo test) may be at risk for toxic exposure. Also at risk for silver exposure are stained glass makers, glassblowers (silver, silver chloride, and nitrate), and metalworkers (silver fumes).

Routes of Exposure: Inhalation and ingestion. Occupational exposures are mostly by inhalation of dusts, metal fumes, and mists.

Symptoms of Exposure: Inhalation of silver oxide fumes causes metal fume fever, a flulike illness whose symptoms include a metallic taste in the mouth; eye, nose, and throat irritation; cough; difficulty breathing; fatigue; fever; chills; sweating; nausea; vomiting; muscle aches; and weakness. Those exposed often recover in one to two days if not reexposed. At some point during continuous exposure to silver oxide fumes, tolerance develops (the fumes no longer cause symptoms). However, over the weekend or after a period without exposure, the tolerance is lost, and "Monday morning fever" may occur.

Contact with silver can cause skin, mouth, nose, and eye irritation.

Ingesting a toxic dose of silver nitrate causes burning mouth pain; blackening of the skin, mucous membranes, and throat; salivation; vomiting of black material; diarrhea; no urine output; shock; convulsions; coma; and death.

Long-term, or chronic, exposure to silver through skin or mucous membrane absorption or ingestion causes argyria, a blue-black or gray permanent discoloration of the skin, nails, mouth, and eyes. Workers chronically exposed to silver have experienced decreased night vision.

OSHA/NIOSH STANDARDS: The OSHA standard (PEL) for silver and its compounds is 0.01 mg/m^3.

Styrene

Styrene is a colorless to yellow, opaque, oily liquid with a sweet, floral odor. Styrene is a building block for polystyrene, a plastic that is one of the most widely used chemicals in industry.

SOURCES OF EXPOSURE: Exposure to styrene occurs primarily in the workplace.

Hobbyists who silk-screen, paint, refinish furniture, dye, and sculpt with plastic may be exposed to styrene in their materials.

Polystyrene is used to make many everyday items, such as combs, brushes, eyeglasses, toys, soap dishes, watering cans, dinnerware, picnic coolers, small appliances, food containers, loose-fill packaging, and audio and videocassettes.

ROUTES OF EXPOSURE: Inhalation, skin absorption, and accidental ingestion.

SYMPTOMS OF EXPOSURE: Exposure to styrene may cause eye, nose, and throat irritation; wheezing; shortness of breath; chest tightness; nausea; drowsiness; light-headedness; dizziness; difficulty in concentrating; impaired balance; incoordination; and memory loss.

Prolonged skin contact can cause chapped skin, rash, and an allergic reaction.

Long-term, or chronic, exposure to styrene causes "styrene sickness": headache, fatigue, nausea, loss of appetite, and depression. Hearing loss and nerve damage in the limbs are also associated with styrene exposure.

PREGNANCY AND REPRODUCTIVE ALERTS: A study has reported birth defects in children of styrene-exposed mothers, and another study of Finnish styrene workers showed an increased number of miscarriages. No conclusive evidence of reproductive outcome of styrene workers exists.

Styrene's ability to damage chromosomes may affect fertility.

OSHA/NIOSH STANDARDS: OSHA standard (PEL) is a TWA of 50 ppm (215 mg/m^3) with a STEL of 100 ppm (425 mg/m^3).

Thallium

Thallium is a soft, white metal found in the earth's crust and in trace amounts in the body. It is extremely toxic.

SOURCES OF EXPOSURE: Thallium-containing rodenticides were an important source of poisoning until 1965, when it was banned for use in the United States. Zinc and lead smelting releases thallium. It is used in various manufacturing processes. Thallium can be found in some homeopathic medicines. It is also used in nontoxic, miniscule doses in blood flow studies of the heart.

Hobbyists who dye, garden, and make jewelry may be at risk for exposure to thallium.

ROUTES OF EXPOSURE: Accidental ingestion, skin absorption, and inhalation.

SYMPTOMS OF EXPOSURE: Loss of hair and pain in the limbs are the major complaints. Initially, nausea, vomiting, diarrhea, stomach pain, and fever occur; a few hours or days later, lethargy, jumbled speech, tremors, muscle spasms, disorientation, loss of sensation or painful sensation in the palms of hands and soles of the feet, hair loss, difficulty walking, and problems with vision may appear. Two to four weeks after exposure, hair loss and Mees' lines (horizontal white bands across the nails) appear. Difficulty breathing may precede death in severe poisoning.

Long-term, or chronic, exposure from ingestion or skin absorption of thallium may cause hair loss, skin problems, brittleness and splitting of the nails, Mees' lines, excess saliva, and a blue gumline.

PREGNANCY AND REPRODUCTIVE ALERTS: A fetus can be affected by thallium crossing the placenta from the mother.

Thallium appears to have some association with difficulty in conceiving due to the lack of sperm in exposed males and menstrual irregularities in exposed females.

OSHA/NIOSH STANDARDS: The federal standard (PEL) for soluble thallium compounds is 0.1 mg/m^3.

Tin

Tin is a soft, silver-white metal. Tin forms many organic and inorganic compounds with differing levels of toxicity. Like lead, it is a heavy metal.

Tin is used widely in industry because it is easily melted and alloys with other metals. Presently, its largest applications are as solders. The more toxic organotins are used as heat stabilizers, catalytic agents, and biocidal compounds to control the growth of many fungi and bacteria.

SOURCES OF EXPOSURE: Tin is used to coat food and beverage cans and in silverware and household utensils. Pewter is composed of 91 percent tin. Stannous fluoride, a tin compound, is used in toothpaste. Tin is used in many industries to produce fungicides, insecticides, paints, ceramics, glass, and inks.

Organotin is used as an additive to polyvinyl chloride (PVC) plastic. PVC products include pipes, bottles, insulation, and dental and medical devices. Organotin has been shown to leach into liquid foods from PVC containers and into bodily fluids from PVC tubing and medical devices. Disposable plastic products may add organotin to the environment or food chain from landfills, composting, and incineration (solid waste management).

Hobbyists who make ceramics (tin oxide is used as a glaze ingredient), dye (organotin), garden (organotin), make glass (stannous chloride is used for iridescence and tin oxide, for polishing), enamel, print (organotin), paint (organotin), or solder may also be at risk for exposure to tin and its compounds.

ROUTES OF EXPOSURE: Inhalation (tin dust), and inhalation, ingestion, and skin absorption of organotins.

SYMPTOMS OF EXPOSURE: Certain tin compounds may irritate the skin and eyes.

Inhalation of tin oxide fumes causes metal fume fever, a flulike illness whose symptoms include a metallic taste in the mouth; eye, nose, and throat irritation; cough; difficulty breathing; fatigue; fever; chills; sweating; nausea; vomiting; muscle aches; and weakness. Those exposed often recover in one to two days if not reexposed. At some point during continuous exposure to tin oxide fumes, tolerance develops (the fumes no longer cause symptoms). However, over the weekend or after a period without exposure, the tolerance is lost, and "Monday morning fever" may occur.

Long-term, or chronic, exposure to dust or fumes of inorganic tin may cause stannosis, a depositing of tin in the lungs, usually without symptoms.

Organotin exposure may cause headache, nausea, dizziness, tinnitus (ringing in the ears), deafness, memory loss, abnormal sensitiveness to light, blurred vision, vomiting, disorientation, psychosis, retention of urine, weakness and paralysis of the limbs, coma, and death.

OSHA/NIOSH STANDARDS: The OSHA standard (PEL) for inorganic tin compounds (excluding the oxides) is 2.0 mg/m^3; and organotin compounds 0.1 mg/m^3.

Toluene

Toluene is a clear, colorless, flammable liquid with a sweet pungent smell. It is a widely used organic solvent.

SOURCES OF EXPOSURE: Toluene is a solvent for paint, lacquers, thinners, coatings, and glue. It is used in industry in many chemical processes and as a motor and aviation fuel.

Hobbyists at risk include painters, paint strippers, printers, silk-screeners, and woodworkers.

ROUTES OF EXPOSURE: Inhalation, skin absorption, and accidental ingestion.

SYMPTOMS OF EXPOSURE: Mild exposure from inhalation or ingestion causes dizziness, weakness, euphoria, headache, nausea, vomiting, tightness in the chest, and staggering. More intense exposure causes blurred vision, tremors, shallow and rapid breathing, violent excitement, delirium, unconsciousness, and convulsions. Exposure may be fatal.

Skin contact with toluene causes irritation, scaling, and cracking.

Long-term, or chronic, exposure from inhalation of toluene begins with headache, loss of appetite, drowsiness, nervousness, and pale skin. Petechiae (a rash due to hemorrhaging under the skin) and abnormal bleeding may also occur. Brain damage after repeated intoxications displays these symptoms: incoordination, tremors, hearing loss, emotional instability, and dementia.

Sudden death due to heartbeat irregularities has occurred in glue sniffers.

CHILD ALERT: Toluene has become a substance of abuse because of its euphoria-producing effect. It is the usual ingredient in rubber or plastic cement abused for glue sniffing. Children using these glues in projects may be inadvertently exposed to toluene. Use arts and crafts materials labeled specifically for use by children.

PREGNANCY ALERT: A recent study found that mothers who sniffed large amounts of toluene while pregnant gave birth to infants with head and limb defects.

REPRODUCTIVE ALERT: Toluene has been linked to adverse effects of both the male and female reproductive capacity.

OSHA/NIOSH STANDARDS: Federal standard (PEL) is a TWA of 100 ppm (375 mg/m^3) with a STEL of 150 ppm (560 mg/m^3).

Trichloroethylene

Trichloroethylene (TCE) is a clear, colorless, easily evaporating liquid with a sweet odor that is chemically classified as a halogenated hydrocarbon compound. It is used widely in industry and is a suspected carcinogen.

SOURCES OF EXPOSURE: TCE is used as a solvent in many industrial applications; as a degreaser for metal parts; in some typewriter correction fluids; and as a cleaner for walls, clothing, and rugs in the household.

TCE is used as an anesthetic by veterinarians. Substance abusers inhale TCE because of its ability to cause intoxication and euphoria.

Hobbyists who work in a darkroom or refinish furniture may also be exposed to TCE.

ROUTES OF EXPOSURE: Inhalation, skin absorption (but typically not in sufficient amounts to cause toxicity), and ingestion.

SYMPTOMS OF EXPOSURE: Depending on the concentration, symptoms of TCE exposure range from dizziness, drowsiness, weakness, headache, blurred vision, nausea, vomiting, stomach cramps, tremor, confusion, depression, insomnia, and loss of coordination to excitement, progressing to loss of consciousness. Victims may have an irregular pulse and difficulty breathing. A toxic dose may result in coma, liver and kidney failure, and death.

Long-term, or chronic, exposure to TCE from inhalation or skin absorption may lead to weight loss, nausea, loss of appetite, fatigue, visual impairment, facial numbness, pain in the joints, skin inflammation, and wheezing.

TCE may aggravate hearing loss from exposure to loud noise.

CANCER ALERT: TCE is a suspected carcinogen. Liver tumors have been reported in mice exposed to TCE. NIOSH considers TCE to be an occupational carcinogen.

Child Alert: Several cases of sudden death have been reported in adolescents sniffing typewriter correction fluid.

OSHA/NIOSH Standards: The current OSHA standard (PEL) is a TWA of 50 ppm (270 mg/m^3) with a STEL of 200 ppm (1080 mg/m^3). NIOSH considers TCE an occupational carcinogen and recommends a TWA of 25 ppm.

Trinitrotoluene and Dinitrotoluene

Trinitrotoluene (TNT) and dinitrotoluene (DNT) are chemically classified as aromatic nitro compounds with a ring of carbon and hydrogen atoms attached to nitrogen and oxygen atoms. TNT is a crystalline solid that exists in five different forms (isomers) based upon its shape. TNT is a relatively stable explosive; DNT is also used in explosives.

Sources of Exposure: TNT is an explosive used in shells, bombs, and mines. DNT is used to produce dyes and explosives and in organic synthesis.

Routes of Exposure: For TNT: Inhalation of dust, fumes, or vapor and skin absorption from dust or ingestion. For DNT: Ingestion, inhalation, and skin absorption.

Symptoms of Exposure: Exposure to TNT causes irritation of the eyes, nose, and throat; sneezing; coughing; inflammation of the skin; and yellow to orange discoloration of the skin, hair, and nails.

Symptoms of exposure to a toxic dose of TNT include cyanosis (blue skin discoloration), paleness, nausea, loss of appetite, decreased or no urine output, and an enlarged liver. In the latest stages of TNT poisoning, nails may show purpura (a change in color caused by hemorrhaging under their surface, in which the nails turn red, then purple, then brownish yellow and then discoloration disappears), and convulsions, coma, and death may occur.

Exposure to a toxic dose of DNT causes headache, irritability, dizziness, weakness, nausea, vomiting, difficulty breathing, drowsiness, unconsciousness, and possibly death.

Long-term, or chronic, exposure to TNT causes the same symptoms as above for TNT exposure. Long-term, or chronic, exposure to DNT may cause anemia whose symptoms include fatigue, pallor, shortness of breath, rapid heart rate, headache, dizziness, fainting, ringing in the ears, irritability, difficulty sleeping or concentrating, sensitivity to cold, loss of appetite, indigestion, nausea, bowel movement irregularity, abnormal menstruation, and loss of libido or impotence. A yellow discoloration of the nails may occur.

Cancer Alert: NIOSH has recommended that DNT be considered a potential workplace carcinogen.

Reproductive Alert: Long-term or chronic exposure to DNT is linked to abnormal menstruation and loss of libido or impotence.

OSHA/NIOSH Standards: The OSHA standard (PEL) for DNT is a TWA of 1.5 mg/m^3; and TNT, 0.5 mg/m^3. NIOSH considers DNT an occupational carcinogen and recommends that exposure to DNT be reduced to the lowest feasible level.

Turpentine

Turpentine is derived from the resin of pine trees. Gum turpentine is a yellow sticky substance, and oil of turpentine is a colorless liquid that evaporates easily at room temperature.

Sources of Exposure: Turpentine is used widely in the chemical industry to produce floor, furniture, shoe, and car polishes; paint thinners; resins; and other products.

Hobbyists who paint (using turpentine to thin paint and varnish), make lithographs, and blow glass may be at risk for exposure.

ROUTES OF EXPOSURE: Inhalation, skin absorption, and ingestion.

SYMPTOMS OF EXPOSURE: Ingestion of turpentine may cause stomach burning, nausea, vomiting, diarrhea, difficult or painful urination, blood in the urine, unconsciousness, difficulty breathing, convulsions, and death.

Vapors are irritating to the eyes, nose, and respiratory system. Inhaling turpentine causes headache, dizziness, anxiety, excitement, mental confusion, tinnitus (ringing in the ears), difficulty breathing, rapid heart rate, unconsciousness, and convulsions.

Skin contact with turpentine is irritating and may cause eczema (an itching or burning inflammation of the skin).

Long-term, or chronic, exposure has caused eczema and subungual hyperkeratosis (a buildup of dead skin under the nails). Repeated exposure to high vapor concentrations causes a predisposition to pneumonia as well as kidney and bladder damage with blood in the urine.

OSHA/NIOSH STANDARDS: The federal standard (PEL) is 100 ppm (560 mg/m^3).

Ultraviolet Radiation

Ultraviolet (UV) radiation is a type of invisible energy emitted in waves of a specific length. It is produced both naturally (from the sun) and artificially (from arcs operated at high temperatures). See Chapter 16, "Radiant Energy," for more information.

SOURCES OF EXPOSURE: The sun is the most common source of UV radiation. Suntanning beds also emit UV energy.

In industry, UV overexposure may occur while working with arc welding and plasma torches and from germicidal and blacklight lamps, carbon arcs, electric arc furnaces, mercury-vapor lamps, hot-metal operations, and laboratory equipment.

ROUTE OF EXPOSURE: Absorption by skin and the lens of the eye.

SYMPTOMS OF EXPOSURE: Because UV radiation does not penetrate deeply into the body, the eye and skin are the main organs affected.

Excess UV exposure causes irritation of the eye (a gritty feeling), sensitiveness to light, tearing, spasmodic winking, pain in the eye, visual impairment, and red, swollen eyelids. These symptoms disappear within forty-eight hours. Intense UV exposure may also cause cataracts (cloudy lens) and may possibly damage the center of the retina (the back of the eye), which impairs vision.

UV radiation to the skin can cause redness (sunburn), swelling, fever, and blistering. Some substances, such as certain foods, drugs, and coal tar, are activated by or work in combination with UV radiation to cause skin reactions. See Chapter 4, "Skin Ailments," and Chapter 16, "Radiant Energy," for more information.

Long-term, or chronic, exposure to UV radiation can cause cataracts, which may lead to decreased vision. Effects on the skin include pigmentation, thickening, accelerated aging, and greater likelihood of developing skin cancer.

CHILD ALERT: Because the effects of UV radiation accumulate throughout life, it is important to protect children from overexposure to the sun, even in infancy. Sunscreen with a skin protection factor (SPF) of at least 15 should be used, even on young infants, when spending time outdoors. Many manufacturers make special lotions that are particularly gentle on sensitive baby skin.

CANCER ALERT: The incidence of skin cancers increases with increased exposure to the sun. Industrial exposure to UV sources and its relation to skin cancer has not yet been fully studied.

OSHA/NIOSH Standards: The OSHA standard (PEL) is 10 mW/cm^2 averaged over any 0.1-hour period. NIOSH has set an exposure limit of 1.0 mW/cm^2 for periods of more than 1,000 seconds and 1,000 mW/cm^2 (1.0 J/cm^2) for periods of less than or equal to 1,000 seconds.

Vanadium

Vanadium is a naturally occurring metal and exists in the pure form as a light gray or white powder or a hard lump. Vanadium is found in small amounts in the earth's crust, fuel oils, the body, and foods, including shellfish. Vanadium and its compounds are used widely in industry.

Sources of Exposure: Vanadium is an alloying agent in the steel industry and used to produce lightweight titanium alloys. It is used as a catalyst in the chemical industry and in the manufacture of synthetic rubber, dyes, glass, ink, and pesticides. It is found in the ash from fossil-fuel boilers.

Inhalation of vanadium pentoxide at work is the most common source of exposure.

Hobbyists who make ceramics, particularly wall tiles, may be exposed if they use certain vanadium-containing glazes, such as the zircon vanadium blues. Painters, printers, textile dyers, photographers, and gardeners may also be at risk for exposure to vanadium.

Route of Exposure: Inhalation.

Symptoms of Exposure: Exposure to vanadium dusts and fumes may irritate the eyes and respiratory tract, causing redness and inflammation of the eyes, skin irritation, runny nose, nose bleeds, sneezing, coughing, a metallic taste in the mouth, sore chest, wheezing, shortness of breath, and weakness.

Inhalation of vanadium oxide fumes causes symptoms of metal fume fever, a flulike illness whose symptoms can include fever; chills; sweating; headache; nausea; vomiting; difficulty breathing; chest pain; eye, nose, and throat irritation; cough; a metallic taste in the mouth; headache; and weakness. Those exposed often recover in one to two days if not reexposed. At some point during continuous exposure to the fumes, tolerance develops (the fumes no longer cause symptoms). However, over the weekend or after a period without exposure, the tolerance is lost, and "Monday morning fever" may occur.

Long-term, or chronic, exposure to vanadium and its compounds may cause chronic bronchitis, pneumonia, and eye irritation. Some workers with heavy exposure have developed a green-black discoloration of the tongue and a metallic taste in the mouth. Changes in the sense of smell have also been reported.

OSHA/NIOSH Standards: The federal standard (PEL) for vanadium pentoxide dust is a ceiling of 0.5 mg/m^3; fumes, a ceiling of 0.05 mg/m^3; and ferrovanadium, a TWA of 1 mg/m^3 with a STEL of 1 mg/m^3 and a STEL of 3 mg/m^3.

Vinyl Chloride

Vinyl chloride (chlorethylene, chlorethene, and monochloroethylene) is a human-made colorless gas at room temperature. However, it is usually stored under pressure and used as a liquid. Its mild, sweet odor is detectable at concentrations too high to serve as an adequate warning of danger. It is used primarily to produce polyvinyl chloride (PVC), a plastic used extensively to make pipes, coatings, and many consumer products.

Sources of Exposure: Vinyl chloride is used mostly to make PVC, a resin used widely in building and construction; furniture; records; toys; packaging; clothing; and car mats, upholstery, and tops. It is also used as a solvent and in chemical reactions.

Consumers may be exposed to small amounts of vinyl chloride as it is released from PVC plastic in new car interiors, the packaging of foods and drinks, and pipes carrying drinking water.

Routes of Exposure: Inhalation and skin absorption.

Symptoms of Exposure: Vinyl chloride irritates the skin and eyes. It may cause lightheadedness, dizziness, nausea, loss of muscle coordination, convulsions, and imbalance. Severe exposure may cause death.

Long-term, or chronic, exposure causes the occupational disease acroosteolysis: disintegration of the bones of the fingers, thickening and atrophy of the skin of the hands and forearms, abnormal sensations in the hands (such as tingling and burning), fatigue, joint and muscle pain, and decreased gripping strength. Broadening and thickening of the ends of the fingers may occur. The nails may grow around these ends.

Vinyl chloride-induced liver disease may cause vague symptoms such as abdominal pain, weakness, fatigue, and weight loss.

Cancer Alert: Vinyl chloride is a carcinogen. Tumors of the liver are the primary finding, however, some studies have reported an increased incidence of cancers of the brain, breast, skin, lung, thyroid, lymph system, and blood components.

Pregnancy Alert: One study found an increased reporting of miscarriages by the wives of vinyl chloride-exposed workers. The conclusions of the study, however, were disputed. Other laboratory studies on microbes and mammal systems have shown vinyl chloride to be able to mutate cells but have not shown teratogenicity (the ability to produce major congenital abnormalities) in animals.

Reproductive Alert: The ability of vinyl chloride to damage DNA may cause difficulty in conceiving.

OSHA/NIOSH Standards: OSHA has set a PEL of vinyl chloride in workplace air as a TWA of 1 ppm with a STEL ceiling of 5 ppm. NIOSH recommends that there be zero exposure (lowest reliably detectable concentration) due to the potential for causing cancer in exposed workers.

Vitamin A

Vitamin A is a fat-soluble vitamin stored primarily in the liver. It plays a role in vision, especially night vision, growth, bone development, and reproduction. Unlike water-soluble vitamins, it is not excreted in the urine but accumulates in the body; doses over 25,000 IU per day can cause symptoms after one month. Vitamin A consists of the following components: vitamin A (formerly fat-soluble vitamin A), retinol, retinol 2, retinal, dehydroretinol, retinoic acid, and beta-carotene.

Sources of Exposure: Preformed vitamin A is found in animal meats, particularly liver, and other animal products. The components needed to build vitamin A (such as beta-carotene) are found in vegetables.

People at risk of toxic exposure include anyone taking large doses for treatment of skin conditions, such as acne, who continues taking it without doctor's supervision; food faddists taking large daily doses of fat-soluble vitamin preparations; and anyone eating foods with high vitamin A content, such as animal liver.

Route of Exposure: Ingestion.

Symptoms of Exposure: Accidental massive ingestion is generally seen in infants and young children. They become drowsy; irritable; show bulging at their fontanel, the soft spot on the top of an infant's head; followed by the skin sloughing off after one to three days.

Although adult overdose is rare (1 to 2 million IU of vitamin A must be ingested), it does occur in people who take large doses of vitamin A for treatment of skin conditions and who are not medically supervised. Adult symptoms are headache, nausea, and vomiting.

Long-term, or chronic, exposure may lead to headaches, blurred and/or double vision, loss of appetite, fatigue, fever, malaise, weakness, and weight loss. Hair loss, brittle nails, fissures at the corners of the mouth, dry peeling skin, rash, orange skin discoloration, and itching may also occur. Muscle pain; bone tenderness; and eye irritation, ulceration, and bulging have also been reported. Mental problems can also result.

CHILD ALERT: Megadose toxicity from vitamin A usually occurs in infants and children from a single ingestion of over 350,000 IU of a medicinal preparation.

PREGNANCY ALERT: Pregnant women should avoid large doses of vitamin A because it may adversely affect the process of organ development in the fetus.

Vitamin D

Vitamin D is a fat-soluble vitamin involved in the body's regulation of calcium.

SOURCES OF EXPOSURE: Vitamin D is found in vitamin supplements and vitamin D_3 is a component of certain rodenticides.

People at risk of toxic exposure include people taking vitamin D to prevent or treat osteoporosis and food faddists taking large daily doses of fat-soluble vitamin preparations.

ROUTE OF EXPOSURE: Ingestion.

SYMPTOMS OF EXPOSURE: Excessively high doses of vitamin D may cause muscle weakness, apathy, headache, loss of appetite, smell distortion, nausea, vomiting, diarrhea, and bone pain.

Long-term, or chronic, exposure to high doses of vitamin D may lead to increased urination, deposits of calcium in the cornea of the eye, and, less frequently, eye alignment deviation (exophtha), and cataracts.

CHILD ALERT: Children may be exposed to vitamin D-containing rodenticides placed on floors where they play.

PREGNANCY ALERT: Congenital heart defects and mental retardation may be caused by excessively high doses of vitamin D taken during pregnancy.

Xylene

Xylene is a highly flammable, clear, colorless liquid with a sweet, pungent smell. It is an organic solvent, in the same chemical class (aromatic hydrocarbons) as toluene and benzene.

SOURCES OF EXPOSURE: Xylene is a constituent of paint, lacquers, varnishes, adhesives and cements, dyes, inks, and cleaning fluids. It is used in the manufacture of many products including plastics, synthetic textiles, quartz-crystal oscillators, perfumes, insect repellents, and pharmaceuticals. Xylene is used as a component in aviation fuel and in various chemical processes.

Hobbyists who print, silk screen, and use solvent-based markers or colored inks may be at risk for exposure to xylene.

ROUTES OF EXPOSURE: Inhalation, skin absorption, and ingestion.

SYMPTOMS OF EXPOSURE: Mild exposure from inhalation or ingestion causes dizziness, weakness, euphoria, headache, nausea, vomiting, tightness in the chest, and staggering. More intense exposure can cause blurred vision, tremors, shallow and rapid breathing, violent excitement, delirium, unconsciousness, convulsions, coma, and sometimes death.

Skin contact causes irritation, scaling, and cracking.

Long-term, or chronic, exposure from inhalation begins with headache, loss of appetite, drowsiness, nervousness, and pale skin. Brain damage after repeated intoxications displays these symptoms: incoordination, tremors, hearing loss, and emotional instability.

REPRODUCTIVE ALERT: Xylene exposure is associated with adverse effects on both male and female reproductive capacity.

CHILD ALERT: Sudden death due to heartbeat irregularities has occurred in glue sniffers.

OSHA/NIOSH STANDARDS: The OSHA permissible exposure limit is a TWA of 100 ppm (435 mg/m^3) with a STEL of 150 ppm (655 mg/m^3).

Zinc

Zinc is a silver-white metal whose compounds, zinc chloride and zinc oxide, are used widely in industry. Zinc chloride is composed of white crystals that dissolve in water and organic solvents. Zinc oxide is an odorless, white or yellow powder that does not dissolve well in water.

SOURCES OF EXPOSURE: Zinc is found in the alloys brass, bronze, aluminum, and nickel. Heating these metals may release zinc oxide fumes, which may cause metal fume fever. Zinc is also applied to iron and steel to stop corrosion in a process known as galvanizing.

Zinc chloride is used to preserve wood; as a soldering flux; and in batteries, dyes, deodorants, solutions for embalming and disinfecting, textile finishing, rubber processing, oil and gas well operations, paper making, taxidermy, and military smoke screens.

Zinc oxide is used as a white pigment in rubber and in sunblock creams. It is used in photocopying, paints, lacquers and varnishes, chemicals, pharmaceuticals, and plastics.

Hobbyists at risk of exposure include those who make ceramics, jewelry, and stained glass (zinc chloride is used as an acid flux), who paint (zinc yellow and zinc white are pigments), who use lacquer, do metalwork (zinc oxide fumes from metal casting), or who blow glass (zinc compounds are used to color and decorate glass).

ROUTES OF EXPOSURE: Inhalation (of dust and fumes) and ingestion.

SYMPTOMS OF EXPOSURE: Inhalation of zinc oxide fumes causes metal fume fever, a flulike illness whose symptoms include a metallic taste in the mouth; eye, nose, and throat irritation; cough; difficulty breathing; fatigue; fever; chills; sweating; nausea; vomiting; muscle aches; and weakness. Those exposed often recover in one to two days. At some point during continuous exposure to zinc oxide fumes, tolerance develops (the fumes no longer cause symptoms). However, over the weekend or after a period without exposure, the tolerance is lost, and "Monday morning fever" may occur.

Zinc chloride is the most toxic form of zinc. No industrial inhalation symptoms have been reported. In military accidents, it irritates the nose, throat, and chest and causes difficulty breathing. Deaths have been reported from severe lung damage. Zinc chloride corrodes the skin on contact and also the digestive tract if swallowed causing vomiting, stomach pain, and vomiting of blood.

Zinc oxide may cause oxide pox, an area of itching, red, pustules.

Long-term, or chronic, exposure does not cause chronic poisoning.

OSHA/NIOSH STANDARDS: The OSHA standard (PEL) for zinc chloride fume is 1 mg/m^3 with a STEL of 2 mg/m^3, and zinc oxide fume, 5 mg/m^3 with a STEL of 10 mg/m^3.

THE TWENTY COMMON SYMPTOMS AND EXPOSURES IN THE WORKPLACE

The following chart relates twenty common symptoms of exposure to some broad occupational groups.

In the first column is an alphabetical listing of occupations, in the second column is one or more of the twenty common symptoms of exposure presented earlier, and in the third column are some of the environmental agents present within that occupation that can cause the symptoms.

This chart is neither an exhaustive nor encyclopedic account. Not included here are the many other agents often at the worksite that can also cause these twenty symptoms. Similarly, there are many other symptoms of serious ailments that commonly occur in a particular occupation but which are not listed here. Some significant, even classic symptoms of common occupationally related diseases, such as cancer, do not appear in this list.

Using this chart can help readers to understand the scope of the problem of workplace exposures, now ranked by the EPA as number one among the top environmental hazards. There are many substances hidden at a worksite—not just the obviously dangerous ones—that can affect health. This chart can demonstrate how very common symptoms sometimes occur as the result, not of common ailments, but of exposure to environmental hazards in the workplace.

Readers can turn to the information sheets and chapters in this book for a more specific understanding of these substances (please note that substances that are listed in *italics* are *not found* in the information sheet listing: all others are described in pp. 359–421).

If You Work in These Occupations	And Are Experiencing	You May Be at Risk from These Agents
Adhesive manufacturer/worker	Conception Difficulty	Benzene, carbon disulfide, formaldehyde, n-hexane, styrene, toluene, xylene
	Cough	Diisocyanates
	Dizziness	Benzene, carbon disulfide, carbon tetrachloride and other halogenated hydrocarbon solvents, cyanide, ethanol, hydrogen sulfide, ketones,

(continued)

If You Work in These Occupations	And Are Experiencing	You May Be at Risk from These Agents
		methanol, petroleum distillates, styrene, trichloroethylene, xylene
	Fever/Chills	Petroleum distillates
	Headache	Benzene; carbon disulfide; carbon tetrachloride, trichloroethylene, and other halogenated hydrocarbon solvents; cyanide; ethanol; ethylene glycol; hydrogen sulfide; methanol; petroleum distillates; styrene; toluene; xylene
	Hearing Changes	Carbon disulfide or trichloroethylene in combination with noise; styrene; toluene; xylene
	Irritation or Dryness of Eyes, Nose, Sinuses, Mouth, or Throat	Toluene diisocyanate
	Memory Loss, Concentration Changes, and Confusion	Cyanide, halogenated hydrocarbon solvents including carbon tetrachloride and trichloroethylene, methanol, n-hexane petroleum distillates, styrene, toluene, xylene
	Nail Abnormalities	Acrylics, methanol
	Numbness and Weakness in the Arms and Legs	Carbon disulfide, carbon tetrachloride and other halogenated hydrocarbon solvents, ethanol, hydrogen sulfide, methyl *n*-butyl ketone, petroleum distillates, styrene
	Rash	Acrylics, epoxy resins, halogenated hydrocarbon solvents, petroleum distillates, phenolic resins, rosin
	Smell Disturbances	Benzene or other petroleum distillates, carbon disulfide, cyanide, halogenated hydrocarbon solvents, hydrogen sulfide
	Tremor	Carbon disulfide; carbon tetrachloride, trichloroethylene, and other halogenated hydrocarbon solvents; ethanol; toluene; xylene

(continued)

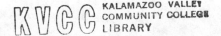

If You Work in These Occupations	And Are Experiencing	You May Be at Risk from These Agents
Adhesive manufacturer/worker (*continued*)	Vision Changes	Benzene, carbon disulfide, carbon tetrachloride, cyanide, halogenated hydrocarbon solvents, hydrazine, hydrogen sulfide, methanol, toluene, trichloroethylene, xylene
	Weakness, Depression	Benzene; carbon disulfide; carbon tetrachloride, trichloroethylene, and other halogenated hydrocarbon solvents; cyanide; ethanol; hydrogen sulfide; petroleum distillates; styrene; toluene; xylene
Aerosol packager	Headache; Tremor	Carbon dioxide
Agricultural worker	Conception Difficulty	Arsenic, carbon disulfide, chlorinated hydrocarbon insecticides, dibromochloropropane, ethylene dibromide, ethylene oxide, mercury, nicotine, paraquat and diquat, polycyclic aromatic hydrocarbons, xylene
	Cough	*Bacteria* and *fungi* in moldy compost, *grain dust*, *hops*, irritant gases, paraquat, phenol, *pink-rot fungus* (celery pickers), *soybean flour* and *dust*
	Diarrhea	Arsenic, benzene hexachloride, copper, paraquat, pesticides, phenol, infections (bacterial and parasitic)
	Dizziness	Arsenic; carbon disulfide; carbon monoxide; chlorinated hydrocarbon insecticides; cyanide; hydrazines; hydrogen sulfide; irritant gases; organic mercury; methyl bromide, chloride, and iodide; nicotine, nitrites and nitrates; pesticides; petroleum distillates; pyrethrums, pyrethrins, and pyrethroids; organic tin; xylene

(continued)

If You Work in These Occupations	And Are Experiencing	You May Be at Risk from These Agents
	Fever/Chills	Certain dinitro derivatives of phenol and cresol, grain dust, paraquat and diquat, petroleum distillates
	Hair Loss	Arsenic
	Headache	Carbon dioxide; carbon disulfide; carbon monoxide; chlorinated hydrocarbon insecticides; copper; cyanide; dinitro derivatives of phenol and cresol; grain dust; hydrogen sulfide; irritant gases; mercury; methyl bromide, chloride, and iodide; nicotine; nitrites and nitrates; noise; paraquat and diquat; pesticides; petroleum distillates; organic tin; xylene
	Hearing Changes	Arsenic; carbon disulfide in combination with noise; carbon monoxide; mercury; nicotine; noise; organic tin; *vibration;* xylene
	Irritation or Dryness of Eyes, Nose, Sinuses, Mouth, or Throat	Arsenic; copper; grain dust; hydrogen sulfide; irritant gases; methyl bromide, chloride, and iodide; paraquat; phenol; tin; ultraviolet radiation
	Memory Loss, Concentration Changes, and Confusion	Arsenic; carbon monoxide; chlorinated hydrocarbon insecticides; cyanide; mercury; methyl bromide, chloride, and iodide; nicotine; pesticides; petroleum distillates; organic tin; xylene
	Nail Abnormalities	Arsenic; dinobuton; dinitro-o-cresol; paraquat and diquat; handling walnuts, pecans, and coffee can stain the nails
	Nausea	Arsenic, hydrazines, paraquat, pesticides, phenol, xylene

(continued)

If You Work in These Occupations	And Are Experiencing	You May Be at Risk from These Agents
Agricultural worker (*continued*)	Numbness and Weakness in the Arms and Legs	Arsenic; carbon disulfide; carbon monoxide; chlorinated hydrocarbon insecticides; hydrogen sulfide; organic mercury; methyl bromide, chloride, and iodide; pesticides; petroleum distillates; phosphorus; organic tin
	Rash	Agricultural chemicals, including pesticides (among the pesticides, the most common contact allergens are carbamates); ammoniated mercury; *animal hair; captans;* chemicals in rubber; fertilizers; *germicidal agents; lanolin;* organomercurials; *parabens;* petroleum distillates; *plants and seeds;* poison ivy/oak/sumac; potassium dichromate; *saliva and secretions; thiurams;* triazines and pyrethrums, including the chemicals used in them; methanol
	Smell Disturbances	Cresol, cyanide, hydrazines, hydrogen sulfide, methyl bromide, petroleum distillates
	Tremor	Arsenic; carbon dioxide; carbon disulfide; carbon monoxide; chlorinated hydrocarbon insecticides; mercury; methyl bromide, chloride, and iodide; nicotine; pesticides; phosphorus; xylene
	Urine Color Changes	Carbon monoxide, copper, dinitro derivatives of phenol and cresol, hydrazines, phenol and phenolic compounds
	Pain on Urination	Mercury; methyl bromide, chloride, and iodide; paraquat and diquat; tin
	Vision Changes	Arsenic; carbon disulfide; carbon monoxide; cyanide; dinitro

(continued)

If You Work in These Occupations	And Are Experiencing	You May Be at Risk from These Agents
		derivatives of phenol and cresol; hydrogen sulfide; methylmercury; methyl bromide, chloride, and iodide; pesticides; ultraviolet radiation; xylene
	Weakness, Depression	Carbon disulfide; carbon monoxide; chlorinated hydrocarbon insecticides; cyanide; dinitro derivatives of phenol and cresol; hydrogen sulfide; mercury; methyl bromide, chloride, and iodide; nitrites; pesticides; petroleum distillates; tin; xylene
Aircraft personnel (crewman, mechanic)	Dizziness	Cyanide, microwaves
	Fever/Chills	Metal oxides such as aluminum, cobalt, magnesium, tin
	Headache	Noise
	Memory Loss, Concentration Changes, and Confusion	Cyanide
	Nausea	Dimethylformamide
	Rash	Chromates, cobalt, epoxy resins
	Smell Disturbances	Cyanides, chromium, halogenated hydrocarbon solvents, vanadium
	Tremor	Vanadium
	Vision Changes	Cyanide, ionizing radiation, laser light, ultraviolet radiation
	Weakness, Depression	Fumes of aluminum, cyanide, magnesium, tin
Alloy maker	Conception Difficulty	Arsenic, cadmium, lead, manganese
	Cough	Cobalt dust, vanadium
	Diarrhea	Aluminum, antimony, arsenic, boron, cadmium, iron, lead, magnesium, nickel, thallium

(continued)

If You Work in These Occupations	And Are Experiencing	You May Be at Risk from These Agents
Alloy maker (*continued*)	Dizziness	Arsenic, lead
	Fever/Chills	Metal oxides such as aluminum, antimony, arsenic, cadmium, cobalt, copper, iron, lead, magnesium, manganese, nickel selenium, silver, thallium, tin, zinc
	Hair Loss	Arsenic, thallium
	Headache	Antimony, boron, cadmium, chromium, copper, lead, manganese, nickel
	Hearing Changes	Arsenic, lead, mercury
	Memory Loss, Concentration Changes, and Confusion	Arsenic, lead, thallium
	Nail Abnormalities	Arsenic, thallium
	Numbness and Weakness in the Arms and Legs	Arsenic, lead, manganese, thallium
	Smell Disturbances	Benzene or other petroleum distillates, cadmium, chromium, hydrogen cyanide or its salts, irritant gases, mercury, nickel, nuisance dusts, vanadium
	Tremor	Arsenic, lead, manganese, thallium, vanadium
	Urine Color Changes	Copper
	Pain on Urination	Boron, cadmium, chromium, lead, tin
	Vision Changes	Arsenic, lead, silver, thallium
	Weakness, Depression	Aluminum, antimony, arsenic, boron, cadmium, cobalt, copper, iron, lead, magnesium, manganese, nickel, selenium, thallium, tin, zinc
Animal handler	Cough; rash	*Hair, mites, skin scales, small insects, urine protein*
Antioxidant manufacturer	Headache; Weakness, Depression	Cresol

(continued)

If You Work in These Occupations	And Are Experiencing	You May Be at Risk from These Agents
Antiseptic manufacturer	Conception Difficulty; Headache; Weakness, Depression	Boric acid, ethanol
	Dizziness; Numbness and Weakness in the Arms and Legs; Tremor	Ethanol
	Hair loss	Boric acid
Artist (See Chapter 20, "Art and Hobbyist Materials")		
Assembly line worker	Dizziness	Halogenated hydrocarbon solvents, including trichloroethylene
	Headache	Trichloroethylene and other halogenated hydrocarbon solvents, noise
	Hearing Changes	Trichloroethylene in combination with noise
	Numbness and Weakness in the Arms and Legs	Halogenated hydrocarbon solvents, vibration
	Smell Disturbances	Halogenated hydrocarbon solvents, petroleum distillates
	Tremor	Trichloroethylene and other halogenated hydrocarbon solvents
	Vision Changes; Weakness, Depression	Halogenated hydrocarbon solvents, trichloroethylene
Athlete	Rash	*Adhesive tapes;* carbamates, *mercaptobenzothiazole, isopropyl*-p-*phenylenediamine,* and *thiurams* in rubber; ethylenediamine dihydrochloride in medications (rarely); formaldehyde in medications and shampoos; *fragrances, parabens,* and *wood alcohols* in creams and lotions; nickel sulfate; rosin; *soaps and detergents*
Automobile mechanic/worker (includes service station attendant)	Conception Difficulty	Cadmium, ethylene glycol ethers, lead, polycylclic aromatic hydrocarbons

(continued)

If You Work in These Occupations	And Are Experiencing	You May Be at Risk from These Agents
Automobile mechanic/worker (includes service station attendant) (continued)	Diarrhea	Cadmium, lead
	Dizziness	Carbon monoxide, ketones, lead, petroleum distillates
	Fever/Chills	Metal oxides such as aluminum, cadmium, cobalt, lead, petroleum distillates, tin
	Headache	Cadmium, carbon monoxide, chromium, lead, noise, petroleum distillates
	Hearing Changes	Carbon Monoxide, lead, noise, trichloroethylene, vibration
	Irritation or Dryness of Eyes, Nose, Sinuses, Mouth, or Throat	Chromium, epoxy resins, lead, tin
	Memory Loss, Concentration Changes, and Confusion	Carbon monoxide, lead, petroleum distillates, solvent mixtures
	Nail Abnormalities	Acrylics; contact with sulfuric acid from batteries can cause paronychia
	Nausea	Carbon monoxide, chromium, lead
	Numbness and Weakness in the Arms and Legs	Carbon monoxide, lead, petroleum distillates
	Rash	Acrylics; antifreezes; carbamates, mercaptobenzothiazole, isopropyl-p-phenylenediamine, and thiurams in rubber; cobalt; epoxy resin; formaldehyde, lanolin and parabens in creams; greases; lubricants; nickel sulfate; petroleum distillates; phenolic resins; potassium dichromate; soaps and detergents; solvents; wood alcohols in creams and soaps
	Smell Disturbances	Cadmium, chromium, halogenated hydrocarbon solvents, petroleum distillates
	Tremor	Carbon monoxide, lead

(continued)

If You Work in These Occupations	And Are Experiencing	You May Be at Risk from These Agents
	Urine Color Changes	Carbon monoxide
	Pain on Urination	Chromium
	Vision Changes	Carbon monoxide; carbon tetrachloride; lead, methanol, microwaves; solvents
	Weakness, Depression	Aluminum; carbon monoxide; lead; petroleum distillates; tin; solvents
Baker, cook, food processor	Cough	*Flour, grain dust*
	Rash	*Antioxidants* for lards and grease; *benzoyl peroxide* in flour bleaching agents; carbamates, *mercaptobenzothiazole, isopropyl-p-phenylenediamine,* and *thiurams* in rubber; *flour;* formaldehyde; *fragrances and flavoring agents; lanolin* in hand cleaners; *moisture; parabens* in candies, jellies, etc.; nickel sulfate; potassium dichromate; *soaps and detergents; sorbic acid* in preservatives; vegetable and fruit juices; methanol in creams
	Vision Changes	Ionizing radiation; microwaves; ultraviolet radiation
Bartender	Rash	*Flavorings, fruit juices, water, soaps* and *detergents*
Battery maker	Conception Difficulty	Benzene, cadmium, lead, manganese, mercury
	Dizziness	Benzene, lead
	Headache	Benzene, cadmium, copper, lead, manganese, mercury, nickel
	Hearing Changes	Arsenic, lead, mercury
	Memory Loss, Concentration Changes, and Confusion	Lead, mercury
	Nail Abnormalities	Arsenic, silver; contact with acids may cause softening and nail damage

(continued)

If You Work in These Occupations	And Are Experiencing	You May Be at Risk from These Agents
Battery maker (*continued*)	Numbness and Weakness in the Arms and Legs	Lead, manganese
	Rash	Carbamates, *mercaptobenzothiazole*, *isopropyl*-p-*phenylenediamine*, and *thiurams* in rubber; fibrous glass; mercury; nickel; phosphoric acid; potassium hydroxide and sodium hydroxide in electrolyte solutions; sulfuric acid; zinc chloride
	Smell Disturbances	Cadmium, irritant gases, mercury, nickel
	Tremor	Lead, manganese, mercury
	Vision Changes	Benzene, lead, silver
	Weakness, Depression	Benzene, lead, magnesium, manganese, mercury, nickel
Bearing maker	Conception Difficulty	Cadmium
	Headache	Cadmium
Beekeeper	Cough	*Bee toxin, pollen, scales and hairs*
Beverage manufacturer, brewery worker	Cough	*Hops*
	Dizziness	Carbon monoxide, ethanol, hydrogen sulfide, irritant gases
	Headache	Benzene; cadmium; carbon dioxide; carbon monoxide; copper; fluorides; hydrogen sulfide; irritant gases; lead; manganese; mercury; nickel
	Hearing Changes	Carbon monoxide
	Memory Loss, Concentration Changes, and Confusion	Carbon monoxide
	Nail Abnormalities	Formaldehyde, hydrofluoric acid; contact with acids may cause softening and nail damage
	Numbness and Weakness in the Arms and Legs	Carbon monoxide; ethanol; fluorides; hydrogen sulfide

(continued)

If You Work in These Occupations	And Are Experiencing	You May Be at Risk from These Agents
	Smell Disturbances	Formaldehyde, hydrogen sulfide gas, sulfur dioxide
	Tremor	Carbon dioxide; carbon monoxide; ethanol
	Vision Changes	Carbon monoxide, hydrogen sulfide
	Weakness, Depression	Carbon monoxide, ethanol; hydrogen sulfide
Bird breeder	Cough	*Proteins* in dried excreta of caged birds, *mycobacteria*
Blacksmith	Conception Difficulty	Lead
	Dizziness	Carbon monoxide, lead
	Headache	Carbon monoxide, lead, noise
	Hearing Changes	Carbon monoxide, lead
	Memory Loss, Concentration Changes, and Confusion	Carbon monoxide, lead
	Numbness and Weakness in the Arms and Legs	Carbon monoxide, lead
	Tremor	Carbon monoxide, lead
	Vision Changes	Carbon monoxide, cyanide, lead
	Weakness, Depression	Carbon monoxide, lead
Bleacher	Dizziness	Irritant gases
	Headache	Irritant gases, fluorides
	Numbness and Weakness in the Arms and Legs	Fluorides
	Smell Disturbances	Chromium, irritant gases
Bookbinder	Headache; Memory Loss, Concentration Changes, and Confusion	Methanol
	Vision Changes	Arsenic, lead, methanol, solvents
Bottling plant worker	Headache; Hearing Changes	Noise

(*continued*)

If You Work in These Occupations	And Are Experiencing	You May Be at Risk from These Agents
Brick, cement worker	Conception Difficulty	Lead
	Cough	Chromium; silica and nuisance dusts
	Dizziness; Hearing Changes	Carbon monoxide, lead
	Hair Loss	Thallium
	Headache	Carbon monoxide, chromium, fluorides, lead
	Memory Loss, Concentration Changes, and Confusion	Carbon monoxide, lead, thallium
	Nail Abnormalities	Arsenic; formaldehyde; hydrofluoric acid (contact with acids may cause softening and nail damage); thallium
	Numbness and Weakness in the Arms and Legs	Carbon monoxide, lead, phosphorus, thallium
	Rash	Carbamates, *mercaptobenzothiazole*, *isopropyl*-p-*phenylenediamine*, and *thiurams* in rubber; nuisance dusts including glass fibers and cement; petroleum distillates; potassium dichromate; *water*; *work cement*
	Vision Changes	Carbon monoxide, lead, thallium, ultraviolet radiation
	Weakness, Depression	Carbon monoxide, lead, thallium
Butcher	Rash	*Water*; *soaps* and *detergents*; carbamates, *mercaptobenzothiazole*, *isopropyl*-p-*phenylenediamine*, and *thiurams* in rubber gloves; *foods* that can cause contact urticaria
Cabinet maker (see Woodworker)		
Carpenter (see Woodworker)		
Cable manufacturer, splicer	Conception Difficulty	Cadmium, lead, polychlorinated biphenyls (PCBs)
	Headache	Cadmium, lead

(continued)

If You Work in These Occupations	And Are Experiencing	You May Be at Risk from These Agents
	Hearing Changes	Lead
	Vision Changes	Lead, solvents
Camphor maker	Changes in Hearing	*Camphor*, turpentine
Cannery worker	Headache; Memory Loss, Concentration Changes, and Confusion	Methanol
	Rash	Carbamates, *mercaptobenzothiazole*, *isopropyl-p-phenylenediamine*, and *thiurams* in rubber; *juices; soaps and detergents; water*
Cellophane producer, sealer	Conception Difficulty	Carbon disulfide, ethylene glycol ethers
	Dizziness; Numbness and Weakness in the Arms and Legs; Vision Changes; Weakness, Depression	Carbon disulfide, hydrogen sulfide
	Headache	Carbon disulfide, glycols, hydrogen sulfide
	Hearing Changes	Carbon disulfide in combination with noise
	Tremor	Carbon disulfide
Celluloid maker, film maker	Conception Difficulty	Ethylene glycol ethers
	Dizziness	Dinitrobenzene, ketones
	Headache	Dinitrobenzene, glycols
	Nail Abnormalities	Dinitrobenzene
Ceramics worker, potter	Conception Difficulty	Arsenic, boric acid, cadmium, lead, manganese, mercury
	Cough	Arsenic, fluorocarbons, mercury, nickel, silica, silver
	Diarrhea	Antimony, arsenic, boric acid, cadmium, copper, lead, magnesium, mercury, nickel
	Dizziness	Arsenic, fluorocarbons, lead

(continued)

If You Work in These Occupations	And Are Experiencing	You May Be at Risk from These Agents
Ceramics worker, potter (*continued*)	Fever/Chills	Cadmium; metal oxides such as antimony, arsenic, cadmium, chromium, cobalt, copper, lead, magnesium, nickel, manganese, mercury, silver, tin, zinc
	Hair Loss	Arsenic, boric acid
	Headache	Antimony, boric acid, cadmium, chromium, copper, fluorides, lead, manganese, mercury, nickel
	Hearing Changes	Arsenic, carbon monoxide, lead, mercury
	Irritation or Dryness of Eyes, Nose, Sinuses, Mouth, or Throat	Arsenic, cadmium, chromium, cobalt, copper, lead, magnesium, manganese, nickel, oxalic acid, selenium, tin, vanadium, zinc
	Memory Loss, Concentration Changes, and Confusion	Arsenic, carbon monoxide, lead, mercury
	Nausea	Arsenic, boric acid, cadmium, chromium, fluorides, hydrazines, lead, mercury
	Nail Abnormalities	Arsenic, chromium salts, hydrofluoric acid
	Numbness and Weakness in the Arms and Legs	Arsenic, lead, manganese
	Rash	*Acids and alkalis*, chloride, *clay dust*, cobalt, mercury, nickel, potassium dichromate, *soaps and detergents*, turpentine, *wet clay*
	Smell Disturbances	Cadmium, chromium, irritant gases, mercury, nickel, nuisance dusts, selenium, vanadium
	Tremor	Arsenic, boric acid, fluorocarbons, lead, manganese, mercury
	Weakness, Depression	Aluminum, antimony, arsenic, boric acid, cadmium, cobalt, copper, lead, magnesium, manganese, mercury, nickel, selenium, tin, zinc

(continued)

If You Work in These Occupations	And Are Experiencing	You May Be at Risk from These Agents
	Vision Changes	Arsenic, carbon monoxide, lead, silver
Cheese maker	Cough	*Penicillum fungus and other mold fungi*
Chemical industry worker	Conception Difficulty	Arsenic, benzene, carbon disulfide, epichlorohydrin, ethylene oxide, formaldehyde, lead, manganese, mercury, styrene, toluene, vinyl chloride, xylene
	Cough	*Azo dyes*, carbon monoxide, chromium, *ethylenediamine*, formaldehyde, *p-phenylenediamine*, phenol, *piperazine* formaldehyde, sulfathiazole, *sulfonechloramides*, *tannic acid*, toluene
	Diarrhea	Antimony, arsenic, formaldehyde, halogenated hydrocarbon solvents, phenol, thallium
	Dizziness	Aniline; arsenic; benzene; diborane; carbon disulfide; carbon monoxide; carbon tetrachloride, trichloroethylene, and other halogenated hydrocarbon solvents; cresol or styrene; cyanide; dinitrobenzene; dinitrotoluene; ethanol; formaldehyde; hydrazine; hydrogen sulfide; irritant gases; lead; methanol; methyl bromide, chloride, or iodide; nickel carbonyl; toluene; vinyl chloride; xylene
	Fever/Chills	Diborane, certain dinitro derivatives of phenol and cresol
	Hair Loss	Arsenic, selenium, thallium
	Headache	Aniline; antimony; benzene; carbon dioxide; carbon disulfide; carbon monoxide; carbon tetrachloride; chromium; cresol; cyanide; dinitrobenzene; dinitro

(continued)

If You Work in These Occupations	And Are Experiencing	You May Be at Risk from These Agents
Chemical industry worker (*continued*)		derivatives of phenol and cresol; dinitrotoluene; ethanol; fluorides; formaldehyde; halogenated hydrocarbon solvents including trichloroethylene; hydrogen sulfide; irritant gases; lead; manganese; methanol; mercury; methyl bromide, chloride, and iodide; nickel; styrene; toluene, vinyl chloride; xylene
	Hearing Changes	Arsenic; carbon disulfide in combination with noise; carbon monoxide; cresol; lead; mercury; styrene; toluene; trichloroethylene in combination with noise; xylene
	Irritation or Dryness of Eyes, Nose, Sinuses, Mouth, or Throat	Antimony; arsenic; chromium; cobalt, ethylenediamine; fluorocarbons; formaldehyde; halogenated hydrocarbon solvents; hydrogen selenide; hydrogen sulfide; irritant gases; lead, magnesium; manganese; methyl bromide, chloride and iodide; naphthalene; oxalic acid; styrene; vanadium
	Memory Loss, Concentration Changes, and Confusion	Arsenic; carbon monoxide; cresol; cyanide; halogenated hydrocarbon solvents including carbon tetrachloride and trichlorethylene; lead; mercury; methanol; methyl bromide, chloride, and iodide; napthalene; styrene; thallium; toluene; xylene
	Nail Abnormalities	Aniline, chromium salts, dinitrobenzene, formaldehyde, hydrofluoric acid, silver, vinyl chloride
	Nausea	Arsenic, benzene, carbon monoxide, dinitrobenzene, dimethylformamide, dinitrophenol, dinitrotoluene, fluorides, formaldehyde, mercury, phenol, selenium

(continued)

If You Work in These Occupations	And Are Experiencing	You May Be at Risk from These Agents
	Numbness and Weakness in the Arms and Legs	Arsenic; carbon disulfide; carbon monoxide; carbon tetrachloride and other halogenated hydrocarbon solvents; ethanol; fluorides; hydrogen sulfide; lead; manganese; methyl bromide, chloride, and iodide; phosphorus; styrene; thallium; vinyl chloride
	Smell Disturbances	Acetates (butyl acetate, ethyl acetate, and PGMEA[a]); cadmium; carbon disulfide; chromium; cresol; cyanide; DMSO; formaldehyde; halogenated hydrocarbon solvents; hydrazine; hydrogen selenide; hydrogen sulfide; irritant gases; mercury; methyl bromide; nickel; nuisance dusts; vanadium
	Tremor	Arsenic; carbon dioxide; carbon disulfide; carbon monoxide; carbon tetrachloride, trichloroethylene, and other halogenated hydrocarbon solvents; ethanol; lead; manganese; mercury; methyl bromide, chloride, and iodide; phosphorus; thallium; toluene; vanadium; xylene
	Pain on Urination	Aniline; chromium; dinitrophenol; formaldehyde; halogenated hydrocarbons; mercury; methyl bromide, chloride, and iodide; naphthalene; phenol and its derivatives; toluene
	Urine Color Changes	Carbon monoxide, dinitro derivatives of phenol and cresol, hydrazines, naphthalene, phenol and phenolic compounds
	Vision Changes	Arsenic; benzene; carbon disulfide; carbon monoxide; carbon tetrachloride; cyanide; dinitro derivatives of phenol and cresol; halogenated hydrocarbon solvents;

(continued)

If You Work in These Occupations	And Are Experiencing	You May Be at Risk from These Agents
Chemical industry worker (*continued*)		hydrogen sulfide; lead; methanol; methyl bromide, chloride, and iodide; silver; thallium; toluene; trichloroethylene; ultraviolet radiation; xylene
	Weakness, Depression	Aniline; benzene; diborane; carbon disulfide; carbon monoxide; carbon tetrachloride, trichloroethylene, and other halogenated hydrocarbon solvents; cresol; cyanide; dinitro derivatives of phenol and cresol; ethanol; hydrogen sulfide; lead; magnesium and manganese oxide; mercury; methyl bromide, chloride, and iodide; nickel; styrene; thallium; toluene; vinyl chloride; xylene; zinc
Chimney sweep	Conception Difficulty	Polycyclic aromatic hydrocarbons
	Dizziness; Headache; Hearing Changes; Memory Loss, Concentration Changes, and Confusion; Numbness and Weakness in the Arms and Legs; Vision Changes; Weakness, Depression	Carbon monoxide
Cleaner, maintenance worker (includes cleaners of pipelines, tanks, septic tanks, wells, degreasers, parts and tool cleaners)	Conception Difficulty	Carbon disulfide
	Dizziness	Carbon disulfide; carbon tetrachloride, trichloroethylene, and other halogenated hydrocarbon solvents; cresol; fluorocarbons; irritant gases; petroleum distillates
	Fever/Chills	Petroleum distillates
	Hair Loss	Arsenic; boric acid
	Headache	Borax; carbon dioxide; carbon disulfide; carbon monoxide from methylene chloride; carbon

(continued)

If You Work in These Occupations	And Are Experiencing	You May Be at Risk from These Agents
		tetrachloride, trichloroethylene, and other halogenated hydrocarbon solvents; cresol; fluorides; glycols; hydrogen sulfide; irritant gases; methyl bromide; petroleum distillates
	Hearing Changes	Carbon disulfide in combination with noise; cresol; trichloroethylene in combination with noise
	Irritation or Dryness of Eyes, Nose, Sinuses, Mouth, or Throat	Boric acid; borax; chlorine; cresol; glutaraldehyde; halogenated hydrocarbon solvents; irritant gases
	Memory Loss, Concentration Changes, and Confusion	Carbon monoxide from methylene chloride, halogenated hydrocarbon solvents including carbon tetrachloride and trichloroethylene, methyl bromide (wool degreaser), petroleum distillates
	Numbness and Weakness in the Arms and Legs	Carbon disulfide; carbon monoxide from methylene chloride; carbon tetrachloride and other halogenated hydrocarbon solvents; wool degreasers: methyl bromide, chloride, and iodide, petroleum distillates
	Tremor	Carbon disulfide; carbon monoxide (released in the blood from exposure to methylene chloride); carbon tetrachloride, trichloroethylene, and other halogenated hydrocarbon solvents; fluorocarbons; methyl bromide (wool degreasers)
	Urine Color Changes	Halogenated hydrocarbon solvents, phenol and phenolic compounds
	Vision Changes	Carbon disulfide, carbon tetrachloride, halogenated hydrocarbon solvents, methyl

(continued)

If You Work in These Occupations	And Are Experiencing	You May Be at Risk from These Agents
Cleaner, maintenance worker (includes cleaners of pipelines, tanks, septic tanks, wells, degreasers, parts and tool cleaners) (continued)		bromide (wool degreaser), trichloroethylene; ultraviolet radiation
	Weakness, Depression	Borax; carbon disulfide; carbon monoxide (from methylene chloride); carbon tetrachloride, trichloroethylene, and other halogenated hydrocarbon solvents; cresol; methyl bromide; (wool degreaser); petroleum distillates
	Smell Disturbances	Carbon disulfide; cresol; halogenated hydrocarbon solvents; irritant gases; petroleum distillates
Coal tar worker, roofer	Dizziness	Aniline; cresol; hydrogen sulfide; petroleum distillates
	Fever/Chills	Petroleum distillates
	Headache	Aniline; cresol; hydrogen sulfide; petroleum distillates
	Hearing Changes	Cresol
	Memory Loss, Concentration Changes, and Confusion	Cresol; naphthalene; petroleum distillates
	Nail Abnormalities	Aniline
	Numbness and Weakness in the Arms and Legs	Hydrogen sulfide
	Smell Disturbances	Cresol; hydrogen sulfide; irritant gases
	Weakness, Depression	Aniline; cresol; hydrogen sulfide; petroleum distillates
Coatings manufacturer	Conception Difficulty	Polychlorinated biphenyls (PCBs), styrene, toluene
	Cough	Diisocyanates, certain acid anhydrides
	Dizziness	Fluorocarbons, ketones, styrene, toluene
	Fever/Chills	Fluorocarbon polymers

(continued)

If You Work in These Occupations	And Are Experiencing	You May Be at Risk from These Agents
	Headache	Fluorides, styrene, toluene
	Hearing Changes; Memory Loss, Concentration Changes, and Confusion	Styrene, toluene
	Tremor	Fluorocarbons, toluene
	Vision Changes	Toluene
	Weakness, Depression	Fluorocarbon polymers, styrene, toluene
Coffee worker	Cough	*Green coffee dust*
Coke oven worker	Conception Difficulty	Polycyclic aromatic hydrocarbons, *elevated temperatures*
	Dizziness; Headache	Carbon monoxide, cyanide, irritant gases
	Memory Loss, Concentration Changes, and Confusion; Weakness, Depression	Carbon monoxide, cyanide
	Numbness and Weakness in the Arms and Legs	Carbon monoxide
Communications worker	Vision changes	Laser light, microwaves
Construction worker, renovator, demolition worker	Conception Difficulty	Lead, polycyclic aromatic hydrocarbons
	Cough	Asbestos, *fungi, wood dusts*
	Fever/Chills	Petroleum distillates
	Headache	Lead, noise, petroleum distillates
	Hearing Changes	Arsenic, cresol, lead, noise, *vibration*
	Irritation or Dryness of Eyes, Nose, Sinuses, Mouth, or Throat	Acrylics
	Memory Loss, Concentration Changes, and Confusion	Lead, petroleum distillates
	Nail Abnormalities	Arsenic, acrylics, *paint products, fiberglass*

(continued)

If You Work in These Occupations	And Are Experiencing	You May Be at Risk from These Agents
Construction worker, renovator, demolition worker (continued)	Numbness and Weakness in the Arms and Legs	Lead, petroleum distillates, vibration
	Rash	Carbamates, mercaptobenzothiazole, isopropyl-p-phenylenediamine, and thiurams in rubber; hot asphalt; nuisance dust; petroleum distillates; potassium dichromate; rosin; water
	Smell Disturbances	Halogenated hydrocarbon solvents, hydrogen sulfide, nuisance dusts, petroleum distillates
	Vision Changes	Arsenic, hydrogen sulfide, laser light, lead, solvents, ultraviolet radiation
Contact lens maker	Nail Abnormalities	Acrylics
Cosmetics worker; cosmetologist, manicurist	Cough	Ethylene diamine; hair spray lacquers that contain vegetable gums, synthetic gum polyvinyl pyrrolidone, carboxymethyl-cellulose, polyvinyl alcohol, or denatured alcohol; orris root; phenylenediamine; powders such as talc or selenium; volatile or essential oils, including eucalyptus, sage, turpentine, and pine
	Irritation or Dryness of Eyes, Nose, Sinuses, Mouth, or Throat	Dye exposure; acrylics
	Nail Abnormalities	Acrylics, ethylenediamine, formaldehyde, and p-phenylenediamine (preservatives)
	Rash	Acrylics; depilatories; formaldehyde; fragrances; glycerol monothioglycolate in permanent wave preparations; hair dyes; hair tints and bleaches; nickel sulfate; p-phenylenediamine in hair dyes, nail polishes, and nail glues; soaps, detergents, and shampoos; water; wave solutions
Data processor	Dizziness; Vision Changes	Video display terminals

(continued)

If You Work in These Occupations	And Are Experiencing	You May Be at Risk from These Agents
Defense worker	Vision Changes	Microwaves
Degreaser (see Cleaner, maintenance worker)		
Dental worker, dental assistant, amalgam maker	Conception Difficulty	Cadmium, ethylene oxide, ionizing radiation, mercury
	Headache	Cadmium, mercury
	Hearing Changes	Mercury
	Irritation or Dryness of Eyes, Nose, Sinuses, Mouth, or Throat	Acrylics, cadmium, epoxy resins, silver, ultraviolet radiation, zinc
	Memory Loss, Concentration Changes, and Confusion	Mercury
	Nail Abnormalities	Acrylics
	Nausea	Cadmium, mercury
	Rash	*Abrasives; amalgam mixtures; benzoyl peroxide* in catalysts; bis-GMA and bisphenol A (epoxy resin); carbamates, *mercaptobenzothiazole, isopropyl-p-phenylenediamine*, and *thiurams* in rubber; formaldehyde; *fragrances; germicidal solutions;* mercury; methyl methacrylate; nickel sulfate; *soaps and detergents; solvents*
	Smell Disturbances	Cadmium, mercury
	Tremor	Mercury
	Pain on Urination	Cadmium, mercury
	Vision Changes	Ionizing radiation (X rays), silver, ultraviolet radiation
	Weakness, Depression	Mercury, nitrous oxide
Detergent industry worker	Conception Difficulty	Benzene, ethanol, ethylene oxide
	Cough	*Bacillus subtilis*
	Dizziness	Benzene, ethanol
	Headache	Benzene, ethanol

(continued)

If You Work in These Occupations	And Are Experiencing	You May Be at Risk from These Agents
Detergent industry worker (*continued*)	Numbness and Weakness in the Arms and Legs; Tremor	Ethanol
	Weakness, Depression	Benzene, ethanol
	Vision Changes	Benzene
Diesel engine operator	Dizziness; Headache; Memory Loss, Concentration Changes, and Confusion; Numbness and Weakness in the Arms and Legs; Tremor; Weakness, Depression	Carbon monoxide
Disinfectant maker	Conception Difficulty	Ethylene oxide; ethylene glycol ethers; formaldehyde; manganese; mercury
	Dizziness	Aniline, cresol, formaldehyde, irritant gases, organic tin, trichloroethylene
	Headache	Aniline, cresol, formaldehyde, fluorides, irritant gases, manganese, mercury, organic tin, trichloroethylene
	Hearing Changes	Organic tin; trichloroethylene in combination with noise
	Memory Loss, Concentration Changes, and Confusion	Cresol, mercury, organic tin, trichloroethylene
	Nail Abnormalities	Aniline, formaldehyde, hydrofluoric acid
	Numbness and Weakness in the Arms and Legs	Fluorides, manganese, organic tin
	Smell Disturbances	Cresol, formaldehyde, irritant gases, mercury
	Tremor	Manganese, mercury, trichloroethylene
	Vision Changes	Methylmercury, silver, trichloroethylene
	Weakness, Depression	Aniline, cresol, mercury, tin, trichloroethylene

(*continued*)

If You Work in These Occupations	And Are Experiencing	You May Be at Risk from These Agents
Distiller	Dizziness; Tremor; Weakness, Depression	Ethanol
	Headache	Carbon dioxide, hydrogen sulfide
Diver, caisson worker	Dizziness	Hydrogen sulfide, nitrogen
	Headache	Carbon dioxide, hydrogen sulfide
	Numbness and Weakness in the Arms and Legs	Hydrogen sulfide
	Tremor	Carbon dioxide
	Vision Changes	Hydrogen sulfide
	Weakness, Depression	Carbon monoxide from contaminated air; *decompression sickness;* hydrogen sulfide
Dry cleaner	Conception Difficulty	Benzene, carbon disulfide, ethylene glycol ethers
	Cough	Fluorocarbons, irritant gases, petroleum distillates
	Dizziness	Benzene; carbon disulfide; carbon tetrachloride, trichloroethylene, and other halogenated hydrocarbon solvents; fluorocarbons; irritant gases; methanol; petroleum distillates
	Fever/Chills	Petroleum distillates
	Headache	Carbon disulfide, carbon tetrachloride, glycols, halogenated hydrocarbon solvents, irritant gases, fluorides, methanol, petroleum distillates, trichloroethylene
	Hearing Changes	Carbon disulfide in combination with noise, trichloroethylene in combination with noise, turpentine
	Irritation or Dryness of Eyes, Nose, Sinuses, Mouth, or Throat	Carbon tetrachloride, fluorocarbons, irritant gases, nuisance dusts

(continued)

If You Work in These Occupations	And Are Experiencing	You May Be at Risk from These Agents
Dry cleaner (*continued*)	Memory Loss, Concentration Changes, and Confusion	Halogenated hydrocarbon solvents including carbon tetrachloride and trichloroethylene, methanol, petroleum distillates
	Nausea	Benzene, carbon disulfide, carbon tetrachloride, fluorocarbon, halogenated hydrocarbon solvents, trichloroethylene
	Numbness and Weakness in the Arms and Legs	Carbon disulfide, carbon tetrachloride and other halogenated hydrocarbon solvents; petroleum distillates
	Rash	Carbamates; *mercaptobenzothiazole, isopropyl*-p-*phenylenediamine,* and *thiurams* in rubber; *cleaning agents;* formaldehyde; halogenated hydrocarbon solvents; petroleum distillates
	Smell Disturbances	Benzene, carbon disulfide, halogenated hydrocarbon solvents, irritant gases (chlorine and phosgene), nuisance dusts
	Tremor	Carbon disulfide; carbon tetrachloride, trichloroethylene, and other halogenated hydrocarbon solvents; fluorocarbons
	Urine Color Changes	Carbon tetrachloride, halogenated hydrocarbon solvents
Dry ice handler	Headache; Tremor	Carbon dioxide
Dye or ink producer, user	Conception Difficulty	Arsenic; benzene; boric acid; carbon disulfide; ethylene glycol ethers; formaldehyde; manganese; mercury; polychlorinated biphenyls (PCBs); xylene
	Cough	Phenylenediamine
	Dizziness	Aniline; arsenic; benzene; carbon disulfide; carbon tetrachloride; cresol; dinitrobenzene;

(continued)

If You Work in These Occupations	And Are Experiencing	You May Be at Risk from These Agents
		dinitrotoluene; ethanol; formaldehyde; hydrazines; hydrogen sulfide; irritant gases; ketones; lead; methanol; methyl bromide, chloride, and iodide; petroleum distillates; organic tin; trichloroethylene; turpentine; xylene
	Fever/Chills	Certain dinitro derivatives of phenol and cresol, petroleum distillates
	Hair Loss	Arsenic, boric acid, thallium
	Headache	Aniline; antimony; benzene; boric acid; carbon disulfide; carbon tetrachloride; chromium; cresol; dinitrobenzene; dinitro derivatives of phenol and cresol; dinitrotoluene; ethanol; fluorides; formaldehyde; glycols; hydrogen sulfide; irritant gases; lead; manganese; mercury; methanol; methyl bromide, chloride and iodide; nickel; petroleum distillates; organic tin; trichloroethylene; turpentine; xylene
	Hearing Changes	Arsenic; cresol; lead; mercury; organic tin; trichloroethylene in combination with noise; turpentine
	Memory Loss, Concentration Changes, and Confusion	Arsenic; carbon tetrachloride; cresol; lead; mercury; methanol; methyl bromide, chloride, and iodide; naphthalene; petroleum distillates; thallium; organic tin; trichloroethylene; xylene
	Nail Abnormalities	Aniline; arsenic; chromium salts; dinitrobenzene; dinitro-o-cresol; formaldehyde; hydrofluoric acid; silver; turpentine
	Numbness and Weakness in the Arms and Legs	Arsenic; carbon disulfide; carbon tetrachloride; ethanol; hydrogen

(continued)

If You Work in These Occupations	And Are Experiencing	You May Be at Risk from These Agents
Dye or ink producer, user (*continued*)		sulfide; lead; manganese; methyl bromide, chloride, and iodide; methyl *n*-butyl ketone; petroleum distillates; thallium; organic tin
	Rash	Cobalt, *disperse orange 3, disperse red 1, disperse yellow 3 and 64*, ethylenediamine, formaldehyde, mercury, nickel, p-*phenylenediamine*, p-*aminoazobenzene*, p-*aminophenol*, petroleum distillates, turpentine
	Smell Disturbances	Acetates (butyl acetate, ethyl acetate, and PGMEA[a]); benzene and other petroleum distillates; chromium; cresol; cyanides; formaldehyde; halogenated hydrocarbon solvents; hydrazine; hydrogen sulfide; irritant gases; mercury; methyl bromide; vanadium
	Tremor	Arsenic; carbon tetrachloride; ethanol; lead; manganese; mercury; methyl bromide, chloride, and iodide; thallium; trichloroethylene; vanadium
	Pain on Urination	Aniline, carbon tetrachloride, formaldehyde, glycols, lead, tin, turpentine
	Vision Changes	Arsenic; benzene; carbon disulfide; carbon tetrachloride; dinitro derivatives of phenol and cresol; halogenated hydrocarbon solvents; hydrogen sulfide; lead; methanol[b], methyl bromide, chloride, and iodide; silver; thallium; trichloroethylene
	Weakness, Depression	Aniline; benzene; boric acid; carbon disulfide; carbon tetrachloride; cresol; dinitro derivatives of phenol and cresol; ethanol; halogenated hydrocarbon

(continued)

If You Work in These Occupations	And Are Experiencing	You May Be at Risk from These Agents
		solvents; hydrogen sulfide; lead; mercury; methyl bromide, chloride, and iodide; nickel; petroleum distillates; perchloroethane; thallium; tin; trichloroethylene; xylene; zinc
Electrician, radio technician	Cough	Aluminum soldering flux with aminoethylethanolamine; asbestos
	Dizziness	Arsenic; organic tin
	Headache; Memory Loss, Concentration Changes, and Confusion; Nail Abnormalities	Methanol
	Rash	Acids; carbamates, *mercaptobenzothiazole*, *isopropyl*-p-*phenylenediamine*, and *thiurams* in rubber; epoxy resins; plating chemicals (nickel); rosin; *soldering flux; solvents*
	Vision Changes	Ultraviolet radiation; methanol; microwaves
Electrical equipment manufacturer	Conception Difficulty	Arsenic
	Cough	Aluminum soldering flux with aminoethylethanolamine, asbestos; fumes of metal oxides such as cadmium
	Dizziness	Arsenic
	Numbness and Weakness in the Arms and Legs	Arsenic
	Rash	Acids; carbamates, mercaptobenzothiazole, isopropyl-p-phenylenediamine, and thiurams in rubber; epoxy resins; rosin; plating chemicals (nickel); soldering flux; solvents
	Smell Disturbances	Nickel, nuisance dusts, selenium
	Vision Changes	Ionizing radiation (X rays); silver; solvents

(continued)

If You Work in These Occupations	And Are Experiencing	You May Be at Risk from These Agents
Electronics industry worker (see Semiconductor, microchip producer)		
Electroplater	Conception Difficulty	Arsenic, benzene, cadmium, carbon disulfide, lead, mercury
	Cough	Chromium, *platinum*
	Dizziness	Benzene, carbon disulfide, cyanide, hydrazines, irritant gases, lead, nickel carbonyl, petroleum distillates
	Fever/Chills	Boron compounds, petroleum distillates
	Hair Loss	Boric acid
	Headache	Benzene, boric acid and boron compounds, cadmium, carbon disulfide, chromium, copper, cyanide, irritant gases, lead, mercury, nickel, petroleum distillates
	Hearing Changes	Arsenic; carbon disulfide in combination with noise; lead; mercury
	Memory Loss, Concentration Changes, and Confusion	Cyanide, lead, mercury, petroleum distillates
	Nail Abnormalities	Arsenic, chromic acid, hydrofluoric acid, silver, sulfuric acid
	Numbness and Weakness in the Arms and Legs	Arsenic, carbon disulfide, lead, petroleum distillates
	Rash	Carbamates, *mercaptobenzothiazole*, *isopropyl*-p-*phenylenediamine*, and *thiurams* in rubber; cobalt; mercury; *metal cleaners;* nickel sulfate; petroleum distillates; *pickling and plating solutions;* potassium dichromate and chromic acid fumes

(continued)

If You Work in These Occupations	And Are Experiencing	You May Be at Risk from These Agents
	Smell Disturbances	Benzene, cadmium, carbon disulfide, chromium, cyanide, hydrazine, mercury, nickel, nuisance dusts, sulfuric acid
	Tremor	Carbon disulfide, lead, mercury
	Vision Changes	Arsenic, benzene, carbon disulfide, cyanide, hydrazines, lead, silver
	Weakness, Depression	Benzene, boric acid and boron compounds, carbon disulfide, cyanide, lead, mercury, nickel, petroleum distillates, tin, zinc
Embalmer, mortician	Conception Difficulty	Formaldehyde, ionizing radiation, mercury
	Cough	Formaldehyde, phenol
	Dizziness; Headache; Smell Disturbances	Formaldehyde, organic mercury
	Hearing Changes; Memory Loss, Concentration Changes, and Confusion; Weakness, Depression	Mercury
	Nail Abnormalities	Formaldehyde
	Numbness and Weakness in the Arms and Legs	Organic mercury
	Rash	Carbamates, *mercaptobenzothiazole*, *isopropyl*-p-*phenylenediamine*, and *thiurams* in rubber; formaldehyde and ammoniated mercury in embalming fluids; *soaps and detergents; water*
	Vision Changes	Ionizing radiation, methylmercury
Enameler	Conception Difficulty	Arsenic, lead
	Cough	Hydrofluoric acid, silica
	Diarrhea	Arsenic, fluoride, lead, nickel
	Dizziness	Arsenic, cresol, lead, methanol
	Fever/Chills	Metal oxides such as arsenic, cobalt, lead, nickel, tin

(*continued*)

If You Work in These Occupations	And Are Experiencing	You May Be at Risk from These Agents
Enameler (*continued*)	Hair Loss	Arsenic
	Headache	Antimony, cresol, fluorides, lead, methanol, nickel
	Hearing Changes	Arsenic, lead
	Memory Loss, Concentration Changes, and Confusion	Arsenic, cresol, lead, methanol
	Nail Abnormalities	Arsenic, chromium, hydrofluoric acid
	Numbness and Weakness in the Arms and Legs	Arsenic, fluorides, lead
	Smell Disturbances	Chromium, irritant gases (or acid mists), nickel
	Tremor	Arsenic, lead
	Vision Changes	Arsenic, lead, methanol[b]
	Weakness, Depression	Antimony, arsenic, cobalt, cresol, lead, nickel, tin
Engraver, etcher	Conception Difficulty	Cadmium
	Headache	Cadmium, chromium
	Numbness and Weakness in the Arms and Legs	Arsenic
	Rash	*Adhesives, etching acids, gold chloride,* nickel sulfate, *paint removers,* potassium dichromate *solvents*
	Smell Disturbances	Cadmium, halogenated hydrocarbon solvents, irritant gases (or acid mists), potassium cyanide
Explosives, fireworks manufacturer; ammunition and detonator workers	Conception Difficulty	Arsenic; benzene; cadmium; carbon disulfide; mercury
	Dizziness	Arsenic; benzene; carbon disulfide; dinitrobenzene; dinitrotoluene; ethanol; hydrazines; irritant gases; ketones; nitrites and nitrates

(continued)

If You Work in These Occupations	And Are Experiencing	You May Be at Risk from These Agents
	Diarrhea	Aluminum; antimony; arsenic; mercury; phosphorus; salts
	Fever/Chills	Certain dinitro derivatives of phenol and cresol
	Hair Loss	Thallium
	Headache	Antimony; benzene; cadmium; carbon dioxide; carbon disulfide; dinitrobenzene; dinitro derivatives of phenol and cresol; dinitrotoluene, glycols; irritant gases; nitrites and nitrates; trinitrotoluene
	Hearing Changes	Mercury
	Irritation or Dryness of Eyes, Nose, Sinuses, Mouth, or Throat	Antimony; arsenic
	Memory Loss, Concentration Changes, and Confusion	Arsenic; mercury; thallium
	Nail Abnormalities	Dinitrobenzene, trinitrotoluene
	Nausea	Arsenic; dinitrotoluene
	Numbness and Weakness in the Arms and Legs	Arsenic; carbon disulfide; ethanol; phosphorus; thallium
	Smell Disturbances	Cadmium, hydrazine, irritant gases, mercury
	Tremor	Arsenic, carbon dioxide, ethanol, mercury, phosphorus, thallium
	Pain on Urination	Cadmium; trinitrotoluene
	Vision Changes	Arsenic; benzene; dinitrophenol; hydrazines; phenol; thallium
	Weakness, Depression	Benzene, carbon disulfide, dinitro derivatives of phenol and cresol, ethanol, mercury, nitrites
Fat, oil and wax processor	Conception Difficulty	Carbon disulfide, ethylene glycol ethers, ethylene dibromide, n-hexane

(continued)

If You Work in These Occupations	And Are Experiencing	You May Be at Risk from These Agents
Fat, oil and wax processor (continued)	Dizziness	Carbon disulfide, carbon tetrachloride, hydrogen sulfide, ketones, methyl bromide, methylene chloride, turpentine
	Headache	Carbon disulfide, carbon monoxide, carbon tetrachloride, glycols, hydrogen sulfide, methyl bromide, nickel, turpentine
	Numbness and Weakness in the Arms and Legs	Carbon disulfide; carbon tetrachloride; hydrogen sulfide; methyl n-butyl ketone; methyl bromide, chloride and iodide; methylene chloride
	Tremor	Carbon disulfide, carbon tetrachloride, methyl bromide, methylene chloride
	Vision Changes	Carbon disulfide, carbon tetrachloride, hydrogen sulfide, methyl bromide
	Weakness, Depression	Carbon disulfide, carbon tetrachloride, hydrogen sulfide, methyl bromide, methylene chloride, nickel
Feather worker	Cough	Uncleaned feathers, mites, moths
Felt, felt hat maker	Conception Difficulty	Mercury
	Dizziness	Carbon monoxide, hydrogen sulfide, irritant gases, methanol
	Headache	Carbon monoxide, hydrogen sulfide, irritant gases, methanol, mercury
	Hearing Changes; Tremor	Carbon monoxide, mercury
	Memory Loss, Concentration Changes, and Confusion	Carbon monoxide, mercury, methanol
	Numbness and Weakness in the Arms and Legs	Carbon monoxide, hydrogen sulfide
	Smell Disturbances	Hydrogen sulfide gas, irritant gases, mercury

(continued)

If You Work in These Occupations	And Are Experiencing	You May Be at Risk from These Agents
	Vision Changes	Carbon monoxide, hydrogen sulfide, methanol
	Weakness, Depression	Carbon monoxide, hydrogen sulfide, mercury
Fertilizer manufacturer, user	Conception Difficulty	Arsenic, cadmium, formaldehyde, manganese
	Dizziness	Cyanide, formaldehyde, hydrogen sulfide, irritant gases, nitrites and nitrates
	Headache	Cadmium, cyanide, fluorides, formaldehyde, hydrogen sulfide, irritant gases, manganese, nitrites and nitrates
	Memory Loss, Concentration Changes, and Confusion	Cyanide
	Nail Abnormalities	Acids, arsenic, formaldehyde
	Numbness and Weakness in the Arms and Legs	Fluorides, hydrogen sulfide, manganese
	Smell Disturbances	Cadmium, hydrogen cyanide and its salts, formaldehyde, irritant gases and mists (ammonia, nitrogen oxides, and sulfuric acid)
	Tremor	Manganese
	Vision Changes	Arsenic, cyanide, hydrogen sulfide
	Weakness, Depression	Cyanide, hydrogen sulfide, nitrites
Fiberglass maker	Headache	Borates
	Weakness, Depression	Borates, styrene and other organic solvents
Firefighter, fire extinguisher manufacturer	Dizziness	Carbon monoxide, carbon tetrachloride, cyanide, fluorocarbons, irritant gases
	Headache	Carbon dioxide, fluorides

(continued)

If You Work in These Occupations	And Are Experiencing	You May Be at Risk from These Agents
Firefighter, fire extinguisher manufacturer (*continued*)	Hearing Changes	Carbon monoxide, noise
	Irritation or Dryness of Eyes, Nose, Sinuses, Mouth, or Throat	Carbon tetrachloride, irritant gases
	Memory Loss, Concentration Changes, and Confusion	Carbon monoxide, carbon tetrachloride, cyanide
	Nausea	Carbon monoxide
	Numbness and Weakness in the Arms and Legs	Carbon monoxide, carbon tetrachloride, phosphorus
	Rash	Carbamates, *mercaptobenzothiazole, isopropyl-p-phenylenediamine,* and *thiurams* in rubber; *water*
	Smell Disturbances	Cyanide, irritant gases
	Tremor	Carbon dioxide, carbon monoxide, carbon tetrachloride, fluorocarbons, phosphorus
	Urine Color Changes	Carbon monoxide, carbon tetrachloride
	Vision Changes	Carbon monoxide, carbon tetrachloride, cyanide
	Weakness, Depression	Carbon monoxide, carbon tetrachloride, cyanide
Fisherman (commercial), fish processor	Cough	*By-products of decaying marine and fish products*
	Dizziness; Headache; Numbness and Weakness in the Arms and Legs; Smell Disturbances; Weakness, Depression	Hydrogen sulfide
	Vision Changes	Hydrogen sulfide, ultraviolet radiation
Flight attendant	Cough	Ozone
Floor covering installers	Nail Abnormalities	Acrylics, methanol
	Rash	Acrylics; carbamates, *mercaptobenzothiazole, isopropyl-p-phenylenediamine,* and

(continued)

If You Work in These Occupations	And Are Experiencing	You May Be at Risk from These Agents
		thiurams in rubber; *cement;* dirt and nuisance dust; *floor strippers;* petroleum distillates; potassium dichromate; rosin; *soaps and detergents; solvents*
Florist	Rash	Carbamates, *mercaptobenzothiazole, isopropyl-p-phenylenediamine,* and *thiurams* in rubber; *irritating plants;* soaps and detergents
Food processor, preserver, technologist	Conception Difficulty	Ionizing radiation
	Cough	*Papain*
	Dizziness	Fluorocarbons, methyl bromide, nitrites and nitrates
	Headache	Carbon dioxide, *licorice,* methyl bromide, nitrites and nitrates, oil of peppermint
	Memory Loss, Concentration Changes, and Confusion	Methyl bromide
	Smell Disturbances	Acetates, methyl bromide, oil of peppermint, phosgene, and sulfur dioxide
	Tremor	Carbon dioxide, fluorocarbons, methyl bromide
	Weakness, Depression	Methyl bromide, nitrites
	Vision Changes	Ionizing radiation, microwaves, ultraviolet radiation
Forestry worker	Conception Difficulty; Dizziness; Hair Loss	Arsenic
	Cough	*Fungi* in wood pulp; *wood dust*
	Headache; Hearing Changes	Noise, *vibration*
	Memory Loss, Concentration Changes, and Confusion; Nausea; Tremor; Vision Changes	Arsenic
	Numbness and Weakness in the Arms and Legs	Arsenic, *vibration*

(continued)

If You Work in These Occupations	And Are Experiencing	You May Be at Risk from These Agents
Forestry worker (*continued*)	Rash	Carbamates, *mercaptobenzothiazole*, *isopropyl*-p-*phenylenediamine*, and *thiurams* in rubber; *pesticides and fungicides;* insects (including those that cause Lyme disease); poison ivy/oak/sumac and other plants; *stains; water; wood*
Forging press operator	Hearing Changes	Noise, *vibration*
Foundry, furnace worker (includes blast-furnace maker and precision caster)	Conception Difficulty	Formaldehyde, lead, manganese, polycyclic aromatic hydrocarbons, *elevated temperatures*
	Cough	Coke oven fumes; fumes of metal oxides such as antimony, aluminum, arsenic, cadmium, chromium, cobalt, copper, iron, lead, magnesium, manganese, mercury, nickel, selenium, silver, tin, and zinc; nuisance dusts, silica
	Diarrhea	Aluminum, formaldehyde, iron, lead, magnesium, nickel
	Dizziness	Carbon monoxide; cresol; cyanide; formaldehyde; hydrogen sulfide; irritant gases; lead; methanol; nickel carbonyl
	Fever/Chills	Metal oxides such as aluminum, iron, lead, magnesium, manganese, nickel, tin, zinc
	Headache	Carbon dioxide; carbon monoxide; cresol; cyanide; formaldehyde; hydrogen sulfide; irritant gases; lead; manganese; methanol; nickel
	Hearing Changes	Carbon monoxide; cresol; lead; noise; *vibration*
	Memory Loss, Concentration Changes, and Confusion	Carbon monoxide; cresol; cyanide; methanol
	Nail Abnormalities	Formaldehyde; acids may soften and damage nails

(*continued*)

If You Work in These Occupations	And Are Experiencing	You May Be at Risk from These Agents
	Numbness and Weakness in the Arms and Legs	Carbon monoxide, hydrogen sulfide, lead, manganese, *vibration*
	Rash	Chromate, cobalt, formaldehyde, heat, nuisance dust, phenolic resins, rosin, *sand, soaps and detergents, water*
	Smell Disturbances	Cresol, hydrogen cyanide, formaldehyde, hydrogen sulfide, nickel, nuisance dusts, sulfur dioxide
	Tremor	Carbon dioxide, carbon monoxide, lead, manganese
	Urine Color Changes	Phenolic compounds
	Pain on Urination	Formaldehyde, phenol and its derivatives
	Vision Changes	Carbon monoxide, cyanide, hydrogen sulfide, lead, methanol, ultraviolet radiation
	Weakness, Depression	Fumes of aluminum, carbon monoxide, cresol, cyanide, hydrogen sulfide, iron, lead, magnesium, manganese, nickel, tin, zinc
Fuel handler (see Petroleum industry worker)		
Furniture finisher, polisher	Conception Difficulty	Benzene, formaldehyde
	Dizziness	Benzene; carbon tetrachloride, methylene chloride, trichloroethylene, and other halogenated hydrocarbon solvents; ethanol; formaldehyde; methanol; petroleum distillates
	Memory Loss, Concentration Changes, and Confusion	Methanol
	Nausea	Benzene, carbon monoxide, halogenated hydrocarbon solvents

(continued)

If You Work in These Occupations	And Are Experiencing	You May Be at Risk from These Agents
Furniture finisher, polisher (*continued*)	Numbness and Weakness in the Arms and Legs	Carbon tetrachloride and other halogenated hydrocarbon solvents; methylene chloride; petroleum distillates
	Vision Changes	Benzene, halogenated hydrocarbon solvents, methanol
	Weakness, Depression	Benzene; carbon tetrachloride and other halogenated hydrocarbon solvents; methylene chloride; petroleum distillates
Furrier, fur dyer	Cough	*Animal hair dust*, p-*phenylenediamine*
Gardener	Conception Difficulty	Arsenic, benzene, chlorinated hydrocarbon insecticides, nicotine
	Diarrhea	Arsenic, benzene hexachloride, pesticides
	Dizziness	Arsenic, benzene, chlorinated hydrocarbon insecticides, nicotine, pesticides, petroleum distillates, organic tin
	Fever/Chills	Certain dinitro derivatives of phenol and cresol
	Headache	Carbon monoxide, chlorinated hydrocarbon insecticides, dinitro derivatives of phenol and cresol, fluorides, pesticides, petroleum distillates, organic tin
	Hearing Changes	Organic tin
	Memory Loss, Concentration Changes, and Confusion	Arsenic, chlorinated hydrocarbon insecticides, nicotine, pesticides, petroleum distillates, thallium, organic tin
	Nausea	Arsenic, pesticides
	Numbness and Weakness in the Arms and Legs	Arsenic, carbon disulfide, chlorinated hydrocarbon insecticides, halogenated hydrocarbon solvents, pesticides, petroleum distillates, thallium, organic tin

(continued)

If You Work in These Occupations	And Are Experiencing	You May Be at Risk from These Agents
	Tremor	Arsenic, chlorinated hydrocarbon insecticides, pesticides, vanadium
Gas producer, worker (natural gas)	Dizziness; Headache	Cyanide, hydrogen sulfide
	Numbness and Weakness in the Arms and Legs	Hydrogen sulfide
	Smell Disturbances	Hydrogen cyanide, hydrogen sulfide
	Vision Changes	Cyanide, hydrogen sulfide
Glass, stained glass, or glassware manufacturer, polisher	Conception Difficulty	Arsenic, cadmium, lead, manganese, *elevated temperatures*
	Diarrhea	Antimony, arsenic, cadmium, lead, magnesium, thallium
	Dizziness	Arsenic, carbon monoxide, hydrogen sulfide, irritant gases, lead, methanol, organic tin, turpentine
	Fever/Chills	Metal oxides such as antimony, arsenic, cadmium, cobalt, lead, magnesium, manganese, nickel, selenium, silver, thallium, tin
	Hair Loss	Arsenic, selenium, thallium
	Headache	Antimony, cadmium, carbon monoxide, chromium, fluorides, hydrogen sulfide, irritant gases, lead, manganese, methanol, nickel, organic tin, turpentine
	Hearing Changes	Arsenic, carbon monoxide, lead, organic tin, turpentine
	Irritation or Dryness of Eyes, Nose, Sinuses, Mouth, or Throat	Antimony, arsenic, cadmium, chromium, cobalt, fluoride, hydrogen sulfide, irritant gases, magnesium, manganese, nickel, selenium, tin, turpentine
	Memory Loss, Concentration Changes, and Confusion	Arsenic, carbon monoxide, lead, methanol, organic tin

(continued)

If You Work in These Occupations	And Are Experiencing	You May Be at Risk from These Agents
Glass, stained glass, or glassware manufacturer, polisher (*continued*)	Nail Abnormalities	Acids, arsenic, carbon monoxide, hydrofluoric acid, turpentine
	Nausea	Cadmium, chromium, hydrogen sulfide, lead
	Numbness and Weakness in the Arms and Legs	Arsenic, carbon monoxide, fluorides, hydrogen sulfide, lead, manganese, thallium, organic tin
	Smell Disturbances	Cadmium, chromium, hydrogen sulfide, irritant gases, nickel, selenium, vanadium
	Tremor	Arsenic, carbon monoxide, lead, manganese, thallium, vanadium
	Pain on Urination	Cadmium, chromium, lead, tin
	Vision Changes	Arsenic, carbon monoxide, hydrogen sulfide, lead, methanol, microwaves, silver, thallium, ultraviolet radiation
	Weakness, Depression	Fumes of antimony, arsenic, carbon monoxide, hydrogen sulfide, lead, magnesium, manganese, nickel, selenium, thallium, tin
Grain elevator worker, fumigator	Conception Difficulty	Ethylene oxide
	Cough	*Flour, grain dust, grain weevil*
	Fever/Chills	Grain dust
	Headache	Carbon dioxide, grain dust
	Tremor	Carbon dioxide; methyl bromide, chloride, and iodide; phosphorus
Gunsmith, hunter, marksman	Fever/Chills	Petroleum distillates
	Headache	Cyanide, lead, noise, petroleum distillates
Gunshot, gun barrel manufacturer	Conception Difficulty	Lead

(*continued*)

If You Work in These Occupations	And Are Experiencing	You May Be at Risk from These Agents
Hairdresser, barber, beautician (see also cosmetologist, manicurist)	Cough	Ammonium persulfate salts, which release ozone and sulfuric acid on contact with water; fluorocarbons; *henna; human hair; orris root; powders*
	Headache	Lead
	Irritation or Dryness of Eyes, Nose, Sinuses, Mouth, or Throat	*Dye exposure*
	Rash	Acrylics; *depilatories;* formaldehyde; *fragrances; glycerol monothioglycolate* in permanent wave preparations; hair dyes; *hair tins and bleaches;* nickel sulfate; *p*-phenylenediamine in hair dyes, nail polishes, and nail glues; *soaps, detergents, and shampoos; water; wave solutions*
	Tremor	Lead
	Vision Changes	Lead, silver, ultraviolet radiation
Health care worker	Conception Difficulty	Ethylene oxide; formaldehyde; ionizing radiation; toluene
	Cough	Bacteria; formalin; glutaraldehyde; hexachlorophene; latex; nitrous oxide; pesticides (pyrethins); microorganisms from ventilating systems; viruses
	Nail Abnormalities	Acrylics
	Rash	Water; soaps and detergents; benzylkonium chloride in disinfectants; chemicals added to rubber in gloves; latex; mercaptobenzothiazole, isopropyl-*p*-phenylenediamine and thiurams in rubber; chlorhexidine; medications; powder; talc
	Vision Changes	Ionizing radiation; laser light; microwaves; ultraviolet radiation
Hydraulic fluid maker	Conception Difficulty	Ethylene glycol ethers

(continued)

If You Work in These Occupations	And Are Experiencing	You May Be at Risk from These Agents
Instrument maker	Hearing Changes; Smell Disturbances; Weakness, Depression	Mercury
	Nail Abnormalities	Thallium
Insulation, enamel manufacturers, workers	Cough	Asbestos, diisocyanates, *fiberglass*, formaldehyde
	Dizziness	Cresol, formaldehyde
	Headache	Formaldehyde, solvents (chlorinated hydrocarbons, toluene)
	Irritation or Dryness of Eyes, Nose, Sinuses, Mouth, or Throat	Toluene diisocyanate
	Memory Loss, Concentration Changes, and Confusion	Cresol
	Smell Disturbances	Cresol, formaldehyde, selenium
Jeweler, jewelry manufacturer	Conception Difficulty	Arsenic, benzene, cadmium, lead, mercury
	Diarrhea	Arsenic, cadmium, lead, mercury, nickel
	Dizziness	Arsenic, benzene, cyanide, irritant gases, lead, methanol
	Fever/Chills	Metal oxides such as aluminum, arsenic, cadmium, lead, mercury, nickel, selenium, silver, thallium, zinc
	Hair Loss	Thallium
	Headache	Benzene, cadmium, cyanide, irritant gases, lead, mercury, methanol, nickel
	Hearing Changes	Arsenic, lead, mercury
	Irritation or Dryness of Eyes, Nose, Sinuses, Mouth, or Throat	Arsenic, cadmium, epoxy resins, irritant gases, nickel, selenium, silver
	Memory Loss, Concentration Changes, and Confusion	Arsenic, cyanide, lead, mercury, methanol, thallium

(continued)

If You Work in These Occupations	And Are Experiencing	You May Be at Risk from These Agents
	Nail Abnormalities	Acids, arsenic, silver, thallium
	Nausea	Arsenic, benzene, cadmium, lead, mercury, selenium
	Numbness and Weakness in the Arms and Legs	Arsenic, lead, thallium
	Rash	Acrylics, *adhesives*, epoxy resin, *gold chloride*, hydrofluoric acid, mercury, *metal cleaners and polishes*, nickel sulfate, potassium dichromate, *solvents*
	Smell Disturbances	Cadmium, chromium, hydrogen cyanide, irritant gases, mercury, nickel
	Tremor	Arsenic, lead, mercury, thallium
	Pain on Urination	Cadmium, lead, mercury
	Vision Changes	Benzene, cyanide, laser light, lead, methanol, silver, thallium
	Weakness, Depression	Fumes of aluminum, arsenic, benzene, cadmium, cyanide, lead, mercury, nickel, selenium, thallium, zinc
Laboratory worker, pathologist	Conception Difficulty	Ethylene, oxide, formaldehyde, ionizing radiation, mercury, n-hexane, toluene, xylene
	Cough	*Animal dander*, glutaraldehyde, *hair*, *mites*, *skin scales*, *small insects*, *urine protein*
	Dizziness	Aniline, cyanide, ethanol, formaldehyde, xylene
	Fever/Chills	Dimethyl sulfoxide
	Headache	Aniline, cyanide, ethanol, formaldehyde, mercury, *potassium*, *sodium*, xylene
	Hearing Changes	Mercury, xylene

(continued)

If You Work in These Occupations	And Are Experiencing	You May Be at Risk from These Agents
Laboratory worker, pathologist (*continued*)	Irritation or Dryness of Eyes, Nose, Sinuses, Mouth, or Throat	Acrylics, epichlorohydrin, formaldehyde, glutaraldehyde, ultraviolet radiation
	Memory Loss, Concentration Changes, and Confusion	Cyanide, mercury, xylene
	Nail Abnormalities	Acrylics, aniline, formaldehyde
	Nausea	Xylene
	Numbness and Weakness in the Arms and Legs	Ethanol, organic mercury
	Rash	*Acetone; acids;* acrylics; carbamates, *mercaptobenzothiazole, isopropyl-p-phenylenediamine,* and *thiurams* in rubber; chromates; epoxy resins; formaldehyde; *formalin;* mercury; *p*-phenylenediamine; *water*
	Smell Disturbances	Cyanide, DMSO, formaldehyde, irritant gases, mercury
	Tremor	Ethanol, mercury, xylene
	Pain on Urination	Aniline, formaldehyde
	Vision Changes	Cyanide, ionizing radiation, methylmercury, ultraviolet radiation, xylene
	Weakness, Depression	Aniline, cyanide, ethanol, mercury, xylene
Laundry worker	Cough	Enzymes from bacteria (*Bacillus subtilis*)
	Rash	*Bleaches;* carbamates, *mercaptobenzothiazole, isopropyl-p-phenylenediamine* and *thiurams* in rubber; fabric softeners; soaps and detergents; spray starch and solvents; stain removers
Lamp manufacturer	Headache	Cadmium, mercury
	Hearing Changes	Mercury

(continued)

If You Work in These Occupations	And Are Experiencing	You May Be at Risk from These Agents
	Smell Disturbances	Cadmium, mercury
Leather worker, tanner, fur processor	Conception Difficulty	Arsenic, benzene, boric acid, formaldehyde, mercury, xylene
	Cough	Chromium, irritant gases
	Diarrhea	Antimony, arsenic, boric acid, borax, carbon tetrachloride, fluorocarbons, halogenated hydrocarbon solvents, magnesium
	Dizziness	Aniline; arsenic; benzene; carbon tetrachloride, trichloroethylene, dimethylformamide, and other halogenated hydrocarbon solvents; cresol; cyanide; formaldehyde; hydrogen sulfide; irritant gases; methanol; petroleum distillates; organic tin, xylene
	Fever/Chills	Petroleum distillates
	Hair Loss	Arsenic, boric acid
	Headache	Aniline; antimony; benzene; boric acid and borax; carbon dioxide; carbon tetrachloride; chromium; cresol; cyanide; fluorides; formaldehyde; glycols; halogenated hydrocarbon solvents, including trichloroethylene; hydrogen sulfide; irritant gases; mercury; methanol; petroleum distillates; organic tin; xylene
	Hearing Changes	Arsenic, lead, mercury, organic tin, trichloroethylene in combination with noise, xylene
	Irritation or Dryness of Eyes, Nose, Sinuses, Mouth, or Throat	Acrylics, antimony, arsenic, carbon tetrachloride, halogenated hydrocarbon solvents, irritant gases, magnesium
	Memory Loss, Concentration Changes, and Confusion	Arsenic; cyanide; cresol; halogenated hydrocarbon solvents including carbon tetrachloride and

(continued)

If You Work in These Occupations	And Are Experiencing	You May Be at Risk from These Agents
Leather worker, tanner, fur processor (*continued*)		trichloroethylene; mercury; methanol; naphthalene; petroleum distillates; organic tin; xylene
	Nail Abnormalities	Acids, acrylics, aniline, arsenic, chromium salts, formaldehyde, hydrofluoric acid, methanol
	Nausea	Benzene, boric acid, carbon tetrachloride, dimethylformamide, halogenated hydrocarbon solvents, trichloroethylene, xylene
	Numbness and Weakness in the Arms and Legs	Arsenic, carbon tetrachloride and other halogenated hydrocarbon solvents, hydrogen sulfide, petroleum distillates, organic tin
	Rash	*Acids and alkalis;* acrylics; carbamates, *mercaptobenzothiazole, isopropyl*-p-*phenylenediamine,* and *thiurams* in rubber; formaldehyde; tanning agents (glutaraldehyde); halogenated hydrocarbon solvents; *lime;* mercury; petroleum distillates; potassium dichromate; *resorcinol; vegetable tannins* from plants
	Smell Disturbances	Benzene, chromium, cyanide-containing compounds, formaldehyde, halogenated hydrocarbon solvents, hydrogen sulfide gas, irritant gases and mists (ammonia, hydrogen chloride, sulfur dioxide, and sulfuric acid), mercury, vanadium
	Tremor	Carbon dioxide, carbon tetrachloride, mercury, trichloroethylene, vanadium, xylene
	Urine Color Changes	Halogenated hydrocarbon solvents
	Vision Changes	Arsenic, benzene, carbon tetrachloride, cyanide, halogenated

(*continued*)

If You Work in These Occupations	And Are Experiencing	You May Be at Risk from These Agents
		hydrocarbon solvents, hydrogen sulfide, methanol, phenol, trichloroethylene, xylene
	Weakness, Depression	Aniline, benzene, boric acid and boron compounds, carbon tetrachloride, cresol, cyanide, hydrogen sulfide, mercury, petroleum distillates, tin, trichloroethylene, xylene
Lens, prism manufacturer	Nail Abnormalities; Weakness, Depression	Thallium
Linoleum manufacturer, worker	Conception Difficulty	Benzene
	Cough	Diisocyanates, petroleum distillates
	Dizziness	Benzene, carbon tetrachloride, methanol, petroleum distillates
	Fever/Chills	Petroleum distillates
	Headache	Carbon tetrachloride, methanol, petroleum distillates
	Irritation or Dryness of Eyes, Nose, Sinuses, Mouth, or Throat	Toluene diisocyanate
	Memory Loss, Concentration Changes, and Confusion	Carbon tetrachloride, methanol, petroleum distillates
	Nausea	Benzene, carbon tetrachloride
	Numbness and Weakness in the Arms and Legs	Carbon tetrachloride, petroleum distillates
	Tremor	Carbon tetrachloride
	Vision Changes	Benzene, carbon tetrachloride, methanol
	Weakness, Depression	Benzene, carbon tetrachloride, petroleum distillates
Lithographer	Conception Difficulty	Arsenic, benzene, lead
	Dizziness	Arsenic, benzene, hydrogen sulfide, lead, methanol, petroleum distillates, turpentine

(continued)

If You Work in These Occupations	And Are Experiencing	You May Be at Risk from These Agents
Lithographer (*continued*)	Headache	Benzene, cadmium, chromium, copper, hydrogen sulfide, lead, methanol, petroleum distillates, turpentine
	Memory Loss, Concentration Changes, and Confusion	Arsenic, lead, methanol, petroleum distillates
	Numbness and Weakness in the Arms and Legs	Arsenic, hydrogen sulfide, lead, petroleum distillates
	Tremor	Arsenic, lead
	Vision Changes	Arsenic, benzene, hydrogen sulfide, lead, methanol[b], ultraviolet radiation
	Weakness, Depression	Benzene, hydrogen sulfide, lead, petroleum distillates
Livestock farmer	Cough	*Grain dust, fungi, bacteria, moldy hay, silo disease*
	Fever/Chills	Grain dust
Longshoreman	Cough; Fever/Chills; Headache	*Grain dust*
Lubricant worker	Fever/Chills; Weakness, Depression	Fluorocarbon polymers
Lumber mill worker, logger	Cough	*Fungi* in wood pulp; wood dust
	Hearing Changes	Noise, vibration
	Rash	Carbamates, *mercaptobenzothiazole, isopropyl-*p-*phenylenediamine,* and *thiurams* in rubber; *pesticides and fungicides;* insects (including those that cause Lyme disease); poison ivy/oak/sumac and other plants; *stains; water; wood*
Machinist	Headache	Halogenated hydrocarbon solvents
	Rash	Carbamates, *mercaptobenzothiazole, isopropyl-*p-*phenylenediamine,* and *thiurams* in rubber; chromates; halogenated hydrocarbon solvents; *tert-butylphenol* in greases;

(continued)

If You Work in These Occupations	And Are Experiencing	You May Be at Risk from These Agents
		p-*chloro-m-xylenol* in cutting fluids; rosin
	Tremor	Halogenated hydrocarbon solvents
	Vision Changes	Halogenated hydrocarbon solvents
	Weakness, Depression	Halogenated hydrocarbon solvents
Military personnel	Conception Difficulty	Ionizing radiation
	Headache	Noise
	Hearing Changes	Noise, *vibration*
	Vision Changes	Ionizing radiation, ultraviolet radiation
Miller	Cough	*Flour, grain dust, grain weevil,* silica
	Fever/Chills	Grain dust
	Headache	Grain dust, noise
Miner	Conception Difficulty	Arsenic, cadmium, ionizing radiation, lead, manganese, mercury
	Cough	Coal dust, chromium, hydrogen sulfide, silica
	Diarrhea	Antimony, cadmium, lead, nickel
	Dizziness	Carbon monoxide, hydrogen sulfide, lead, nitrites and nitrates, nitrogen (in coal miners)
	Headache	Antimony, cadmium, carbon dioxide, carbon monoxide, chromium, cresol, cyanide, fluorides, hydrogen sulfide, irritant gases, lead, manganese, mercury, nickel, nitrites and nitrates
	Hearing Changes	Arsenic, carbon monoxide, cresol, lead, mercury, noise, *vibration*
	Irritation or Dryness of Eyes, Nose, Sinuses, Mouth, or Throat	Chromium, hydrogen sulfide, iron dusts and fumes, nickel, nuisance dusts, tin

(continued)

If You Work in These Occupations	And Are Experiencing	You May Be at Risk from These Agents
Miner (*continued*)	Memory Loss, Concentration Changes, and Confusion	Arsenic, carbon monoxide, cresol, cyanide, lead, mercury, thallium
	Nail Abnormalities	Arsenic, hydrofluoric acid, thallium
	Numbness and Weakness in the Arms and Legs	Carbon monoxide, hydrogen sulfide, lead, manganese
	Smell Disturbances	Cadmium, chromium, cresol, cyanide salts, hydrogen selenide gas, hydrogen sulfide, irritant gases, mercury, nickel, nuisance dusts, selenium, vanadium
	Pain on Urination	Cadmium, chromium, lead, mercury, tin
	Vision Changes	Carbon monoxide, hydrogen sulfide, ionizing radiation, lead, ultraviolet radiation
	Weakness, Depression	Carbon monoxide, hydrogen sulfide, lead, mercury, nickel, nitrites, radon, tin
Mirror manufacturer	Conception Difficulty	Benzene, formaldehyde, lead
	Dizziness; Headache	Benzene, cyanide, formaldehyde, irritant gases, lead
	Hearing Changes	Lead, mercury
	Memory Loss, Concentration Changes, and Confusion	Cyanide, lead
	Nail Abnormalities	Formaldehyde, silver
	Numbness and Weakness in the Arms and Legs; Tremor	Lead
	Smell Disturbances	Cyanide, formaldehyde, halogenated hydrocarbon solvents, irritant gases, mercury
	Vision Changes	Benzene, cyanide, lead, silver
	Weakness, Depression	Benzene, cyanide, lead
Moth repellent worker	Memory Loss, Concentration Changes, and Confusion	Naphthalene

(*continued*)

If You Work in These Occupations	And Are Experiencing	You May Be at Risk from These Agents
Mushroom worker	Cough	*Bacterial allergens* found in moldy compost
Musician	Headache; Hearing Changes	Noise
	Rash (hematoma)	Nickel; rosin; *woods* including ebony, rosewood, cocobolo, and African blackwood
Nail polish manufacturer	Conception Difficulty	Ethylene glycol ethers
Navigator	Vision Changes	Microwaves
Nuclear industry worker	Conception Difficulty	Cadmium, ionizing radiation
	Dizziness	Hydrogen sulfide
	Headache	Hydrogen sulfide
	Nausea	Cadmium, hydrogen sulfide
	Numbness and Weakness in the Arms and Legs	Hydrogen sulfide
	Smell Disturbances	Cadmium, hydrogen sulfide
	Tremor	Vanadium
	Vision Changes	Hydrogen sulfide, ionizing radiation
	Weakness, Depression	Hydrogen sulfide
Office worker	Dizziness	Video display terminals
	Rash	Carbamates, *mercaptobenzothiazole, isopropyl-p-phenylenediamine, and thiurams* in rubber; inks; low humidity in modern office buildings can cause itchy, red, scaly patches on the skin; nickel sulfate; *papers*, especially carbonless paper; *soaps and detergents*
	Vision Changes	Video display terminals
	Weakness, Depression	Solvents in correction fluids and in copy machine toner
Oil extractors	Cough	*Castor bean meal, cotton seed, linseed*

(continued)

If You Work in These Occupations	And Are Experiencing	You May Be at Risk from These Agents
Oil well prospector, oil field worker	Conception Difficulty	Ionizing radiation
	Weakness, Depression	Hydrogen sulfide
	Vision Changes	Hydrogen sulfide, ionizing radiation, ultraviolet radiation
Oil, wax preparer	Memory Loss, Concentration Changes, and Confusion	Carbon monoxide from methylene chloride; methyl bromide
Optical lens, prism maker	Hair Loss; Vision Changes	Thallium
Paint, lacquer, pigment, or varnish user, remover, or manufacturer	Conception Difficulty	Arsenic, benzene, boric acid, cadmium, carbon disulfide, epichlorohydrin, ethylene glycol ethers, formaldehyde, lead, manganese, mercury, polychlorinated biophenyls (PCBs), styrene, toluene, xylene
	Cough	Diisocyanates, *dimethyl ethanolamine*, petroleum distillates, silica
	Diarrhea	Boric acid, cadmium, carbon tetrachloride, halogenated hydrocarbon solvents, lead, turpentine
	Dizziness	Aniline; arsenic; benzene; carbon disulfide; carbon monoxide; carbon tetrachloride, trichloroethylene, and other halogenated hydrocarbon solvents; cresol; ethanol; formaldehyde; irritant gases; ketones; lead; methanol; petroleum distillates; styrene; organic tin; toluene; turpentine; xylene
	Fever/Chills	Petroleum distillates
	Hair Loss	Arsenic, boric acid, selenium, thallium
	Headache	Aniline; benzene; boric acid; cadmium; carbon disulfide; carbon monoxide; chromium; copper;

(continued)

If You Work in These Occupations	And Are Experiencing	You May Be at Risk from These Agents
		cresol; ethanol; formaldehyde; glycols; halogenated hydrocarbon solvents including carbon tetrachloride and trichloroethylene; irritant gases; lead; manganese; mercury; methanol; nickel; petroleum distillates; styrene; organic tin; toluene; turpentine; xylene
	Hearing Changes	Arsenic; carbon monoxide (paint stripper); carbon disulfide in combination with noise; cresol; lead; mercury; styrene; organic tin; toluene; trichloroethylene in combination with noise; turpentine; xylene
	Irritation or Dryness of Eyes, Nose, Sinuses, Mouth, or Throat	Acrylics, arsenic, cadmium, carbon tetrachloride, chromium, diisocyanates, epoxy resins, halogenated hydrocarbon solvents, irritant gases, toluene diisocyanate, turpentine
	Memory Loss, Concentration Changes, and Confusion	Arsenic; carbon monoxide; cresol; halogenated hydrocarbon solvents including carbon tetrachloride and trichloroethylene; lead; mercury; methanol; petroleum distillates; *solvent mixtures;* styrene; thallium; organic tin; toluene; xylene
	Nail Abnormalities	Acrylics, aniline, arsenic, chromium salts, formaldehyde, thallium, turpentine
	Nausea	Arsenic, benzene, cadmium, carbon disulfide, chromium, halogenated hydrocarbon solvents
	Numbness and Weakness in the Arms and Legs	Arsenic, carbon disulfide, carbon monoxide, carbon tetrachloride and other halogenated hydrocarbon solvents, ethanol, methyl *n*-butyl ketone, lead, manganese, petroleum distillates, styrene, thallium, organic tin

(continued)

If You Work in These Occupations	And Are Experiencing	You May Be at Risk from These Agents
Paint, lacquer, pigment, or varnish user, remover, or manufacturer (*continued*)	Smell Disturbances	Acetates (butyl acetate, ethyl acetate, and PGMEA[a]), benzene and other petroleum distillates, cadmium, carbon disulfide, chromium, cresol, formaldehyde, halogenated hydrocarbon solvents, hydrazine, hydrogen cyanide, hydrogen sulfide, irritant gases (ammonia, chlorine, phosgene, and ozone), mercury, methyl bromide, nickel, selenium, vanadium
	Rash	Acrylics; chromates; cobalt; epoxy resin; halogenated hydrocarbon solvents; mercury; nickel; *paint pigments*, including chloro-*p*-nitraniline, F4R red, hansa yellow, para red, and toluidine red; *paint removers and strippers*; petroleum distillates; phenolic resins; *p*-phenylenediamine; potassium dichromate; rosin; *soaps and detergents*; solvents; turpentine; water
	Tremor	Arsenic, carbon disulfide, carbon monoxide (released as a by-product of metabolism of methylene chlorine), carbon tetrachloride, ethanol, lead, manganese, mercury, thallium, toluene, trichloroethylene, vanadium, xylene
	Urine Color Changes	Turpentine
	Vision Changes	Arsenic, benzene, carbon disulfide, carbon monoxide (paint stripper), carbon tetrachloride, halogenated hydrocarbon solvents, lead, methanol, thallium, toluene, trichloroethylene, ultraviolet radiation, xylene

(continued)

If You Work in These Occupations	And Are Experiencing	You May Be at Risk from These Agents
	Weakness, Depression	Benzene; boric acid; carbon disulfide, carbon monoxide; carbon tetrachloride, trichloroethylene, and other halogenated hydrocarbon solvents; cresol; ethanol; lead; mercury; nickel; petroleum distillates; styrene; thallium; tin; toluene; xylene
Paper, pulp manufacturer, worker	Conception Difficulty	Formaldehyde, mercury, polychlorinated biphenyls (PCBs)
	Dizziness	Carbon monoxide, formaldehyde, hydrogen sulfide, irritant gases, ketones, organic tin
	Fever/Chills	Dimethyl sulfoxide
	Headache	Carbon monoxide, chromium, formaldehyde, hydrogen sulfide, irritant gases, mercury, organic tin
	Hearing Changes	Carbon monoxide, lead, mercury, noise, organic tin
	Memory Loss, Concentration Changes, and Confusion	Carbon monoxide, mercury, organic tin
	Nail Abnormalities	Acrylics, chromium salts, hydrofluoric acid, formaldehyde; acids and alkalis may damage nails
	Numbness and Weakness in the Arms and Legs	Carbon monoxide, hydrogen sulfide, organic tin
	Smell Disturbances	Chromium, DMSO[b], formaldehyde, hydrogen sulfide, irritant gases (ammonia, chlorine, and sulfur dioxide), mercury
	Tremor	Carbon monoxide, mercury
	Vision Changes	Carbon monoxide, hydrogen sulfide, microwaves
	Weakness, Depression	Carbon monoxide, hydrogen sulfide, mercury, tin

(continued)

If You Work in These Occupations	And Are Experiencing	You May Be at Risk from These Agents
Parking attendant	Dizziness; Headache	Carbon monoxide; irritant gases; lead
	Hearing Changes; Memory Loss, Concentration Changes, and Confusion; Numbness and Weakness in the Arms and Legs; Tremor	Carbon monoxide, lead
	Vision Changes; Weakness, Depression	Carbon monoxide
Perfume maker	Conception Difficulty	Toluene, xylene
	Dizziness	Aniline, cresol, ethanol, toluene, trichloroethylene, xylene
	Headache	Aniline, cresol, ethanol, glycols, toluene, trichloroethylene, xylene
	Hearing Changes	Trichloroethylene in combination with noise; toluene; xylene
	Irritation or Dryness of Eyes, Nose, Sinuses, Mouth, or Throat	Acetate
	Memory Loss, Concentration Changes, and Confusion	Toluene, trichloroethylene, xylene
	Nail Abnormalities	Aniline
	Numbness and Weakness in the Arms and Legs	Ethanol
	Smell Disturbances	Acetates (PGMEA[b], butyl acetate, and ethyl acetate)
	Tremor	Ethanol, toluene, trichloroethylene, xylene
	Pain on Urination	Aniline
	Vision Changes	Toluene, trichloroethylene, xylene
	Weakness, Depression	Aniline, cresol, ethanol, toluene, trichloroethylene, xylene
Pesticide manufacturer, applicator	Conception Difficulty	Arsenic; benzene; boric acid; cadmium; carbon disulfide; chlorinated hydrocarbon

(continued)

If You Work in These Occupations	And Are Experiencing	You May Be at Risk from These Agents
		insecticides; dibromo-chloropropane; ethylene dibromide; mercury; nicotine; paraquat and diquat; polychlorinated biphenyls (PCBs)
	Cough	Pyrethrins
	Dizziness	Arsenic; benzene; carbon disulfide; carbon tetrachloride, trichloroethylene, and other halogenated hydrocarbon solvents; chlorinated hydrocarbon insecticides; cresol; cyanide; hydrazines; irritant gases; organic mercury; methyl bromide, chloride, and iodide; nicotine; pesticides; petroleum distillates; pyrethrum, pyrethrins, and pyrethroids; organic tin; turpentine
	Fever/Chills	Certain dinitro derivatives of phenol and cresol, paraquat and diquat, petroleum distillates
	Hair Loss	Arsenic, boric acid, selenium, thallium
	Headache	Benzene; boric acid and boron compounds; cadmium; carbon dioxide; carbon disulfide; chlorinated hydrocarbon insecticides; copper; cyanide; dinitro derivatives of phenol; fluorides; halogenated hydrocarbon solvents including carbon tetrachloride and trichloroethylene; irritant gases; mercury; methyl bromide; chloride, and iodide; nicotine; paraquat and diquat; pesticides; petroleum distillates; organic tin
	Hearing Changes	Arsenic; carbon disulfide in combination with noise; mercury; nicotine; organic tin;

(*continued*)

If You Work in These Occupations	And Are Experiencing	You May Be at Risk from These Agents
Pesticide manufacturer, applicator (*continued*)		trichloroethylene in combination with noise; turpentine
	Memory Loss, Concentration Changes, and Confusion	Arsenic; chlorinated hydrocarbon insecticides; cyanide; halogenated hydrocarbon solvents including carbon tetrachloride and trichloroethylene; mercury; methyl bromide, chloride, and iodide; nicotine; pesticides; petroleum distillates; thallium; organic tin
	Nail Abnormalities	Arsenic, dinitro-*o*-cresol, dinobuton, fluoride, hydrofluoric acid, paraquat and diquat, turpentine
	Nausea	Arsenic, benzene, cadmium, dimethylformamide, fluoride, pesticides (such as paraquat and diquat)
	Numbness and Weakness in the Arms and Legs	Arsenic; carbon disulfide; carbon tetrachloride and other halogenated hydrocarbon solvents; chlorinated hydrocarbon insecticides; fluorides; organic mercury; methyl bromide, chloride, and iodide; pesticides; petroleum distillates; phosphorus; thallium; organic tin
	Rash	Carbamates, *mercaptobenzothiazole*, *isopropyl*-p-*phenylenediamine*, and *thiurams* in rubber; ethylenediamine; formaldehyde; *fumigants;* halogenated hydrocarbons; mercury; nuisance dust; *pesticides;* petroleum distillates; *plants and woods; soap and detergents;* turpentine
	Smell Disturbances	Cadmium, carbon disulfide, cresol, halogenated hydrocarbon solvents, hydrazine, hydrogen cyanide and its salts, irritant gases (phosgene and sulfur dioxide), methyl bromide, nicotine, selenium, vanadium

(continued)

If You Work in These Occupations	And Are Experiencing	You May Be at Risk from These Agents
	Tremor	Arsenic; carbon dioxide; carbon disulfide; carbon tetrachloride; chlorinated hydrocarbon insecticides; mercury; methyl bromide, chloride, and iodide; nicotine; pesticides; phosphorus; thallium; vanadium
	Vision Changes	Arsenic; benzene; carbon disulfide; carbon tetrachloride; cyanide; dinitro derivatives of phenol and cresol; methylmercury; methyl bromide, chloride, and iodide; nicotine; pesticides; thallium
	Weakness, Depression	Benzene; boric acid and boron compounds; carbon disulfide; carbon tetrachloride, trichloroethylene, and other halogenated hydrocarbon solvents; chlorinated hydrocarbon insecticides; cyanide; dinitro derivatives of phenol and cresol; mercury; methyl bromide, chloride, and iodide; pesticides; petroleum distillates; thallium; tin
Petroleum industry worker (includes fuel and propellant manufacturers, handlers, and refiners)	Conception Difficulty	Arsenic; benzene; carbon disulfide; ethanol; ethylene oxide; ionizing radiation; lead; manganese; styrene; toluene; xylene
	Diarrhea	Aluminum; decaborane; halogenated hydrocarbon solvents; pentaborane
	Dizziness	Arsenic; benzene; decaborane and pentaborane; carbon monoxide; carbon disulfide; ethanol; fluorocarbons; halogenated hydrocarbon solvents; hydrazines; hydrogen sulfide; irritant gases; lead; methyl chloride; nickel carbonyl; petroleum distillates; styrene; toluene; turpentine; xylene
	Fever/Chills	Diborane; petroleum distillates

(continued)

If You Work in These Occupations	And Are Experiencing	You May Be at Risk from These Agents
Petroleum industry worker (includes fuel and propellant manufacturers, handlers, and refiners (continued)	Hair Loss	Arsenic
	Headache	Aniline; benzene; carbon monoxide; carbon disulfide; fluorides; halogenated hydrocarbon solvents; hydrogen sulfide; irritant gases; lead; manganese; methyl chloride; nickel; petroleum distillates; styrene; toluene; xylene
	Hearing Changes	Arsenic; carbon disulfide in combination with noise; lead; styrene; toluene; turpentine; xylene
	Memory Loss, Concentration Changes, and Confusion	Arsenic, carbon monoxide; decaborane and pentaborane; halogenated hydrocarbon solvents; lead; methyl chloride; petroleum distillates; styrene; toluene; xylene
	Nail Abnormalities	Aniline; arsenic; hydrofluoric acid
	Nausea	Fluoride; halogenated hydrocarbon solvents; hydrogen sulfide; xylene
	Numbness and Weakness in the Arms and Legs	Arsenic; carbon disulfide; carbon monoxide; ethanol; halogenated hydrocarbon solvents; hydrogen sulfide; lead; manganese; methyl bromide, chloride, and iodide; petroleum distillates; styrene
	Smell Disturbances	Benzene and other petroleum distillates; carbon disulfide; halogenated hydrocarbon solvents; hydrazine; hydrogen sulfide; irritant gases; metal carbonyl dusts
	Tremor	Arsenic; carbon disulfide; carbon monoxide; ethanol; fluorocarbons; halogenated hydrocarbon solvents; lead; manganese; methyl chloride; toluene; xylene
	Urine Color Changes	Halogenated hydrocarbon solvents

(continued)

If You Work in These Occupations	And Are Experiencing	You May Be at Risk from These Agents
	Vision Changes	Arsenic; benzene; carbon disulfide; halogenated hydrocarbon solvents; hydrogen sulfide; ionizing radiation; lead; methyl chloride; toluene; xylene
	Weakness, Depression	Aniline; benzene; carbon disulfide; ethanol; halogenated hydrocarbon solvents; hydrogen sulfide; lead; methyl chloride; nickel; petroleum distillates; styrene; toluene; xylene; zinc
Pharmaceutical chemist, manufacturer	Conception Difficulty	Arsenic, benzene, cadmium, ethylene dibromide, ionizing radiation, manganese, mercury, xylene
	Cough	Antibiotics: *ampicillin, cephalosporins, penicillin, spiramicin, tetracycline*; biological enzymes: *bromelin, flaviastase, pancreatin, pepsin, trypsin; methyldopa; psyllium*
	Dizziness	Aniline, arsenic, benzene, ethanol, fluorocarbons, hydrazines, irritant gases, ketones, organic mercury, methyl chloride, nitrites and nitrates, trichloroethylene, turpentine, xylene
	Headache	Aniline, antimony, benzene, cadmium, carbon dioxide, ethanol, fluorides, irritant gases, manganese, methyl chloride, nitrites and nitrates, trichloroethylene, turpentine, xylene
	Hearing Changes	Arsenic; mercury; styrene; trichloroethylene in combination with noise; turpentine; xylene
	Irritation or Dryness of Eyes, Nose, Sinuses, Mouth, or Throat	Acetate, cadmium, ethylenediamine, fluorocarbons, hydrazines, magnesium, phenol, ultraviolet radiation

(continued)

If You Work in These Occupations	And Are Experiencing	You May Be at Risk from These Agents
Pharmaceutical chemist, manufacturer (*continued*)	Memory Loss, Concentration Changes, and Confusion	Arsenic; mercury; methyl chloride; thallium; trichloroethylene; xylene
	Nail Abnormalities	Aniline, arsenic, hydrofluoric acid, microwaves, thallium, turpentine
	Numbness and Weakness in the Arms and Legs	Arsenic; ethanol; manganese; organic mercury; methyl bromide, chloride, and iodide; thallium
	Rash	Chemicals in rubber gloves, such as carbamates, *mercaptobenzothiazole, isopropyl*-p-*phenylenediamine*, and *thiurams;* cobalt; ethylenediamine; mercury; *p*-phenylenediamine; turpentine
	Smell Disturbances	Acetates (butyl acetate, ethyl acetate, and PGMEA[a]), cadmium, hydrazine, irritant gases
	Tremor	Arsenic; carbon dioxide; ethanol; fluorocarbons; manganese; mercury; methyl chloride; thallium; trichloroethylene; xylene
	Vision Changes	Arsenic, benzene, ionizing radiation, methyl chloride, methylmercury, microwaves, silver, thallium, trichloroethylene, ultraviolet radiation, xylene
	Weakness, Depression	Aniline, benzene, ethanol, mercury, methyl chloride, nitrites, thallium, trichloroethylene, xylene
Photographic chemical manufacturer, photographer, film processor	Conception Difficulty	Benzene, boric acid, cadmium, formaldehyde, lead, mercury
	Cough	*Ethylenediamine*, *p*-phenylenediamine, *platinum*, selenium, silver
	Diarrhea	Boric acid, cadmium, fluoride, lead, mercury

(*continued*)

If You Work in These Occupations	And Are Experiencing	You May Be at Risk from These Agents
	Dizziness	Aniline, benzene, carbon monoxide, cresol, cyanide, formaldehyde, hydrazines, irritant gases, ketones, lead, methylene chloride, trichloroethylene
	Fever/Chills	Certain dinitro derivatives of phenol and cresol
	Hair Loss	Selenium
	Headache	Aniline, benzene, boric acid, cadmium, carbon monoxide, chromium, cresol, cyanide, dinitro derivatives of phenol, fluorides, formaldehyde, irritant gases, lead, mercury, trichloroethylene
	Hearing Changes	Lead, mercury, trichloroethylene
	Memory Loss, Concentration Changes, and Confusion	Carbon monoxide, cresol, cyanide, lead, mercury, trichloroethylene
	Nail Abnormalities	Acids and alkalis, aniline, chromium salts, fluorides, formaldehyde, methanol, silver; photographic developer
	Nausea	Benzene, boric acid, cadmium, fluoride, mercury, trichloroethylene
	Numbness and Weakness in the Arms and Legs	Carbon monoxide from methylene chloride, lead
	Rash	*Acids, alkalis, water;* chemicals in rubber gloves, such as carbamates, *mercaptobenzothiazole, isopropyl-p-phenylenediamine,* and *thiurams;* chromates; cobalt; *color developers CD-2, -3, and -4;* ethylenediaminetetra-acetic acid; formaldehyde; *hydroquinone* in developers; mercury
	Smell Disturbances	Acetates (butyl acetate, ethyl acetate, and PGMEA[a]), cadmium, chromium, cyanide compounds,

(continued)

If You Work in These Occupations	And Are Experiencing	You May Be at Risk from These Agents
Photographic chemical manufacturer, photographer, film processor (continued)		formaldehyde, halogenated hydrocarbon solvents, hydrazine, irritant gases, mercury, vanadium
	Tremor	Carbon monoxide, lead, methylene chloride, mercury, trichloroethylene, vanadium
	Pain on Urination	Cadmium, chromium, formaldehyde, lead, mercury
	Vision Changes	Benzene, cyanide, dinitro derivatives of phenol and cresol, lead, methanol, silver, trichloroethylene
	Weakness, Depression	Aniline, benzene, boric acid, cresol, cyanide, dinitro derivatives of phenol and cresol, lead, mercury, methylene chloride, trichloroethylene
Plastics, resin, and polyurethane manufacturer, worker	Conception Difficulty	Benzene; carbon disulfide; ethylene glycol ethers; ethylene dibromide; ethylene oxide; epichlorohydrin; formaldehyde; ionizing radiation; lead; polybrominated biphenyls (PBBs); styrene; vinyl chloride; xylene
	Cough	*Anhydrides*, diisocyanates, *epoxy resins*, formaldehyde
	Diarrhea	Aluminum
	Dizziness	Aniline; benzene; carbon disulfide; cresol; cyanide; fluorocarbons; formaldehyde; hydrazines; irritant gases; ketones; lead; methylene chloride; polybrominated biphenyls (PBBs); organic tin; styrene; trichloroethylene; turpentine; vinyl chloride; xylene
	Fever/Chills	Fluorocarbon polymers; metal oxides such as aluminum, cobalt, nickel, selenium, tin, zinc

(continued)

If You Work in These Occupations	And Are Experiencing	You May Be at Risk from These Agents
	Hair Loss	Selenium
	Headache	Aniline; benzene; cadmium; carbon disulfide; carbon monoxide; fluorides; formaldehyde; glycols; irritant gases; nickel; organic tin; styrene; trichloroethylene; turpentine; vinyl chloride; xylene
	Hearing Changes	Cresol, styrene, organic tin, xylene
	Irritation or Dryness of Eyes, Nose, Sinuses, Mouth, or Throat	Aluminum; cresol; diisocyanates; *fluorocarbons;* phenolic resins; selenium; tin; toluene diisocyanate; zinc
	Memory Loss, Concentration Changes, and Confusion	Carbon monoxide; cresol; cyanide; naphthalene; organic tin; styrene; trichloroethylene; xylene
	Nail Abnormalities	Acrylics (plexiglass); aniline; hydrofluoric acid; formaldehyde; turpentine; vinyl chloride
	Nausea	Dimethylformamide, polytetrafluoroethylene (Teflon, Silverstone)
	Numbness and Weakness in the Arms and Legs	Carbon disulfide; lead; methylene chloride; methyl *n*-butyl ketone; styrene; organic tin; vinyl chloride
	Rash	Catalysts; cobalt; epoxy resins; ethylenediamine; phenolic resins; rosin; turpentine
	Smell Disturbances	Acetates (PGMEA[a], butyl acetate, and ethyl acetate), carbon disulfide, cresol, formaldehyde, hydrogen cyanide, hydrazine, irritant gases (ammonia and chlorine), nickel, selenium
	Tremor	Carbon disulfide; fluorocarbons; methylene chloride; trichloroethylene; xylene
	Pain on Urination	Aniline, formaldehyde, glycols, phenol and its derivatives, tin

(*continued*)

If You Work in These Occupations	And Are Experiencing	You May Be at Risk from These Agents
Plastics, resin, and polyurethane manufacturer, worker (*continued*)	Vision Changes	Carbon disulfide; cyanide; ionizing radiation; microwaves; trichloroethylene; ultraviolet radiation; xylene
	Weakness, Depression	Aniline; benzene; carbon disulfide; cresol (phenol and phenolic compounds); cyanide; fluorocarbon polymers; fumes of aluminum, cadmium, cobalt, nickel, selenium, tin, zinc; methylene chloride; polybrominated biphenyls (PBBs); styrene; trichloroethylene; vinyl chloride; xylene
Plumber	Conception Difficulty; Diarrhea	Arsenic, lead
	Cough	Asbestos
	Dizziness	Arsenic, carbon monoxide, lead
	Fever/Chills	Fumes of metal oxides such as arsenic, copper, lead
	Headache	Carbon monoxide, copper, lead
	Hearing Changes	Lead, methylene chloride
	Irritation or Dryness of Eyes, Nose, Sinuses, Mouth, or Throat	Arsenic
	Memory Loss, Concentration Changes, and Confusion	Arsenic, carbon monoxide, lead
	Nail Abnormalities	Solvents; acids and alkalis may also damage nails
	Nausea	Arsenic, carbon monoxide, copper, lead, zinc (from solder); hydrogen sulfide (from sewage)
	Numbness and Weakness in the Arms and Legs	Arsenic, carbon monoxide, lead
	Rash	Chemicals in rubber such as carbamates, *mercaptobenzothiazole, isopropyl*-p-*phenylenediamine,* and *thiurams;* epoxy resin; formaldehyde; *hand cleaners;* rosin;

(continued)

If You Work in These Occupations	And Are Experiencing	You May Be at Risk from These Agents
		metal cleaners; soaps and detergents; sodium hydroxide in drain openers; *soldering flux; water*
	Tremor	Arsenic, carbon monoxide, lead
	Urine Color Changes	Carbon monoxide
	Vision Changes	Arsenic, carbon monoxide, lead, solvents
	Weakness, Depression	Carbon monoxide, lead, hydrogen sulfide
Police officer	Conception Difficulty	Lead
	Hearing Loss	Noise, vibration
	Memory Loss, Concentration Changes, and Confusion	Lead
	Rash	Nickel sulfate, potassium dichromate
Polish manufacturer	Headache; Weakness, Depression	Cyanide
	Hearing Changes; Nail Abnormalities	Turpentine
Postal worker	Rash	Carbamates, *mercaptobenzothiazole, isopropyl-p-phenylenediamine,* and *thiurams* in rubber; formaldehyde; *paper; p*-phenylenediamine in stamp ink; potassium dichromate; rosin
Precision Caster (see Forging press operator)		
Preservative manufacturer, user, food preserver	Conception Difficulty; Dizziness; Tremor; Weakness, Depression	Carbon disulfide
	Headache	Carbon disulfide, copper, irritant gases
	Numbness and Weakness in the Arms and Legs	Carbon disulfide; methyl bromide, chloride, and iodide
	Vision Changes	Carbon disulfide, dinitro derivatives of phenol and cresol, ionizing radiation (X rays), methylmercury, methyl bromide

(continued)

If You Work in These Occupations	And Are Experiencing	You May Be at Risk from These Agents
Printer, lithographer	Conception Difficulty	Benzene, ethylene glycol ethers, lead, mercury, polycyclic aromatic hydrocarbons, toluene, xylene
	Cough	*Gum arabic, gum tragacanth*
	Dizziness	Aniline; benzene; carbon tetrachloride, trichloroethylene, and other halogenated hydrocarbon solvents; cyanide; lead; methanol; petroleum distillates; organic tin; toluene; xylene
	Fever/Chills	Petroleum distillates
	Headache	Aniline; benzene; cyanide; glycols; halogenated hydrocarbon solvents including carbon tetrachloride and trichloroethylene; lead; mercury; methanol; noise; petroleum distillates; organic tin; toluene; xylene
	Hearing Changes	Noise in combination with lead, mercury, organic tin, styrene, toluene, trichloroethylene, turpentine, xylene
	Memory Loss, Concentration Changes, and Confusion	Cyanide; halogenated hydrocarbon solvents including carbon tetrachloride and trichloroethylene; lead; mercury; methanol; petroleum distillates; organic tin; toluene; xylene
	Nail Abnormalities	Alkalis, aniline, methanol, solvents, turpentine
	Numbness and Weakness in the Arms and Legs	Carbon tetrachloride, lead, petroleum distillates, organic tin
	Rash	*Beeswax;* chemicals in rubber gloves such as carbamates, *thiurams, mercaptobenzothiazole, isopropyl-p-phenylenediamine,* chromates; *color developers* CD-2 and CD-3; formaldehyde; *inks;*

(continued)

If You Work in These Occupations	And Are Experiencing	You May Be at Risk from These Agents
		mercury; nickel sulfate; *paper*; petroleum distillates; potassium dichromate; turpentine
	Smell Disturbances	Benzene, chromium, cyanide, halogenated hydrocarbon solvents, mercury
	Tremor	Carbon tetrachloride, lead, mercury, toluene, trichloroethylene, xylene
	Vision Changes	Benzene, carbon tetrachloride, cyanide, lead, methanol, toluene, trichloroethylene, ultraviolet radiation, xylene
	Weakness, Depression	Aniline, benzene, carbon tetrachloride, cyanide, lead, mercury, petroleum distillates, tin, toluene, trichloroethylene, xylene
Propellant manufacturer, user (see also Explosives maker)	Dizziness	Carbon tetrachloride and other halogenated hydrocarbon solvents, fluorocarbons, methyl chloride, methylene chloride, nitrites and nitrates
	Headache	Carbon monoxide, carbon tetrachloride, fluorides, methyl chloride, nitrites and nitrates
	Memory Loss, Concentration Changes, and Confusion	Carbon monoxide, carbon tetrachloride, methyl chloride
	Nail Abnormalities	Arsenic; aniline; hydrofluoric acid
	Numbness and Weakness in the Arms and Legs	Carbon monoxide; carbon tetrachloride and other halogenated hydrocarbon solvents; methyl bromide, chloride, and iodide
	Tremor	Carbon tetrachloride, fluorocarbons, methyl chloride, methylene chloride
	Vision Changes	Carbon tetrachloride, halogenated hydrocarbon solvents, methyl chloride

(continued)

If You Work in These Occupations	And Are Experiencing	You May Be at Risk from These Agents
Propellant manufacturer, user (see also Explosives maker) (*continued*)	Weakness, Depression	Carbon tetrachloride, methyl chloride, methylene chloride, nitrites
Railway boxcar loader, shop or track worker	Cough	*Grain dust*
	Fever/Chills	Grain dust
	Vision Changes	Ultraviolet radiation
Refiner, ore processor, metal worker, scrap metal recycler, smelting industry workers	Conception Difficulty	Arsenic, cadmium, ionizing radiation, lead, manganese, mercury
	Cough	Acrolein; fumes of metal oxides such as cobalt and nickel; tungsten carbide; vanadium trioxide; nickel sulfide; platinum salts; vanadium pentoxide
	Diarrhea	Aluminum, antimony, arsenic, boric acid, boron, copper, halogenated hydrocarbon solvents, lead, magnesium, mercury, nickel
	Dizziness	Arsenic; carbon monoxide; carbon tetrachloride, trichloroethylene, and other halogenated hydrocarbon solvents; cyanide; fluorocarbons; irritant gases; lead; methanol; nickel carbonyl; petroleum distillates
	Fever/Chills	Metal oxides such as aluminum, antimony, arsenic, cadmium, cobalt, copper, iron, lead, magnesium, manganese, mercury, nickel, selenium thallium, tin, and zinc; fluorocarbon polymers; petroleum distillates
	Hair Loss	Arsenic; boric acid; selenium; thallium
	Headache	Antimony; boric acid and boron compounds; cadmium; carbon monoxide; chromium; copper;

(*continued*)

If You Work in These Occupations	And Are Experiencing	You May Be at Risk from These Agents
		cresol; cyanide; fluorides; glycols; halogenated hydrocarbon solvents including carbon tetrachloride and trichloroethylene; hydrogen sulfide; irritant gases; lead; manganese; mercury; methanol; nickel; nitrites and nitrates; noise; petroleum distillates
	Hearing Changes	Arsenic; carbon monoxide; cresol; lead; mercury; noise; trichloroethylene in combination with noise; vibration
	Irritation or Dryness of Eyes, Nose, Sinuses, Mouth, or Throat	Aluminum, arsenic, boron, chromium, cobalt, copper, epoxy resins, *fluorocarbons*, iron dusts and fumes, irritant gases, magnesium, nickel, nuisance dusts, tin, vanadium, zinc
	Memory Loss, Concentration Changes, and Confusion	Arsenic; carbon monoxide; cresol; cyanide; halogenated hydrocarbon solvents including carbon tetrachloride and trichloroethylene; lead; mercury; methanol; petroleum distillates; thallium
	Nail Abnormalities	Arsenic; hydrofluoric acid; methanol; acids may soften and damage nails; thallium
	Nausea	Arsenic, lead, mercury
	Numbness and Weakness in the Arms and Legs	Arsenic; carbon monoxide; carbon tetrachloride and other halogenated hydrocarbon solvents; ethanol; fluorides; lead; manganese; petroleum distillates; phosphorus; thallium
	Rash	*Acids, alkalis*, cobalt, epoxy resin, halogenated hydrocarbon solvents, mercury, nickel sulfate, petroleum distillates, potassium dichromate, rosin, *solvents*

(continued)

If You Work in These Occupations	And Are Experiencing	You May Be at Risk from These Agents
Refiner, ore processor, metal worker, scrap metal recycler, smelting industry workers (*continued*)	Smell Disturbances	Cadmium; chromium; cresol; cyanide; halogenated hydrocarbon solvents; hydrogen sulfide; hydrogen selenide gas; irritant gases; mercury; nickel; nuisance dusts; petroleum distillates; selenium; vanadium
	Tremor	Arsenic; carbon monoxide; carbon dioxide; fluorocarbons; lead; manganese; mercury; phosphorus; thallium; vanadium
	Urine Color Changes	Carbon monoxide, copper
	Pain on Urination	Boron, glycols, halogenated hydrocarbons, lead, mercury
	Vision Changes	Arsenic; carbon monoxide; cyanide; halogenated hydrocarbon solvents; hydrogen sulfide; ionizing radiation; laser light; lead; methanol; trichloroethylene; thallium; ultraviolet radiation
	Weakness, Depression	Fumes of aluminum, antimony, arsenic, cadmium, cobalt, copper, cyanide, iron, lead, magnesium, manganese, mercury, nickel, selenium, tin, thallium, zinc; boric acid and boron compounds; carbon monoxide; carbon tetrachloride, trichloroethylene, and other halogenated hydrocarbon solvents; cresol; cyanide; fluorocarbon polymers; mercury; petroleum distillates
Refrigeration worker, refrigerant or propellant manufacturer	Conception Difficulty	Formaldehyde
	Cough	Fluorocarbons (freon)
	Dizziness	Carbon monoxide, carbon tetrachloride and other halogenated hydrocarbon solvents, fluorocarbons, formaldehyde,

(*continued*)

If You Work in These Occupations	And Are Experiencing	You May Be at Risk from These Agents
		irritant gases, methyl bromide and chloride
	Headache	Carbon dioxide, carbon monoxide, carbon tetrachloride, fluorides, formaldehyde, irritant gases, methyl bromide and chloride
	Memory Loss, Concentration Changes, and Confusion	Carbon monoxide, carbon tetrachloride, methyl bromide and chloride
	Numbness and Weakness in the Arms and Legs	Carbon monoxide; carbon tetrachloride and other halogenated hydrocarbon solvents; methyl bromide, chloride, and iodide
	Smell Disturbances	Halogenated hydrocarbon solvents, irritant gases (ammonia, chlorine, sulfur dioxide, and ozone), methyl bromide, nuisance dusts
	Tremor	Carbon dioxide, carbon monoxide, carbon tetrachloride, fluorocarbons, methyl bromide and chloride
	Vision Changes	Carbon monoxide, carbon tetrachloride, halogenated hydrocarbon solvents, methyl bromide and chloride
	Weakness, Depression	Carbon monoxide, carbon tetrachloride, methyl chloride
Restaurant worker	Nail Abnormalities	Microwaves
Rubber worker (latex worker)	Conception Difficulty	Arsenic, benzene, carbon disulfide, chloroprene, formaldehyde, lead, polychlorinated biphenyls (PCBs), polycyclic aromatic hydrocarbons, styrene, vinyl chloride
	Cough	Diisocyanates, silica
	Dizziness	Aniline; arsenic; benzene; decaborane and diborane (boric acid and boron compounds);

(continued)

If You Work in These Occupations	And Are Experiencing	You May Be at Risk from These Agents
Rubber worker (latex worker) (continued)		carbon disulfide; carbon tetrachloride and other halogenated hydrocarbon solvents; cresol, cyanide, ethanol, formaldehyde, hydrazines, hydrogen sulfide, irritant gases, ketones, lead, methanol, methyl chloride, petroleum distillates, styrene, organic tin, turpentine, vinyl chloride
	Fever/Chills	Diborane; metal oxides such as aluminum, antimony, arsenic, cobalt, lead, magnesium, selenium, tin, zinc; petroleum distillates
	Hair Loss	Arsenic, chloroprene, selenium
	Headache	Aniline, antimony, benzene, carbon disulfide, carbon tetrachloride and other halogenated hydrocarbon solvents, cresol, cyanide, ethanol, fluorides, formaldehyde, hydrogen sulfide, irritant gases, lead, methanol, methyl chloride, petroleum distillates, styrene, organic tin, turpentine, vinyl chloride
	Hearing Changes	Arsenic; carbon disulfide in combination with noise; cresol; lead; styrene, organic tin; turpentine
	Irritation or Dryness of Eyes, Nose, Sinuses, Mouth, or Throat	Toluene diisocyanate
	Memory Loss, Concentration Changes, and Confusion	Arsenic, decaborane, carbon tetrachloride, cresol, cyanide, lead, methanol, methyl chloride, petroleum distillates, styrene, organic tin
	Nail Abnormalities	Aniline, arsenic, formaldehyde, methanol, turpentine, vinyl chloride

(continued)

If You Work in These Occupations	And Are Experiencing	You May Be at Risk from These Agents
	Numbness and Weakness in the Arms and Legs	Arsenic; carbon disulfide; carbon tetrachloride and other halogenated hydrocarbon solvents; ethanol; fluorides; hydrogen sulfide; lead; methyl bromide, chloride, and iodide; petroleum distillates; styrene; organic tin; vinyl chloride
	Rash	Carbamates, *mercaptobenzothiazole*, *isopropyl*-p-*phenylenediamine*, and *thiurams* in rubber; cobalt; ethylenediamine; formaldehyde; halogenated hydrocarbon solvents; petroleum distillates; phenolic resins; turpentine
	Smell Disturbances	Benzene, carbon disulfide, chromium, cresol, cyanide, formaldehyde, halogenated hydrocarbon solvents, hydrazine, hydrogen sulfide gas, irritant gases (nitrogen oxides, sulfur dioxide, and hydrogen chloride), nuisance dusts, selenium, vanadium
	Tremor	Arsenic, carbon disulfide, carbon tetrachloride, ethanol, lead, methyl chloride, vanadium
	Vision Changes	Arsenic, benzene, carbon disulfide, carbon tetrachloride, cyanide, halogenated hydrocarbon solvents, hydrogen sulfide, lead, methanol, methyl chloride, microwaves, solvents
	Weakness, Depression	Aniline; arsenic; benzene; diborane (boric acid and boron compounds); carbon disulfide; carbon tetrachloride and other halogenated hydrocarbon solvents; cresol (phenol and phenolic compounds); cyanide; ethanol; fumes of aluminum, antimony, cobalt, lead, magnesium, selenium, tin, zinc; hydrogen sulfide; methyl chloride;

(*continued*)

If You Work in These Occupations	And Are Experiencing	You May Be at Risk from These Agents
Rubber worker (latex worker) (continued)		petroleum distillates; styrene; vinyl chloride
Sandblaster	Cough	Silica
	Smell Disturbances	Nuisance dusts
Seed handler	Numbness and Weakness in the Arms and Legs	Organic mercury
	Vision Changes	Methylmercury
Semiconductor, microchip producer	Conception Difficulty	Arsenic
	Dizziness	Arsenic; arsine gas; borane; halogenated hydrocarbon solvents; organic tin
	Hair Loss	Arsenic, selenium, thallium
	Headache	Fluorides
	Hearing Changes	Arsenic; organic tin
	Memory Loss, Concentration Changes, and Confusion	Arsenic, thallium
	Nail Abnormalities	Arsenic; hydrofluoric acid; methanol; selenium; silver; thallium
	Nausea	Arsenic, fluoride, selenium, thallium
	Numbness and Weakness in the Arms and Legs	Arsenic, thallium; organic tin
	Rash	Acids; carbamates, *mercaptobenzothiazole*, *isopropyl*-p-*phenylenediamine*, and *thiurams* in rubber; epoxy resins; plating chemicals (nickel); rosin; *soldering flux; solvents*
	Smell Disturbances	Nickel; nuisance dusts; selenium
	Tremor	Arsenic, phosphorus, thallium
	Vision Changes	Arsenic, thallium

(continued)

If You Work in These Occupations	And Are Experiencing	You May Be at Risk from These Agents
Septic tank cleaner, sewer worker	Dizziness	Carbon monoxide, hydrogen sulfide, irritant gases
	Headache	Carbon monoxide, hydrogen sulfide, irritant gases
	Hearing Changes	Carbon monoxide
	Memory Loss, Concentration Changes, and Confusion	Carbon monoxide
	Numbness and Weakness in the Arms and Legs	Carbon monoxide, hydrogen sulfide
	Smell Disturbances	Hydrogen sulfide and other irritant gases
	Tremor	Carbon monoxide
	Vision Changes	Carbon monoxide, hydrogen sulfide
	Weakness, Depression	Carbon monoxide, hydrogen sulfide
Shipbuilder, shipyard	Conception Difficulty	Lead, styrene
	Cough	Diisocyanates, dusts of certain woods
	Dizziness; Headache; Hearing Changes; Memory Loss, Concentration Changes, and Confusion; Weakness, Depression	Lead, styrene and other solvents
	Irritation or Dryness of Eyes, Nose, Sinuses, Mouth, or Throat	Toluene diisocyanate
	Numbness and Weakness in the Arms and Legs	Lead, styrene, *vibration*
Shoemaker, repairer	Conception Difficulty	Benzene
	Dizziness	Benzene; carbon tetrachloride, trichloroethylene, and other halogenated hydrocarbon solvents; irritant gases; ketones; methanol; petroleum distillates
	Fever/Chills	Petroleum distillates

(continued)

If You Work in These Occupations	And Are Experiencing	You May Be at Risk from These Agents
Shoemaker, repairer (*continued*)	Headache	Benzene, halogenated hydrocarbon solvents including carbon tetrachloride and trichloroethylene, irritant gases, methanol, petroleum distillates
	Hearing Changes	Trichloroethylene in combination with noise
	Irritation or Dryness of Eyes, Nose, Sinuses, Mouth, or Throat	Acetate, carbon tetrachloride, irritant gases, phenolic resins
	Memory Loss, Concentration Changes, and Confusion	Halogenated hydrocarbon solvents including carbon tetrachloride and trichloroethylene, methanol, petroleum distillates
	Numbness and Weakness in the Arms and Legs	Carbon tetrachloride and other halogenated hydrocarbon solvents, petroleum distillates
	Rash	Carbamates, *mercaptobenzothiazole*, *isopropyl*-p-*phenylenediamine*, and *thiurams* in rubber; *cements*; epoxy resin; formaldehyde; halogenated hydrocarbon solvents; petroleum distillates; phenolic resins; *polishes and dyes*; potassium dichromate; rosin; *solvents*; *stains*
	Smell Disturbances	Acetates (butyl acetate, ethyl acetate, and PGMEA[a]), benzene, halogenated hydrocarbon solvents, irritant gases
	Tremor	Carbon tetrachloride, trichloroethylene
	Urine Color Changes	Carbon tetrachloride
	Pain on Urination	Carbon tetrachloride, p-phenylenediamine
	Vision Changes	Benzene, carbon tetrachloride, halogenated hydrocarbon solvents, methanol, trichloroethylene

(continued)

If You Work in These Occupations	And Are Experiencing	You May Be at Risk from These Agents
	Weakness, Depression	Benzene, halogenated hydrocarbon solvents including trichloroethylene, petroleum distillates
Slaughterhouse worker	Dizziness; Headache; Vision Changes; Weakness, Depression	Hydrogen sulfide
Soap maker	Dizziness; Headache; Vision Changes; Weakness, Depression	Hydrogen sulfide
Solder manufacturer, worker	Conception Difficulty	Arsenic, cadmium, lead
	Cough	Flux that contains aminoethylethanolamine, phosgene
	Dizziness	Arsenic, cyanide, hydrazines, lead
	Fever/Chills	Fumes of metal oxides such as antimony, cadmium, copper, lead, magnesium, silver, zinc
	Headache	Cadmium, copper, cyanide, lead
	Hearing Changes	Arsenic, lead
	Memory Loss, Concentration Changes, and Confusion	Arsenic, cyanide, lead
	Numbness and Weakness in the Arms and Legs	Arsenic, lead
	Rash	*Acids and salts*, nickel sulfate, potassium dichromate, rosin
	Smell Disturbances	Cadmium, cyanide, hydrazine, nuisance dusts
	Tremor	Arsenic, lead
	Vision Changes	Arsenic, cyanide, lead, silver
Solvent worker	Conception Difficulty	Carbon disulfide, epichlorohydrin, *n*-hexane, styrene, toluene, xylene
	Dizziness	Carbon disulfide; carbon tetrachloride, trichloroethylene, and other halogenated hydrocarbon solvents; ethanol; fluorocarbons;

(continued)

If You Work in These Occupations	And Are Experiencing	You May Be at Risk from These Agents
Solvent worker (*continued*)		ketones; styrene; toluene; turpentine; xylene
	Headache	Carbon disulfide, ethanol, fluorides, halogenated hydrocarbon solvents including carbon tetrachloride and trichloroethylene, styrene, toluene, turpentine, xylene
	Hearing Changes	Carbon disulfide in combination with noise; styrene; toluene; trichloroethylene in combination with noise; turpentine; xylene
	Memory Loss, Concentration Changes, and Confusion	Halogenated hydrocarbon solvents including carbon tetrachloride and trichlorethylene, styrene, toluene, xylene
	Numbness and Weakness in the Arms and Legs	Carbon disulfide, carbon tetrachloride, ethanol, methyl *n*-butyl ketone, styrene
	Tremor	Ethanol, fluorocarbons, trichloroethylene and other halogenated hydrocarbon solvents, toluene, xylene
	Vision Changes	Carbon tetrachloride, halogenated hydrocarbon solvents, toluene, trichloroethylene, xylene
	Weakness, Depression	Carbon disulfide; carbon tetrachloride, trichloroethylene, and other halogenated hydrocarbon solvents; ethanol; styrene; toluene; xylene
Spice worker	Cough	*Garlic powder, molds, papain, spices, trypsin*
Stone worker	Cough	Silica
	Smell Disturbances	Nuisance dusts
Sugar refiner	Headache	Irritant gases
Synthetic fabric maker	Nausea	Dimethylformamide

(*continued*)

If You Work in These Occupations	And Are Experiencing	You May Be at Risk from These Agents
Taxidermist	Conception Difficulty	Arsenic, mercury
	Dizziness; Hair Loss; Nail Abnormalities	Arsenic
	Headache	Mercury
	Hearing Changes; Memory Loss, Concentration Changes, and Confusion	Arsenic, mercury
	Nausea	Arsenic, *decaying matter*, formaldehyde, mercury
Tea maker, worker	Cough	*Tea fluff, green leaf tea*
Textile mill worker, textile printer, textile worker	Conception Difficulty	Arsenic, boric acid, cadmium, carbon disulfide, ethylene glycol ethers, ethylene oxide, flame retardants [tris-(2, 3-dibromopropyl) phosphate], formaldehyde, xylene
	Cough	Carbon monoxide; *cotton, flax*, and *hemp* dusts; diisocyanates; petroleum distillates
	Dizziness	Arsenic; carbon disulfide; carbon tetrachloride, trichloroethylene, and other halogenated hydrocarbon solvents; cresol; formaldehyde; hydrazines; hydrogen sulfide; irritant gases; ketones; methylene chloride; petroleum distillates; organic tin; xylene
	Hair Loss	Arsenic, boric acid, selenium
	Headache	Antimony, boric acid, cadmium, carbon dioxide, carbon disulfide, carbon monoxide, chromium, copper, cresol, formaldehyde, glycols, halogenated hydrocarbon solvents including carbon tetrachloride and trichloroethylene, hydrogen sulfide, irritant gases, nickel, noise, petroleum distillates, organotin compounds, xylene

(*continued*)

If You Work in These Occupations	*And Are Experiencing*	*You May Be at Risk from These Agents*
Textile mill worker, textile printer, textile worker (*continued*)	Hearing Changes	Noise in combination with arsenic; carbon disulfide in combination with noise; noise; organic tin; trichloroethylene; xylene
	Irritation or Dryness of Eyes, Nose, Sinuses, Mouth, or Throat	Acrylics, antimony, arsenic, cadmium, carbon tetrachloride, copper, diisocyanates, formaldehyde, hydrogen sulfide, irritant gases, magnesium, naphthalene, nickel, oxalic acid, phenolic resins, selenium, tin, toluene diisocyanate, zinc
	Memory Loss, Concentration Changes, and Confusion	Arsenic, carbon monoxide, cresol, halogenated hydrocarbon solvents including carbon tetrachloride and trichloroethylene, naphthalene, petroleum distillates, organic tin, xylene
	Nail Abnormalities	Acrylics, aniline, arsenic, chromium salts, formaldehyde
	Numbness and Weakness in the Arms and Legs	Arsenic, carbon disulfide, carbon tetrachloride and other halogenated hydrocarbon solvents, hydrogen sulfide, methyl *n*-butyl ketone, methylene chloride, petroleum distillates, organic tin
	Rash	Acrylics; carbamates, *mercaptobenzothiazole*, and *isopropyl*-p-*phenylenediamine*, and *thiurams* in rubber; *detergents*; dyes; formaldehyde; halogenated hydrocarbons; nickel sulfate; petroleum distillates; phenolic resins; resins; rough fibers
	Smell Disturbances	Benzene, cadmium, carbon disulfide, chromium, formaldehyde, halogenated hydrocarbon solvents, hydrazine,

(continued)

If You Work in These Occupations	And Are Experiencing	You May Be at Risk from These Agents
		hydrogen sulfide and other irritant gases, nuisance dusts, vanadium
	Tremor	Arsenic, carbon dioxide, carbon disulfide, carbon tetrachloride, methylene chloride, trichloroethylene, vanadium, xylene
	Vision Changes	Arsenic, carbon disulfide, carbon tetrachloride, halogenated hydrocarbon solvents, hydrogen sulfide, microwaves, trichloroethylene, ultraviolet radiation, xylene
	Weakness, Depression	Boric acid and boron compounds; carbon disulfide; carbon tetrachloride, trichloroethylene, and other halogenated hydrocarbon solvents; cresol; hydrogen sulfide; methylene chloride; nickel; petroleum distillates; tin; xylene; zinc
Theatrical artist	Rash	Adhesives; carbamates, *mercaptobenzothiazole*, *isopropyl*-p-*phenylenediamine*, and *thiurams* in rubber; formaldehyde; fragrance; o-*nitro*-p-*phenylenediamine*, m-*phenylenediamine*, *resorcinol*, and p-*toluenediamine* in hair dyes; *quarternium* 15 and *paraben* mix in cosmetics; rosin; soaps and detergents
Thermometer maker	Hair Loss	Thallium
	Vision Changes	Methyl chloride, thallium
Tobacco processor	Conception Difficulty	Ethylene oxide, nicotine
	Cough	*Green leaf tobacco*
	Dizziness	Nicotine, trichloroethylene
	Headache	Glycols, nicotine, trichloroethylene

(continued)

If You Work in These Occupations	And Are Experiencing	You May Be at Risk from These Agents
Tobacco processor (*continued*)	Hearing Changes	Nicotine, trichloroethylene in combination with noise
	Memory Loss, Concentration Changes, and Confusion	Nicotine, trichloroethylene
	Smell Disturbances	Nicotine, nuisance dusts
	Tremor	Nicotine, trichloroethylene
	Vision Changes	Nicotine, trichloroethylene, ultraviolet radiation
	Weakness, Depression	Trichloroethylene
Tunnel worker, well digger	Dizziness	Carbon monoxide, hydrogen sulfide, nitrites and nitrates, nitrogen
	Headache	Carbon monoxide, hydrogen sulfide, nitrites and nitrates
	Hearing Changes	Carbon monoxide, lead
	Memory Loss, Concentration Changes, and Confusion	Carbon monoxide
	Numbness and Weakness in the Arms and Legs	Carbon monoxide, hydrogen sulfide
	Smell Disturbances	Hydrogen sulfide, nuisance dusts
	Tremor	Carbon monoxide
	Vision Changes	Carbon monoxide, hydrogen sulfide
	Weakness, Depression	Carbon monoxide, hydrogen sulfide, nitrites
Typesetter	Diarrhea; Headache	Antimony
Vacuum tube maker	Headache; Tremor	Carbon disulfide
Varnish, stain worker, manufacturer	Weakness, Depression	Aniline
	Tremor	Ethanol
Vat worker	Headache; Tremor	Carbon dioxide

(*continued*)

If You Work in These Occupations	And Are Experiencing	You May Be at Risk from These Agents
Veterinarian	Conception Difficulty	Ionizing radiation
	Nail Abnormalities	Acrylics
	Rash	*Animal hair;* carbamates, *mercaptobenzothiazole, isopropyl-p-phenylenediamine,* and *thiurams* in rubber; ethylenediamine; germicidal solutions; insecticides; *medications;* potassium dichromate; rosin; soaps and detergents
	Vision Changes	Ionizing radiation; laser light; microwaves; ultraviolet radiation
Videotape producer	Headache	Chromium
Water treatment worker	Conception Difficulty	Manganese
	Dizziness	Hydrazine, irritant gases
	Headache	Carbon dioxide, copper, irritant gases, manganese
	Tremor	Carbon dioxide, manganese
	Vision Changes	Silver
Weld inspector	Conception Difficulty	Ionizing radiation
	Vision Changes	Arsenic, benzene, halogenated hydrocarbon solvents, ionizing radiation, lead, ultraviolet radiation
Welder	Conception Difficulty	Arsenic, benzene, cadmium, ionizing radiation, lead, manganese
	Cough	Chromium hydrofluoric acid, manganese, nickel, nitrogen dioxide, ozone, phosgene
	Diarrhea	Aluminum, antimony, arsenic, cadmium, copper, halogenated hydrocarbon solvents, iron, lead, magnesium, nickel, phosphine
	Dizziness	Arsenic, benzene, halogenated hydrocarbon solvents, irritant gases, lead

(continued)

If You Work in These Occupations	And Are Experiencing	You May Be at Risk from These Agents
Welder (*continued*)	Fever/Chills	Fumes of metal oxides such as aluminum, antimony, arsenic, cadmium, chromium, cobalt, copper, iron, lead, magnesium, manganese, nickel, zinc
	Headache	Antimony, benzene, cadmium, carbon dioxide, chromium, copper, halogenated hydrocarbon solvents, irritant gases, lead, manganese, nickel
	Hearing Changes	Arsenic, carbon monoxide, lead, mercury, trichloroethylene
	Irritation or Dryness of Eyes, Nose, Sinuses, Mouth, or Throat	Aluminum, antimony, arsenic, cadmium, chromium, cobalt, copper, halogenated hydrocarbon solvents, iron dusts and fumes, irritant gases, lead, magnesium, manganese, nickel, vanadium, wood, zinc
	Memory Loss, Concentration Changes, and Confusion	Arsenic, halogenated hydrocarbon solvents, lead
	Nail Abnormalities	Arsenic
	Nausea	Arsenic, benzene, cadmium, halogenated hydrocarbon solvents, lead
	Numbness and Weakness in the Arms and Legs	Arsenic, halogenated hydrocarbon solvents, lead, manganese, phosphorus
	Rash	Carbamates, *mercaptobenzothiazole*, *isopropyl*-p-*phenylenediamine*, and *thiurams* in rubber; cobalt; halogenated hydrocarbon solvents; nickel; potassium dichromate; ultraviolet radiation
	Smell Disturbances	Cadmium, chromium, halogenated hydrocarbon solvents, irritant gases, mercury, nickel, nuisance dusts, selenium

(continued)

If You Work in These Occupations	And Are Experiencing	You May Be at Risk from These Agents
	Tremor	Arsenic, carbon dioxide, halogenated hydrocarbon solvents, lead, manganese, phosphorus, vanadium
	Urine Color Changes	Copper, halogenated hydrocarbon solvents
	Pain on Urination	Cadmium, chromium, halogenated hydrocarbons, lead
	Weakness, Depression	Fumes of aluminum, antimony, arsenic, cadmium, cobalt, copper, iron, lead, magnesium, manganese, nickel, tin, zinc; benzene; halogenated hydrocarbon solvents
	Vision Changes	Arsenic, benzene, halogenated hydrocarbon solvents, ionizing radiation, lead, ultraviolet radiation
Wire coating worker	Cough	Diisocyanates
	Irritation or Dryness of Eyes, Nose, Sinuses, Mouth, or Throat	Toluene diisocyanate
Woodworker, furniture manufacturer, refinisher, preserver	Conception Difficulty	Arsenic, boric acid, dioxins, formaldehyde, *n*-hexane, mercury, polycyclic aromatic hydrocarbons, toluene
	Cough	Adhesives containing diisocyanates, formaldehyde, *fungicides, fungi and fungal spores, sawmill dust*
	Diarrhea	Boric acid
	Dizziness	Arsenic; carbon tetrachloride, trichloroethylene and other halogenated hydrocarbon solvents; cresol; formaldehyde; irritant gases; organic mercury; methanol; petroleum distillates; organic tin; toluene
	Fever/Chills	Certain dinitro derivatives of phenol and cresol, petroleum distillates

(continued)

If You Work in These Occupations	And Are Experiencing	You May Be at Risk from These Agents
Woodworker, furniture manufacturer, refinisher, preserver (*continued*)	Hair Loss	Boric acid
	Headache	Benzene, boric acid and borax, chromium, cresol, dinitro derivatives of phenol and cresol, fluorides, formaldehyde, halogenated hydrocarbon solvents including carbon tetrachloride and trichloroethylene, irritant gases, mercury, methanol, noise, petroleum distillates, organotin compounds, toluene
	Hearing Changes	Arsenic, cresol, mercury, noise, organic tin, *vibration*
	Memory Loss, Concentration Changes, and Confusion	Arsenic, cresol, halogenated hydrocarbon solvents including carbon tetrachloride and trichloroethylene, mercury, methanol, petroleum distillates, organic tin
	Nail Abnormalities	Arsenic, chromium salts, formaldehyde; *ebony* and *mahogany* woods, *paints*, *stains*, and *varnishes* may also discolor the nail
	Nausea	Arsenic, boric acid, carbon tetrachloride, fluorides, formaldehyde, phenol
	Numbness and Weakness in the Arms and Legs	Arsenic, carbon tetrachloride and other halogenated hydrocarbon solvents, fluorides, organic mercury, petroleum distillates, organic tin
	Rash	Carbamates, *mercaptobenzothiazole*, *isopropyl*-p-*phenylenediamine*, and *thiurams* in rubber; epoxy resins; formaldehyde; halogenated hydrocarbon solvents; petroleum distillates; phenolic resins; *p-tert-butylphenol*, ammoniated mercury, and potassium

(continued)

If You Work in These Occupations	And Are Experiencing	You May Be at Risk from These Agents
		dichromate in preservatives; resins; rosin in varnishes, adhesives, solvents, wood bleaches, shellacs, lacquers, varnishes, soaps, and bleaches; sawdust and other nuisance dusts
	Smell Disturbances	Acetates, benzene, chromium, cresol, formaldehyde, halogenated hydrocarbon solvents, irritant gas (ozone), mercury, nuisance dusts
	Tremor	Arsenic, carbon tetrachloride, mercury
	Vision Changes	Arsenic, benzene, carbon tetrachloride, creosote and cresols, dinitro derivatives of phenol and cresol, halogenated hydrocarbon solvents, lead, methanol, methylmercury, microwaves, toluene, trichloroethylene, ultraviolet radiation
	Weakness, Depression	Boric acid and boron compounds; carbon tetrachloride, trichloroethylene, and other halogenated hydrocarbon solvents; cresol; dinitro derivatives of phenol and cresol; mercury; petroleum distillates; tin; toluene
Wool degreaser, scourer	Smell Disturbances	Cresol, irritant gases (sulfur dioxide and phosgene), methyl bromide
X-ray worker, tube maker	Conception Difficulty	Ionizing radiation

[a] Abbreviations used: PGMEA, propylene glycol monomethyl ether acetate; DMSO, dimethylsulfoxide.

Note: Agents listed in italics are not listed in the information sheets, pp. 359–421.

The Sources of Environmental Health Hazards

CHAPTER 13

Water

O f the many compounds necessary for life, none rivals water in importance. Several primitive organisms do not need oxygen, but no life form survives without water. Our bodies are composed of about 65 percent water by weight. Losing just 1 percent of that bodily water makes us feel thirsty; losing 15 percent will kill us.

Water is a collection of molecules, each molecule containing two atoms of hydrogen and one atom of oxygen. Water is nature's universal solvent and has an extraordinary capacity to pick up other substances with which it comes into contact. Pure water, consisting solely of H_2O molecules, exists nowhere in nature.

Water's attraction for other chemicals is vital. Life depends on water's ability to transport nutrients within our cells and to carry away cellular wastes. Some chemicals found naturally in drinking water (e.g., the minerals calcium and magnesium and the metals copper and iron) contribute to nutrition.

Unfortunately, water's affinity for chemicals extends to pollutants as well, and the consequences of that attraction often create headlines.

• In the early 1980s, more than 1,000 private wells and five community water supplies in Suffolk County, New York, were found to exceed recommended guidelines for the pesticide Aldicarb. Aldicarb, which can impair the central nervous system, had been applied to potato crops and then seeped into groundwater. The state health department recommended that residents buy bottled water or install water-filtration systems capable of removing organic pollutants.

• Between 1964 and 1973, the Velsicol Chemical Company buried 200,000 drums of pesticide wastes in shallow pits at a farm it owned near Toone, Tennessee. The chemicals leaked out and contaminated the wells of nearby residents, many of whom developed nausea, breathing problems, severe fatigue, and diseases of the liver and kidney. One well that supplied drinking water to six families had levels of carbon tetrachloride that were 2,400 times the maximum allowed by the U.S. Environmental Protection Agency (EPA). In 1986, a Tennessee court awarded the residents $5 million in medical and property compensation and $7.5 million in punitive damages.

• In 1988, the *Lansing* (Michigan) *State Journal* commissioned independent tests of drinking water provided to Lansing homes. The tests found that half the homes tested had lead levels that exceed the EPA's proposed lead standard of 10 parts per billion.

Similar cases of polluted drinking water crop up regularly. It is not surprising that many Americans—nearly 70 percent, according to a 1989 national survey—are worried about drinking-water quality.

SOURCES OF WATER POLLUTION

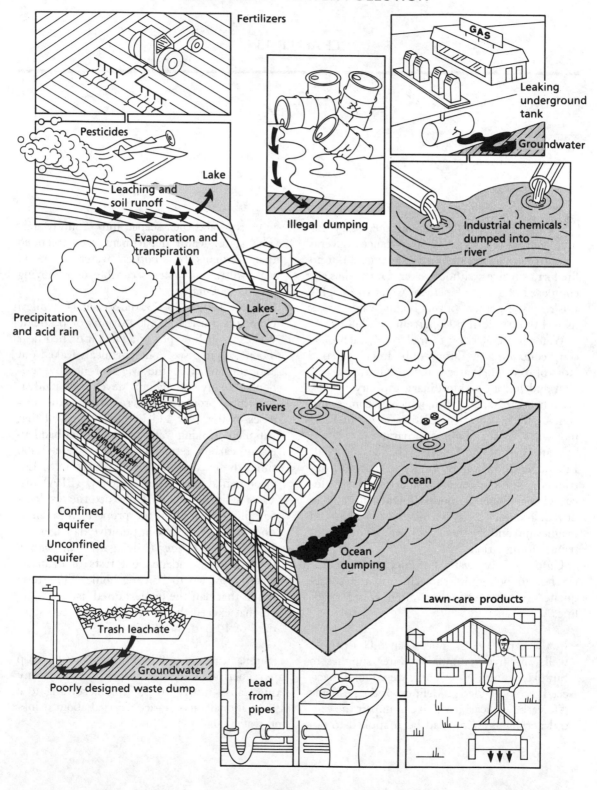

Fertilizers

Pesticides

Leaching and soil runoff

Lake

Illegal dumping

GAS

Leaking underground tank

Groundwater

Industrial chemicals dumped into river

Evaporation and transpiration

Lakes

Precipitation and acid rain

Groundwater

Rivers

Confined aquifer

Unconfined aquifer

Ocean

Ocean dumping

Lawn-care products

Trash leachate

Groundwater

Poorly designed waste dump

Lead from pipes

SOURCES OF WATER AND RISK OF POLLUTANTS

About half the population gets its drinking water from surface water, and the other half gets it from groundwater. The likelihood of having a water-pollution problem and the nature of that problem depends to a large extent on where your drinking water comes from (see Figure 13.1).

Surface water includes the lakes, rivers, reservoirs, and streams that provide the water to most major cities (for example, the Ohio and Mississippi rivers and Great Lakes are major surface sources of drinking water). Groundwater is drawn from underground aquifers—vast stretches of underground rock formations that are saturated with water. Most groundwater users are residents of rural areas who tap into groundwater from private wells.

Surface water generally contains a greater variety of contaminants and greater number of bacterial and organic pollutants than does groundwater. This is because it is exposed to acid rain, storm water runoff from cities, pesticide runoff from agricultural areas, and industrial waste.

On the other hand, when pesticides and other toxic organic chemicals find their way into groundwater, their concentrations can be hundreds of times higher than in surface waters. Pesticides and fertilizers spread on the land can seep through the earth and into groundwater. Hazardous wastes may seep from poorly maintained landfills or waste-storage sites. Industrial wastes disposed through injection into the ground, leaking underground gasoline storage tanks, or carelessly discarded household chemicals are all sources of groundwater contamination.

Whether it comes from surface water or groundwater, the risk of becoming ill from consuming contaminated drinking water is very small. For the 87 percent of Americans who are served by large municipal water systems, the risk of illness is even lower.

Water from public systems generally undergoes a series of treatments. In the first step, known as primary treatment, water sits in storage ponds to allow silt and other organic matter to settle out. Next the water is filtered through beds of sand and then disinfected, usually with chlorine, to kill potentially harmful microorganisms. Municipal water may receive other treatments as well, including filtration and aeration.

As a result of this monitoring and treatment, customers of large municipal water systems generally drink safe water. However, other water users, those living in small communities or who have their own private wells, may need to be more vigilant.

Sixty-four percent of America's nearly 60,000 water systems serve fewer than 500 people. For the most part, small public systems are expected to meet the same quality standards as large municipal systems. However, the EPA has estimated that 9,000 public water systems—almost all of them small—cannot meet federal regulations without improving their facilities and equipment.

The 40 million Americans who use private wells have even less protection. Unlike public water systems, private well water is generally not tested or treated at all. The source of well water—the groundwater from underground aquifers—can be contaminated in a variety of ways. For this reason, private well users should test their drinking water yearly for contaminants (see Box 13.2).

Figure 13.1 SOURCES OF WATER POLLUTION.

Surface water becomes contaminated by acid rain, urban storm water runoff, pesticide runoff, and industrial waste. Groundwater becomes contaminated by pesticides and fertilizers, hazardous wastes, industrial wastes, leaking underground gasoline storage tanks, or discarded household chemicals.

Box 13.1   FLUORIDATED WATER: HOW SAFE?

Sodium fluoride has been added to municipal water supplies since 1945 to prevent tooth decay. (It is added to toothpastes and mouth rinses for the same reason). Today, about half of all Americans drink fluoridated water.

The public health benefits of sodium fluoride are well established. Children in communities with fluoridated water have been shown to have between 25 and 65 percent less tooth decay than children in communities where the water supply is not fluoridated.

Some groups, such as the National Health Federation and the Safe Water Foundation, have objected to fluoridation of public water supplies, contending that fluoride is a toxic and possibly carcinogenic chemical. Congress ordered the U.S. Public Health Service and National Toxicology Program to conduct an animal study investigating such concerns in 1977.

For two years, groups of male and female mice and rats were given water containing either no fluoride or varying amounts of it. While none of the mice or female rats developed cancer, some of the male rats did. One of the fifty male rats drinking the water containing the medium fluoride dose (45 parts per million) developed bone cancer. Four rats drinking the water containing the high fluoride dose (79 parts per million) developed bone cancer. These fluoride levels are many times higher than the level of 1 part per million in fluoridated water.

These preliminary results, released in 1989, reignited the fluoridation controversy. When the National Toxicology Program's Board of Scientific Counselors' Technical Reports Review Panel evaluated the results of the study in April 1990, they found the evidence "equivocal"—too weak to attribute the bone cancers to fluoride. Pointing out that no cancers occurred in mice or in female rats receiving the same dose of fluoride and that only a few of the male rats were affected, the panel decided the cancers in the male rats could have occurred by chance rather than because of the fluoride.

The results of many epidemiologic studies comparing cancer rates of people living in fluoridated-water and nonfluoridated-water communities have been reassuring. The National Institute of Environmental Health Sciences summed up its position: "After 45 years of water fluoridation involving scores of human epidemiological studies both in the United States and in other countries, there has not been any evidence that shows a relationship between fluoridation and cancer or other diseases in humans."

The resurgence of controversy surrounding fluoridation prompted the U.S. Public Health Service to conduct an in-depth study on the benefits versus risks of fluoride in water. Released in 1991, the report concluded that animal and epidemiologic studies fail to demonstrate a link between fluoridated water and cancer and advised that fluoridation continue because of its proven dental health benefits.

Box 13.2   FINDING OUT IF YOUR WATER IS SAFE

The color, taste, or odor of drinking water cannot tell you if it is safe. It must be analyzed using scientific instruments.

Federal law requires most public water companies to test their water regularly and to make the results available to their customers free of charge. Contact your local water utility and ask for the last complete analysis. Contact a state or local public health official if the analysis is not available.

This analysis will tell you the quality of the water when it left the treatment plant, not necessarily as it comes out of your tap. For example, lead enters water after it has left the utility on its journey to your tap. If you suspect a particular problem and want to test for lead or want reassurance on the quality of your water, you can have your water analyzed.

What to Test

An analysis can be tailored to the pollutant or pollutants about which you are concerned. If you are served by a municipal utility, you may just want to find out about lead.

If your source is a private well, you run a greater risk of having unsafe water than people served by large utilities. You should contact the public health department to find out about groundwater contamination in your area. If you use well water, it would be wise to test drinking water at least once each year for bacteria, radon, and inorganic chemicals, such as nitrates. If there is a landfill, gasoline station, refinery, military base, or chemical plant within a mile or two, also test for possible contamination by organic chemicals. If your well is in a rural area, have the water tested for nitrates and pesticides.

Whether your drinking water comes from groundwater or surface water, consider testing your water for lead if anyone in the household is under age six, pregnant, your house is more than thirty years old or brand new, or if the plumbing pipes are joined with lead solder.

Where to Have It Tested

It is best not to have your water tested by a company that sells water-treatment equipment, even if it offers a free or low-cost water analysis as part of its sales effort; the results may not be objective. Instead, look in the phone directory under Laboratories—Testing for an independent state-certified laboratory.

Another possibility is a mail-order laboratory. Mail-order test results are generally accurate, but no single analysis is perfect. If a test report says that a particular pollutant is present at high levels, have your water tested by a second laboratory before taking costly remedial action. Two mail-order laboratories given good ratings in 1988 by Consumers Union are the following:

• Suburban Water Testing Laboratories, 4600 Kutztown Road, Temple, PA 19560. Telephone 1-800-433-6595.

(continued)

Box 13.2   FINDING OUT IF YOUR WATER IS SAFE (*continued*)

• National Testing Laboratories, 6151 Wilson Mills Road, Cleveland, OH 44143. Telephone 1-800-458-3330.

Both mail-order laboratories will send you a kit that contains collection bottles and detailed instructions. You collect your water in bottles and then ship the bottles back by overnight package delivery. In two to three weeks, the laboratories will send you the test results and an explanation of the numbers.

If your drinking water is polluted, you can choose from several types of water treatment devices to help solve the problem as described in Box 13.3.

POLLUTANTS THAT MATTER MOST

Often what causes people to become concerned about their water is its appearance, taste, or smell. Unfortunately, these attributes are not the only crucial ones: Water that poses a health hazard often looks, tastes, and smells just fine.

For example, manganese and iron in well water often produce offensive tastes and odors and can also stain clothes and household fixtures. These two metals have no known adverse health effects at levels generally found in water. But lead, another metal commonly found in drinking water, is tasteless, odorless, and colorless at levels that can be toxic (on the order of 5 or 10 parts per billion).

The federal government regulates 62 (as of 1993) contaminants that may appear in your drinking water under the Safe Drinking Water Act of 1974 (see Box 13.4 and Table 13.1).

Microorganisms

Microorganisms are the oldest and most lethal health threat in drinking water. It was only at the turn of the century with the introduction of disinfection of water supplies, mainly through chlorination, that the death toll from the epidemics of such water-borne diseases as cholera and typhoid fever was brought under control. Despite impressive gains, illnesses from microbes in drinking water remain a problem: Between 1971 and 1982, water-borne microorganisms caused more than 47,000 documented cases of illness in the United States and the actual toll is probably much higher. Most of these illnesses arose either due to lack of water treatment or to inadequate treatment of water sources.

Although most water-borne microbial outbreaks involve surface water, groundwater may also be a culprit. Private wells can become contaminated with bacteria and viruses due to leaking septic tanks or animal feedlot wastes that seep into the ground.

To prevent disease outbreaks, water utilities are required to monitor water monthly for coliform bacteria, which are present in fecal matter. Coliforms are *indicator* organisms—often harmless in themselves, their presence in a water supply suggests that the water may have been contaminated by other disease-causing microbes.

The coliform test has helped keep water-borne disease outbreaks at a low level in the United States. However, the absence of coliforms does not guarantee the absence of harmful microbes. A number of organisms, including the polio and Norwalk viruses; bacteria such as *Legionella*, and various protozoa, including *Giardia lamblia*, can survive the disinfection methods that effectively kill coliforms.

Box 13.3   TREATING YOUR WATER

Home water-treatment equipment has turned into a booming business: Sales of these devices are expected to exceed $1 billion a year by 1995, and there are now some 400 manufacturers trying to interest consumers in their water-treatment systems.

Let the buyer beware: Before purchasing any equipment, first determine that you do, indeed, have a problem (see Box 13.2).

Do not be seduced by the "sludge test" that a water-treatment salesperson may run on your tap water: Seconds after adding a few drops of an anonymous chemical to your tap water, an unsightly sludgelike residue forms at the bottom of the bottle to convince you that your water is not "pure." The chemical was probably a flocculating agent, a substance that precipitates out dissolved minerals in the water and exaggerates the quantity of these minerals—most of which are harmless.

If testing by an independent laboratory (one that does not sell water-treatment equipment) indicates that your water should be treated, there are four types of devices from which to choose. Base your choice on the kinds of contaminants present in your water.

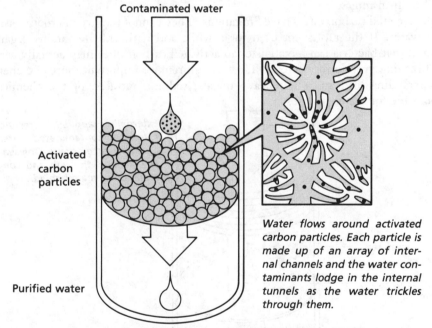

Water flows around activated carbon particles. Each particle is made up of an array of internal channels and the water contaminants lodge in the internal tunnels as the water trickles through them.

Figure 13.2   A GRANULAR ACTIVATED CARBON FILTER.

Granular Activated Carbon Filters

These are the most popular and versatile treatment devices, capable of removing many of the contaminants found in drinking water. They are quite effective against

(continued)

Box 13.3 TREATING YOUR WATER (*continued*)

taste and odor problems, chlorine, all organic chemicals that may result from chlorination, as well as pesticides.

Activated carbon is charcoal that is honeycombed with tiny channels. As water passes through this labyrinth, chemicals stick to the walls of the channels and are filtered out. The more charcoal, the more water a filter can treat before it begins to lose its effectiveness. Charcoal filters work best when water trickles through them slowly. The longer the water remains in contact with the carbon, the more contaminants will be trapped inside the filter. Large high-volume filters generally have cartridges that are ten inches high and three inches in diameter. These cartridges generally contain enough charcoal to treat about 1,000 gallons of water. The cartridges will then become clogged and must be replaced.

Some high-volume filters mount under a sink cabinet, while others sit on the countertop. Both types dispense filtered water from their own faucet, which is mounted on the sink or countertop.

Smaller carbon filters are much less efficient at removing contaminants. They include small filters that fit on the end of a sink faucet and water pitchers that have small built-in filters.

All activated carbon filters have limitations. They cannot remove microorganisms from water. If the tap is not used for a while and if the filter contains organic material that bacteria can metabolize, an activated carbon filter may actually serve as a breeding ground for bacteria. They cannot remove important inorganic chemicals including lead and other heavy metals, sodium, nitrates, or the chemicals responsible for water hardness.

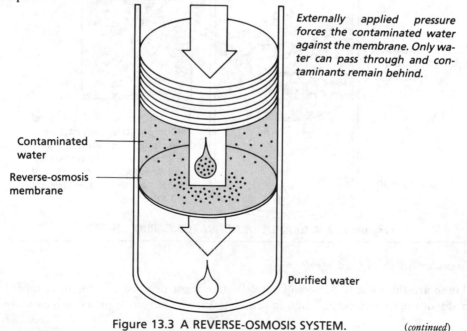

Externally applied pressure forces the contaminated water against the membrane. Only water can pass through and contaminants remain behind.

Contaminated water

Reverse-osmosis membrane

Purified water

Figure 13.3 A REVERSE-OSMOSIS SYSTEM.

(*continued*)

Box 13.3   TREATING YOUR WATER (*continued*)

Reverse-Osmosis Systems

In these filters, pressure in the water line forces water through a cellophanelike plastic sheet known as a semipermeable membrane. The membrane holds back large molecules and charged particles but allows water and small organic molecules to pass through.

Reverse-osmosis can remove salt and most other inorganic chemicals from water. They are especially useful in treating brackish (salty) water and water with excess amounts of lead or other heavy metals, nitrates, and fluoride.

Home treatment units work slowly, however, producing just a few gallons a day for drinking or cooking. They also waste a lot of water: Only 10 to 25 percent of the water passing through a unit comes out the spigot; the rest goes down the drain.

A typical reverse-osmosis unit consists of a sediment filter, the reverse-osmosis membrane, a storage tank, and an activated carbon filter. Prices vary widely depending on differences in capacity and complexity of design.

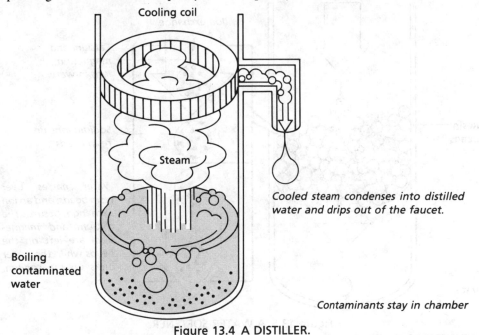

Cooling coil

Steam

Cooled steam condenses into distilled water and drips out of the faucet.

Boiling contaminated water

Contaminants stay in chamber

Figure 13.4   A DISTILLER.

Distillers

Rather than filtering pollutants from water, a distiller removes water from its pollutants. A distiller boils water and then cools the steam until it condenses. The

(*continued*)

Box 13.3   TREATING YOUR WATER (*continued*)

condensed water drips into a collection jug, while everything else stays behind in the boiling chamber.

Distillers are excellent for treating brackish water. They are also quite useful—even better than reverse-osmosis systems—in cleansing water that is contaminated with heavy metals.

An important drawback to distillers is their ineffectiveness against volatile organics. This large group of chemicals, which includes chloroform and benzene, frequently contaminates groundwater. In a distiller, volatile organics tag along with water boiling away.

Boiling water kills microorganisms but, so far, manufacturers are not referring to their distillers as sterilizers. The National Sanitation Foundation, which sets performance standards for water-treatment devices, has developed a new certification procedure that will allow certain distillers to be classified as sterilizers.

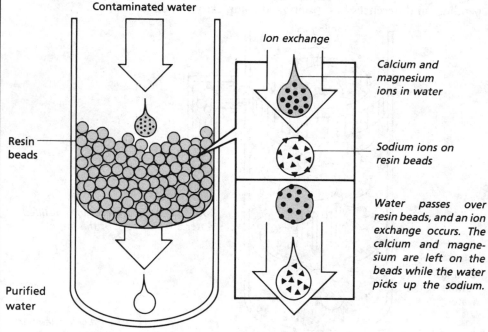

Figure 13.5 A WATER SOFTENER.

Water Softeners

These devices, which have been sold for more than sixty years, play no role in making water safer. They are designed to remove calcium and magnesium—the two hard minerals that make water "hard," leading to soap-curd deposits in bathtubs and sinks, dull-looking laundry, and scaly deposits on faucets and showerheads and inside water heaters and pipes.

(*continued*)

Box 13.3 TREATING YOUR WATER (*continued*)

Water softeners work on the principle of ion exchange. Hard water flows through a tank filled with synthetic resin beads, each of which has millions of sodium ions loosely attached to it. The water exchanges its "hardness" ions—mainly calcium and magnesium—for the "soft" sodium ions, and then it flows on to the faucets.

The resin eventually becomes saturated with hardness ions and must then be regenerated. That is accomplish by allowing salt from a brine tank to flow through the resin. The resin then gives up its hardness ions in exchange for the sodium ions. The brine containing the hardness ions goes down the drain.

Organic Chemicals

Many of the pesticides, herbicides, and industrial solvents that contaminate our drinking supplies are organic chemicals. This chemical family also includes the by-product substances formed during chlorination, such as chloroform and other trihalomethanes, that have become the focus of public controversy.

At high doses, many organic chemicals can cause acute illness or death. Such high levels do occur in drinking water, as exemplified by the polluted Tennessee wells mentioned earlier. Much more common, however, are situations where organic chemicals are found in drinking water in very dilute amounts—typically in concentrations expressed in parts per billion. For most of these substances, clear evidence of a hazard at the low levels usually found in drinking water is lacking. However, the possibility cannot be ruled out that, even at low levels, toxic chemicals if ingested over many years could result in chronic health effects such as cancer, birth defects, and nervous system disorders.

Organic contamination stems from a variety of sources. Most of these chemicals occur naturally, such as those formed by the decay of animal and vegetable matter such as bark, leaves, and soil deposited in the water. Naturally occurring organics populate surface water more than groundwater, because surface water is exposed to this matter more often than groundwater.

Other organic chemical pollutants are synthetic chemicals, such as pesticides and herbicides, that seep into groundwater, as well as the potent industrial solvents and hazardous wastes that are released into waterways or seep through waste sites.

The more important types of organic water pollutants include the following:

Chlorination by-products (trihalomethanes).

The concern over chlorination of our water supplies evolved when it was discovered in the 1970s that when chlorine reacts with naturally occurring organic matter, such as dead leaves, it gives rise to chemicals called trihalomethanes (THMs). The principal THM that is worrisome is chloroform, a suspected human carcinogen.

Because chlorination is so widely used, many public water supplies contain low levels of THMs as well as other chemicals formed as by-products of chlorination. The health risk from ingesting these chemicals is not clear. In high doses, chloroform has been shown to cause cancer in laboratory animals. Some epidemiological studies suggests that, collectively, the THMs and other chlorination by-products cause a slight increase in cancer risk, although the studies are neither conclusive nor completely consistent.

Chlorination remains one of the most important means for ridding our water supplies of microorganisms, and its importance as a means of preventing disease still markedly outweighs any

Box 13.4   THE SAFE DRINKING WATER ACT

Federal protection of drinking water began at the turn of the century when the U.S. Public Health Service set the first standards for limiting bacteria in water. The modern age of drinking-water protection began in 1974 when Congress passed the Safe Drinking Water Act (SDWA). The SDWA was prompted by growing concern that the nation's drinking-water quality was deteriorating. Congressional approval was spurred by the release of a major study of New Orleans drinking water that found elevated levels of many organic chemicals. The purpose of the SDWA was to "assure that water supply systems serving the public meet minimum national standards for the protection of public health." The law covers all public water systems that serve twenty-five or more people.

The EPA is charged with implementing and enforcing the SDWA. One of the EPA's main responsibilities under the law is to establish maximum contaminant levels (MCLs) for drinking-water pollutants that may pose a health risk. So far, the EPA has issued MCLs for 62 contaminants (see Table 13.1) and plans to issue a total of 83 by 1994. Most of the sixty-two pertain to organic chemical contaminants. Any state may regulate contaminants for which MCLs have not yet been set.

To ensure that MCLs are met, the EPA requires public water systems to monitor water quality and maintain records. The systems must regularly test for all contaminants for which the EPA has issued MCLs.

A major provision of the SDWA requires water-system operators to notify their customers when the system violates a health standard or monitoring requirement. A recent study of EPA computer records, however, found that many operators ignore this provision: Customers were not told they were drinking substandard water in 94 percent of the cases where systems violated the law.

---

risks of its use. It is nonetheless desirable to keep levels of these chemicals as low as possible. The EPA requires that water-supply systems serving more than 10,000 people keep THM levels below 100 parts per billion. The agency does not set limits for THMs in small water-supply systems, partly because such systems have experienced disease outbreaks from inadequate chlorination.

Chlorinated hydrocarbons. Many of the chemicals in this group are widely used in industry as solvents, degreasers, and raw materials. Common examples include trichloroethylene, 1,1-dichloroethylene, 1,1,1-trichloroethane, 1,2-dichloroethane, and tetrachloroethylene. PCBs are also members of this group.

Chlorinated hydrocarbons frequently find their way into our waterways, discharged into rivers, lakes, and oceans as part of industrial effluents. Some of the same properties that make them attractive to industry cause problems once they enter the environment.

Because they are solvents, they migrate readily through soil and into groundwater. They usually cause localized problems involving groundwater contaminated by a toxic waste site, landfill, or military base. (In fact, chlorinated hydrocarbons are routinely found as contaminants at Superfund hazardous waste sites [see p. 571].)

In high doses, chlorinated hydrocarbons can cause nervous system damage, many are toxic to the liver and kidney, and they may cause cancer.

Table 13.1 NATIONAL PRIMARY DRINKING-WATER STANDARDS

Contaminants	Health Effects	MCL[a]	Sources
ORGANIC CHEMICALS			
Acrylamide[b]	Probable cancer, nervous system	TT[c]	Flocculents in sewage/wastewater treatment
Alachlor[b]	Probable cancer	0.002	Herbicide on corn and soybeans; under review for cancellation
Aldicarb[d]	Nervous system	0.003	Insecticide on cotton, potatoes; restricted in many areas due to groundwater contamination
Aldicarb sulfone[d]	Nervous system	0.002	Degraded from aldicarb by plants
Aldicarb sulfoxide[d]	Nervous system	0.004	Degraded from aldicarb by plants
Atrazine[b]	Reproductive and cardiac	0.003	Widely used herbicide on corn and on noncrop land
Benzene	Cancer	0.005	Fuel (leaking tanks); solvent commonly used in manufacture of industrial chemicals, pharmaceuticals, pesticides, paints, and plastics
Carbofuran[b]	Nervous system and reproductive system	0.04	Soil fumigant/insecticide on corn/cotton; restricted in some areas
Carbon Tetrachloride	Possible cancer	0.005	Commonly used in cleaning agents, industrial wastes from manufacture of coolants
Chlordane	Probable cancer	0.002	Soil insecticide for termite control, corn; potatoes; most uses cancelled in 1980
2,4-D[b] (Current MCL = 0.1)	Liver, kidney, nervous system	0.07	Herbicide for wheat, corn, rangelands
Dibromochloropropane (DBCP)[b]	Probable cancer	0.0002	Soil fumigant on soybeans, cotton; cancelled in 1977
Dichlorobenzene p-	Possible cancer	0.075	Used in insecticides, moth balls, air deodorizers

(continued)

Table 13.1 NATIONAL PRIMARY DRINKING-WATER STANDARDS (*continued*)

Contaminants	Health Effects	MCL[a]	Sources
Dichlorobenzene o-[b]	Nervous system, lung, liver, kidney	0.6	Industrial solvent; chemical manufacturing
Dichloroethane (1,2-)	Possible cancer	0.005	Used in manufacture of insecticides, gasoline
Dichloroethylene (1,1-)[b]	Liver/kidney effects	0.007	Used in manufacture of plastics, dyes, perfumes, paints, SOCs (Synthetic Organic Chemicals)
Dichloroethylene (cis-1,2-)[b]	Nervous system, liver, circulatory	0.07	Industrial extraction solvent
Dichloroethylene (trans-1,2)[b]	Nervous system, liver, circulatory	0.1	Industrial extraction solvent
Dichloropropane (1,2)[b]	Probable cancer, liver, lungs, kidney	0.005	Soil fumigant; industrial solvent
Endrin[e]	Nervous system/kidney effects	0.0002	Insecticide used on cotton, small grains, orchards (cancelled)
Epichlorohydrin[b]	Probable cancer, liver, kidney, lungs	TT[c]	Epoxy resins and coatings, flocculents used in treatment
Ethylbenzene[b]	Kidney, liver, nervous system	0.7	Present in gasoline and insecticides; chemical manufacturing
Ethylene dibromide (EDB)[b]	Probable cancer	0.00005	Gasoline additive; soil fumigant; solvent cancelled in 1984; limited uses continue
Heptachlor[b]	Probable cancer	0.0004	Insecticide on corn; cancelled in 1983 for all but termite control
Heptachlor epoxide[b]	Probable cancer	0.0002	Soil and water organisms convert heptachlor to the epoxide
Lindane[b] (Current MCL = 0.004)	Nervous system, liver, kidney	0.0002	Insecticide for seed/lumber/livestock pest control; most uses restricted in 1983
Methoxychlor[b] (Current MCL = 0.1)	Nervous system, liver, kidney	0.04	Insecticide on alfalfa, livestock
Monochlorobenzene[b]	Kidney, liver, nervous system	0.1	Pesticide manufacturing; metal cleaner, industrial solvent

(*continued*)

Table 13.1 NATIONAL PRIMARY DRINKING-WATER STANDARDS (*continued*)

Contaminants	Health Effects	MCL[a]	Sources
Pentachlorophenol[b]	Probable cancer, liver, kidney	0.001	Wood preservative and herbicide; nonwood uses banned in 1987
Polychlorinated biphenyls (PCBs)[b]	Probable cancer	0.0005	Electrical transformers, plasticizers; banned in 1979
Styrene[b]	Liver, nervous system	0.1	Plastic manufacturing; resins used in water treatment equipment
Tetrachloroethylene	Probable cancer	0.005	Dry cleaning/industrial solvent
Toluene[b]	Kidney, nervous system, lung	1	Chemical manufacturing; gasoline additive; industrial solvent
Total Trihalomethanes (TTHM) (chloroform, bromoform, bromo-dichloromethane, dibro-mochloromethane)	Cancer risk	0.1	Primarily formed when surface water containing organic matter is treated with chlorine
Toxaphene[b] (Current MCL = 0.005)	Probable cancer	0.003	Insecticide/herbicide for cotton, soybeans; cancelled in 1982
2-4-5-TP (Silvex)[b] (Current MCL = 0.01)	Nervous system, liver, kidney	0.05	Herbicide on rangelands, sugar cane, golf courses; cancelled in 1983.
Trichloroethane (1,1,1)	Nervous system problems	0.2	Used in manufacture of food wrappings, synthetic fibers
Trichloroethylene (TCE)	Possible cancer	0.005	Waste from disposal of dry cleaning materials and manufacturing of pesticides; paints, waxes, and varnishes; paint stripper; metal degreaser
Vinyl chloride	Cancer risk	0.002	Polyvinyl chloride pipes and solvents used to join them; industrial waste from manufacture of plastics and synthetic rubber

(*continued*)

Table 13.1 NATIONAL PRIMARY DRINKING-WATER STANDARDS (continued)

Contaminants	Health Effects	MCL[a]	Sources
Xylenes[b]	Liver, kidney, nervous system	10	Paint/ink solvent; gasoline refining by-product; component of detergents
INORGANIC CHEMICALS			
Arsenic[f]	Dermal and nervous system toxicity effects	0.05	Geological, pesticide residues, industrial waste, and smelter operations
Asbestos[b]	Benign tumors	7 MFL[g]	Natural mineral deposits; also in asbestos/cement pipe
Barium[d] (Current MCL = 1.0 mg/l)	Circulatory system	2	Natural mineral deposits; oil/gas drilling operations; paint and other industrial uses
Cadmium[b]	Kidney	0.005	Natural mineral deposits; metal finishing; corrosion product plumbing
Chromium[b] (Current MCL = 0.05)	Liver/kidney, skin, and digestive system	0.1	Natural mineral deposits; metal finishing, textile, tanning, and leather industries
Copper[j]	Stomach and intestinal distress; Wilson's disease	TT[c]	Corrosion of interior household and building pipes
Fluoride	Skeletal damage	4	Geological; additive to drinking water; toothpaste; foods processed with fluorinated water
Lead[j] (Current MCL = 0.05)	Central and peripheral nervous system damage; kidney; highly toxic to infants and pregnant women	TT[c]	Corrosion of lead solder and brass faucets and fixtures; corrosion of lead service lines
Mercury	Kidney, nervous system	0.002	Industrial/chemical manufacturing; fungicide; natural mineral deposits
Nitrate	Methemoglobinemia "blue-baby syndrome"	10	Fertilizers, feedlots, sewage; naturally in soil, mineral deposits

(continued)

Table 13.1 NATIONAL PRIMARY DRINKING-WATER STANDARDS (*continued*)

Contaminants	Health Effects	MCL[a]	Sources
Nitrite[b]	Methemoglobinemia "blue-baby syndrome"	1	Unstable, rapidly converted to nitrate; prohibited in working metal fluids
Total (Nitrate and Nitrite)[b]	Not applicable	10	Not applicable
Selenium	Nervous system	0.05	Natural mineral deposits; by-product of copper mining/smelting
RADIONUCLIDES			
Beta particle and photon activity	Cancer	4 mrem/yr[b]	Radioactive waste, uranium deposits, nuclear facilities
Gross alpha particle activity	Cancer	15 pCi/L[i]	Radioactive waste, uranium deposits, geological/natural
Radium 226/228	Bone cancer	5pCiL[i]	Radioactive waste, geological/natural
MICROBIOLOGICAL			
Giardia lamblia	Stomach cramps, intestinal distress (giardiasis)	TT[c]	Human and animal fecal matter
Legionella	Legionnaires' disease (pneumonia), Pontiac fever	TT[c]	Water aerosols such as vegetable misters
Total coliforms	Not necessarily disease-causing themselves, coliforms can be indicators of organisms that can cause gastroenteric infections, dysentery, hepatitis, typhoid fever, cholera, and other. Also, coliforms interfere with disinfection.	See note[k]	Human and animal fecal matter
Turbidity	Interferes with disinfection	0.5–1.0 NTU (nephelometric turbidity unit)	Erosion, runoff, discharges
Viruses	Gastroenteritis (intestinal distress)	TT[c]	Human and animal fecal matter

(*continued*)

Table 13.1 NATIONAL PRIMARY DRINKING-WATER STANDARDS (*continued*)

Contaminants	Health Effects	MCL[a]	Sources
OTHER SUBSTANCES			
Sodium	Possible increase in blood pressure in susceptible individuals	None (20 mg/l reporting levels)[l]	Geological, road salting

Source: EPA 570/9 - 91 - 012FS (August 1991).

[a]Maximum Contaminant Level in milligrams per liter, unless otherwise noted. [b]Effective date, July 30, 1992. [c]TT: Treatment technique requirement in effect. [d]Effective date, January 1, 1993. [e]Phase V proposes changing MCL for endrin to 0.002. [f]MCL for arsenic currently under review. [g]Million fibers per liter, with fiber length greater than 10 microns. [h]"Rem" means the unit of dose equivalent from ionizing radiation to the total body of any internal organ or organ system. A "millirem (mrem)" $\frac{1}{1000}$ of a rem. [i]"Picocurie (pCi)" means the quantity of radioactive material producing 2.22 nuclear transformations per minute. [j]Effective date, December 7, 1992. [k]For large systems (40 or more routine samples per month) no more than 5.0% of the samples can be positive. For small systems (39 or fewer routine samples per month) no more than one sample can be positive. [l]Monitoring is required and data is reported to health officials to protect individuals on highly restricted sodium diets.

PCBs, which were extensively used for decades as insulating liquids in electrical equipment, were banned in the 1970s after studies found them to be extremely toxic and probable human carcinogens. They persist in our environment because they are extremely insoluble; having been dumped into waterways, they settled into the sediment, and were also taken up by bottom-dwelling fish. PCBs collect in the tissues of these fish and are then passed onto humans in worrisome quantities when the fish are eaten, through the process of bioaccumulation (see Chapter 17, "Food Safety," and Figure 17.1, pp. 600–601).

At high concentrations, PCBs can affect the liver and skin. They cause both acute and chronic liver damage and possibly liver cancer, as well as the skin disease chloracne. Although the EPA has not yet set a maximum contaminant level for PCBs, the preliminary standard is 0 milligrams per liter, which means that there is *no* detectable level of PCBs considered to be safe.

Aromatic hydrocarbons. This chemical group includes toluene, xylene, and benzene, a proven human carcinogen. All aromatic hydrocarbons can affect fetal development at high concentrations.

Both groundwater and surface water contain aromatic hydrocarbons released via industrial effluents, leaky gasoline storage tanks, and homeowner activities, such as the improper disposal of various cleaning fluids.

Box 13.5 COLIFORM WATER TEST

Public health officials rely on the coliform test for assessing other types of water as well as drinking water. Beach closings usually occur because of a positive coliform test.

To perform the test, a technician pours water into a petri dish containing a culture medium on which coliform bacteria can grow. For drinking water, the average number of coliforms per test (averaged over a month) must be less than one per 100 milliliters of water.

Box 13.6 THE INCREASING THREAT OF VIRUS AND PROTOZOA

Although chlorination effectively eliminates many types of harmful bacteria, many viruses and protozoa escape this type of disinfection. The polio virus; the Norwalk virus, which causes gastroenteritis; and the protozoan *Giardia lamblia* are three examples of microorganisms that can—and do—survive chlorination.

Public health officials are concerned about a rise in the incidence of both of these types of disease-causing microbes and of new strains of chlorine-resistant bacteria in our water supplies.

• *Giardia lamblia* was identified 300 years ago, but only recently have researchers appreciated its importance as a cause of water-borne illness. Over the past ten years, *Giardia lamblia* has become one of the leading causes of water-borne-disease outbreaks in the United States. Once swallowed, the protozoan attaches itself to the intestinal wall and causes giardiasis, characterized by diarrhea, nausea, weight loss, and weakness. Beavers and other small animals are often the sources of contamination, which is why giardiasis is sometimes called "beaver fever." Many hunters, backpackers, and fishermen have made the mistake of drinking water directly from pristine-looking rivers and lakes and contracted giardiasis as a result.

Most giardiasis outbreaks have involved surface-water systems where the only treatment was disinfection. Giardia cysts are extremely tough and resist disinfection, but filtering water can greatly reduce their numbers. The EPA now proposes that utilities use filtration as well as disinfection in the purification process in order to reduce the threat of giardiasis.

• Forty percent of the nonbacterial gastroenteritis outbreaks that occurred between 1976 and 1980 have been traced to the Norwalk virus. In many of these outbreaks, the major route of transmission was drinking water from local water supplies that were inadequately disinfected or were contaminated with sewage.

Benzene made headlines in February 1990 when trace levels of the substance were found in the bottled mineral water Perrier. The contamination led to the voluntary recall of 72 million bottles of the water. Benzene is ordinarily present in the carbon dioxide added to Perrier to provide carbonation. Although it is generally removed by filtration, in this instance the filters had become saturated with the chemical, allowing the benzene to enter the water. Because of this disclosure, the U.S. Food and Drug Administration (FDA) has ordered Perrier to remove the claim "naturally sparkling" from its labels.

The FDA's limit of benzene in bottled water is 5 parts per billion.

Pesticides and herbicides. These organic chemicals most often cause problems in agricultural areas due to runoff into surface water or seepage into groundwater. In high doses, they can cause liver, kidney, and nervous system damage and possibly cancer (see pp. 97 and 607–615).

Heavy Metals

Low levels of a number of potentially toxic heavy metals—lead, cadmium, mercury, chromium, and copper—often are detected in drinking water. Leaking landfills may be to blame when heavy metals contaminate groundwater.

Box 13.7 COASTAL POLLUTION

In the summer of 1988, New York area beaches were befouled with medical wastes—used syringes, dressings, and other material—causing many of the beaches to be temporarily closed to the public. The incident focused attention on the widespread problem of coastal pollution.

Much of the nation's wastes, including sewage, industrial waste, and agricultural runoff, end up in coastal water. For example, when the oil tanker *Exxon Valdez* ran aground in March 1989, it spilled 11 million gallons of crude oil into Alaska's Prince William Sound, devastating the ocean and coastal environment (see Figure 13.6). Even oil-vessel spills that originate in the ocean may eventually find their way toward land. The contaminants usually remain near the coastline for years, with only about 10 percent ever reaching deep water.

Untreated or partially treated sewage can be a particularly serious problem. In addition to offending the senses, sewage poses the threat of infection with hepatitis A and other ailments. Most sewage-caused illnesses result when people eat shellfish pulled from sewage-contaminated areas. Swimmers and boaters can also be affected; simply swimming in sewage-polluted waters can cause illness from ingesting sufficient numbers of any of the intestinal pathogens, including salmonella and shigella bacteria and rotaviruses.

Sewage sludge is blamed for many of the illnesses that occur when people eat shellfish contaminated with bacteria or viruses. Such contamination over the years has prompted state officials to close what had been some of the nation's best shellfish beds.

Fish caught in coastal waters may be tainted with organic chemicals from industrial effluents. Fatty fish from such waters are especially vulnerable. Salmon and trout from the Great Lakes often contain high levels of polychlorinated biphenyls, (PCBs), DDT, and dieldrin, an insecticide. The fish become contaminated from ingesting the smaller fish that constitute their diet; the pollutants accumulate along the food chain, especially in fat, which is why fatty coastal fish such as striped bass and bluefish may contain high PCB levels (see Figure 17.1, pp. 600–601).

Women of childbearing age should avoid fish that may have high levels of PCBs; PCBs may harm fetuses, and because they are stored in breast tissue, they can be passed to infants through breast milk. Mercury, another pollutant, is also toxic to fetuses. A pregnant woman who eats lots of large deep-ocean fish such as swordfish and tuna, as well as other large freshwater fish, may exceed safe levels for mercury intake (see p. 223).

Metal-finishing operations that discharge waste waters into sewers may contaminate surface waters. Or, as is often the case with cadmium, copper, and lead, metals may reach drinking water from the corrosion of pipes.

Even small quantities of some heavy metals are unhealthy, interfering with the proper functioning of enzymes, chemicals essential to various biologic and metabolic processes. Because many enzymes may be affected by a particular metal, toxic exposure can result in a variety of physiological effects from permanent damage to

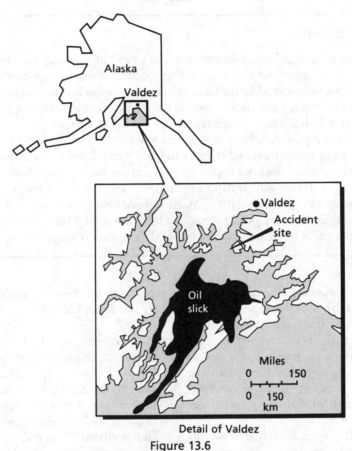

Alaska

Valdez

•Valdez
Accident site

Oil slick

Miles
0   150

0   150
km

Detail of Valdez
Figure 13.6

As shown here, the migration of the spill of the *Exxon Valdez* graphically demonstrated oil's devastating impact on the ocean environment.

the brain and nervous system to kidney damage and even infertility in men.

Fetuses and infants are particularly sensitive to the toxic effects of heavy metals. Of all the heavy metals, the one that ranks as the most important public health threat is lead.

Lead. Lead has been used since ancient times and is thought to have contributed to the decline of the Roman Empire. Ancient Romans used lead acetate to sweeten their wine and applied lead-containing glazes to their pottery, which then leached into the wine. Their daily lead intake may have been substantial—perhaps enough to kill or debilitate.

In high doses, lead can cause severe brain damage and death. Chronic low-level exposure—the kind associated with lead-contaminated drinking water—mainly threatens fetuses, infants, and children because their developing nervous systems are particularly vulnerable to lead's toxic effects. Recent studies show that lead exposure at a young age can cause permanent learning disabilities and hyperactive behavior (see Chapter 5, "The Brain and Nervous System," and Chapter 12, "Of Special Concern: Infants and Children"). Pregnant women also should be concerned about lead in their drinking water (see Chapter 11, "Reproductive Effects and Prenatal Exposures").

Box 13.8   DIOXIN

Dioxin is so toxic that one-millionth of a gram can kill a guinea pig. In addition, studies involving mice and rats suggest that dioxin is also a potent carcinogen.

Dioxin is an unintended by-product of several processes: incineration; the manufacture of chlorinated chemicals, such as the disinfectant hexachlorophene, herbicides, and pesticides; and chlorine bleaching of pulp and paper.

Tests over the past decade have detected low levels of dioxin, in the parts-per-trillion range, in some rivers and streams and in the fish living in them. Fortunately, dioxin found in water does not appear to pose a major health risk. However, it may accumulate in fish downstream from paper mills and become a threat to humans who eat them. In April 1990, the EPA announced that dioxin released as a water pollutant in this way may pose a threat, and it is preparing regulations that would require paper mills to reduce the amount of dioxin they release.

In the last decade, two developments underscored the potent health problem posed by lead: Surveys determined that lead-contaminated drinking water is much more widespread than had been assumed, and much lower levels of lead than previously considered harmful were found to pose a significant threat to health—particularly the health of fetuses, infants, and children.

In 1986, the EPA estimated that some 40 million Americans were drinking water that contained potentially hazardous lead levels. It has ranked lead as one of the most worrisome drinking-water pollutants. Although our total lead exposure is considered much lower than it was a decade ago—since lead-based paints were banned, lead was removed from gasoline, and lead solder has largely disappeared from food cans—the relative importance of drinking water as a source of lead contamination has increased.

Unlike other pollutants, lead contamination of the water itself is not the significant problem, although lead from automobile or industrial emissions, when it falls to the ground, may sometimes contaminate surface water. Lead becomes a problem mainly as water passes through piping on the way to the sink. There are three main sources for this contamination: service pipes from water mains, leaded solder in plumbing, and brass faucets.

- If your home was built between about 1910 and 1940, there is a significant chance that it has lead service pipes (the pipes connecting your house to the water main in the street). Newer houses may also have lead pipes, especially in colder regions, such as the Northeast and northern Midwest, that favor lead pipes because they resist cracking due to freezing and thawing.
- The plumbing in most households consists of copper pipes connected by solder that is half lead and half tin. A federal law passed in 1986 prohibited the further use of leaded solder in pipes that carry drinking water.
- Most chrome-plated bathroom or kitchen faucets are made of brass, which contains from 3 to 8 percent lead.

If your water is soft, or acidic, it is likely to corrode plumbing and fixtures, making it easier for lead to leach into it on its journey to your pipes. According to the EPA, about 80 percent of public water utilities deliver water that is moderately or highly corrosive.

To minimize lead in drinking water, the EPA sought to require utilities to make their water

Box 13.9 IS BOTTLED WATER ANY PURER?

According to industry experts, Americans have turned to bottled water primarily for one reason: concern about the safety of public drinking water. However, bottled water, which costs almost 1,000 times as much as tap water, contains its fair share of contaminants.

A 1989 published study analyzed thirty-seven brands of domestic and imported mineral waters, measuring levels of numerous minerals and other chemicals as well as acidity. Twenty-four of the thirty-seven brands had one or more values that were not in compliance with U.S. drinking-water standards. The authors' conclusion: "It is unlikely that a survey of community water supplies would find as high a degree of noncompliance."

Bottled water need not originate from a spring or other pristine source. It is required only to come from an "approved source"—meaning a source that meets drinking-water standards. That source may be the local community water supply.

At the national level, bottled water is regulated by the FDA, which applies the same health-protection standards to bottled water that the EPA applies to tap water. The FDA adjusts those standards as EPA regulations change. Bottled water should be as good as tap water, but there is no requirement that it be better.

Sales of bottled water in the United States have soared over the last fifteen years. Americans spent $2.2 billion on bottled water in 1990, a 700 percent increase over 1975. One in twenty Americans now drinks bottled water—one in six in California. The various types of bottled water available include the following:

- *Still water.* Still water is any bottled water without carbonation, which is usually sold in 1- or 5-gallon containers. It can originate from a spring or municipal source and can be natural or processed.
- *Sparkling water.* Sparkling water contains carbon dioxide, either present naturally or added to the water. Examples include seltzer water and club soda.
- *Spring water.* Spring water comes from a natural spring, such as an artesian well. A product sold as "natural" spring water has not been processed. Carbonation can be natural or from the addition of carbon dioxide. If carbon dioxide is added, it must come from a natural source if the word *natural* is on the label.
- *Mineral water.* Mineral water usually contains high amounts of dissolved mineral salts, such as sodium, calcium, magnesium, and iron salts. All waters have some minerals unless they are distilled. Some commercial mineral waters consist of tap water to which minerals and carbon dioxide have been added.
- *Distilled water.* Distilled water is purged of most of its minerals by heating the water and condensing the vapor.

less corrosive. The agency implemented regulations, effective December 7, 1992, requiring all public water systems to use treatment techniques that limit lead to 15 parts per billion, down from the agency's prior limit of 50 parts per billion. However, it is still a good idea for

---

Box 13.10   HOW TO MINIMIZE LEAD IN YOUR DRINKING WATER

It is important to test drinking water for lead if your household includes children under six or a woman who is pregnant or likely to become pregnant (see Box 13.2 for information on testing water).

Lead levels should not exceed 5 parts per billion. If they do or if you do not know the lead content of your water (it is prudent to assume it contains some lead), the following steps can help minimize some of the lead in your drinking water.

- Never use hot water for cooking or drinking. Hot water tends to dissolve more lead from pipes. Use cold water, especially when preparing baby formula.
- Do not drink the first water that comes out of your tap in the morning. Lead concentrations are highest in water that has sat in pipes for several hours. When you use the tap for the first time, let the water run for two to five minutes or until it is as cold as possible. Flush the toilet or run the shower to help rid the piping system of stagnant water.
- Let the water run for a few seconds before drinking when you use the tap during the day.

---

consumers to take a few simple measures described in Box 13.10 to minimize the amount of lead in drinking water.

Radon

Officials of the EPA estimate that water-borne radon, the naturally occurring radioactive gas formed during the radioactive decay of uranium, may cause more cancer deaths than all other drinking-water contaminants combined. Radon is odorless and invisible, found everywhere in the earth's crust, and can accumulate to dangerously high levels inside buildings, where it probably poses a greater health risk than any other indoor pollutant (see p. 558 for a more detailed discussion of radon).

The EPA estimates that inhaled indoor radon causes between 5,000 and 20,000 lung cancer deaths each year. Most of these deaths result from radon that percolates up from the earth and enters houses through holes and cracks in the foundation. Some fraction of these deaths—between 100 and 1,800 per year—are attributed to radon from household water. Radon dissolved in the water escapes into the indoor air when the water is sprayed in showers, washing machines, and other mechanisms.

The EPA estimates that at least 8 million people may have undesirably high radon levels in their water supply. The risk is limited to people using groundwater: The radon from subterranean rock formations leaches into the groundwater and cannot escape into the atmosphere. Water from surface sources such as rivers or reservoirs is not a problem because the radon will bubble out into the atmosphere before arriving at the faucet.

Groundwater users most at risk from water-borne radon use private wells or community water systems serving fewer than 500 people. Larger systems generally provide water treatment that aerates the water and disperses any radon gas that it contains.

Elevated levels of radon have been found in sections of all of the states thus far surveyed by the Environmental Protection Agency, not just in those areas formerly considered to be radon

Box 13.11 THE ASBESTOS HAZARD

Asbestos commonly occurs in the nation's water supplies, entering through cement distribution pipes or through natural contamination. The clear link between inhaled asbestos and lung cancer has aroused concern about the health effects of ingested asbestos through contaminated drinking water. Numerous animal studies have not found that ingested asbestos poses a cancer hazard, but until the matter is settled definitively, asbestos in water remains a safety concern.

For this reason, in 1985, the residents of Woodstock, New York, were instructed not to use their community's water for drinking or showering. The town's aged water pipes, which were made of asbestos and cement, had started to disintegrate, and large quantities of asbestos fibers were turning up in the town's water. Agitation of water can cause asbestos fibers to become airborne, turning them into a potential cancer-causing hazard.

In 1981, the EPA compiled national data on asbestos in water. The agency found levels below the detection limit in 117 cities, levels of less than 1 million fibers per liter in 216 cities, 33 cities with levels between 1 and 10 million fibers per liter, and 40 cities with asbestos levels greater than 10 million fibers per liter. The agency has proposed that utilities with an asbestos problem should limit the concentration to less than 7 million fibers per liter.

If you are concerned about asbestos in your water, have your water tested for the presence of asbestos fibers (see Box 13.3).

"hot spots." The only way to determine reliably if there is a radon problem in a particular home is to test the air. (Inexpensive detection devices are available and are discussed in more detail in Box 14.8, p. 559.) If the air level is low, you do not have to worry about radon in your water. If your indoor radon level is high and you use groundwater, you should test the water.

Some state programs will test water for radon for a modest cost (about $10 to $15). Commercial laboratories, including mail-order companies, charge about $25. Results of the test are expressed in picocuries of radon per liter of water.

Experts disagree on what level of water-borne radon should be considered hazardous. Groundwater radon levels typically range from 200 to 600 picocuries per liter. Levels greater than 100,000 picocuries per liter have been found in some private wells. EPA officials say you should definitely take action if your water's radon level is 10,000 picocuries per liter or higher. (A level

of 10,000 picocuries per liter in water is estimated to produce 1 picocurie per liter in the indoor air.)

If your water merits attention, simple measures such as ventilating your bathroom, laundry, or kitchen may suffice. If you need water treatment, you will have to treat all the water entering the house, not just the tap water. Treatment options include granular activated carbon units or home aerators.

Nitrates

Nitrates are primarily a contaminant of groundwater. They mainly threaten infants less than six months old, who may become seriously ill with methemoglobinemia from drinking water high in nitrates.

Drinking water usually provides only about 1 percent of a person's daily intake of nitrates, with most of the rest coming from vegetables.

However, some water—mainly from private wells in farming areas—contains excessively high levels of nitrates. High levels of nitrates are usually caused by agricultural activities. Chemical fertilizers and manure from animal feedlots are rich sources of nitrogen compounds, which are transformed to nitrates in the soil and enter groundwater. Wastes that leak from septic tanks are also a major contributor of nitrates to groundwater.

EPA officials report that nitrate pollution in rural areas seems to be worsening. Surveys have found that 3 percent of the rural population— about 600,000 households—use well water that exceeds the EPA nitrate standard of 10 parts per million.

Infants are mainly threatened when nitrate-rich water is mixed with formula. Bacteria in infants' digestive tracts convert the relatively harmless nitrates into nitrites. The nitrites in turn combine with some of the hemoglobin in the blood to form methemoglobin, a compound that cannot transport oxygen. The resulting condition, methemoglobinemia, can deprive vital organs of oxygen, but severe cases can cause dangerous shortness of breath and weakness (all evidence of shortage of oxygen). Some adults, including pregnant women, may also have an increased tendency to develop methemoglobinemia.

Rural families with infants or pregnant women should test their wells regularly for nitrates (see Box 13.2). High levels of nitrates may be a sign that other contaminants—agricultural pesticides or bacteria and viruses from septic tanks—are also in the water.

CHAPTER 14

Air

On a Thursday morning in October 1948, residents of Donora, Pennsylvania, stepped out of their houses into a world covered with a heavy gray fog that seeped into their lungs, making it hard to breathe. Soon, one after the other, members of the community became ill with respiratory problems, burning eyes and throats, and headaches. Six days later, when the air-pollution episode ended, 6,000 people—almost one-half of the community— had become sick, and 20 were dead.

Although air pollutants were not measured at the time of the 1948 deadly Donoran fog, estimates made after the event suggest that no one chemical in the air ever reached levels that, by itself, should have been so toxic. Instead, the fog's capacity to choke the residents appears to have arisen from a particularly lethal mixture of pollutants that formed as a result of a freak long-lasting temperature inversion.

Surrounded by hills, Donora is in a basin, rendering it vulnerable to temperature inversions. Under normal conditions, warm air rises to the cooler air above, carrying pollutants with it and dispersing them into the atmosphere. During a temperature inversion, however, the opposite occurs: A warm layer of air acts as a lid that traps cooler and more dense polluted air near the ground. Usually, temperature inversions last just a few hours; in the case of Donora, it lasted

for days, allowing pollutants at ground level to build up to harmful concentrations.

Much the same circumstances were behind the greatest of all air-pollution disasters, which occurred in 1952 in London, England; this five-day temperature inversion trapped airborne pollutants released from the heavily concentrated smoke-emitting industries and coal-burning residences in the area, allowing them to concentrate into a deadly "pea soup" fog that killed 4,000 by the time it lifted.

For decades, foul polluted air was something most communities willingly endured as a necessary evil accompanying a town's industrial vitality. The deadly episode of air pollution in Donora—the first major air-pollution disaster in the United States—was a watershed in ending this type of environmental innocence.

In the United States, the air today is measurably cleaner than it was at the century's midpoint. There are fewer factory stacks emitting plumes of black smoke or sulfurous fumes, and few houses still rely upon burning coal for domestic heat, the chief culprits in the Donora fog and the London "pea soupers." Largely because of enforcement of the Clean Air Act of 1970 and its amendments (see Box 14.3), industries have reduced their use of soft coal and heavy oil, and plants that do have stacks now employ devices to control airborne emissions of pollutants.

SOURCES OF OUTDOOR AIR POLLUTION

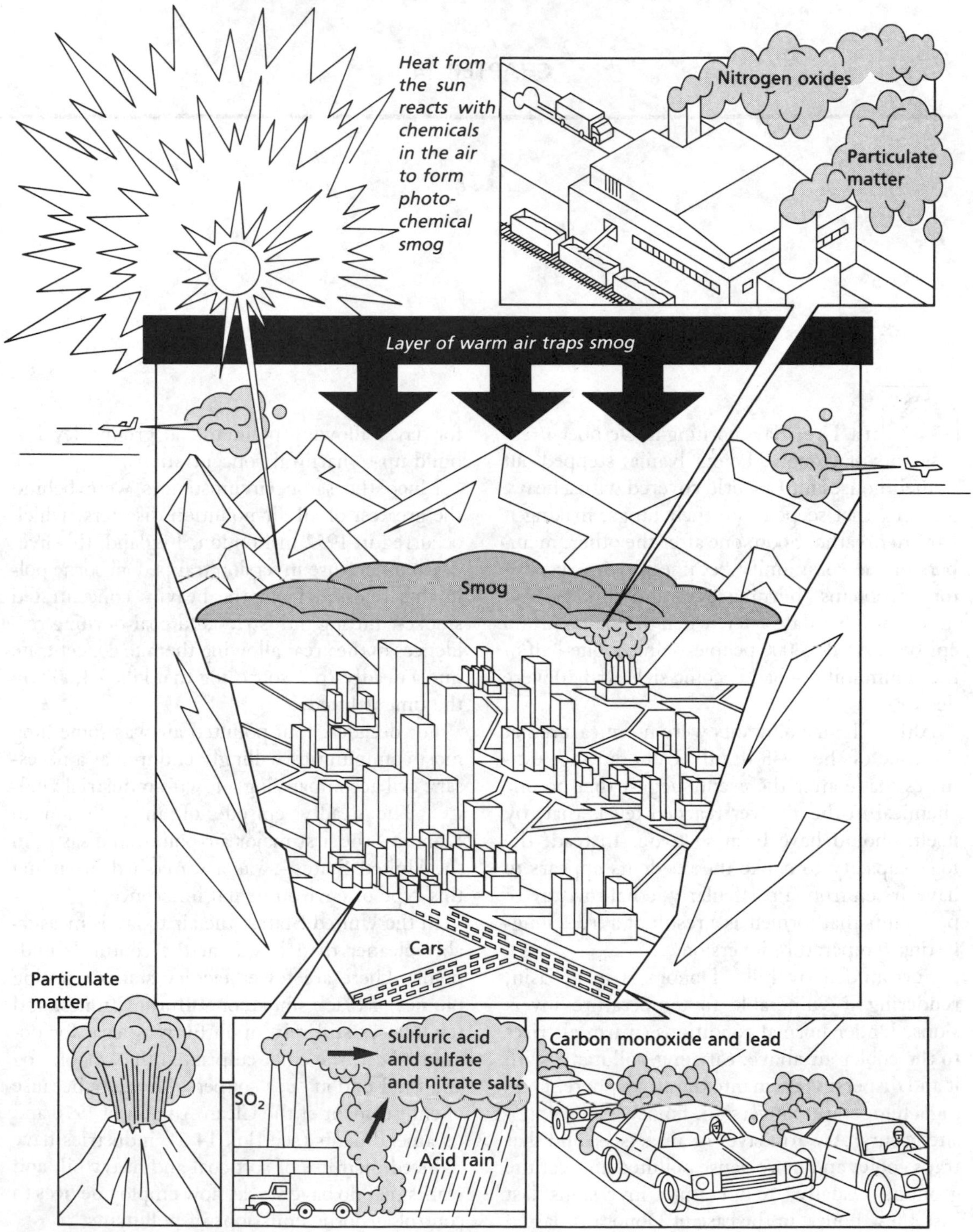

Heat from the sun reacts with chemicals in the air to form photo-chemical smog

Nitrogen oxides

Particulate matter

Layer of warm air traps smog

Smog

Cars

Particulate matter

SO₂

Sulfuric acid and sulfate and nitrate salts

Acid rain

Carbon monoxide and lead

The geographic and weather conditions that led to the toxic buildup of pollutants in the air over Donora and London remain, however, and continue to be a potent factor in efforts to provide urban residents with clean, breathable air (see Box 14.1). Ubiquitous to all countries, air pollution is virtually impossible to avoid, for no matter how toxic, unattractive, or foul smelling the air may be, we cannot live without it.

As we move toward the next century, air pollution remains one of the world's most pressing environmental challenges. The Global Environment Monitoring System (GEMS), set up by the United Nations and working in conjunction with the World Health Organization, estimates that 1.2 billion inhabitants of cities across the globe are exposed to air pollutants at levels sufficient to damage their health. Exposure to damaging pollutants is not equally shared, however: The United States and some of the other more developed nations have made significant progress in curbing airborne pollutants, whereas less developed countries, including China, and poorer developed nations—the countries that formerly comprised the Soviet Union, Poland, and some other East European countries—have levels of urban outdoor pollutants that both far exceed recommended limits to maintain health and that are still rising.

The range of air-pollutant effects on human life and health is wide. Depending upon the specific concentrations and combinations of the agents, air pollution is linked to many human ailments, some transient (irritated throats, red eyes, skin rashes, headaches, nausea, dizziness, and an increased incidence of upper respiratory symptoms) and some chronic and serious (respiratory diseases, such as emphysema, bronchitis, and asthma, and cancer).

Although everyone can be affected by foul air, some people are more vulnerable than others; for instance, people over the age of sixty-five, infants and young children, and people who suffer respiratory ailments or cardiovascular disease. These were the groups of people who accounted for most of the hospitalizations and deaths during the lethal London fog episode and in other incidents of air-pollution disasters.

Air pollution imperils the environment in local and in unexpectedly far-reaching ways as well, threatening to destroy both the beauty and the balance of nature: Passengers in a plane flying low over many urban areas may not be surprised to find the city lights obscured by a layer of pollution, but visitors to the Grand Canyon are often stunned when they arrive on a day when visibility is limited. Rather than standing at the rim of this great wonder of nature and seeing all the way to the horizon, these unlucky tourists may see a mere five or ten miles, the view obscured by air pollution "imported" by the wind from distant industrialized parts of Arizona and neighboring states.

The contribution of air pollutants to acidic deposition, commonly called acid rain, similarly degrades the view, eroding monuments and building facades, and damages the ecology of areas outside the immediate sources of pollution.

Figure 14.1 SOURCES OF OUTDOOR AIR POLLUTION.

Outdoors, the major primary air pollutants are carbon oxides; sulfur oxides; nitrogen oxides; volatile organic compounds, such as hydrocarbons, benzene, tetrachloroethylene, carbon tetrachloride, and chlorofluorocarbons; and particulate matter. The major secondary pollutants include ozone and photochemical oxidants, as well as particulates in solid form or liquid form, such as sulfuric acid (H_2SO_4) and nitric acid (HNO_3).

Emissions of sulfur dioxide (SO_2) and nitrogen dioxide, emitted in tall stacks by electric power plants and industrial plants burning coal or oil contribute to acid rain formation.

In places where air is trapped over a city, perhaps due to surrounding mountains, automotive and industrial emissions can be trapped near the ground and, in the glare of the sun, can turn into photochemical smog.

Box 14.1 MEXICO CITY

Mexico City is a classic, and chilling, example of a city in which geography and weather conspire to create particularly dangerous conditions. Like Donora, it is surrounded by mountains, which subject the city to thermal inversions, trapping its automotive and industrial emissions near the ground. Under the glare of the brilliant sun, the chemicals turn into photochemical smog.

Leaded gasoline is still in wide use in Mexico City, and this compounds the unhealthy effects: Pollution in Mexico City is so severe that women diplomats are urged to return to their native cities during pregnancy, as lead can affect the development of fetuses and young children.

As part of the efforts to control pollution, cars have been banned one day a week, sulfur is to be removed from diesel oil, and the lead content of gasoline is to be cut in half. Yet, in March 1992, levels of ozone reached the highest levels in the city's history, forcing schools to close and local industries to cut back their production to reduce emissions. The mayor of Mexico city has warned major industries to cut emissions or move out of the city.

Perhaps the greatest ecologic hazards attributed to our fouling of the air are those that affect the entire world, such as ozone depletion and the rise of greenhouse gases. Ozone depletion, a gradual thinning of the protective layer of ozone that shields the earth, and us, from the harmful rays of the sun, is increased through releases of such airborne substances as chemical chlorofluorocarbons (CFCs); these leak into the air from refrigerators and air-conditioners, from evaporation of industrial solvents, and by manufacturing processes. The loss of the protective ozone shield increases exposure to ultraviolet rays and that leads to the development of skin cancers and cataracts as well as to the threat to the stability of ecologic systems.

Greenhouse gases include carbon dioxide (produced mainly as a by-product of the burning of fossil fuels and of deforestation), methane (produced by bacteria decaying organic matter), CFCs, nitrous oxide (released by the breakdown of nitrogen fertilizers in soil, livestock wastes, and groundwater contaminated with nitrates), and ozone. Increasing levels of these gases in the atmosphere act similarly to the panes of windows in a greenhouse, reflecting back to earth heat that otherwise would dissipate into the atmosphere; the net effect is an elevation in the surface temperature of the earth. In the last half of the twentieth century, levels of greenhouse gases have increased significantly, and while scientists debate the rate of their increase and how quickly (or slowly) they will contribute to a higher thermometer reading in our backyards, the potential exists for ecologic and economic disaster.

Both ozone depletion and the rise of greenhouse gases are air-pollution problems of sufficient magnitude to affect the global habitat and will require international cooperation in order to be addressed effectively.

SOURCES OF AIR POLLUTION

Natural forces, such as volcanoes and forest fires, release hazardous gases and particles into the atmosphere, but by far the chief sources of today's air-pollution problems—both indoors and out—are the result of human activity.

Most of the major air pollutants are released

Box 14.2   THE TWO TYPES OF SMOG

The term *smog* was coined in generations past to describe the smoke, ashes, soot and other particulate matter, sulfur dioxide, and droplets of sulfuric acid created by the burning of soft coal and heavy oil in industry. Controlled and limited use of these fuels has greatly reduced this gray industrial smog in the United States, although it is still a major problem in such countries as Poland and Czechoslovakia.

In the United States today, the term *smog* refers to photochemical smog, a mixture formed when some of the pollutants emitted directly into the atmosphere chemically react in the presence of sunlight to form a mixture containing other chemical combinations as well. The most significant component of smog is ozone.

Although the general public often uses the term *smog* generically to refer to the many substances that make up urban air pollution, the Environmental Protection Agency (EPA) and state and local governments use the term as a synonym for ozone; high ozone levels prompt "smog alerts" when people, particularly the elderly and those with heart or lung diseases, are warned to remain indoors.

---

into the atmosphere from the combustion of fossil fuels. By far the greatest contributor to these emissions are fossil fuel–burning vehicles, such as cars, as well as power and industrial plants.

Outdoors, the major primary air pollutants are carbon oxides (CO, CO_2); sulfur oxides (SO_2, SO_3); nitrogen oxides (NO); volatile organic compounds (VOCs), such as hydrocarbons, benzene, tetrachloroethylene, carbon tetrachloride, and chlorofluorocarbons (CFCs); and particulate matter (PM).

Secondary pollutants are formed in the air through chemical reactions between a primary pollutant and one or more chemicals. The major secondary pollutants include ozone (O_3) and photochemical oxidants, as well as particulates in solid or liquid form, such as sulfuric acid (H_2SO_4) and nitric acid (HNO_3).

Airborne agents are released, in quantities that stagger the mind, both from stationary sources, such as residences, industries and power plants that burn fossil fuels, and mobile sources, such as automobiles and trucks: According to EPA estimates, billions of pounds of about 15,000 airborne chemicals that are suspected of causing harm to human health are released by industry every year. Equally troubling is the hefty amount of polluting chemicals emit-

ted from 198 million vehicles in which Americans travel more than 2 trillion miles a year.

All of the major categories of outdoor air pollutants are regulated under the Clean Air Act (see Box 14.3). This is not the case, however, when it comes to indoor air pollutants; the concentrations of airborne substances that contaminate air within buildings remains largely unregulated, yet, according to public health officials and the EPA, rival or surpass outdoor air pollutants in terms of damage to human health.

Indoor air pollution is by and large the product of human activity, modern invention, and attempts to conserve energy by making buildings airtight. Radon, a naturally occurring gas found in many homes in this country, is considered by the EPA to constitute one of the greatest health threats (see Chapter 3, "How We Perceive Risks and How Scientists Measure Them"). Indoor contaminants, released from numerous human-made products, range from tobacco smoke—the leading contributor to indoor air pollution—to fumes, vapors, and gases released from cleaning agents and disinfectants; the padding under rugs; materials used to build cabinets, walls, and furniture; gas stoves; wood stoves; and other consumer products such as paints, paint strippers, and air fresheners. In ad-

Box 14.3   REGULATING CLEAN AIR

Laws to eliminate the burning of soft coal date back to thirteenth-century England, but they were all too often flouted. The medieval laws were strict—a merchant was tortured and hanged in 1306 for burning and selling soft coal—but soft-coal burning continued. A high tax on coal also failed to serve as a deterrent. By the seventeenth century the English were suffering with the "great stinking fogs" and attributing to them an observed increase in respiratory illnesses and in deaths.

In the United States, the Walsh–Healey Act of 1936, although not exclusively an air-pollution act, was the first to deal with this hazard on a nationwide basis. The Occupational Safety and Health Act, passed in 1970, set health standards for air pollutants in the workplace, notably for such toxic chemicals as arsenic, asbestos, benzene, carbon monoxide, formaldehyde, and mercury.

The Clean Air Act

Improvements in air quality in the U.S. largely result from the Clean Air Act of 1970. The Clean Air act was passed in 1970—a watershed year in terms of environmental legislation—largely in response to increasing episodes of health-damaging air pollution that occurred in urban centers, such as New York City and Los Angeles, during the 1960s. It completely changed the U.S. air-pollution control

Table 14.1 NATIONAL AMBIENT AIR QUALITY STANDARDS

Pollutant	Averaging Time	Standard Level of Concentration [a]
Small particulates	Annual arithmetic mean	0.05 mg/m^3
	24 hr	0.15 mg/m^3
Sulfur dioxide	Annual arithmetic mean	0.03 ppm[b] (0.08 mg/m^3)
	24 hr[c]	0.14 ppm (0.365 mg/m^3)
Carbon monoxide	8 hr[c]	9 ppm (10 mg/m^3)
	1 hr[c]	35 ppm (40 mg/m^3)
Nitrogen dioxide	Annual arithmetic mean	0.053 ppm (0.1 mg/m^3)
Ozone	Maximum daily 1-hr average[d]	0.12 ppm (0.235 mg/m^3)
Lead	Maximum quarterly average	0.0015 mg/m^3

[a] Abbreviations used: ppm, parts per million of air; mg, milligram. [b] Values in parentheses are an approximately equivalent concentration. [c] Not to be exceeded more than once per year. [d] The standard is attained when the expected number of days per calendar year with maximum hourly average concentrations above 0.12 ppm is equal to or less than 1.

(continued)

Box 14.3 REGULATING CLEAN AIR (*continued*)

picture, setting National Ambient (Outdoor) Air Quality Standards for six "criteria pollutants—carbon monoxide, nitrogen dioxide, lead, sulfur dioxide, ozone, and particulates—the pollutants that are encountered most often, contribute the most to outdoor air pollution, and have a measurable adverse effect on public health and welfare (see Table 14.1).

The act set "primary" standards that mandated the maximum amount of each pollutant to be permitted in the air over a specific time period. The standard was based on scientific studies designed to reveal the dose or threshold level of a substance required to produce a harmful response. When the standards were established, they incorporated a margin of safety, ranging from 10 to 50 percent above the threshold or dose levels, a margin intended to protect infants, the elderly, and others unusually susceptible to ill effects of air pollution.

In order to achieve these primary standards, the act called for industries and automotive manufacturers to achieve a 90 percent reduction in emissions of the criteria pollutants by 1975 through the use of pollutant control devices. The reduction failed to materialize in many regions, and so, in 1977, the act was amended to require states to establish emission inspection programs in areas where air did not meet the quality standards.

The Clean Air Act Amendments of 1990 introduced regulations more comprehensive than any in the past, with the stated goal of removing 56 billion pounds of pollutants annually.

Air Toxins

In addition to reaffirming the primary standards for criteria pollutants, the Clean Air Act Amendments of 1990 placed 189 chemicals in the separate category of hazardous pollutants, or air toxics. These chemical compounds and mixtures are released by such stationary sources of pollution as chemical factories, steel mills, power plants, pulp and paper mills, dry cleaners, and mobile sources such as automobiles and trucks. According to the EPA, exposure to air toxics in doses above the threshold level is implicated in causing or contributing to an increased number of fatalities or serious irreversible or incapacitating illnesses, including cancer, birth defects, lung disease, nervous system disorders, and liver damage.

Before the 1990 amendments, emission standards had been set for only seven toxins: asbestos, beryllium, mercury, vinyl chloride, benzene, arsenic, and radionuclides. Under the 1990 amendments, these and 182 others are to be further investigated and regulated within ten years.

An important aspect of the regulation is the establishment of standards for the technology that will be required to control emissions of pollutants. Between now and the year 2000, emission standards for all 189 substances will be set through the use of the best pollution control technologies available, known as maximum achievable technologies. Once that is accomplished, the program will enter a second phase

(*continued*)

Box 14.3   REGULATING CLEAN AIR (*continued*)

in which more stringent emission standards will be set if the remaining residual risks of exposure are judged to be too high.

There are an estimated 30,000 major industrial sources of air pollution, each with the potential for emitting 10 or more tons of any one air toxin or 25 tons of a combination of toxins a year. Even though the EPA has yet to set standards for all but seven of the air toxins, industries have been ordered to begin reducing their total emissions year by year, starting now.

---

dition, concentrations of dusts, fibers, and microorganisms such as fungi, bacteria, molds, and viruses contribute to the indoor pollution tally.

Harmful airborne substances can concentrate within the confines of buildings to reach levels ten to forty times the levels measured outdoors.

Because, on average, Americans spend increasing amounts of time indoors, there is a high likelihood of being affected by indoor air pollutants. (The shift in population has been from rural into urban areas, and city dwellers spend 70 to 90 percent of their time indoors.)

OUTDOOR (AMBIENT AIR) POLLUTION

Outdoor, or ambient air, pollution arises largely from the burning of fossil fuels, vehicle emissions, and emissions from power plants, factories, and smelters, as well as from natural sources such as pollens and fungi.

Over the past decades since the Clean Air Act of 1970 was passed, the air in this country has improved. Overall, the average American breathes air that contains no more than the permissible levels of many of the major pollutants: There are notable declines in the amounts of lead, carbon monoxide, sulfur dioxide, and nitrogen dioxide spewed into the atmosphere, although there are still problematic levels of two other important pollutants—ozone and suspended particulate matter.

Of course, "averages" do not tell the whole story: Despite the significant declines, the EPA estimates that six out of ten urban Americans live in cities that have air that does not meet safety standards (see Table 14.1). For example, nationwide averages of carbon monoxide, a colorless and odorless gas that is emitted from the tailpipes of cars and trucks and from industry, are well below the allowable limits set by the EPA; however, in forty-one cities located in the Northeast and on the West Coast, carbon monoxide is present in levels above the standard at least some of the time. (There are two maximum exposure levels for carbon monoxide—35 parts per million of air for a one-hour exposure and 9 parts per million for an eight-hour exposure. In tunnels and underground garages, exposure levels can routinely rise to as high as 87 parts per million, and in small enclosed spaces, such as a running car in an unvented garage, carbon monoxide levels can increase to concentrations that can cause fatalities.)

Ozone levels in ninety-six cities widely scattered throughout the country are above the regulatory standard. In over seventy-two cities—ranging in size from large centers, such as Los Angeles, Denver, Phoenix, and Las Vegas, to smaller urban areas, such as Pagosa Springs, Colorado, and Presque Isle, Maine—there are excessive amounts of suspended particulate matter in the air as well.

A significant dent has been made in curbing some of the other pollutants, such as nitrogen dioxide (nationwide, levels of this gas have been

Box 14.4 THE DAMAGE WROUGHT BY ACID DEPOSITION

Acid rain results when emissions of sulfur dioxide and nitrogen dioxide, emitted in tall stacks by electric power plants and industrial plants burning coal or oil, reach high into the atmosphere, combining with other chemicals to form droplets containing solutions of sulfuric acid and sulfate and nitrate salts. The droplets are carried by winds in the upper atmosphere across the region, falling to earth as acid-contaminated dry or wet (in snow, fog, or rain) deposits. Such acidic deposition is a widespread problem in many parts of the world.

Acid rain directly threatens the soils upon which it falls, for instance, by upsetting the delicate ecological balance of the microorganisms that reside under the soil's surface. Alkaline soils, such as those containing high amounts of limestone, called buffered soils, can tolerate higher amounts of acid rain than can poorly buffered soils.

The soil is stripped of such nutrients as calcium, potassium, and magnesium that are vital for the growth of healthy trees and other vegetation. For example, the red spruce growing in the high elevations in the northern Appalachians are showing the harmful effects of exposure to acid. Without trees to hold it down, soil is eroded into the waterways, adding impurities and reducing the amount of land available for agriculture.

Acid rain takes an aesthetic toll on the world as well. Over the past two decades, acid rain in Athens, Greece, has so badly damaged some of the statues in the Parthenon that they have been replaced by models.

Acid rain, snow, and fog can be widely dispersed by the wind to distances far from the original source of emissions. In Canada, for example, gases produced by a smelter at Sudbury deposited acid rain and acid particulates in a lake more than 50 miles away, severely affecting the population of fish.

In the United States, acid rain is a major problem in Ohio, Indiana, New York, Pennsylvania, Illinois, Missouri, West Virginia, and Tennessee. As countries around the world become more highly industrialized, sulfur dioxide becomes a greater threat. In China, for example, monitored emissions of sulfur dioxide are three to five times as high as anywhere on this continent, according to GEMs. The elevated levels are due to a marked increase in the burning of fossil fuels that occurred between 1979 and 1985.

cut in half) and sulfur dioxide (levels have dropped by a third), although the gases still remain problematic in terms of environmental effects.

The most significant, and impressive, reduction has been in the levels of airborne lead, a pollutant that can damage the nervous system and is particularly hazardous to infants and young children (see Chapter 5, "The Brain and Nervous System"; Chapter 11, Reproductive Effects and Prenatal Exposures"; and Chapter 12, "Of Special Concern: Infants and Children"). Lead levels are now a fraction—less than one-tenth—of the amounts allowed under air-pollution statutes, largely due to the elimination of lead emissions from the tail pipes of cars. Since 1975, the phaseout of leaded gasoline and the equipping of cars with catalytic control devices have reduced lead emissions by 99 percent in less than two decades. (Lead remains an im-

---

Box 14.5 "GOOD" OZONE, "BAD" OZONE

The fact that ozone is injurious to human health may come as a surprise, as you have read in the newspapers and in this book that the depletion of ozone is endangering the world. This is a case of "good" ozone versus "bad" ozone.

Ozone (O_3) is a particular molecular configuration of oxygen produced by ultraviolet light acting on oxygen (O_2) in the presence of volatile organic compounds and nitrogen oxides.

"Good" ozone in the upper atmosphere miles above earth (the stratosphere) serves as a protective shield, filtering damaging ultraviolet radiation and keeping it from reaching the earth. A reduction in this protective ozone layer will allow more of the sun's ultraviolet rays to reach the earth. Increased exposure to this damaging form of radiant energy will lead to a rise in skin cancers, cataracts, and damage to animal and plant life.

"Bad" ozone is present in the troposphere, the lower layer of the atmosphere—the air we breathe. An increase in bad ozone is associated with the adverse health effects discussed in this chapter.

---

portant hazard in soil, water, and products such as paint. For more information on lead, see the Lead information sheet, p. 392).

Significant Pollutants

Sulfur Dioxide and Acid Rain. Pollution control devices and cuts in the sulfur component of fuel have reduced the amount of sulfur dioxide in the air, but large amounts are still being produced in the burning of fossil fuels by electric utilities, oil refineries, pulp and paper mills, and nonferrous smelters. The Clean Air Act Amendments of 1990 call for a reduction by the year 2000 of one-half of the 20 million tons of sulfur dioxide still being emitted annually.

Sulfur dioxide, like all air pollutants, causes breathing difficulties, which are particularly hazardous for people with chronic lung diseases and those who are prone to asthma during exercise (see Chapter 6, "Respiratory Ailments"). Heart disease may also be aggravated.

Harmful enough in its own right, sulfur dioxide can be transformed into a major component of one of the most prevalent air-to-soil contaminants, acid rain (see Box 14.4). Some studies suggest that acid rain may aggravate such lung diseases as bronchitis (particularly in children and the elderly) and asthma, but, to date, there is no conclusive proof that acid rain directly affects human health. There is no question, however, that it damages the ecology.

Nitrogen Dioxide. This gas is a lung irritant that contributes to the onset of bronchitis and pneumonia and lowers resistance to such respiratory infections as influenza. Produced by the combustion of fuel (in power plants, diesel engines, and various industrial processes, such as metal smelting), it is emitted from automobiles and trucks as well. A highly reactive gas, nitrogen dioxide is a component of the aerosols that fall to earth as acid rain and a major participant in the reactions that create ozone.

Ozone. This major component of photochemical smog is formed when pollutants, such as nitrogen oxides and hydrocarbon, emitted in great quantities by automobile exhausts and emissions from electric utilities, oil refineries, and chemical plants react chemically in the presence of sunlight (see Box 14.2). More ozone forms at high temperatures than at low, so the hotter the

---

Box 14.6   WHAT TO DO DURING A SMOG ALERT

When ozone levels rise, many communities issue smog alerts. In the Los Angeles area, for example, 178 smog alerts were issued during the parching summer of 1988. To cope with days of excessively high ozone levels:

- *Reduce activity*. It is the quantity of ozone that reaches the lungs rather than its actual concentration in the air that makes the difference and the more you work or play, the greater your intake of air.
- *Shut out ozone*. Smog alerts ordinarily advise people to remain indoors, but if the windows are left open, the indoor levels of ozone can match those outdoors.
- *Make sure your office is properly ventilated*. Even in buildings with closed windows, indoor levels can be excessively high, depending upon how well ventilated the building is. Make sure your building has and uses a filtering system that removes ozone.

---

day and the longer a heat wave lasts, the greater the buildup of ozone and smog (see Box 14.2).

Unlike other air pollutants that are harmful mostly to unhealthy individuals, ozone injures everyone. Exposure to excessive levels produces coughing and painful breathing and, over time, can damage the lungs. When researchers at the University of Southern California performed autopsies on Los Angeles inner-city youths who had died in homicides or traffic accidents, they already found signs that the fourteen- to twenty-five-year-olds had subtle but significant lung damage; the researchers attributed the damage to three factors: exposure to tobacco smoke, past respiratory infections, and chronic exposure to high levels of ozone, a finding buttressed by animal evidence showing that primates exposed to high levels of ozone show identical changes.

Most vulnerable to the ill effects are people who have chronic respiratory ailments, such as asthma, emphysema, bronchitis, or cardiovascular disease, and children. Running, engaging in active sports, and other forms of exercise compound the likelihood of experiencing the ill effects of ozone, as air intake increases during these activities. People who exercise can experience coughing, wheezing, labored breathing, shortness of breath, throat dryness, pain during

deep breathing, chest tightness and pain, fatigue, headache, and nausea. (See p. 745 for information on exercising in urban areas to avoid peak ozone levels.) However, even sedentary individuals are affected, often feeling too poorly to get through a normal day in a normal manner.

In many regions of the United States, ozone levels remain too high: Between one-quarter to one-half of the population, living mostly in ninety-six cities, is, at some point in the year, exposed to peak ozone levels ranging from 0.13 to 0.36 parts per million; this is well above the EPA standard of 0.12 parts per million for a one-hour average ozone concentration (the peak ozone levels vary, depending upon the temperatures and weather conditions of a given year). In some cities, such as Los Angeles, ozone peak levels have exceeded allowable limits over one hundred days during the year.

Although the standard is set for a one-hour exposure, even brief exposures to ozone at levels above the standard can affect a person. Some scientists believe that the 0.12-part-per-million regulatory level is too high to be safe and that future research will lead to the setting of a lower maximum, even though many cities are still having difficulty in meeting the requirement as it stands.

SOURCES OF INDOOR AIR POLLUTION

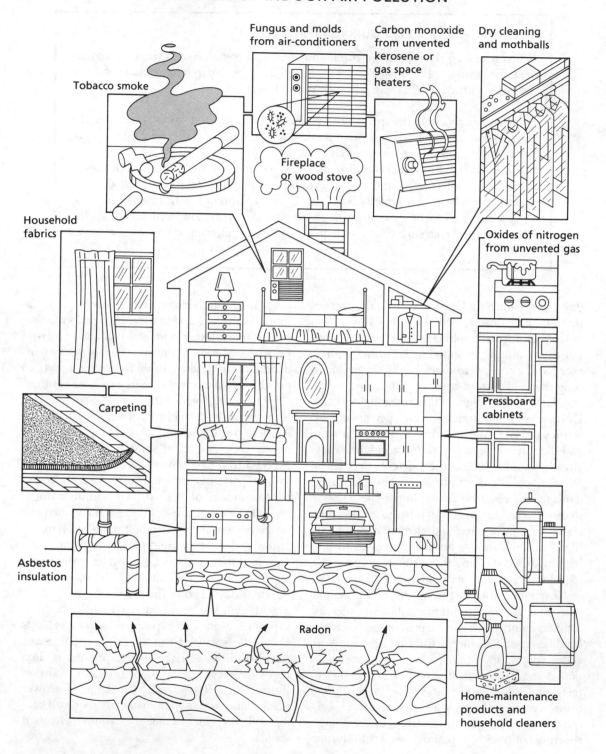

Tobacco smoke

Fungus and molds from air-conditioners

Carbon monoxide from unvented kerosene or gas space heaters

Dry cleaning and mothballs

Fireplace or wood stove

Household fabrics

Oxides of nitrogen from unvented gas

Carpeting

Pressboard cabinets

Asbestos insulation

Radon

Home-maintenance products and household cleaners

Efforts to curb the formation of ozone by reducing the automotive emissions that are the primary source of pollutants contributing to it have only made a dent: Despite significant decreases in the pollutants released by each car, overall the number of cars in urban areas, such as Los Angeles, remains too high to effectively solve this problem.

Improvements are possible, however. Many people viewed it as folly when the 1984 Olympics were held in Los Angeles, the city with the highest ozone levels in the United States (from 1984 to 1986, the EPA standard was exceeded on an average of 154 days each year). To the surprise of many, however, the city mobilized so effectively to keep vehicles off the roads during the critical period of competition that ozone levels dropped—an indication of what can be done when the stakes are high enough.

Suspended Particulate Matter. Suspended particulate matter, or particulates, are tiny solid or liquid particles made up of smoke, dust, fog, soot, and condensed chemical and metallic fumes. When breathed in, they can have serious effects on the respiratory system, because the smaller particulates manage to evade its defenses. As is true of other pollutants, people with bronchitis, asthma, and other respiratory disease and cardiovascular problems are particularly susceptible to their effects. The smaller they are in size, the more potentially damaging particulates are because the fine particulates can evade many of the respiratory tract's defenses. Suspended particulate matter (PM) that is less than 10 micrometers in diameter, known as PM_{10}, are the ones listed in the Clean Air Act as comprising a criteria pollutant index.

A recently completed decade-long study in Philadelphia by researchers from the EPA and Harvard School of Public Health found that as levels of particulates increased in the area there was a corresponding increase in the number of cases of illness and death.

In both Philadelphia and Seattle, harmful effects occurred when levels of particulates were well below current EPA standards. Further discoveries about the dangers of particulates may eventually lead to changes in the regulations.

INDOOR AIR POLLUTION

Because the indoor environment is largely closed, harmful substances cannot diffuse in the air as they might outdoors; particularly in tightly sealed, energy-efficient homes and offices, pollutants can be found at levels several times higher indoors than in the air outside.

Sources of indoor air pollutants range from those that occur naturally, such as the radioactive, cancer-causing gas radon, and microorganisms (bacteria, molds, and fungi), to those produced by human activity. Many of the consumer products and appliances used in the home can introduce harmful agents not found, or found in smaller amounts, in outdoor air. These indoor-air contaminants include carbon monoxide and gas fumes from poorly vented stoves,

Figure 14.2 SOURCES OF INDOOR AIR POLLUTION.

Radon gas, environmental tobacco smoke, asbestos, and formaldehyde are the four most dangerous indoor air pollutants according to the EPA and public health officials. Other indoor air contaminants include carbon monoxide from unvented gas; microorganisms such as bacteria, molds, and fungi; unvented fumes from gas and wood heaters; fumes from the residue of dry-cleaning products or mothballs; asbestos dusts; volatile organic chemicals and gases emanating from common consumer products; and gases, fibers, dusts, and chemicals (notably formaldehyde) in building materials such as pressboard, carpet backing, and synthetic tile.

unvented fumes from gas and wood heaters, fumes from the residue of dry cleaning products or mothballs, asbestos dusts, volatile organic chemicals and gases emanating from common consumer products, and an array of other gases, fibers, dusts, and chemicals, including formaldehyde. Humidity can be a factor as well.

Houses and buildings have become more tightly sealed, holding in heat in winter and coolness in summer and trapping increased concentrations of airborne pollutants all year round. Gases and particulate matter from these indoor sources can become highly concentrated in such buildings. The reliance on synthetic materials—pressboard, plywood, and plastics in construction materials and synthetic fibers in wall-to-wall carpeting, furniture construction, and drapery—has increased concentrations of numerous potentially damaging vapors, fumes, and gases as well.

- Indoor levels of volatile organic chemicals (VOCs)—carbon-based chemicals, such as hydrocarbons, that are released from common household products—can accumulate to dangerously high concentrations. Many of the volatile organic chemicals not only irritate the eyes, nose, and throat but can induce headaches, depression, irritability, and general malaise—the characteristics of sick-building syndrome. Levels of hydrocarbons were found to be one hundred times higher indoors than outdoors, according to an EPA study of indoor air in seven cities including Greensboro, North Carolina; Pittsburgh, Pennsylvania; and Los Angeles, California, each of which has measurably high ambient air levels of volatile organic compounds at least some of the time. The highest concentrations were found in newer more tightly sealed buildings (see Box 14.7).
- Tobacco smoking is the single largest source of indoor air pollution. Exposure to environmental tobacco smoke (also called passive or sidestream smoke) is implicated in respiratory problems and chronic ear infections in children and in almost 4,000 lung cancer deaths each year. Tobacco smoke is the most common

source of exposure to the carcinogen benzene as well as numerous other carcinogens and substances that can cause reproductive, respiratory, or other health impairments (see pp. 139, 235, and Box 22.3, p. 730 for more information on health effects).
- Homes with gas stoves or unvented kerosene heaters can develop indoor concentrations of nitrogen dioxide, a by-product of high-temperature combustion, that exceed the EPA's limit of 63 parts per billion in outdoor air.
- The EPA and the New Jersey State Health Department estimate that almost one-third of the homes in New Jersey have enough radon seeping into their basements to pose a greater than one in one hundred lifetime risk of lung cancer, yet fewer than 5 percent of New Jersey homeowners have tested their homes for the presence of this dangerous indoor air pollutant.

As with outdoor air pollution, the people most vulnerable to exposure to indoor airborne contaminants are the elderly, the young, people who are sick, women who are pregnant, people who already suffer chronic respiratory or heart disease, and workers who spend large amounts of time indoors in factories and offices. In most cases, the pollutants encountered in the workplace are the same as those encountered at home or on the streets, but exposures may be many times more concentrated.

The Most Dangerous Pollutants

The EPA and public health officials list environmental tobacco smoke, radon, asbestos, and formaldehyde as the four most dangerous indoor air pollutants.

Environmental Tobacco Smoke. Also known as side-stream or passive smoke, environmental tobacco smoke is that which is released into the air from the burning end of a cigarette without going through the filter. Smoking is the largest single source of indoor pollution (as well as the

+---+
| **Box 14.7   SICK-BUILDING SYNDROME AND BUILDING-RELATED ILLNESSES** |
| |
| The EPA estimates that as many as one-third of the buildings in the United States |
| suffer from *sick-building syndrome*, which means that the air they contain causes |
| nonspecific symptoms in people such as dizziness, lethargy, headaches, stuffed-up |
| sinuses, coughing, sneezing, runny noses, burning eyes, upper respiratory infec- |
| tions, or flulike symptoms. Most sufferers of sick-building syndrome recover upon |
| leaving the building because their symptoms are direct reactions to pollutants in the |
| building's air. |
| |
| Sick-building syndrome (or tight-building syndrome) arises from a combination |
| of faulty ventilation, the presence of air pollutants, and tight energy-conserving |
| construction that seals windows closed and limits the exchange of indoor air with |
| outdoor air—factors that conspire to trap and accumulate indoor airborne agents. |
| |
| In 1987, the National Research Council distinguished this syndrome from |
| building-related illnesses, which are not specific ailments unto themselves but dis- |
| eases due to exposure to a chemical or biological agent in a building. (Examples of |
| building-related illnesses include Legionnaires' Disease, "humidifier fever," and hy- |
| persensitivity pneumonia.) Unlike sick-building syndrome, the symptoms of |
| building-related illnesses are relatively clear-cut and, once diagnosed, must be |
| treated; simply leaving the building will not cure the ailment. However, once the |
| source of the illness is eradicated, the outbreaks cease. |
| |
| Humidity seems to be a factor contributing to building-related illnesses, partic- |
| ularly among children who seem to suffer more frequent bouts of respiratory ill- |
| nesses when living in damp homes. Many biological agents that can cause disease or |
| trigger allergic symptoms prefer moist environments, such as mold and allergen- |
| shedding dust mites, which thrive where the relative humidity exceeds 70 percent. |
| Outbreaks of Legionnaires' Disease were directly related to microorganisms that |
| grew in the presence of a moist environment (see Box 1.3, p. 27). |
+---+

greatest preventable cause of death and disease), and smokers endanger not only themselves, but those around them. An estimated 3,800 deaths from lung cancer are attributed to exposure to environmental tobacco smoke.

The smoke from a typical tobacco cigarette contains numerous dangerous chemicals, including benzene (see Figure 22.2, p. 734). The EPA calculates that more cases of leukemia result from household exposure to benzene than industrial exposure, with exposure to tobacco smoke the major source of indoor benzene. A smoker may inhale 600 micrograms of benzene a day, whereas a person exposed to environmental tobacco smoke is likely to be inhaling 17 micrograms. The effect of that much benzene expo-

sure on the U.S. population could result in a minimum of 500 leukemias a year in smokers, 50 in those inhaling side-stream smoke; in fact, a 1993 study linked environmental tobacco smoke to as much as one-third of all adult leukemias.

Children appear to be particularly susceptible to adverse effects from environmental tobacco smoke. A number of studies have linked parents' smoking to health problems in children, notably respiratory problems and chronic ear infections. The children may also have an increased risk of lung cancer. Nearly 70 percent of children live in homes where there is at least one smoker, according to a large-scale study carried out by the Harvard School of Public Health (see Chapter 12, "Of Special Concern: Infants and Children," and Chapter 6, "Repiratory Ailments").

Recent studies connect environmental tobacco smoke with harmful effects on pregnancy and increased probability of bearing low-birth-weight babies (see Chapter 11, "Reproductive Effects and Prenatal Exposures").

Radon. Although the public is relatively apathetic about the risks posed by radon, a naturally occurring radioactive gas, the EPA ranks indoor exposure to radon at the top of its list of risks, tied for first place with chemicals in the workplace as a cause of cancer (see p. 44).

Radon gas is released by the decay of uranium-238 in rocks and soil. It seeps into houses through cracks in the foundation, basement, and floors. The radon gas itself decays, like all radioactive substances, forming very small particles called radon daughters or progeny. These attach to dust particles in the air that are inhaled and deposited deep within the lungs. As the radon daughters continue to decay, they damage the cells that line the airways.

An estimated 5,000 to 20,000 cancers a year are attributed to exposure to radon indoors. In the past, radon outdoors has not been viewed as a serious hazard because of its wide diffusion in outdoor air.

Radon is measured in picocuries per liter of air. (A picocurie is one-trillionth of a curie, which is a unit of measurement for radioactivity.) The EPA has set 4 picocuries per liter of air as the highest acceptable level within the home, a guideline based on calculations of the lowest level that can readily be attained with existing technology, not the dose at which there is no observable adverse effect. The EPA estimates that at exposure levels of 15 picocuries per liter of air the risk of developing cancer becomes comparable to that faced by the one-pack-a-day smoker. Radon acts synergistically with tobacco smoke, multiplying the risks of developing lung cancer in smokers and smoke-exposed nonsmokers.

In 1984, the Pennsylvania Bureau of Radiation Protection obtained a reading in excess of 2,600 picocuries per liter of air in a home in Bucks County. Although this measurement was exceptional, high levels of radon in the area were not unusual. Extrapolating from the data obtained from a sampling of houses, the researchers estimated that more than 10,000 residents were exposed to levels higher than 100 picocuries per liter of air and that more than 180,000 homes in the state had radon levels above 20 picocuries per liter of air.

While state surveys have identified radon hot spots—regions of the country where many homes exceed the national average—high enough levels of radon to merit concern have been found in every state where homes have been tested. The EPA estimates that 6 percent of houses in the United States have radon levels high enough above 4 picocuries per liter of air to warrant taking corrective action (see Box 14.8), and testing is the only reliable way to determine if a particular house has a problem.

Formaldehyde. As many as 10 to 20 million Americans are affected by chronic respiratory ailments and symptoms characteristic of sick-building syndrome due to exposure to the volatile organic chemical formaldehyde, which is released (outgassed) from products that contain it.

In animal studies, formaldehyde has been associated with cancer. In humans, the epidemiologic evidence of the link to cancer is inconclusive: In one study of morticians and pathologists, professionals who are occupationally exposed to high levels of formaldehyde in embalming fluid, an increase in deaths due to brain cancer and leukemias was found. Another study of workers exposed to formaldehyde in six British chemical plants also found that they had a higher incidence of deaths due to lung cancer than was expected. A 1986 study of industrial workers exposed to low levels of formaldehyde was found by some to show an increase in lung cancer that was too small to be statistically significant. Others felt the increase in lung cancer was significant, especially for workers with the longest exposures.

The sources of formaldehyde are well known: It is used widely in plywood, particle board,

Box 14.8 WHAT TO DO ABOUT RADON

Radon gas is odorless and colorless, and most people do not know they are exposed to it. A complex series of factors help to determine the extent to which any dwelling accumulates radon: Two seemingly identical and adjacent homes can harbor widely different radon concentrations—one reason why the U.S. Public Health Service advises all homeowners to test for radon.

Radon can be measured in the home using a number of relatively inexpensive devices: You can measure the levels with an inexpensive charcoal canister for three to seven days, or with a plastic (alpha-track) detector for two to four weeks, or—the best procedure—for a full year. These devices are provided by some state and local governments and private firms. (To find a private firm, contact your state radiation or environmental protection agency office; they can provide a list of reputable companies—those which have voluntarily submitted to an EPA evaluation of their abilities in measuring and analyzing radon data. Since prices for the services vary, select three companies from that list and choose the one that is most competitive in its price.) Radon levels are highest in the basement, and measurements should be made in the lowest regularly occupied area of the house.

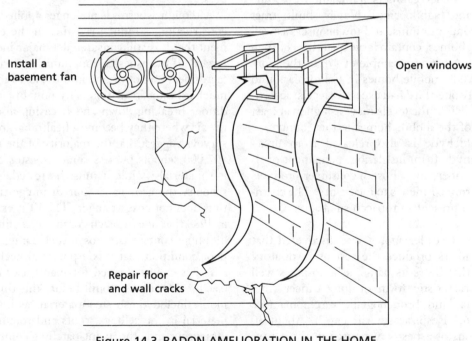

Install a basement fan

Open windows

Repair floor and wall cracks

Figure 14.3 RADON AMELIORATION IN THE HOME.

(continued)

Box 14.8   WHAT TO DO ABOUT RADON (*continued*)

Here are some simple, practical approaches to reducing radon levels in the home:

- Improve ventilation. Open windows on all sides of the house.
- Install a fan in the basement that draws air out from beneath the foundation. According to the EPA, this action can reduce indoor radon levels by 90 percent. Keep vents on all sides of basements and crawl spaces fully open year-round.
- Seal any visible cracks in the basement floor and subsurface walls through which radon can seep into the house. Because cement-block walls can transmit up to ten times more radon than visible cracks, seal walls with latext paint or topcoat.
- Consider facing subsurface basement walls with masonite or particle-board.

For more information about detectors and radon-reduction techniques, contact your EPA regional office or call the hot line at 1-800-SOS-RADON. The EPA provides two useful consumer booklets, "Citizen's Guide to Radon" and "Home Buyers and Sellers Guide."

---

paneling, and fiberboard, materials often used to construct kitchen cabinets and countertops, furniture, and subflooring. Newly built tract homes, condominiums, and townhouses, as well as mobile homes, contain large quantities of such products. A random sample of 470 of the more than 500,000 mobile homes in California found that nearly one-third had excessive levels; according to the EPA, the levels may be high in at least one-half of the mobile homes in this country.

Formaldehyde is also released from urea–formaldehyde foam insulation, permanent press fabrics, rubber, and a host of consumer products ranging from cosmetics to medicines. The chemical is also present in tobacco smoke.

Asbestos. Decades ago, it was discovered that asbestos fibers produce the serious respiratory disorder that bears its name, asbestosis, as well as a characteristic form of lung cancer (mesothelioma) and bronchogenic carcinoma (see Chapter 6, "Respiratory Ailments"). About 30 million tons of asbestos was used in the course of this century in more than 3,000 applications, chiefly because of its excellent properties as an insulating and fireproofing material. Millions of

people were thus exposed to asbestos's toxic fibers.

Although asbestos is no longer applied in new construction, so much remains in the environment that it is still considered a major indoor air hazard. If the asbestos-containing material is intact, fibers do not escape into the air. However, much asbestos insulation is by now in poor condition, breaking down and releasing fibers into the air where they become a health hazard. EPA surveys suggest that the majority of the nation's 107,000 schools possess some asbestos-containing materials; while it must be tested, in most schools, the asbestos is not disintegrating and thus does not pose a danger. The EPA estimated in 1988 that one in seven commercial and public buildings contain asbestos in such comparatively poor condition that it is a potential health risk.

Asbestos was banned for many uses in 1974 (see p. 126). Houses built before this time commonly included asbestos materials as insulating material in the ceilings, roofs and roofing shingles, grout and other paint-patching compounds, boiler-encasing materials, and steam-pipe-insulating material, which may contain as much as 90 percent asbestos. Prior to the mid-1970s,

---

Box 14.9 HOW TO IMPROVE THE AIR IN YOUR HOME

- Do not smoke tobacco.
- Improve ventilation. Open the windows, except during smog alerts; install exhaust fans or air-to-air heat-exchanging devices that draw fresh air in through one duct and expel it through another; and vent stoves and heaters to the outside.
- Keep gas appliances in good repair.
- Check the home for radon. If levels are found to be high, make the recommended changes.
- Determine whether asbestos insulation is in poor condition and if so, call in a specialist for removal.
- Substitute water-based products for hydrocarbon-based cleaners that emit volatile hydrocarbon gases.
- Look for environmentally safer products. Consumer demand has created what manufacturers are calling the "green" phenomenon, requiring them to use alternatives to hazardous materials.
- When purchasing home furnishings, select fabrics that do not have a high pile to concentrate pollutants and dust or that shed irritating fibers.
- Maintain indoor humidity levels between 30 and 50 percent to help prevent water from condensing on building materials. Ventilate the attic and crawl space, and use exhaust fans to remove the moisture that builds up during cooking and bathing. Fill water reservoirs of cool mist or ultrasonic humidifiers daily with distilled water, and clean evaporation trays in air-conditioners and dehumidifiers frequently. Keep the basement dry. Clean and dry water-damaged rugs and carpets within twenty-four hours, if possible, to prevent disease-causing bacteria and mold from taking up residence.
- Do not burn leaves or cook over a backyard fire. These practices are already outlawed in some high-pollution areas.

---

many ovens, dishwashers, and other appliances were wrapped in asbestos insulation. Some manufacturers added it to vinyl or linoleum flooring.

Warning: Should you have reason to believe there is deteriorating asbestos in your home, do not try to remove it yourself. Attempts to do that can result in far higher exposures than leaving it in place. The EPA advocates bringing in specialists to deal with the material. (See Box 6.6, p. 127, for more information.)

In 1989 the EPA ordered virtually all uses of asbestos to be phased out by 1997; however, the order was overturned by an appeals court in 1991. (For details about asbestos regulation and additional facts about its health effects, see the Asbestos information sheet, p. 365, and Chapter 6, "Respiratory Ailments.")

Minimizing Air Pollution in the Home

Identifying an indoor air-pollution problem at home is the first step toward improving it. In many cases, the solution is as simple as opening windows; in others, as when radon or asbestos must be removed, professional help is required.

The most significant change of all can be the most difficult—to give up smoking. (See Chapter 22, "The ABCs of Staying Healthy," for information on smoking-cessation strategies.)

Other steps to improve the air quality in the home are listed in Box 14.9.

CHAPTER 15

Soil

Along with water and air, soil is a critical part of the life-support system for the planet earth. Soil bears the plants that release life-giving oxygen into the atmosphere and holds the nutrients and water that supports the croplands, forests, and grasslands necessary for human and wildlife survival. The groundwater aquifers that supply drinking water are recharged because of the soil's ability to absorb rainwater, and the cycle of life, death, and renewal is fueled by organisms that inhabit the soil, helping to recycle plant and animal remains to the nutrients that will support the next generation of soil life.

Soil can present a health risk to human life, however, by exposing us to contaminants that come to rest in its different layers. Individuals can become exposed, directly or indirectly, to soil toxins in a number of ways. Directly, people come into contact with polluted soil by digging in it, as do gardeners and construction workers; by playing in and around it; by breathing dust raised from it; or even by eating it, as small children sometimes do. Indirectly, people drink water containing pollutants leached from nearby soil, eat vegetables and fruits that have absorbed toxins from the ground, and eat meat contaminated with toxins that accumulate when herds graze in contaminated pastures. The threat of exposure to dangerous substances via contaminated soil is not as great as that posed by tainted water or air; most people do not come in direct contact with contaminated soil in landfills or at chemical dumps, and few actually live or work where radioactive materials are present. However, when the soil in a particular area is contaminated, the threat can be pervasive. It can affect people's surroundings and their food and water supplies, and in extreme situations, it can even force them to move from their homes.

TYPES OF SOIL HAZARDS

Soils have long been used as repositories for residential, industrial, and commercial wastes. Disposal ponds and landfills have traditionally been dumped on top of the soil; more recent landfills have been buried in the surrounding soil (mainly because of complaints about the smell and appearance of mounds of garbage from nearby residents). Tailings from mines, such as ore and coal, have also been dumped on top of surface soil, often depositing heavy metals or acids there. Buried dumps, tanks, and barrels often leak harmful chemicals into the soil.

Other soil pollution is hard to trace to a single source, making it difficult to control or evaluate.

Acid rain can deposit harmful acids in soils as a result of sulfur dioxide and nitrogen dioxide emissions miles away (see Box 14.4, p. 551). Hard-to-trace pollution also results from spills and leaks that wash off parking lots and highways, from "midnight dumping" of pollutants at unauthorized sites or along highways, from backyard pollutants such as used motor oil and chemical fertilizers, and from lead from pre-1978 automotive emissions, which remains settled in soil even today.

The types and sources of soil pollution vary among the layers of the soil at any given site. Within only a few feet of soil, there are a number of layers that differ in their composition and in the types of disturbance and contamination to which they are vulnerable.

Pollutants released into the air can eventually come to rest in the first few inches of soil, sometimes persisting for years after the initial threat has passed. For example, airborne emissions of the heavy metal lead, which settled in urban soils, still threaten city youngsters. Acid rain is one of the most prevalent air-to-soil contaminants. It upsets the delicate ecological balance of the microorganisms that reside under the soil's surface and strips the soil of nutrients vital for the growth of healthy trees and other vegetation (see Chapter 14, "Air"). The soil's uppermost layers can also become laden with agricultural chemicals applied to the surface or with toxic chemicals dumped into an aboveground landfill.

Deeper soil layers are threatened from sources such as underground gasoline tanks; improperly designed waste dumps; natural contaminants, such as the elements arsenic and barium, which are found in certain types of rock and can leach into soil and water; and radioactive elements formed as uranium-containing rock decays, such as radon.

It is difficult to separate soil and water pollution because both are an instrumental part of the earth's balanced water system; the soil can serve as a conduit for toxic elements that percolate through its pores. Pollutants at the deeper levels not only contaminate the soil but can threaten groundwater sources. Risks to water can also develop when the soil is disturbed; for example, at a mine site where the soil is piled outside, as rain seeps through the pile, it can leach out acids and carry them into the local groundwater.

Whether they are contaminated naturally or artificially through our actions, all layers of the fffsoil can present a health risk. Starting at the top and working to deeper layers, here are several ways in which the health risks emerge.

Urban Contamination

The top soil layers in urban areas are plagued with soil contamination problems compounded by the concentration of people and the abundance of toxic materials. Contaminants accrue from used motor oil (which also contains toxic metals such as lead and arsenic), antifreeze, pesticides, and paints, all of which are often poured into drains, gutters, ditches, catch basins, or the corner of a backyard. When enough of the material enters the ground, the contaminants can eventually seep into the groundwater and then into local water supplies.

Playgrounds, city streets, backyards, or drainage ditches where excessive amounts of contaminants were poured present health risks to children as well as people tending urban gardens.

(These materials present an additional health risk beyond those caused through ingesting or breathing in the contaminants: Many of the materials are flammable or corrosive to skin. These materials should be disposed of properly. For information on disposal, see Chapter 19, "Consumer Products.")

Urban lead contamination of soil due to vehicle emissions can pose a direct health hazard to children, despite the phaseout of lead in gasoline in the United States beginning in 1975 (lead is still found in gasoline in other countries, including Great Britain). Lead contamination may also be caused by industrial emissions. Both types of emissions can eventually settle to the ground and contaminate urban soils and, in some areas, even rival other sources of exposure, such as contact

SOURCES OF SOIL POLLUTION

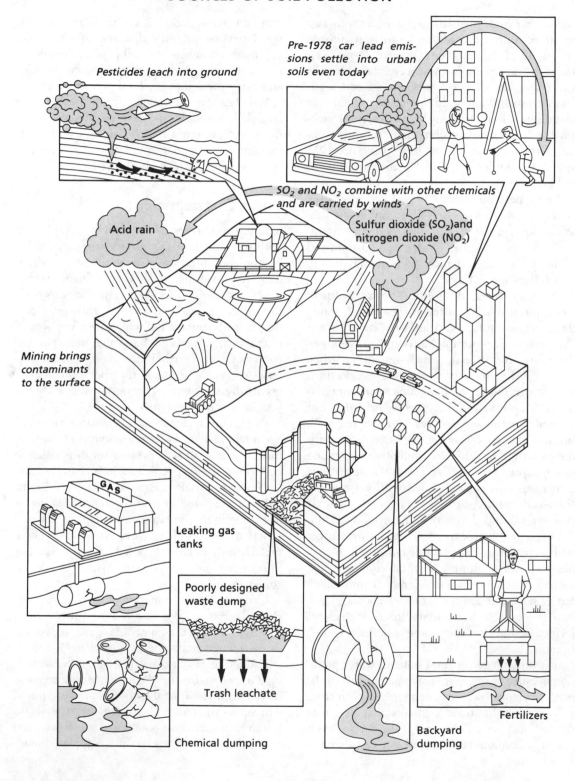

Pesticides leach into ground

Pre-1978 car lead emissions settle into urban soils even today

SO_2 and NO_2 combine with other chemicals and are carried by winds

Sulfur dioxide (SO_2) and nitrogen dioxide (NO_2)

Acid rain

Mining brings contaminants to the surface

GAS

Leaking gas tanks

Poorly designed waste dump

Trash leachate

Chemical dumping

Backyard dumping

Fertilizers

with crumbling lead-based paint. In rural areas, estimated lead levels are 10 to 30 parts per million, whereas in suburban areas levels increase to 100 parts per million and can be as high as 1,000 parts per million in urban areas. Children playing in these contaminated soils are vulnerable to lead poisoning, as they can be exposed by ingesting the soils and inhaling the lead-laden dust blown by the wind or moved by human activity (see Chapter 12, "Of Special Concern: Infants and Children").

Farm and Nonfarm Agricultural Pollutants

Residues of high concentrations of agricultural chemicals, such as pesticides and fertilizers, can make their way into the soil to eventually contaminate both water and food supplies.

Pesticides are composed of chemicals that vary in their level of toxicity to humans and animals. Each of the several classes of pesticides in use has a distinct soil *half-life*, the time it takes for the concentration to be reduced by one-half; this affects the period it persists in the soil or rainwater runoff. Half-life is affected by the properties of the soil, in particular its ability to retard the movement of the pesticide to the groundwater.

In regions that rely on surface water for potable water supplies, limiting pesticide spread is crucial to avoid contamination of streams, rivers, and lakes. Soil erosion can also carry pesticides into the water system. With successive applications, a pesticide with a long soil half-life can build up and remain in the soil for years. This is what happened in areas of the western United States where trace amounts of pesticides used many years ago and currently banned, such as arsenic and copper salts, are still found in the soil of some orchards.

Pesticides also vary in their ability to bind with either water or with fat molecules in animal tissues. This latter characteristic of a pesticide is important because it can determine whether or not a pesticide will accumulate over time to toxic levels in animal tissues. Whereas water-soluble substances are excreted from the body relatively quickly, fat-soluble molecules persist for a month or longer in animal tissues. (See Box 15.3 and Chapter 17, "Food Safety," for a discussion of bioaccumulation.)

Even agricultural chemicals that are not directly toxic to humans or animals may eventually pose a human health risk if applied to soil. For example, fertilizers contain and release harmless nitrates in the soil; the nitrates are converted to potentially harmful nitrites for absorption by plants (nitrites also enter the soil from the fecal matter of farm animals). If excessive amounts of highly soluble nitrates are applied to the earth, they can migrate through the soil, be converted into dangerous nitrites, and enter drinking water supplies. Excessive exposure to nitrites can interfere with the transport of oxygen by hemoglobin in the blood and cause blue-baby syndrome (methemoglobinemia).

Farms are not the only source of soil contamination by agricultural chemicals. Similar chemicals are used to treat 25 million acres of grass each year in the United States, including residential yards; golf courses; industrial park lawns; and other residential, industrial, and commercial lawns. According to a 1991 statement by the Senate Environmental and Public Works Sub-

Figure 15.1 SOURCES OF SOIL POLLUTION.

Soils have long been used as repositories for residential, industrial, and commercial wastes. Disposal ponds and landfills, tailings from mines dumped on the soil's surface, buried dumps, tanks, and barrels that leak—all contribute to soil pollution. Other soil pollution is hard to trace to a single source, such as acid rain, chemicals from spills and leaks that wash off parking lots and highways, and lead from pre-1978 automotive emissions, which remains settled in soil even today.

Box 15.1   WHAT IS SOIL?

Soil is defined as the loose material formed by the physical and chemical disintegration of inorganic material (such as the weathering of rock) and organic material (the bacteria, fungi, wastes, and decay of plants and animals). The soil is a slowly evolving layer of the earth's crust composed of layers (see Fig. 15.2). Soil thickness varies depending on climate and age, because heat and water weather local rock, which adds particles to the soil. As weathering continues, it also breaks the particles down further into their basic elements, thus contributing nutrients to the soil.

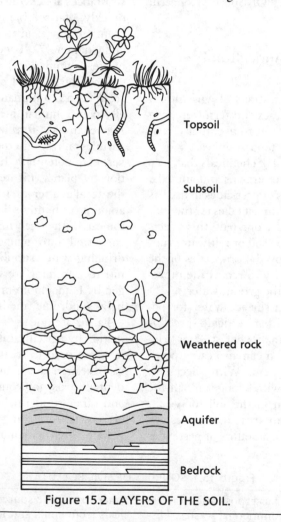

Topsoil

Subsoil

Weathered rock

Aquifer

Bedrock

Figure 15.2 LAYERS OF THE SOIL.

The type and amount of organic matter present is also controlled by climate. Relatively warm, wet regions, such as the northeastern United States, tend to have

(continued)

Box 15.1 WHAT IS SOIL? (*continued*)

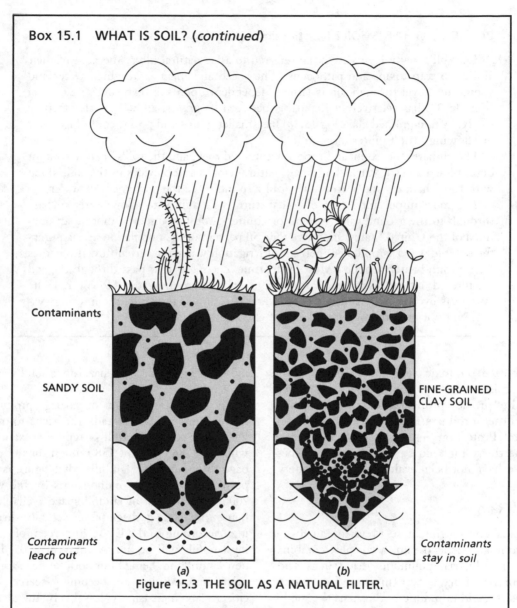

Contaminants

SANDY SOIL

FINE-GRAINED CLAY SOIL

Contaminants leach out

Contaminants stay in soil

(a)   (b)

Figure 15.3 THE SOIL AS A NATURAL FILTER.

a highly varied vegetation and an abundance of animal life. At the opposite extreme, dry regions, such as the desert Southwest, support less vegetation and wildlife. In all types of climate, various types of microorganisms not only help to produce nutrients for plants but chemically weather the soil, decompose organic waste, and detoxify some environmental toxins.

Groundwater aquifers running beneath the rock of a soil can receive pollutants that have managed to make their way past the upper layers of the ground.

(*continued*)

Box 15.1   WHAT IS SOIL? (*continued*)

The soil's many layers are often referred to as a "natural filter," because of their ability to trap toxins and pathogens. The speed and manner in which water and chemicals travel through soil is largely dependent upon soil texture. A sandy soil (Fig. 15.3*a*) has relatively wide spaces between its grains, allowing water to flow freely. A fine-grained clay (Fig 15.3*b*) has smaller grains and pores, confining water or allowing little to filter through.

The climate, the extent and type of weathered rock, and the soil's organic content determine a soil's texture. The small, natural cracks and crevices in the soil, along with root channels and worm holes, can also influence the movement of water.

The most important aspect of soil texture is its ability to allow water to pass through to the groundwater system, or aquifer. Aquifers underlie more than one-third of the United States, and more than 50 percent of the population uses aquifers for potable water supplies; 40 percent of irrigation water for agriculture also comes from groundwater supplies. Most of the time, chemicals that pass through the soil are filtered out, or dissipated, before they reach the groundwater. However, if the system is overloaded, as through the overapplication of fertilizer, the filtering system will not hold the overabundance of chemicals.

---

committee on toxic substances, many of the companies manufacturing these lawn products failed to provide proper warning about the danger of their products. According to the Environmental Protection Agency (EPA), thirty-three of the thirty-four most popular residential pesticides have not been evaluated for their safety.

Acid Rain

Perhaps one of the more prevalent air-to-soil contaminants is acid rain, a complex combination of industrial pollutants that fall as acid-contaminated dry or wet (in snow, fog, or rain) deposits. Acid rain directly threatens the soil by upsetting the delicate ecological balance of the microorganisms that reside under its surface. (see Chapter 14, "Air," for a detailed discussion of acid rain.)

Landfills

Waste disposal and contamination of deeper layers of soils are inseparable issues. Among the most common sources of hazardous solid wastes are landfills.

The increasing amount of garbage produced in the United States already threatens to overwhelm the current landfill system. For example, while in 1986, we sent 158 million tons of garbage to our nation's landfills, that figure is expected to rise to 193 million tons by the year 2000. The amount of landfill space available to house this rising garbage pile is actually shrinking: According to the EPA, 70 percent of existing landfills will be full by the year 2005. Few new landfills are being built both because appropriate, unused sites are becoming scarcer and citizens are increasingly less likely to tolerate landfills in their own neighborhoods. The scarcity of landfills and increased public awareness of their dangers, such as the leaching of dangerous chemicals as water filters through the landfill, have led many consumers to consider alternatives; these include recycling, and the refusal of consumers to purchase heavily packaged or otherwise wasteful goods. Without extensive recycling, reuse, and conservation programs—

Box 15.2   IS THE SOIL AROUND YOUR HOUSE CONTAMINATED?

Testing soil for contaminants is an expensive process, especially since every substance requires a separate test. However, if there is any suspicion, you may want to take the following steps:

- Research your property's history to find out what was on the site before your house was constructed. If it was a manufacturing site, find out what products were made. If it was farmland, find out what crops were grown (different chemicals are used on different crops). This will help you determine whether to have your soil tested and the best soil tests to use.
- Research the general terrain of the area. In particular, find out the direction of groundwater flow (this is particularly relevant for people who have private wells). If there is a manufacturing operation or gas station that is leaking a chemical into the local groundwater, your water and soil may also be affected if your groundwater is located downstream.
- Inform your local county health department of what you find. They may be able to link specific symptoms to certain chemicals or note epidemiological trends, such as a cluster of illnesses in a particular neighborhood. Be sure to mention whether you use a private well or the local municipal water supply.
- Contact your state environmental agency (usually referred to as the Environmental Quality or Environmental Protection Agency) or local health department if you suspect soil contamination. They may be receiving similar complaints from other people in the area and may be able to put together a pattern of contamination. They also will help to determine your best course of action if you do find contamination on your property and can refer you to a reliable soil-testing company.

---

by citizens as well as industry and commercial concerns—we are not likely to stem the overflow of landfills and their subsequent dangers (see Box 15.4).

It is difficult to discuss the hazards posed by landfills in a general way because each site is unique, varying in construction, combination of chemicals, and numerous soil and water characteristics. Today, the health risks associated with living near a landfill depend on several factors: the landfill's age (older landfills tended to be unlined and, therefore, more prone to leaks), its contents, and what—if anything—is leaking into the surrounding area.

The routes of exposure from landfill-contaminated soils are varied and many: Children playing close to a landfill or individuals living in homes built on a buried landfill site are especially high risk of exposure, as are workers who come in direct contact with or move the contaminated soils from site to site. Well-water supplies also are a route of exposure with contaminated water from landfills able to percolate through the soil. (This type of pollution is especially common around unlined landfills or dumps where runoff from rains readily carries contaminants into the soil.)

Dumps and Tanks

Industry makes use of a large number of chemicals known or suspected to pose health hazards to humans and the environment. Some of the contamination of the deeper layers of our soil and water can be traced to the past history of

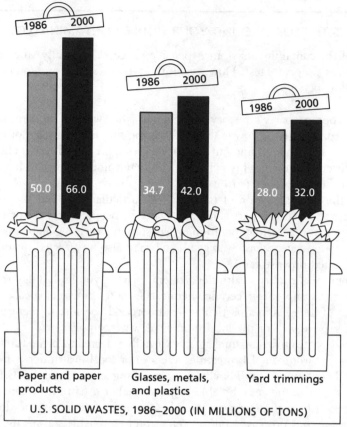

1986   2000

1986   2000

1986   2000

50.0   66.0

34.7   42.0

28.0   32.0

Paper and paper products

Glasses, metals, and plastics

Yard trimmings

U.S. SOLID WASTES, 1986–2000 (IN MILLIONS OF TONS)

Figure 15.4 THE 1986–2000 GARBAGE PILE.

dumping or releasing industrial and chemical manufacturing wastes into the environment.

The health hazards posed by many of these substances have been known or suspected for years. Since the 1950s, for example, scientists have warned of the possible ill effects of dioxins, polychlorinated biphenyls (PCBs), and heavy metals, such as lead and mercury. Despite this knowledge, wastes were routinely buried under the soil, dumped in unused corners of industrial plants, or hauled off the site and deposited in an unlined landfill.

In the 1970s, concern increased over the potential health risks posed by an expanding number of unregistered and unregulated dumps around the country. Many of the chemicals used in manufacturing processes were regulated or banned be-

cause of their potential health risks to humans.

Years of indiscriminate and unregulated dumping have taken their toll: Even after a factory closes or moves, hazardous industrial wastes can remain a problem for the surrounding soils and, in turn, the individuals living nearby. It is difficult to quantify the health risks posed by such soil contaminants. There are reports suggesting contaminated soils may have possible health effects on children and adults who play and work in these areas, but the studies are incomplete.

In many cases, the type, extent, and lasting effect of chemicals used on one-time sites are unknown. For example, in the past, chemical dumps were occasionally "rehabilitated," deemed safe, and then used as locations for hous-

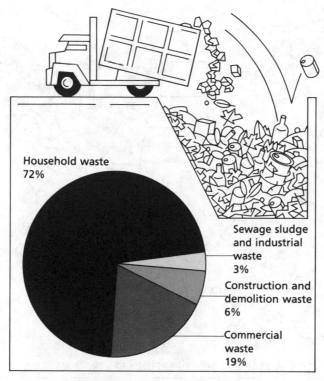

CURRENT MIX OF U.S. LANDFILL WASTES

Source for chart information: U.S. Environmental Protection Agency.

ing developments, playgrounds, or industrial buildings. Love Canal, New York, situated not far from Niagara Falls, is one of the most infamous examples of one such hazardous dump site (see Box 15.5).

Superfund Program. In 1980, Congress established the Superfund Program to identify and clean up a few hundred of the worst contaminated sites around the United States. More than ten years after its inception, this list of former dump and waste sites on the Superfund priority list has grown from the original 400 to 1,207.

Only 63 of the 1,207 identified sites have been cleaned up as of this writing. According to a National Academy of Sciences report, the Superfund Program is hampered by a lack of an inventory of toxic wastes at sites and a systematic method for identifying new sites. Due to a lack of funding, there is a notable dearth of the

needed scientific studies that could establish whether and to what extent Superfund-site contaminants pose a human health risk at low levels of exposure.

Site-specific contaminants may contain heavy metals, such as chromium, cadmium, zinc, nickel, and lead, as well as volatile organic compounds, such as benzene and polychlorinated biphenyls. All of these substances are known to pose health risks to humans.

Tanks. Old, improperly installed, and leaking gasoline tanks under thousands of service stations and on gasoline tank farms are a troublesome source of soil contamination. The bare steel tanks used to store gas often were installed with no protection against corrosion; within a few years of installation, certain soils and water damaged and corroded the tanks until the contents leaked into the surrounding earth. Such

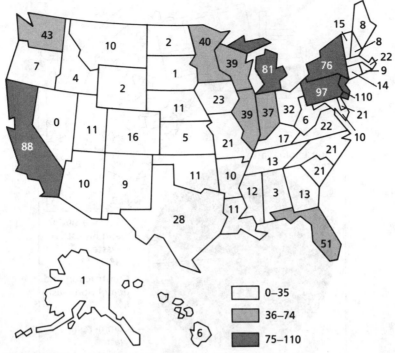

Figure 15.5 A MAP OF THE SUPERFUND PRIORITY SITES.

At the time this book went to press, 1,207 sites were designated for cleanup under the Superfund Program. Approximately 40 million Americans live within four miles of designated Superfund sites. There is no "typical" Superfund site; each contains a different combination of toxic substances as well as different physical characteristics, such as soil texture, that can affect the leakage of pollutants into groundwater or soil.

Source: U.S. Environmental Protection Agency.

Box 15.3 NUCLEAR FALLOUT AND SOIL CONTAMINATION

Radioactive fallout from nuclear accidents and testing of nuclear devices is a rare source of serious top-layer soil contamination. In the 1986 nuclear accident at the Chernobyl power plant in the Ukraine, large quantities of radioactive volatile substances, such as iodine-131 and cesium-134 and -137, were released into the atmosphere in a plume of radioactive smoke that rose 1,500 meters into the air. Winds carried some of these substances to eastern Europe and Scandinavia. Some of these radioactive substances, including radiocesium, have been found in eastern European grasses and soils.

Box 15.4   GARBAGE UNEARTHED

Until the recent push to contain landfills better and reduce the amount of waste by recycling, a wide variety of solid wastes were thrown into massive, all-purpose landfills scattered across the country. A typical batch of waste would contain a mixture of garbage: relatively benign food wastes; products that varied in their ability to decompose, such as paper, glass, metals, and plastic products; and toxic or volatile chemicals, such as paint thinners, contaminated motor oil, and acid and lead from leaky car batteries. Depending on the landfill, the garbage was buried or allowed to decompose naturally. Unfortunately, many of these wastes can last decades before they start to show signs of decomposition.

The Garbage Project at the University of Arizona excavates landfills to find out what happens to the materials buried within them. Their efforts at examining more than 9,000 loads of garbage from the Tucson, Arizona, area and other parts of the United States have unearthed some interesting findings:

- Although landfills were intended as sites where garbage would decay in the soil, they actually *preserve* refuse. Tightly packed and covered garbage often remains hidden from light or moisture—important promoters of decay—and appears to remain relatively intact for long periods of time.
- Thirty percent of the trash by volume is nondegradable plastics.
- Food and yard debris degrade at a very slow rate in landfills—around 25 to 50 percent every ten or fifteen years. Uneaten food was recognizable as long as a quarter of a century after it was thrown away.
- Paper and paper products constitute over one-half of the trash in landfills. The researchers found that much of the paper was, in effect, mummified, with newspapers deep in some landfills legible decades later. This may be positive in some respects: Rapid degradation would allow the release of ink and paint toxins into the surrounding soil.

leaks can go on for years without being detected.

In an effort to minimize leaking gas tanks as a source of soil contamination, the EPA has instituted new regulations and programs requiring the monitoring of such underground systems and mandating that new tanks be made of noncorrosive materials.

Natural Contaminants

In addition to the numerous human-made hazards of soil contamination, natural contaminants occur deep within the layers of earth. Radon is an example of such a contaminant: This natu-

rally occurring element is an odorless, invisible gas derived from natural radioactive decay of radium and uranium. Radon filters through the cracks in the soil and can enter and accumulate in houses and buildings (especially those that are well sealed for energy conservation), potentially exposing the occupants to excessive amounts of the gas. The gas breaks down into "radon daughters," giving off ionizing radiation. Long-term exposure to high levels of radon can contribute to lung cancer in humans.

Radon levels in the soil vary greatly from place to place. According to the EPA, no state is completely free of radon, but some sites are much

---

Box 15.5 LOVE CANAL: A CASE OF HAZARDOUS WASTES

The story of Love Canal, New York, started during the 1940s, when approximately 22,000 tons of chemical manufacturing wastes containing dioxins, polychlorinated biphenyls, and other hazardous compounds were dumped into the canal by industries. When the canal was filled, the hazardous compounds were buried and capped with impermeable clay.

In the 1950s, a housing development was built on the site. By the 1970s, residents noticed unusual odors in their basements and oily puddles on their lawns—the result of the clay cap leaking. Declaring a fifty-block site a disaster area in 1978, the federal government bought the homes of 2,500 residents (about 70 people chose to remain). As there was too much contaminated soil to remove, it was sealed with a newer, more advanced cap. A seventy-acre lot was fenced in and surrounded with monitoring devices to detect any leakage. By 1990, parts of the area were declared fit again for human habitation.

Love Canal is one of hundreds of hazardous wastes sites in the country and the world. Other examples include Times Beach, Missouri, where for ten years the town had contracted to have its dirt streets sprayed with waste oils to keep down the dust. By 1982, it was learned that the oil was contaminated with dioxins that bound to the soil, exposing the residents to the contaminants; the cleanup is planned to continue until 2000. Major sites have also been discovered in Jersey City, New Jersey; Woburn, Massachusetts; St. Louis, Michigan; and Denver, Colorado.

---

more concerned with radon than others because of its proximity to the surface and characteristics of the soil (see Chapter 14, "Air").

A less common soil-related health risk involves NORMs, or naturally occurring radioactive materials, which are the natural radioactive materials brought up from the ground primarily from oil drilling, mining, fertilizer manufactur-

ing, and burning coal for electricity. For example, the element radium is a NORM that collects in pits where oil field wastes are dumped. Officials have found radium readings over sixty times higher than what is considered normal and safe in soil around these pits. The health risks associated with NORMS are usually of concern to mining, drilling, and agricultural workers.

SOLUTIONS TO SOIL CONTAMINATION

Because the potential hazards posed by soil contamination are continually evolving, solutions to soil-related risks are difficult to pinpoint. Further complicating this complex issue is the difficulty that exists when trying to interpret the estimates of how much health risk is posed by soil contamination. For instance, many long-term studies have neither proved nor disproved the potential health risks of soil contaminants

because of conflicting data and because reports of health hazards may be confounded by other existing pollution in an area. In other cases, risk estimates may be revised downward as new information is gathered.

Public perception of a potential soil contaminant also plays a major role in assessing risk. For instance, only when a soil contaminant is found on their own property will some people perceive a soil hazard as "risky" enough to demand removal. For others, the mere presence of a potential hazard anywhere in the same city is perceived as cause for alarm (see Chapter 2, "Illness and the Environment: Finding the Links," and Chapter 3, "How We Perceive Risks and How Scientists Measure Them.")

To understand the real threats, more reliable and far-reaching studies are needed to address the issues of how soil contaminants affect individuals as well as the ecology. Until then, the best route for curbing soil contamination is reform and education. Encouragingly, new regulations for landfills and sites for housing, industry, or playgrounds set by the EPA have led to fewer potential contamination problems. Innovative ways of cleaning or washing the soil and high-temperature incineration of contaminated soil have also reduced potential health risks. In addition, extensive federal and state EPA public education programs on the risks of radon exposure detail comprehensive guidelines for monitoring and reducing elevated radon levels in the home.

Another positive example of education involves the growing emphasis on community recycling efforts and overall awareness. For example, increasing public knowledge of the potential dangers of living on or near contaminated soil has spurred numerous communities to insist that local officials investigate and eventually clean up potentially toxic sites.

Until studies can pinpoint the nature of all soil hazards, there are several wise practices to follow. Although it is not always easy to do, individuals and companies can modify health risks due to soil contamination by:

- Long-term recycling.
- Choosing products that use packaging that reduces waste.
- Confining hazardous wastes with better landfill technology.
- Changing agricultural practices, such as the use of more insect-resistant crops and fewer pesticides.
- Developing strict guidelines for industrial and commercial emissions.
- Identifying previously unknown waste sites and dumps.
- Developing alternative waste technology.
- Proper disposal of personal toxic materials.

CHAPTER 16

Radiant Energy

R adiant energy, commonly referred to as *radiation*, has been part of the earth's environment since the beginning of time. Early in the earth's evolution, before oxygen appeared in the atmosphere, high-energy radiation may have contributed to the formation of the amino acids, alcohols, aldehydes, and hydrocarbons that became the building blocks of living matter. As life evolved, radiation's interaction with living cells may have contributed to the beneficial mutations that led to the evolution of new species, including *Homo sapiens*.

Today, most of the radiation we receive still comes from natural sources, such as heat and light. Higher-energy radiation continues to stream down from the sun and other stars, and such radiation also emanates from naturally occurring radioactive minerals, such as radium, buried in the earth's crust. Some radioactive elements are also deposited in tiny amounts within human tissue. A much smaller amount of the radiation we receive comes from human-made sources such as X-ray machines, radios, heat sources, nuclear power plants, and microwave ovens.

Although most of the radiation we receive comes from nature, most of us still perceive radiation as unnatural. Research indicates that the public tends to overestimate radiation risks, for example, those posed by living near a nuclear power plant, and to underestimate more com-

mon risks, such as the likelihood of dying due to cigarette smoking or an automobile accident. Radiation arouses so much fear in part because it is possible for a person to be unknowingly exposed to it, and individuals feel they have little control over the extent of their exposure to it (see Chapter 3, "How We Perceive Risks and How Scientists Measure Them"). We associate it with dread outcomes such as the horrific 1945 atomic bombings of Hiroshima and Nagasaki and the 1986 explosion at the Chernobyl nuclear reactor complex in what was formerly the Soviet Union.

Radiation can be a deadly force, but it also has many beneficial effects. We would not exist without heat and light from the sun. Radiant energy is used for communications (e.g., radios and televisions), for cooking (e.g., radiant heat and microwaves), in the form of laser beams for surgery, and to power modern telecommunications systems. We use radiant energy to induce mutations in seeds (i.e., to produce new strains of plants with desirable characteristics) and to help diagnose and treat health problems. In high doses, radiation is used to kill unwanted bacteria, molds, and insects, allowing us to preserve food or sterilize surgical instruments.

When most of us think about radiation, we are usually thinking about *ionizing* radiation, the type emitted by X-ray machines and radioactive materials. Ionizing radiation is characterized by sufficiently large amounts of energy to liberate electrons and disrupt the molecular structure of living cells, causing chemical changes that may damage or destroy the cells. Experts agree unequivocally that large doses of ionizing radiation can severely damage tissues and may cause cancer in humans (see Box 16.1).

On the other hand, *nonionizing* radiation, the type harnessed in microwaves, heaters, car phones, and electric blankets, does not impart enough localized energy to break chemical bonds but can have physical effects. For example, infrared radiation can cause damage through its capacity to burn the skin or deeper tissues.

Because of its higher concentration of energy, a given amount of ionizing radiation is more damaging than an equal quantity of nonionizing radiation. Eric J. Hall, the author of *Radiation and Life* (Pergamon Press), illustrates this difference by comparing ionizing and nonionizing radiations to a 1-kilogram rock and a 1-kilogram handful of sand, respectively. Thrown at a rabbit, he says, "the sand would do little damage because the energy would be divided between thousands of tiny particles. By contrast, the rock could have a lethal effect if it hit a vital target."

On the other hand, the total amount of energy emitted in the form of X rays for a diagnostic chest X ray is much smaller than the amount of energy emitted in a short time by an electric heater.

IONIZING RADIATION

Some types of ionizing radiation, such as some of those present in streams of cosmic rays, are so energetic that they pass easily through the human body. Others, such as the alpha radiations from some of the radionuclides released during the Chernobyl nuclear accident, do not have enough energy to penetrate through the skin cells, although they can penetrate the thinner cells lining the lungs and stomach if inhaled or ingested. (After a nuclear explosion, it may be dangerous to breathe the particles suspended in the outdoor air, known as radioactive fallout. People also are advised not to eat contaminated produce grown near nuclear accident sites lest they swallow radioactive particles that have settled on plants. People also are told to avoid drinking milk from those areas, as it can become radioactive when cows graze on contaminated plants in the vicinity of an accident.)

Health Effects of Ionizing Radiation

The biological effects of exposure to ionizing radiation depend on the amount of radiation absorbed and the conditions of exposure. Several different units of measure are used to quantify the dosage of ionizing radiation absorbed by living organisms.

Quantifying the Radiation Dose. The dose that is absorbed in a given cell or tissue is measured in units of rads or grays. One rad is equal to 100 ergs per gram, and one gray is equal to 100 rads or 1 joule per kilogram of energy absorbed (a joule is a measure of work or energy). However, the biological effects of ionizing radiation depend on the *type* of radiation as well as the dose; equal doses of two different kinds of ionizing radiation may produce different effects, which is why scientists commonly multiply the dose by a so-called quality factor (related to the biological effectiveness of that particular type of radiation) to derive the *dose equivalent*, which is expressed in units of rem (an abbreviation for rad equivalents man) or sieverts (1 sievert equals 100 rem). Subunits that are commonly used include the millirem (thousandths of a rem) and millisievert (1 millisievert equals 1/1000th of a sievert). In a year, the average American receives the equivalent of about 100 millirem of ionizing radiation to the whole body and 2,500 millirem to the lung from natural sources.

An added wrinkle in the task of calculating

SOURCES OF EXPOSURE TO IONIZING RADIATION

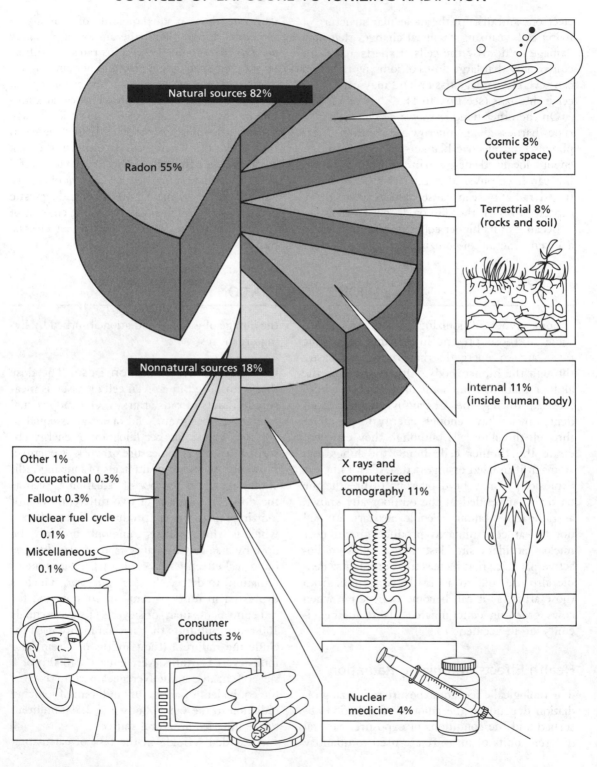

Natural sources 82%

Radon 55%

Cosmic 8%
(outer space)

Terrestrial 8%
(rocks and soil)

Internal 11%
(inside human body)

Nonnatural sources 18%

Other 1%
Occupational 0.3%
Fallout 0.3%
Nuclear fuel cycle
0.1%
Miscellaneous
0.1%

X rays and
computerized
tomography 11%

Consumer
products 3%

Nuclear
medicine 4%

Box 16.1 THE ELECTROMAGNETIC SPECTRUM

Electromagnetic radiation is a broad term encompassing various forms of radiant energy, such as visible light, X rays, and cosmic rays, which are generated by electrical and magnetic fields and travel in waves. The properties of a particular type of wave is determined by its wavelength. Waves are also measured by frequency, which is the number of times a wave repeats itself over a given distance or length of time. Frequency is measured in *hertz*, the number of wave repetitions, or cycles, emitted per second from the source. The frequency is inversely proportional to wavelength; the shorter the wave, the more emitted per second.

Visible light is the most familiar type of electromagnetic radiation. It consists of waves that range in length from 380 to 760 nanometers (billionths of a meter). The shortest waves of visible light appear violet to the human eye, and the longest look red. The invisible waves just shorter than violet light are termed ultraviolet light. Shorter still are the wavelengths of ionizing radiation: X rays, gamma rays, and cosmic rays coming from outer space. The shorter a radiation's wavelength, the higher its energy.

Moving from visible light toward the longer end of the spectrum (left), red light becomes infrared radiation (known for its ability to heat food or activate the remote control of a television) with an increase in wavelength. Beyond infrared are microwaves, radar, and radio and television waves. A television signal might have a wavelength of more than a mile.

biological effects of exposure to ionizing radiation is that within a large group exposed to the same radiation source, some individuals may be more sensitive to the exposure than others. Further complicating the issue is that some types of effects may not be apparent until many years after an initial exposure, making it difficult to establish a causal linkage between them.

Much has been learned about both the short- and long-term health effects of ionizing radiation from epidemiological studies of people who survived the atomic bombings in Japan in 1945. Shortly after those attacks, the U.S. and Japanese governments formed the Joint Commission for the Investigation of the Effects of the Atomic Bombs. Since that time, researchers from both countries have studied a group of about 100,000 survivors who were exposed to a range of radiation doses, the level of exposure depending on how far they were from the blasts and on the shielding effects of buildings. In recent years, these studies—now conducted at the Radiation Effects Research Foundation in Hiroshima—have enabled scientists to en-

Figure 16.1 SOURCES OF EXPOSURE TO IONIZING RADIATION.

This chart is based upon the 1990 report of the National Research Council's committee on the biological effects of ionizing radiation (BEIR). It represents the average percentage of ionizing radiation received from various sources by an individual American, as measured in *effective dose equivalents*, a measure that takes into account both the amount of radiation from a particular source and the likelihood that radiation from that source will produce harm.

Adapted with permission from *Health Effects of Exposure to Ionizing Radiation: BEIR V*, page 19. Copyright 1990 by the National Academy of Sciences. Published by the National Academy Press, Washington, D.C.

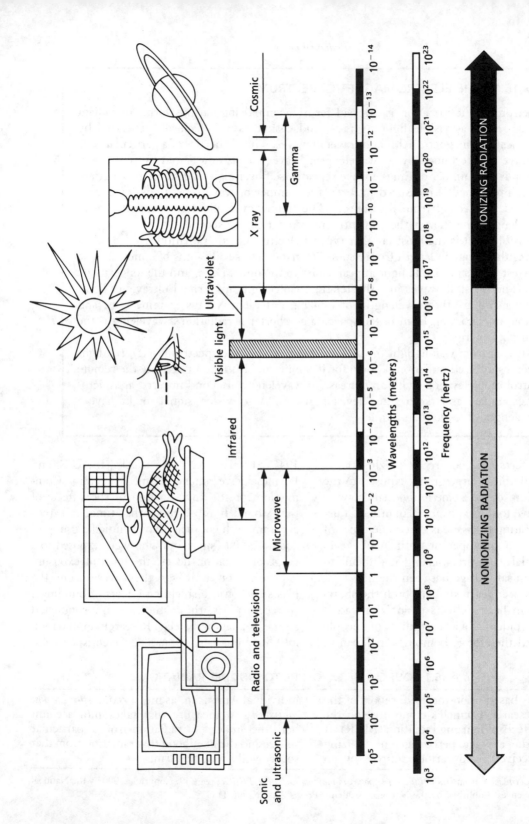

Figure 16.2 THE ELECTROMAGNETIC SPECTRUM.

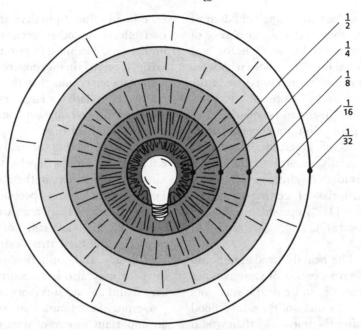

$$\frac{1}{2}$$
$$\frac{1}{4}$$
$$\frac{1}{8}$$
$$\frac{1}{16}$$
$$\frac{1}{32}$$

Figure 16.3 HOW RADIANT ENERGY DROPS OFF OVER DISTANCE.

All forms of electromagnetic radiation—from light to X rays to microwaves—drop off sharply in concentration, or intensity, the farther away they get from their source. You can see an example of this by lighting a candle or light bulb in a dark room; the light source is surrounded by a small bright "halo" that fades rapidly toward its edges. We can best understand the reason for this effect by recalling the origin of the word *radiation;* the waves do in fact "radiate" from their source like the spokes in a wheel. Just as a wheel's spokes are bunched together much more closely at the hub than near the rim, so do electromagnetic waves become less concentrated as they travel. The ratio of radiation intensity to distance from the source is ½^r, where r equals the distance. Thus, if at a certain unit of distance the intensity is one-half the intensity at the source, the intensity becomes one-quarter at two units from the source. At only five units, the intensity drops to one-thirty-second of the original.

large their understanding of radiation's health effects.

Effects on Genes. For years after the Hiroshima and Nagasaki bombings, many people feared that the radiation released would have devastating genetic effects. In Japan, the stigma of being a bomb survivor is so great that some survivors still are reluctant to identify themselves, fearing discrimination against their families. However, scientists have discovered that the radiation released by the bombs has had no discernible effect on survivors' children. Tests comparing more than 30,000 children of survivors with about 40,000 children whose mothers were not exposed have found no increase in birth defects, cancers, or chromosome abnormalities.

Although the test results are not conclusive proof that the radiation caused no genetic effects, they do mean that if any genetic effects were produced, they are too subtle to be detected in this population.

Effects on the Embryo. Although children conceived after the bombings were spared, some who were already in their mothers' wombs were not. Called *pika* children (meaning "children of the flash") in Japan, they had a higher chance of being born with abnormally small heads and later exhibited stunted growth. Those who were exposed to high doses of radiation between the eighth and fifteenth weeks of prenatal development were also more likely to be mentally retarded or to do poorly on intelligence tests. During those weeks of gestation, embryonic brain cells are especially sensitive to radiation. The prenatally irradiated children also have shown an increased risk of getting cancer as adults (see Chapter 11, "Reproductive Effects and Prenatal Exposures").

Links to Cancer. The heavily irradiated bomb survivors have shown an excess of various types of cancers. For example, more of the survivors developed leukemia, a cancer of the white blood cells, in the years after the bombings than would have been expected in an unexposed population. The number of excess leukemia cases increased until about 1960 and then began to taper off, subsiding to more or less normal levels by about 1975. Heavily irradiated bomb survivors also have shown increased rates of cancers of the thyroid gland, breast, lung, stomach, colon, bladder, and esophagus.

The data show that the risk was highest for the group that survived the largest dose, lower for those that received smaller doses, and undetectable at doses approaching those usually associated with natural sources. Altogether, during the first forty years after irradiation, a total of 360 cancers, including 81 cases of leukemia, have been attributed to radiation from the bombs, an increase of about 6 percent in the overall risk of cancer for the survivors of Hiroshima and Nagasaki.

It is noteworthy that some types of cancer do not appear to have increased at all as a result of the bombings, including cancers of the gallbladder, rectum, uterus, bone, pancreas, and testis.

Calculating Low-Level Radiation Risks. In generalizing from the bomb survivors' experience in an effort to understand low-dose radiation effects on other groups, there are many limitations. The most important are that the survivors received their exposure to radiation nearly instantaneously and that the doses received by many were relatively large. For most other people, exposure to radiation is stretched over much longer periods of time.

Also complicating the analysis is the fact that not all ethnic groups develop the same cancers in identical frequencies in the absence of exposure. For example, Japanese people are more prone to stomach cancer than are Americans. Furthermore, scientists are still not sure whether the impact of the blast that destroyed buildings or the dietary and sanitation problems that followed it may also have contributed to the cancers found among survivors and their offspring.

Despite these limitations, survivor studies are an important source of data concerning the effects of radiation on otherwise healthy people of all ages and both sexes. In general, the data are consistent with those derived from studies of other irradiated human populations, such as patients treated with radiation for various diseases and radiation workers. Scientists have had to extrapolate from such data to calculate the risks of low-level ionizing radiation, such as those that are potentially associated with nonnatural sources. In calculating risks, scientists generally take a conservative view and assume that *any* dose of radiation may have some effect. This does not mean that everyone who gets a low dose will get cancer. Rather, it means that a low dose administered to a large group may contribute to the causation of cancer in a few people within the group. Everyone in the group is assumed to be at risk, and the risk of cancer is often assumed to be proportional to the dose received. This is consistent with what is known of radiation effects in both humans and animals.

A National Research Council committee on the biological effects of ionizing radiations (BEIR) recently reassessed the doses that bomb survivors are believed to have received. The committee found that the bombs actually released less radiation than had been believed and that the shielding provided by buildings was better than had been calculated. That means that the cancers were caused by smaller doses of radiation than had been thought previously.

In 1990, the BEIR committee published the fifth in a series of reports detailing the health effects of exposure to low levels of ionizing radiation. The report stated that the risk of cancer from low-level radiation may be three to four times greater than estimated in the committee's 1980 report. The new report estimates that as much as 3 to 5 percent of all cancers in the general population might be attributable to ionizing radiation from all sources combined, including medical exams, nuclear power plants, and natural radiation. The BEIR committee was not able to determine whether there is any "safe" dose of ionizing radiation—a dose so small that it has absolutely no harmful effects on human populations—but neither could it exclude the possibility (see Figure 16.1).

There have been numerous attempts to answer this question by other means, including studies of radiation workers and studies of populations that live in areas of high natural background radiation; however, these are difficult epidemiological studies to perform reliably. Taken together, the studies support the conclusion that such small doses of ionizing radiation as are received from natural background cause no detectable effect, which means that if there is any effect at all, it is so small compared to all the other factors that influence health as to be undetectable. This is consistent with the conclusions obtained by extrapolations from observations on the atomic bomb survivors.

DNA REPAIR. Although the National Research Council's BEIR committee raised its estimates of cancer risk for low doses of radiation received all at once, the committee pointed out that the cancer risk from low doses that are received slowly may be significantly smaller. The idea that prolonged exposure is much less dangerous than rapid exposure to the same dose is based on ex-

perimental studies. In laboratory animals, when a low dose of X rays or gamma rays is spread over a period of weeks or months, the number of resulting cancers is two to ten times smaller than if the dose is given all at once. It is noteworthy in this connection that an instantaneous dose of ionizing radiation causes more total injury to DNA molecules, which may play a role in initiating cancer formation, than the same dose accumulated gradually over a long enough period of time so that the DNA damage is repaired apace with its production. DNA repair is a natural process; at any given time, a significant percentage of cells in the body normally undergo DNA damage from causes other than ionizing radiation (see Box 16.2).

Sources of Exposure to Ionizing Radiation

Figure 16.1, based upon the 1990 report of the National Research Council's committees on the biological effects of ionizing radiation (BEIR), depicts the average percentage of ionizing radiation received from various sources by an individual in the United States.

Natural sources were estimated to account for about 82 percent of the total. Two-thirds of these exposures were attributed to radon, a naturally occurring radioactive gas that emanates from certain rocks and soil, and is now recognized as the largest source of environmental radiation. Other natural sources include: cosmic radiation (8 percent), such as gamma rays, which emanate from outer space; terrestrial sources (8 percent), including radioactive minerals, such as uranium and thorium, common in the earth's crust; internal radiation (11 percent), including naturally occurring isotopes of elements present in food and water that are taken in and assimilated into the body.

Nonnatural sources account for 18 percent of our exposure to ionizing radiation. These sources include: radiation from medical procedures (15 percent), including X rays and computerized tomography (11 percent) and nuclear

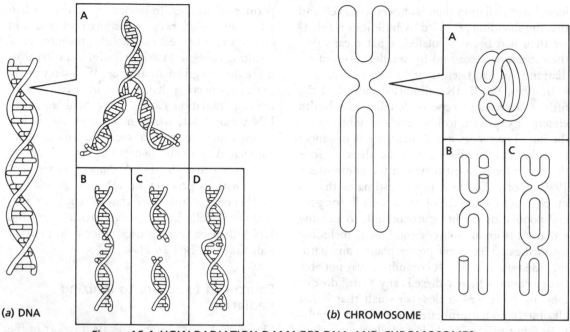

Figure 16.4 HOW RADIATION DAMAGES DNA AND CHROMOSOMES.

medicine (4 percent); consumer products (3 percent), including radon in domestic water supplies, building materials, mining and agricultural products, as well as tobacco smoke; and other sources (less than 1 percent), including occupational exposure and exposure to radioactive fallout or the products of the nuclear fuel cycle.

Natural Background Radiation. Nature is by far the greatest source of radiation. Natural radiations reach us from the sky, the ground, and even from within our own bodies (see Figure 16.1). Because natural radiation is present to some degree in every environment, it is often called *background* radiation.

Scientists estimate that natural sources produce about 82 percent of all ionizing radiation received by human populations, and two-thirds of that comes from radon. Radon is a gas released during the decay of radium, which is itself a by-product of uranium's radioactive decay. Other naturally occurring radioactive minerals found in rocks, soil, and building materials, such

as thorium, also produce background radiation. Radioactive forms of elements such as carbon and potassium, deposited in human tissues in small amounts, produce internal radiation. The remaining natural radiation we are exposed to consists of cosmic rays.

COSMIC RAYS. One-quarter to one-third of our natural whole-body background radiation dose is caused by cosmic radiation from outer space, such as gamma rays. These rays strike everywhere but are most intense at high altitudes, where the atmosphere is thinner. Exposure to cosmic rays doubles for every 2,000-meter increase in altitude. For example, a person living in Denver will receive more than twice as much cosmic radiation as someone living in San Francisco.

Air travel also exposes a person to more cosmic rays. Planes fly much higher now than in the past, so they receive more cosmic radiation, especially the Concorde and some corporate jets, which fly even higher than commercial airliners.

Box 16.2 HOW RADIATION DAMAGES DNA AND CHROMOSOMES

Deoxyribonucleic acid (DNA) molecules (see Figure 16.4*a*) provide the mechanism for cells to reproduce; without them, we would not be able to produce new skin, blood, and reproductive cells. DNA is a complex molecule shaped as a double helix—a spiral "ladder," the rungs of which are made of chemical building blocks. The sequence of chemical blocks acts as a code, specifying an individual's physical characteristics. Each cell has a set of threadlike chromosomes (see Figure 16.4*b*) made from DNA; these chromosomes contain genetic instructions enabling the cell to divide and multiply. When a cell divides, its chromosomes peel open like zippers. New chemical building blocks attach themselves along the exposed halves of the zipper, forming two identical chromosomes in place of one. Thus, each half of the dividing cell receives a full set of chromosomes.

Radiation harms genetic material by damaging or severing DNA strands: it can cause two DNA strands to fuse together (Figure 16.4*a*-A), break one or both strands (B and C), or break DNA "rungs" (D). If DNA damage is sufficient, it can cause chromosomes to form in ring shapes (Figure 16.4*b*-A), with missing sections (B), or with two centers (C); this can hinder or even prevent cell reproduction.

In the embryonic stages of life, when the relatively few cells in the organism are rapidly dividing to form new ones, vulnerability to radiation is high. Later the cells become more numerous and specialized. However, many retain their ability to divide, including blood, skin, intestinal mucosa, and sperm cells. This is why exposing the male gonads to large doses of radiation can cause sterility. The vulnerability of dividing cells also explains why radiation is used to treat cancer: tumor cells, which divide and reproduce incessantly, are generally more susceptible to radiation than the normal cells surrounding them.

Modern planes also fly many intercontinental routes, passing close to the poles, where the earth's magnetic field concentrates the charged particles beaming down from outer space.

Cosmic radiation is most pronounced during solar storms. Solar activity peaks every eleven years; the most recent active period began in 1989. A passenger flying during a single solar flare can receive as much radiation as someone who takes one hundred normal airline flights—enough for a pregnant woman, during just one flight, to exceed the maximum monthly radiation limit for the fetus. To avoid this possibility, some experts are recommending that radiation monitors be installed on planes. If the monitor detected a solar flare, the plane could drop to a lower altitude to reduce the dose received by its occupants. There is no practical way to shield an airplane from cosmic rays.

The radiation dose received during a single cross-country trip is small, but pilots, flight attendants, and frequent fliers are regularly exposed to increased levels of cosmic radiation. In some cases, therefore, flight crews may be exposed to as much radiation as nuclear power plant workers.

RADIOACTIVE MINERALS IN THE EARTH. Naturally occurring radioactive minerals such as uranium and thorium, common in the earth's crust, are unevenly distributed around the globe. Regions in which radioactive minerals are present near the soil surface may have levels of natural radiation many times higher than in other areas.

High levels of radioactive minerals are often found in granite and limestone. Parts of Brazil, India, China, Italy, France, Iran, Madagascar, and Nigeria have high levels of background radiation. (Persons living in areas where background radiation levels are high have not been found to exhibit adverse health effects, but there have been few studies investigating such effects thus far.)

When removed from the soil and concentrated, radioactive minerals can have potent effects. For example, one of the first radioactive elements studied was radium, which is formed during the natural decay of uranium. Radium was discovered by Pierre and Marie Curie almost a century ago, subsequently was widely used as a radiation therapy source to treat cancer. Other sources have since been developed using human-made radioactive material manufactured in reactors, but radium remains an important source in some parts of the world.

Radium's toxicity became apparent in the 1930s, when scientists found an increased incidence of bone cancer in factory workers who painted luminous clock, watch, and instrument dials with paint containing radium. The workers customarily pointed the tips of their fine paintbrushes between their lips, thus ingesting radium each time.

Researchers have recently found that industrial activities—primarily oil drilling, mining, fertilizer manufacturing, and burning coal for electricity—are bringing buried radium to the surface. The public first learned of this problem in 1986, when an oil field worker discovered radioactive pipes in a well in Mississippi. The pipes were contaminated with radium that had leached into water pumped to the surface along with the oil.

Radium has now been found in oil-producing operations in many parts of the United States, especially in the South. Tests of wells in Louisiana and other southern states have found radiation levels up to thirty times higher than the government allows at nuclear power plants. Radium also collects in the pits where oil field wastes are dumped. Officials have found readings as high as 500 picocuries per gram in the soil around these pits. (The normal level is 0.5 to 2 picocuries per gram.)

The government has not set any exposure limits for oil workers, who may be receiving more radiation than nuclear industry workers. Some oil workers breathe radium-contaminated dust, as well as radon, while cleaning sludge out of oil pipes.

Radon: Radon gas emanates from rocks and soil. It accumulates in uranium mines and in the basements, foundations, and ground floors of houses in some geographic areas (see p. 558).

A higher than average incidence of lung cancer has been found in uranium miners, who inhale the radon gas, which accumulates in poorly ventilated mines.

Based on a report by the National Research Council, the U.S. Environmental Protection Agency (EPA) currently estimates that radon gas in homes may be responsible for as many as 16,000 lung cancer deaths a year. According to the EPA, radon is the second leading cause of lung cancer after smoking. However, there is a debate over these estimates, which are based on extrapolations from the experience of the more heavily exposed miners. (See Chapter 14, "Air," for a detailed discussion of radon.)

Internal Radiation. Naturally occurring isotopes of potassium, carbon, hydrogen, and other elements present in food and water are taken up by the body and assimilated into its cells, where they continue to release radiation. About one-third of the whole-body radiation dose we receive is from such internal sources.

The amount of radioactivity in drinking water from different sources varies widely—one glass may contain 10,000 times as much as another. Some foods also contain more radioactive minerals than others. For example, nuts and cereals tend to have more radium than do milk or meat. The total amount in any case, however, is small.

Box 16.3   X RAYS

Like many scientific achievements, Wilhelm Röntgen's discovery of X rays was accidental. On November 8, 1895, Röntgen was conducting an experiment in which he passed an electric current through a glass tube that had been partially evacuated of air. In the darkened laboratory, the tube was covered with black paper, but Röntgen noticed a glow coming from a light-sensitive sheet of paper that, by chance, had been left on his laboratory bench. The glow, he later learned, was produced by X rays emanating from the tube.

In later experiments, Röntgen noticed that the X rays passed easily through a thick book or two decks of cards but were absorbed by metal or other dense materials. When he put his hand between an X-ray tube and a fluorescent screen, Röntgen discovered that he could see the bones inside his hand. He also took a picture of his wife's hand that clearly showed her wedding ring as well as her bones.

Within less than ten years after their discovery, X rays were being used to view bone fractures and healing and to detect bullets lodged in the body. Bones are opaque to X rays because they are composed of relatively heavy elements such as calcium. But X rays pass easily through the body's soft tissues and other materials made of light elements such as hydrogen and carbon.

In modern X-ray equipment, X rays are usually produced by heating a tungsten wire filament to liberate electrons inside a glass vacuum tube. A very large voltage is then used to attract the electrons to a tungsten target producing X rays upon their deceleration. The energy of the X rays depends on the accelerating voltage used.

Ionizing Radiation from Nonnatural Sources. Although the lion's share of our exposure to ionizing radiation comes from natural sources, we are also exposed from a variety of artificial sources.

RADIATION USED IN MEDICINE. For most people, diagnostic medical procedures are the main source of exposure to such radiation. About one-quarter of our total whole-body exposure comes from diagnostic radiography, including X rays and computerized tomography scans, which use X-ray beams to create a three-dimensional picture of a body part. A smaller contribution comes from nuclear medicine, in which radioactive substances such as iodine-131 are injected into the body as imaging agents, helping physicians to make accurate diagnoses. Not included in this estimate is the very small percentage of the population that receives relatively high localized doses of radiation as part of radiation therapy.

Diagnostic Radiography (X Rays): Almost every American has had at least one X-ray examination. According to the American College of Radiology, in 1985 alone, U.S. radiologists performed 265 million X-ray exams.

X rays are used in a variety of examinations. In the most conventional type of exam, a photographic film is exposed to X rays that pass through a part of the body. The X rays create an image on the film in the same way that rays of light create an image on the film used in cameras. Mammograms (special X rays of the breast) and dental images (the most common type of X-ray exam) are made by this method. (See Chapter 22, "The ABCs of Staying Healthy," for guidelines on the use of mammography.)

In a second type of X-ray imaging, known as

fluoroscopy, a fluorescent screen is used instead of photographic film. Fluoroscopy is the technology that allows security guards to examine luggage moving along a conveyor belt at the airport. In medicine, it allows a radiologist to watch moving parts of the body rather than still images. For example, the radiologist can view barium swallowed by the patient—barium is a heavy element that is opaque to X rays—as it passes through the stomach and intestines.

A third type of X-ray imaging technique is known as a computerized tomography scan. In this exam, the patient lies inside a machine shaped like a giant doughnut. X rays are emitted from the "doughnut" so as to cross-fire a slice of the patient's body, and many such slices are combined and processed by a computer to form a cross-sectional picture of the part examined.

The radiation dose from a single X-ray examination is relatively small; for example, a standard chest X ray exposes the skin to about 20 millirem and deeper tissues receive smaller doses (compared with the average American's total annual whole-body exposure to radiation from natural sources of about 100 millirem).

X-ray exams may not be completely risk-free. Pelvimetry studies, involving X rays, used to be performed routinely on pregnant women, but a number of studies suggested that the children of mothers exposed to X rays during pregnancy were more likely to develop leukemia, so this practice was stopped except in cases of medical necessity. Ultrasound methods, which are believed to be without significant risk, have since become available for routine monitoring purposes.

The most prudent guideline regarding exposure to X rays is that no one should have one without a clear medical need. Most dentists agree that adults need not have dental X rays every year, and most doctors no longer perform any X rays on a routine basis.

Radiation Therapy for Cancer: Ever since the discovery of radiation, physicians have used it to treat a variety of diseases. For example, X radiation was used as a treatment for arthritis, acne, ringworm, and enlarged tonsils in the 1930s and 1940s. (These practices were ended because better and safer methods are available.)

Radiation therapy is one of the most effective treatments currently available for many types of malignant tumors. For small tumors of the vocal cords, breast, prostate, and cervix, radiation provides an alternative to surgery or a supplement to extensive surgery. For some types of tumors, radiotherapy is the only form of treatment available. Of course, treatment must be designed to destroy tumors without irreparably damaging adjacent normal tissues; this requires skilled staff and excellent equipment.

NUCLEAR POWER PRODUCTION. The amount of radiation received by the general population from all U.S. nuclear power plants during normal operation is quite small—less than 1 percent of the total annual whole-body radiation dose

---

Box 16.4 MINIMIZING X-RAY RISKS

In all types of X-ray exams, it is important that up-to-date and well-maintained equipment is used and that technicians are well-trained and licensed.

Keep a record of all the X-ray exams you have had. If you move, request that your records be transferred to your new doctor and dentist, so that the exams do not have to be repeated unnecessarily.

Keep in mind that X rays, like drugs and surgery, may carry a small risk. But in most cases, the benefits derived from X rays far outweigh the risks.

received from natural sources (see Figure 16.1). Researchers from the National Cancer Institute reported in 1990 that they were unable to find any increased risk of cancer deaths for people living either in the 107 U.S. counties that have nuclear installations or adjoining counties.

Another study, released a few weeks later, did find a small cluster of leukemia cases among adults living and working in twenty-two communities within ten miles of the Pilgrim nuclear power plant in Massachusetts between 1978 and 1983. That study focused on a much smaller geographic area than did the National Cancer Institute's study, and it tabulated diseases as well as mortality.

Both studies were prompted by a 1987 report in Great Britain that found an increased number of leukemia deaths among children living within ten miles of the Sellafield nuclear-reprocessing plant. A subsequent study reported that children in the Sellafield vicinity who developed leukemia were more likely to be born to men who had worked at the plant. A French study patterned after the British study found no excess cancers, however, and further studies have demonstrated excesses in groups who are not exposed to ionizing radiation. Hence, whether the excesses are attributable to radiation or to other causes, including chance clusters, remains to be determined. These studies also demonstrate the difficulty of the epidemiological approach to investigating these questions, because the rates of the diseases under study are subject to many different factors besides the one of interest (see Chapter 2, "Illness and the Environment: Finding the Links").

NUCLEAR WEAPONS PRODUCTION. Approximately 600,000 Americans have worked in the nuclear weapons industry since its birth in the early 1940s. At its peak, the U.S. government's weapons production program operated at more than one hundred sites in thirty-two states. The Department of Energy, which oversees the nuclear weapons industry, now anticipates a reduced need for nuclear arms in the coming century and has proposed to shut down all but five plants by the year 2015.

In the mid-1980s, the public became aware of the fact that there had been radioactive emissions from weapons plants. That year, the Department of Energy declassified documents showing that radioactive iodine had been released during the 1940s and 1950s from the nation's oldest weapons production facility, the 560-square-mile Hanford Nuclear Reservation in southeastern Washington.

In July 1990, Energy Secretary James D. Watkins announced that doses of radiation released from Hanford had been large enough to increase the risk of certain illnesses, including cancer. The day after Watkins' statement, a panel of scientific experts made public the first part of a five-year $15 million study financed by the Department of Energy. The Secretarial Panel for the Evaluation of Epidemiological Research Activities said that during the largest known radioactive releases, between 1944 and 1947, many persons residing in counties near the Hanford reservation had absorbed levels of radiation higher than those the Department of Energy now considers permissible for people living near its weapons plants.

NUCLEAR WORKERS. More than 1.3 million Americans have jobs that regularly expose them to radiation. These workers include dentists; radiologists; research assistants; miners; and people who work at nuclear power plants, weapons plants, and waste facilities. In the United States, the Nuclear Regulatory Commission sets an upper limit of 5 rem per year for occupational exposure to whole-body radiation, close to fifty times the total amount of whole-body radiation most Americans receive each year from natural sources. (The limits are much lower for pregnant workers). Radiation workers are encouraged to keep their exposure as small as reasonably possible, however, and their exposure is monitored with film badges or other devices.

Because scientists have recently raised their

Box 16.5　RISK PERCEPTION AND NUCLEAR ACCIDENTS

Although advancements in the standard of living, nutrition, and health care have lengthened the average person's life expectancy by some thirty years since the turn of this century, a recent poll indicates that a sizable portion of the population feel they are exposed to a greater array of life-threatening environmental risks than ever before. Clearly, factors beyond a purely numerical estimate of risk are significant in coloring our perceptions of various environmental agents as "risky."

Radiation is a case in point. Although an individual's chance of being killed in an automobile accident are much higher than their odds of being killed by exposure to radiation, we still worry more about the nuclear power plant in the next town than about the risk of driving to that town in our car. Much of this fear of nuclear reactors rests in the fact that they work on the same principle as the atomic bomb, the deadliest weapon ever used.

In the last fifty years, there have been more than 300 accidents that have exposed people to radiation, eight of them involving nuclear reactors. The most serious reactor accident in the United States occurred at Three Mile Island in Pennsylvania in 1979. A presidential panel convened that year concluded that the amount of radiation received from the accident by those residing in the vicinity was small compared with natural radiation levels. A study published in 1990 found no evidence that the accident had caused an increased risk of cancer in neighborhoods within ten miles of the plant.

After the Three Mile Island accident, the presidential panel estimated that the 2 million people living within a 50-mile radius of the plant had collectively received a total of 3,300 person-rem of radiation—a tiny dose (.00165 rem) per person. From this dose, the panelists predicted a risk of less than one additional cancer death compared with 200,000 cancer deaths that would occur in the population from natural causes. In other words, each person living within 50 miles of the plant could say that his or her increased chance of dying of cancer as a result of the accident was about 1 in 2 million.

Let's compare that figure with other risks the same people encountered in 1978, the year before the accident. In that year, the average American's chance of dying of heart disease was 1 in 299; his or her chance of dying of cancer was 1 in 550; and his or her chance of dying in an automobile accident was 1 in 4,164. In fact, a person living near Three Mile Island was ten times more likely to die from being accidentally electrocuted than from radiation, according to one calculation.

Although radiation from Three Mile Island appeared to be less dangerous than more common risks, it received far more attention from the media. Dr. Bernard L. Cohen, a University of Pittsburgh nuclear physicist who studied articles published in *The New York Times* during the four years preceding the accident, found that there were an average of 120 articles per year on highway deaths (one story per 417 deaths) and 240 articles per year on industrial accidents (one story per 240 deaths). During the same period, there were 200 articles on the possibility of fatalities related to nuclear energy, although there was no evidence that a single death from radiation

(continued)

Box 16.5   RISK PERCEPTION AND NUCLEAR ACCIDENTS (*continued*)

had occurred. In fact, the accident at Three Mile Island probably did more damage to the psychological well-being of the people living nearby than to their physical health.

On the other hand, the 1986 accident at Chernobyl in the former Soviet Union looms for some as a powerful image of the potential risks. The worst nuclear accident in history, it released several hundred thousand times as much radiation as the Three Mile Island accident. After the explosion, Soviet officials evacuated about 135,000 people living within 30 kilometers of the reactor complex, but some people living downwind from Chernobyl and outside the evacuated areas may have received more radiation than others living within the 30-kilometer radius.

Two people were killed outright at Chernobyl as a result of burns and radiation injuries, and twenty-nine others died shortly afterward in the hospital. The Soviet government is now monitoring almost 700,000 people who lived near the reactor or who have been involved in cleanup efforts.

estimates of risks from low-level radiation, the International Commission on Radiological Protection recommended in November 1990 that the exposure limit for radiation workers be lowered from 5 rem per year to 10 rem per five years, or an average of 2 rem per year. Approval of the lower limit would not affect most workers, who receive far less radiation than the recommended maximum. The rare job that does expose a worker to the maximum dose could be split up among several employees.

So far, scientists have not found convincing evidence of an increase in cancers among contemporary radiation workers. Some studies have suggested increases in selected cases; other studies have found radiation workers to live longer than other groups, possibly due to improved fitness and health care.

RADIOACTIVE WASTE. There are four basic types of radioactive waste.

1. The first consists of *mill tailings* left over from uranium mining. For example, in Germany, four decades of uranium mining left miles of abandoned shafts and huge slag heaps, which will cost the country an estimated $3.6 billion in cleanup expenses. Mill tailings account for a large percentage of radioactive wastes by volume, but their level of radioactivity is very low. However, they do remain radioactive for more than 100,000 years.

2. The second type is *high-level radioactive waste*, which produces intense radiation and heat. High-level wastes include spent fuel rods from nuclear reactors and liquids created during the reprocessing of reactor fuel to obtain plutonium for nuclear weapons. High-level waste remains radioactive for tens of thousands of years.

The United States alone has more than one hundred sites that were contaminated by nuclear weapons production. From 1946 to 1970, the government also disposed of approximately 50,000 barrels of radioactive waste in the Pacific Ocean, a practice that has now stopped.

A large volume of high-level defense wastes are now stored in underground tanks at three government sites—the Hanford Nuclear Reservation in Washington, the Idaho National Engineering Laboratory near Idaho Falls, and the Savannah River plant near Aiken, South Carolina. These wastes are mainly in the form of liquids, salt cakes, and sludges.

Years ago, some of the metal tanks at the Hanford site deteriorated and leaked liquid wastes.

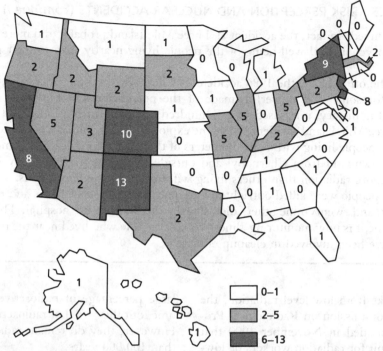

Figure 16.5 HIGH-LEVEL RADIOACTIVE WASTE SITES IN THE UNITED STATES.

Among the aftereffects of the cold war nuclear arms race was the contamination of sites across the United States by activities relating to the weapons program, including radioactive tailings from the mining and milling of uranium, the release of radioactivity at long-used nuclear test sites, contaminated nuclear reactors used by the military, and the dumping of nuclear wastes.

This map provides the number of high-level waste sites per state as identified by the U.S. Department of Energy. Few regions of the country were untouched by contamination; such sparsely populated western states as Colorado and New Mexico, home to a number of uranium mines and testing areas, are among the leaders in nuclear sites of concern.

A study published in 1978 by the National Research Council said that the leaks were contained by the surrounding soil and did not endanger public health. Since then, Hanford's liquid wastes have been put in tanks with double walls to prevent further leaks. However, inside some of the new storage tanks, a crystallized crust has now formed on the surface of the liquid wastes, trapping explosive hydrogen gas beneath it.

Spent fuel rods from commercial nuclear reactors are currently stored on metal racks in pools of water at the reactor sites. These storage

pools were designed for temporary use, but the U.S. Government has not yet found a suitable permanent disposal site for the wastes that have accumulated in the pools. Because the wastes are simply stored at the sites where they are produced, every nuclear power plant in the country is effectively also a radioactive waste storage site.

Officials now hope to build a deep underground repository in which to store the high-level wastes currently held at sites all over the country. Their efforts are focused on a site at Yucca Mountain, Nevada. However, that site's planned opening has already been postponed from 2003 to 2010.

3. A third type of radioactive waste is known as *transuranic waste*. Generated during weapons production, it contains elements, such as plutonium, that have higher atomic numbers than uranium. Current proposals call for transuranics to be buried at a waste isolation pilot plant in Carlsbad, New Mexico; at the time of this writing, however, while the EPA has allowed the Department of Energy to begin testing the site by burying 1 percent of the total material that would eventually be deposited there, the opening of this site is stalled.

4. The final category of radioactive waste, *low-level waste*, is by far the largest in terms of volume—one hundred times that of high-level wastes—but far smaller in terms of radioactivity.

Low-level radioactive wastes can be solid, liquid, or gaseous. Most (about half) of such wastes are produced by commercial nuclear power plants and include compacted trash, bulk waste (dirt, wood, concrete, and steel), spent resins, and solidified wet wastes. According to the International Atomic Energy Agency, about thirty nations use nuclear reactors to generate electricity. More than 500 reactors are now in operation, and another 100 or so are under construction. These plants produced a total of about 370,000 cubic meters of low-level waste in 1990.

Hospitals and research laboratories also contribute to the volume of low-level waste (including contaminated clothing, a variety of equipment, and even the carcasses of laboratory animals) as do pharmaceutical companies and other industries. In general, these wastes are far less radioactive than those from power plants: Within one hundred years or so, most of the radioactivity in these items decays to levels considered safe by government standards.

Currently, low-level wastes must be sent to and buried at approved disposal sites; only four are still open, located in Beatty, Nevada; Barnwell, South Carolina; Richland, Washington; and Clive, Utah. In 1993, the Beatty site was empowered to refuse shipments from other states, and the Barnwell site will follow suit in June, 1994. The Clive, Utah site accepts only certain kinds of low-activity, high-level waste. Several states have plans to establish new sites, but few are likely to open for several years.

Consumer Products. About 3 percent of our annual radiation dose comes from exposure via consumer products. This dose is not distributed equally among the population but depends upon the products used by a consumer. Some of the products that are known to release small amounts of radiation are television sets, smoke detectors, phosphate fertilizers, and building materials (see Chapter 19, "Consumer Products"). Breathing tobacco smoke also can deposit radioactive particles in the lining of the bronchial tract.

NONIONIZING RADIATION

Although scientists have long known of ionizing radiation's harmful and beneficial effects, this is not true of some forms of nonionizing radiation, which include visible light, ultraviolet radiation, and the types of radiation produced by radar antennas, radio and television broadcast towers, power lines, and all electrical appliances (see Figure 16.2).

Ultraviolet Radiation

Most of the ultraviolet (UV) radiation we are exposed to comes from the sun. There are two basic types of UV radiation, UVA radiation and UVB radiation. UVA radiation, which has longer wavelengths than UVB and, therefore, has lower energy, can penetrate the skin and damage underlying connective tissues over time, resulting in wrinkles. UVA and UVB are also implicated in the development of nonmelanomatous and melanomatous skin cancers (see Chapter 4, "Skin Ailments").

The sun's rays are most intense closest to the equator and at higher altitudes, where the thinner atmosphere provides less protection. The ozone layer, which is an effective shield against UV rays, has recently been decreasing; for each 1 percent loss of ozone from the upper atmosphere, there is a 2 percent increase in the amount of UV radiation that reaches the earth and the amount of UV exposure we experience.

Even in areas with high levels of UV radiation, it is possible to protect yourself against exposure. One way is to use sunscreens that block UV radiation. In parts of the world, the broadbrimmed hat is an essential protective garment. However, the rates of skin cancer have alarmingly reached epidemic proportions because of the rise in the popularity of sunbathing.

In addition to causing skin cancers, UVB radiation has also been associated with cataract formation. Cataracts are more common in sunny tropical parts of the world than in temperate regions. People who spend a lot of time in the sun are most likely to get cortical cataracts, which affect the outer part of the eye's lens. Wear UV-blocking sunglasses (which can be prescribed and purchased from a reputable optician) will help protect against cataracts. Sunglasses that do not block these rays should not be used: They can actually increase the eye's UV exposure, because, although blocking visible light, they allow the pupil to open more widely and expose the lens to the harmful rays.

Health Effects of Other Types of Nonionizing Radiation

The type of electric power most commonly used in the United States is derived from an alternating current. Unlike the direct current produced by batteries, which flows steadily in one direction, alternating current flows back and forth at a rate of 60 hertz, or cycles per second. (In Europe, current alternates at a rate of 50 hertz.)

Alternating current produces both electric and magnetic fields, together called electromagnetic fields (EMFs) (see Figure 16.6). Until recently, many scientists found it difficult to believe that the EMFs produced by power lines and appliances could have any biological effects whatsoever. These fields do not impart enough localized energy to break the chemical bonds that hold molecules together. Furthermore, the magnetic field of the earth itself—powerful enough to make a compass work—is at least a hundred times stronger than the magnetic fields generated by devices such as video display terminals.

In 1989, however, three Carnegie Mellon University scientists wrote in a report for the congressional Office of Technology Assessment that "the emerging evidence no longer allows one to categorically assert that there are no risks. But it does not provide a basis for asserting that there is a significant risk." The report called for "prudent avoidance" of EMFs: routing new power transmission lines so that they avoid people, widening rights-of-way, developing new house wiring designs to minimize fields, and redesigning appliances to minimize or eliminate fields.

In 1990, an EPA draft report labeled EMFs "possible" human carcinogens. The report noted that a handful of studies had tentatively linked EMFs to leukemia, lymphoma, and brain cancer in children. Additional studies had also suggested that occupational exposure to EMFs increased the risk of leukemia, brain tumors, and other cancers in adults. The report said that the existing evidence suggested, although it did not prove, a causal link between EMFs and cancer. While in 1991 the EPA's Science Advisory Board reviewed the report and judged it to have overstated the connection between EMFs and cancer, mounting new evidence questions that view.

Low Versus High Levels of EMFs. One difficulty in establishing EMF limits is the fact that the relationship between dose and response isn't clear. Some studies have suggested that certain

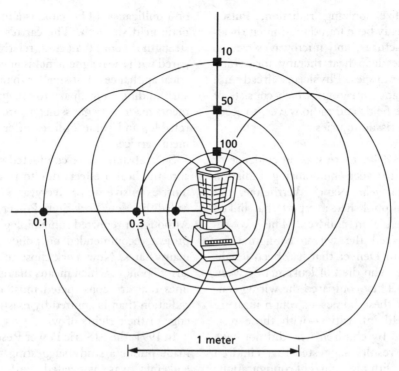

● Magnetic field (in milligauss)

■ Electric field (in volts per meter)

Figure 16.6 ELECTRIC AND MAGNETIC FIELDS OF APPLIANCES.

An electric field, such as that generated by electrical appliances, induces an accompanying magnetic field. The fields line up at right angles to one another. The intensity of a magnetic field is measured in units called gauss. This figure shows the electrical and magnetic fields of a blender. Such small tabletop appliances can have much more powerful magnetic fields than larger appliances, such as televisions, because their motors are often housed in lightweight plastic, which permits the field to escape readily. Other appliances that have relatively strong magnetic fields include electric shavers, hair dryers, and vacuum cleaners.

weak fields may be more dangerous than stronger ones, intermittent or pulsed exposures may be worse than continuous steady exposures, and some frequencies may be more damaging than others. A few researchers have reported that effects appear to occur only in "windows," specific narrow ranges of field intensity and frequency. (Perhaps EMFs of certain frequencies resonate with the natural frequencies of calcium ions in our bodies' cells, speeding up their exit through cell membranes, for example.)

Scientists understand very little about how EMFs interact with human cells. EMFs are not known to cause any chromosomal damage and, thus, they are not thought to *initiate* cancer. However, it is conceivable that EMFs may *promote* the development of cancer by altering the cell's production of proteins that are related to tumor growth, although the mechanism for this is unclear.

It is possible that as scientists learn more about nonionizing radiation they will be able to harness cellular mechanisms for beneficial purposes, just as they have done in developing cancer therapies that utilize ionizing radiation. Pulsed EMFs have already been found to stimulate healing in bone fractures, and microwaves can be used to provide deep heat therapy for aching joints and sore muscles. Physicians already use magnetic resonance imaging, which consists of strong magnetic fields and radio waves, to accurately diagnose tissue injuries.

CANCER. Until 1979, there was no evidence of an association between nonionizing radiation and cancer. That year, Nancy Wertheimer and Edward Leeper published a report that linked EMFs to leukemia in children. The two researchers inspected the wiring configurations outside houses in Denver that had been inhabited by children who died of leukemia between 1950 and 1973. They compared the wiring configurations near these homes—a rough measure of magnetic field intensities—with those near homes inhabited by children who did not have leukemia. The results suggested that children living in homes with high-current configurations were about twice as likely to die of leukemia. (Keep in mind that the normal risk of childhood leukemia is small—about 2 in 2,900 children per year are afflicted.)

A group of researchers led by David Savitz at the University of Colorado Medical School published a follow-up study in 1986. The study took into account factors such as exposure to X rays and pesticides that might have biased the results of the earlier study. However, this study, too, implied a link between power lines and childhood cancer.

To understand the potential scope and significance of this research, keep in mind that, in the United States, there are more than 350,000 miles of transmission lines that carry high-voltage power from generating stations to the communities where electricity is consumed. Another 2 million miles of lower-voltage distribution lines channel the electricity to individual homes.

In most of the studies that have suggested a link between power lines and cancer, differences were observed at radiation levels as low as 2 or 3 milligauss. (The gauss is a measure of magnetic field strength. The earth's magnetic field strength is about 0.5 gauss, relatively large compared with the magnetic fields generated by electrical appliances, but smaller than, say, the field surrounding an ordinary toy magnet.) Measurements made with gaussmeters are generally very reliable, and some utilities offer free measurement services.

Several states have conducted studies to measure the health effects due to power lines. The most extensive was a five-year $5 million study called the New York State Power Lines Project. Although it reported some biological effects, the project recommended no policy changes. Like many states, New York chose to adopt a "similarity" policy, which means that any new power lines that are constructed must not emit more radiation than is emitted by existing lines at the edge of their rights-of-way.

In 1991, the Electric Power Research Institute made public a study suggesting that childhood leukemia was associated with proximity to power lines and certain electric appliances like hair dryers and black-and-white television sets. However, the researcher who conducted the study did *not* find a correlation between childhood cancer and direct indoor measurements of electric and magnetic fields.

A more clear-cut correlation of childhood cancer with exposure was suggested, however, by a study of Swedish children reported in 1992. This case-control study included all children with cancer and all adults with leukemia or brain tumors diagnosed between 1960 and 1985 among nearly half-a-million people who lived within 300 meters of any 220- and 400-kV power lines in Sweden; the researchers found an association between proximity to the power-line magnetic fields and the incidence of childhood leukemia.

In September, 1992, the Swedish National Board for Industrial and Technical Development (NUTEK) announced a new policy that assumes there is a connection between exposure to power frequency magnetic fields and cancer, in particular, as it pertains to children.

Box 16.6 COOKING WITH MICROWAVES

Inside a microwave oven, an electron tube called a magnetron produces microwaves. These beams bounce off the metal surfaces on the oven's interior, and as they volley back and forth, they agitate water molecules in the food to be cooked. The molecular friction produces heat.

Although microwave radiation does not make food radioactive, it can heat human tissue. For that reason, the government requires that every microwave oven be designed to shut off automatically if its door opens. The government has also set a limit on the amount of radiation that can leak out of the door—no more than 1 milliwatt per square centimeter at a distance of approximately two inches.

Some companies sell leakage detectors that allow you to measure how much radiation is escaping from the oven, but the U.S. Food and Drug Administration warns that these devices are unreliable. The best way to avoid radiation is to stand back from the oven while it's in operation, because microwave radiation falls off quickly with distance. At a distance of twenty inches from the oven, the radiation level is one hundred times lower than at a distance of two inches.

Among adults, reports linking EMFs to cancer have been occupational studies. These studies have pointed to an increased risk of leukemia and brain tumors among electrical workers exposed to strong magnetic fields. Workers who may be at risk include electricians, electrical equipment assemblers, aluminum-reduction workers, streetcar and subway motorpeople, radio and radar operators, power station operators, power and telephone linepeople, telephone repairers and installers, welders, and motion picture projectionists.

Further occupational evidence comes from an ongoing study at Johns Hopkins University. Involving more than 50,000 male employees of New York Telephone Company, the study has suggested a higher than expected risk of leukemia for young workers. Cable splicers, the group with the highest exposure to magnetic fields, have shown a leukemia rate seven times higher than employees who do not work on telephone lines. Cable splicers also have appeared more likely to contract cancers of the lymph, lung, prostate, and colon. Parallel findings have been observed in Scandinavian studies reported in 1992, including occupationally exposed Swedish workers (in whom the risk of leukemia and brain tumors also appeared to be increased) and Norwegian workers (in whom the risk of leukemia was increased.)

These findings are only part of the story. The scientific literature also contains a number of "negative" studies—studies that have *not* shown an association between EMFs and cancer. And scientists have criticized the research methods used in some of the "positive" studies. Further research should help explain the contradictory findings of the cancer studies done to date. New occupational and residential studies are currently underway in the United States, Australia, Brazil, Canada, Finland, France, the Netherlands, New Zealand, Sweden, Switzerland, Taiwan, and the United Kingdom. To keep things in perspective, though: Even if electromagnetic radiation does turn out to cause cancer, it is probably far less hazardous than such carcinogens as tobacco smoke and asbestos.

Microwaves. Microwaves have a wide range of uses, from cooking food to relaying telephone calls by satellite. Soviet researchers have long been interested in the effects of microwaves, which they have interpreted to cause changes in brain waves, hallucinations, irritability, depression, and other symptoms. For a period of many years, Soviet researchers beamed microwaves at the U.S. embassy in Moscow. Some U.S. intelligence officers were aware of the radiation, which they called the Moscow Signal, but they did not tell embassy personnel that they were the subjects of a Soviet "experiment." Subsequent studies of these personnel have shown no increases in death or disease rates.

The federal government has set a standard for occupational exposure to microwaves of 10 milliwatts per square centimeter—much higher than the standard for leakage from microwave ovens. Above this level, microwaves are capable of heating human cells.

Consumer Products. Every appliance that uses electrical power also produces nonionizing radiation. Additional radiation is emitted by the wiring in buildings and by electrical currents passing through plumbing and gas lines.

Appliances such as hair dryers, electric razors, and power tools produce very high levels of electromagnetic radiation. However, these appliances are generally used only for short periods of time. Also, the level of radiation emitted drops off dramatically with distance. Of greater potential concern are appliances that are used for hours at a time, particularly video display terminals, cellular and car phones, and electric blankets.

CHAPTER 17

Food Safety

The act of eating, of putting food in our mouths and swallowing it, is intimate and essential. Yet few of us grow our own food or know the farmers and ranchers who do. We only have a vague idea of who makes the cereals, breads, cheeses, candies, or frozen dinners we eat. Instead of a direct relationship, we rely on an integrated food supply system of unprecedented sophistication. For safe, nutritious, and affordable food, we are dependent on the integrity of strangers.

Given these circumstances, it's not surprising that we worry. Food safety concerns consistently rank high in consumer surveys: In the United States, three out of four Americans surveyed in 1991 by the Food Marketing Institute ranked food safety a "very important" concern, and nine out of ten of them ranked it at least "somewhat important."

There are reasons to be concerned about the safety of our food, but our fears may greatly exaggerate the magnitude of the risks. For example, we fear the potential threat from pesticide residues on produce, but avoiding fruits and vegetables may be a greater threat to our health than ingesting pesticides. (There is good evidence that people who do *not* eat at least five servings of fruits and vegetables each day run up to twice the risk of developing cancer as people who eat produce frequently and abundantly.)

Hardly a month passes without a new study or an ominous headline declaring that foods we eat are unsafe. Many consumers are confused by the rash of often conflicting reports. They dismiss food safety issues as being out of their control.

However, there *are* things consumers can do to ensure a safer food supply. This chapter will explore the most common food concerns, including food-borne illness, pesticides, animal drugs, natural toxins, environmental contaminants, irradiation, and food additives, and distinguish the legitimate worries from the overblown concerns. At the same time, it will detail some steps consumers can take to control the safety of their food.

THE REGULATORY SAFETY NET

Although each of us would *like* a simple answer to such basic questions as, Are pesticide residues on my peach? or Are the additives in my breakfast cereal dangerous to my health? the answers are not so readily apparent. Issues of food safety are complex and touch upon personal, cultural, regulatory, and environmental concerns.

Before passage of the federal Pure Food and

THE PROCESS OF BIOACCUMULATION OF PCBS.

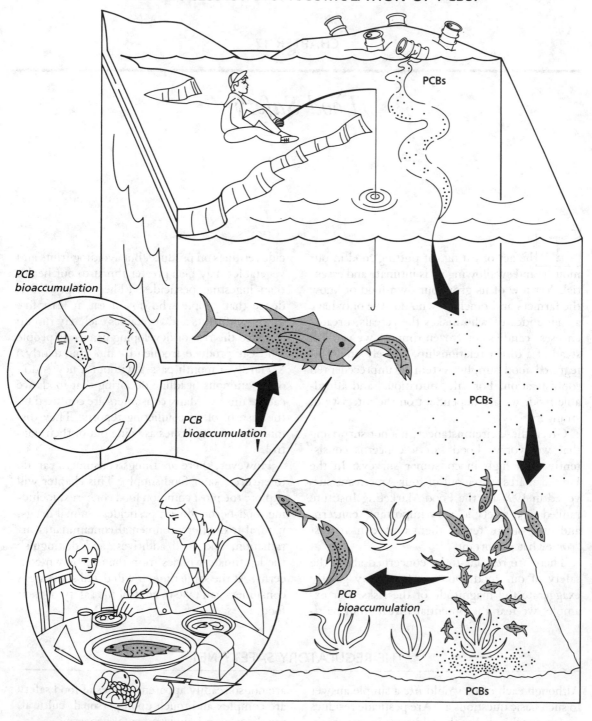

PCBs

PCB bioaccumulation

PCB bioaccumulation

PCBs

PCB bioaccumulation

PCBs

PCBs

Box 17.1 SUMMARY OF THE THREE GOVERNMENTAL GROUPS

Today, three government agencies oversee the U.S. food supply, regularly testing, evaluating, and ensuring that the foods we eat are safe.

The Food and Drug Administration

- Is responsible for the "safety and wholesomeness" of all food, except meat, poultry, and eggs.
- Regulates food additives and veterinary drugs.
- Sets tolerance levels for drug residues in milk, eggs, meat, and poultry and some chemical contaminants in fish.
- Enforces pesticide residue limits in foods and tests all foods (except poultry) for residues and other contaminants.
- Regulates food labeling, except for meat, poultry, eggs, and alcoholic beverages.

The Environmental Protection Agency

- Approves the use and application of pesticides (including herbicides, fungicides, and insecticides).
- Sets tolerance levels for pesticide residues in food.
- Mandates national drinking-water standards.

The U.S. Department of Agriculture

- Is responsible for the safety of meat, poultry, and eggs.
- Inspects meat and poultry products.
- Regulates food and color additives in meat and poultry.
- Inspects eggs and egg products.

Figure 17.1 THE PROCESS OF BIOACCUMULATION OF PCBS.

Polychlorinated biphenyls, or PCBs (shown here), are not soluble in water but are soluble in fat. PCBs discharged into a river persist for years, entering the food chain when they are ingested in very small amounts by phytoplankton (microscopic organisms in water) and accumulate to levels many times greater than that in the surrounding water. When small fish feed on the phytoplankton, the PCBs are passed onto their fatty tissues and concentrate at levels much higher than those found in the phytoplankton. Larger fish feed on these smaller fish, and the levels of PCBs in their fatty tissues accumulate to even higher concentrations of PCBs. Humans eating the larger fish ingest PCBs at a concentration *hundreds of thousands* of times greater than the level at which the chemical originally entered the food chain. In the human body, PCBs are stored in fatty tissues, and may be present in even more highly concentrated amounts in breast milk.

Drug Act and the Meat Inspection Act, both in 1906, American food was routinely adulterated. Chalk was often added to milk to make it whiter, arsenic was added to meat or fish to keep it from spoiling, and toxic copper salts were added to canned vegetables to make them greener.

Today, numerous laws and three federal government agencies—the Environmental Protection Agency (EPA), the Food and Drug Administration (FDA), and the U.S. Department of Agriculture (USDA)—oversee the foods we eat and their additives and ingredients, designed to ensure that all meet specific standards to be safe for consumption (see Box 17.1).

Unfortunately, this vast regulatory safety net still has occasional holes. For example, herbs are regulated as foods rather than the more stringently regulated category of drugs, even though they often act as drugs.

To remedy regulatory dilemmas, government committees and consumer groups have prodded the EPA and the FDA into action. In 1988, a congressional committee directed the EPA to begin a massive reevaluation process (to be completed by 1997) of all registered pesticides to ensure they meet standards set by current safety data. For its part, the FDA plans to streamline the number of steps in its enforcement process, from fifteen to five.

EVALUATING RISKS TO THE FOOD SUPPLY

Despite the rallying cry of consumer groups that much of our food supply is contaminated with dangerous pesticides, additives, preservatives, and hormones, the risk of illness from these substances is actually very small. The greatest food threat to our health, by far, is food-borne illness due to microorganisms or parasites, often referred to as food poisoning. In 1983, the Centers for Disease Control and Prevention (CDC) reported that there were approximately 6 million cases of infectious food-borne disease, 9,000 of which resulted in death. No new statistics have been taken since then, and CDC experts contend that the great majority of infections are probably not even reported. Although bacterial and viral food contamination causes intestinal illness in millions of Americans each year, most vulnerable to the serious consequences from these ailments are the very old, very young, and individuals with compromised immune systems.

More minor are the risks from pesticides, animal drugs, natural toxins, environmental contaminants, additives, and irradiation in that order.

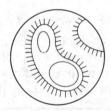

Confronting the Major Food Risks: Microbial Contamination

Beef, poultry, fish, seafood, dairy foods, and eggs are especially susceptible to contamination with disease-causing bacteria. Two major factors contribute to the food-borne illness problem: food production and slaughter methods, and improper handling.

- **Food production and slaughter methods.** Although poultry- and meat-processing plants are periodically inspected by the USDA, microbial or chemical contamination cannot always be detected by sight, which is the current inspection method. What's more, the tremendous problem of fecal contamination, a predominant cause of food poisoning, can result from factory methods of slaughter.

• **Improper handling of foods.** Keeping cold foods cold and hot foods hot prevents microbes from multiplying. This prevents illness, even if a food is contaminated, because there typically must be a large number of organisms present before symptoms will develop. Food left at room temperature for more than two hours is an invitation to trouble. Improper handwashing or sanitation of cooking utensils can introduce bacteria at any point during preparation, storage, or transportation of foods.

Among the microorganisms that can multiply due to improper handling of food is *Salmonella*, which most often results in gastroenteritis, an intestinal disorder with symptoms of nausea and diarrhea. Rarely, it can lead to death, especially in the young, old, and immunocompromised. *Campylobacter jejuni* and *Staphylococcus aureus* also are leading causes of gastroenteritis. *Listeria monocytogenes*, a reasonably rare but potentially fatal food-borne bacteria can multiply over the temperature range that includes refrigeration (2 to 42°).

Refrigerated fresh products that are not cooked after purchase, including such prepared salads as chicken and egg, are especially vulnerable to bacterial proliferation. Prepared food that is kept warm until served (such as meats, soups, and gravies) are prone to microorganisms such as *Clostridium perfringens*.

Cold spots, areas of underheated food, can be trouble in foods cooked in microwave ovens, unless the dishes are rotated carefully while cooking or the food is in closed containers that allow steam to cook the food thoroughly.

Although microbial contamination can affect most any foods, those high in protein are more vulnerable than others.

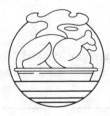

Poultry. According to USDA surveys, one-third to nearly two-thirds of all raw poultry is contaminated with the *Salmonella* bacteria and/or *C. jejuni*. Today's automated processing of poultry may be partially to blame. Water baths to loosen feathers can become a breeding ground for bacteria, and defeathering machines can pound microorganisms into the skin. Evisceration by machine can cause the viscera to break open with fecal matter contaminating the skin and flesh. Although consumer groups urge the government to alter these practices, consumers themselves can reduce the risk of illness by following proper handling techniques (see Box 17.2).

Although proper purchasing, handling, and cooking can minimize the chances of becoming ill, stronger regulations and better self-policing by the poultry, beef, fish and seafood industries are necessary to stem the rise in infected animals. Without industry-wide regulations, for example, a poultry farmer who spends money to protect his or her flock from *Salmonella* puts him- or herself at a competitive disadvantage in the marketplace.

Eggs. *Salmonella* can contaminate cracked or broken eggs. The bacteria also has been found in unbroken, unblemished eggs, thought to be caused when the *Salmonella*-contaminated chicken transmitted the bacteria directly to the eggs while in the ovary. Although only 1 in 10,000 eggs is possibly so contaminated, because of the very real health threat the USDA has nevertheless cautioned against the use of raw eggs in foods such as Hollandaise sauce, Caesar salad, and even undercooked eggs, as in runny scrambled eggs or sunny-side-up fried eggs.

Dairy. Most dairy food problems involve raw unpasteurized milk, a product banned by the FDA for interstate sale because of the greater risk of contamination. Pasteurization kills most disease-causing bacteria. In rare instances, well-refrigerated pasteurized milk has become contaminated with bacteria, usually at the milk-

Box 17.2 REDUCING THE RISK OF MICROBIAL CONTAMINATION

Consumers who understand the many opportunities and situations for microbial overgrowth, as well as the limitations of our federal inspection service, can protect their health with the following tips.

When Preparing Foods . . .

- Before handling food, make sure hands, especially under the fingernails, are clean.
- After touching raw meat, poultry, or fish, always wash hands with soap before touching other foods.
- After cutting raw meat, poultry, or fish, wash the cutting surface and knife with hot, soapy water. Cross-contamination is a common cause of microbial infection; for example, if tomatoes are chopped on a cutting board or with a knife still containing meat juices, the tomatoes can become contaminated as well.
- Avoid defrosting protein foods, raw or cooked, at room temperature. Instead, defrost them overnight in the refrigerator or in the microwave oven.
- Rinse raw chicken under cold water to wash away or cut down the amount of surface bacteria. Then wash the sink with hot, soapy water.
- Use paper towels, not sponges or rags, to wipe surfaces that have hosted meat or poultry.

When Cooking Foods . . .

- Cook meat, poultry, and fish thoroughly. According to the USDA's Meat and Poultry Hot Line (1-800-535-4555), beef, veal, lamb, pork, and poultry should be cooked to a minimum internal temperature of 160°F.
- Keep cold foods cold and hot foods hot. Bacteria thrive in warm, moist places. The danger zone lies between 60 and 125°F. The safety of food becomes questionable if it has been in this zone for more than two hours.
- Make sure foods cooked in a microwave are thoroughly heated. To ensure this, stir foods often or buy a carousel that rotates. Covering food creates a moist, steamy atmosphere that more successfully kills bacteria.
- Make sure hamburger is at least brownish pink, with an internal temperature of 170°F after cooking.
- After barbecuing meat, poultry, or fish, use a clean plate for the cooked food, not the same plate that had raw food on it. The same advice applies to the utensils that were used to handle the raw food.

And the Raw Facts . . .

- Avoid eating raw eggs, including those in foods that are not cooked, such as homemade eggnog, Hollandaise sauce, mayonnaise, or Caesar salad dressing. Un-

(continued)

> **Box 17.2   REDUCING THE RISK OF MICROBIAL CONTAMINATION** (*continued*)
>
> dercooked eggs, such as a runny omelette or fried eggs over easy or sunny-side up, may also pose a *Salmonella* problem.
> - Never eat raw shellfish.
> - Never eat raw meat or fish, such as steak tartare, sushi, or sashimi.

packaging plant. Still, proper refrigeration after the point of contamination will prevent illness.

Fish. Eating raw shellfish is risky business. An estimated 1 in every 250 oysters or clams is contaminated with microbes, often with *Salmonella* or sometimes with the bacteria *Vibrio vulnificus* or the Norwalk virus, not to mention hepatitis A. A 1991 federal Institute of Medicine report, "Seafood Safety," concluded that raw shellfish, particularly bivalve mollusks such as clams and oysters, pose the greatest fish and shellfish threats. With regard to these diseases, properly stored and cooked fish and shellfish can be consumed without worry.

Meat. Hamburger is more likely contaminated with *Salmonella* and other pathogenic bacteria than steak, because it is handled more and has more surface area, which increases the risk of contamination. Contaminated hamburger was the source for the virulent strain of *E. coli* bacteria that caused a 1993 outbreak of dangerous enterohemorrhagic *E. coli* infection that killed at least one child and sickened 400 others.

Parasites. The most infamous parasite is *Trichinella spiralis*, which can be found in raw pork. When the pork is not thoroughly cooked, this parasite can survive and cause trichinosis in humans, an infection with trichina larvae. Once in the intestines, the larvae mature into worms, causing diarrhea, vomiting, fever, and muscle pain. Today, the problem of trichinosis primarily is confined to privately raised pigs that may be fed uncooked garbage and, thus, become infected with the parasite. Proper refrigeration and cooking also has helped curb the disease.

Parasite problems are more common with seafood. For instance, *Anasakis simplex*, a translucent larval worm that can infect herring and other fish, can likewise infect individuals who eat raw fish, such as in sushi. It's best to leave sushi making to the experts. Of the approximately four cases a year of *Anasaki* infection that

Table 17.1 FRESHWATER AND SALTWATER VARIETIES OF FISH

Freshwater Varieties	*Saltwater Varieties*[a]
Catfish, some varieties of clams and mussels, crayfish, pickerel, perch (except ocean perch), some varieties of salmon, some varieties of shrimp, trout	Albacore; anchovy; some varieties of clams and mussels; cod; crab; eel; flounder; game fish, including swordfish and marlin; grouper; haddock; halibut; herring; lobster; mackerel; ocean perch; octopus; oysters; pollock; some varieties of salmon, including Atlantic and Pacific; shark; most varieties of shrimp; snapper; squid; tuna; turbot

[a]Most forms of processed fish, such as breaded fish cakes and fish sticks, are made from saltwater fish, particularly cod, haddock, and pollock.

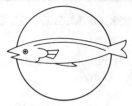

Box 17.3 FISH SAFETY FACTS

Americans are eating more fish than ever before: In the last decade, consumption figures (per person) indicate that people are eating approximately 25 percent more fish.

In 1992, Consumers Union released the findings of a six-month investigation that focused on the quality of fish purchased in supermarkets and specialty shops in several major cities. The results: Approximately 40 percent of the fish sampled was deemed to be of fair or poor quality.

In light of such findings, you might want to rethink the role fish plays in your diet. For the average individual (with the exception of those who are pregnant or very young or old), omitting fish from the diet is probably not necessary. The best advice is to eat a wide variety of seafood, although it may be wise to limit consumption of fish that may be high in contaminants such as polychlorinated biphenyls, mercury, and lead to no more than once a week (examples of such fish include salmon, swordfish, lake whitefish, fresh tuna, and clams).

Consider the following guidelines when purchasing or consuming fish.

- Fish should not smell overly "fishy." If it does, don't buy it. (Freshwater fish sometimes give off an odor similar to that of cucumbers if they are fresh.) Fish should feel firm to the touch and the eyes should be clear with no sign of cloudiness or milkiness.
- The skin of fish should resemble a varnishlike, translucent mucus. Colors should be vivid and bright. If fish has begun to discolor, exhibits depressions, blemishes, or tears in the flesh, or is covered with a sticky yellow-brown mucus, pass it by.
- Look for steaks or filets that are moist and have a translucent sheen. Avoid fish with dried-out flesh.
- Fresh whole fish should have gills that are moist and bright red. Pass it by if the gills are clumped, brown, or covered by mucus.
- Inspect the fish display at the market: Numerous fish piled high under bright lights are ripe for spoiling. If fish are placed in pans surrounded by ice, it may be a sign that the retailer cares about quality. Whole fish should be under ice.
- Purchase only the freshest fish from established stores, not back-of-the-truck operations.
- Avoid reef-feeding predator fish and large game fish unless you've caught it yourself in demonstrably safe waters. Stick to deep-ocean (i.e., tuna, salmon, sea bass, and cod), surface (i.e., mackerel and bluefish), and freshwater fishes (i.e., trout and catfish). (See Table 17.1.)

(continued)

Box 17.3   FISH SAFETY FACTS (*continued*)

- Recreational sportsmen who fish lakes or ponds should only consume their catch if it comes from tested waters that have been deemed safe and contaminant-free.
- When buying such shellfish as clams or mussels, only choose those with tightly closed shells; discard any fish with shells that have opened.
- Keep fish refrigerated at all times. Place fish in its original wrapper in the coldest part of the refrigerator. Cook within one day of purchase.

---

have occurred in the United States since 1980, many have been associated with the consumption of raw fish prepared at home. A trained sushi chef should know how to spot these barely visible worms, although many toxicologists routinely urge people to avoid eating all raw fish as the health risks they pose are too high.

Table 17.2 contains a summary of what you should be aware regarding food-borne illnesses.

DEALING WITH MINOR RISKS

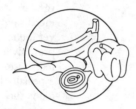

Pesticides

No food safety issue inflames passions as intensely as pesticide use. The American system of agriculture relies heavily on a wide assortment of these potent chemicals to coax higher yields and protect the growth of food crops and livestock.

The EPA is responsible for registering and approving the specific uses of pesticides and to establish the acceptable tolerance levels for pesticide residues on food. The FDA actually enforces these regulations in the marketplace, with the exception of meat and poultry, which are regulated and enforced by the USDA (see Box 17.1).

Before new pesticides are approved for use in the United States, the manufacturers must register them. This process involves testing the chemical's toxicity in animals, looking at its ability to cause cancer, as well as examining other possible toxic effects in animals, such as the ability to cause birth defects or affect the nervous system adversely.

Older pesticides already in use must submit new toxicity data in order to be re-registered. If there is concern about a substance's toxicity, a registration can be withdrawn (this was the case with the pesticide ethylene dibromide, a suspected carcinogen). Unfortunately, only a few pesticides are reexamined each year, and the re-registration procedure is slow (see Box 17.7 for a discussion of the debated issues).

As our measuring tools become more sophisticated for measuring smaller and smaller levels of carcinogenic residues, we find ourselves in a paradox. We can now measure what we couldn't detect before, but we do not know whether these minute amounts of the chemicals actually pose a risk to human health.

Complicating this issue is the Delaney Clause, a section of the Food Additive Amendment passed in 1958, that specifies that no substance that is carcinogenic can be added to food *at any level*.

Currently, industry advocates and the FDA

Table 17.2 FOOD-BORNE ILLNESS FACTS

Illness	Offending Organism	Time of Onset and Symptoms	Method of Transmission and Food Source
Anasakiasis	Anasakis simplex	Symptoms don't appear for a week (confounding diagnosis), then mimic ulcer pain: acute abdominal pain, fever, nausea, vomiting, and diarrhea	Infrequently found in raw fish, such as herring, Pacific salmon, sushi, sashimi, and cerviche; once eaten, if not coughed up or passed in the bowels, larvae can penetrate the stomach lining and cause severe pain. To control: kill by cooking or freezing
Botulism	Clostridium botulinum	Symptoms appear 4–36 hr. after eating: double vision, trouble swallowing and breathing, slurred speech	Rare but deadly; spores are widespread, but only produce toxin when there is no air, such as in cans of food; restaurant foods are increasingly involved, yet foods canned improperly at home are most often to blame, especially low-acid foods such as corn, green beans, and mushrooms, also soups, beets, tuna, olives, luncheon meats, pate, and garlic in oil
Paralytic and neurotoxic shellfish poisonings	Neurotoxins produced by marine dinoflagellates	Within minutes (paralytic type) or hours (neurotoxic type), a sufferer experiences burning of the mouth and extremities, nausea, vomiting, and diarrhea, also muscle weakness, paralysis, and trouble breathing (in paralytic type); symptoms are milder in neurotoxic type	Both caused by toxins found in red tides that contaminate mollusks caught off the Pacific and New England coasts (paralytic type) and off Florida (neurotoxic type)

(continued)

Table 17.2 FOOD-BORNE ILLNESS FACTS (*continued*)

Illness	Offending Organism	Time of Onset and Symptoms	Method of Transmission and Food Source
Food Poisoning	*Clostridium perfringens*	Symptoms typically occur 12 hr. after eating: the abdominal pain and diarrhea are usually mild and last less than a day	Illness results from extensive growth of microbes in food and requires time to grow in intestines, producing spores that release toxin; usually caused by food prepared and kept warm until served, such as with picnics or in food service establishments; will only grow in certain protein-containing foods such as meat, poultry, soups, and gravies
Giardiasis	*Giardia lamblia*	Symptoms appear after an incubation period of 1–2 weeks and include diarrhea, flatulence, nausea, and vomiting	Most often associated with contaminated water, but also uncooked foods
Listeriosis	*Listeria monocytogenes*	Symptoms take from days to weeks to appear and include fever, headache, diarrhea, meningitis, conjunctivitis, and miscarriage	Less common, but often fatal, especially with immunocompromised persons with AIDS or cancer, also elderly, alcoholics, diabetics, and pregnant women; *L. monocytogenes* contaminates many foods and can grow at refrigerator temperatures, but most people appear to resist illness; risky foods for susceptible individuals include soft cheese, pâté, raw milk, uncooked poultry, frozen pork tongue, and seafood

(*continued*)

Table 17.2 FOOD-BORNE ILLNESS FACTS (continued)

Illness	Offending Organism	Time of Onset and Symptoms	Method of Transmission and Food Source
Campylobacteriosis or Campylobacter enteritis	Campylobacter jejuni	Symptoms appear 2 to 5 days after eating: cramping, fever, diarrhea, and bloody stools lasting 7 to 10 days	Growth of organism not required for illness, but bacteria is easily killed by cooking; found most often in raw poultry, hamburger, milk, and mushrooms; increasing in incidence
Ciguatera poisoning		Symptoms begin 6 to 12 hr. after eating: nausea, vomiting, and diarrhea, often followed by slowed heart rate and lowered blood pressure; characterized by severe itching, temperature reversal (cold feels hot), and numbness and tingling of the extremities, which can last just days or for months	Ciguatoxins are produced by algae; toxins are passed from algae to fish; unrelated to mishandling or spoilage; found most often in bottom-dwelling predator fish caught near reefs in the Caribbean and off Florida and Hawaii, such as amberjack, red snapper, sea bass, and surgeonfish; toxin not destroyed by cooking
Enteric E. coli infections (Enterotoxigenic, Enterinvasive, Enterohemorrhagic [0157], Enteropathogenic)	Escherichia coli	Symptoms begin anywhere from hours to a week after eating. They include watery diarrhea; with severe infections, symptoms include bloody diarrhea; symptoms of enterhemorrhagic (0157) infection can include bloody diarrhea and can lead to kidney failure	Most E. coli is transmitted by personal contact, but these strains are food-borne as well; found most often in undercooked ground beef and unpasteurized milk; children are very susceptible to more severe effects of enterohemorrhagic infections
Salmonellosis	Salmonella	Symptoms appear anywhere from 6 to 72 hr. after eating: nausea, cramps, diarrhea, and fever headache	Most severe in the elderly, infants, and the immunocompromised; growth of organism not required for illness, but

(continued)

Table 17.2 FOOD-BORNE ILLNESS FACTS (*continued*)

Illness	Offending Organism	Time of Onset and Symptoms	Method of Transmission and Food Source
			the more bacteria present, the more likely and faster illness will occur; found in raw meat, poultry, fish, dairy products, and eggs; one type, *S. enteritidis*, has been found in the eggs of affected chickens; proper refrigeration and cooking will prevent illness
Scombroid poisoning		Within minutes or hours of ingestion a reaction ensues: flushing, itching, cramps, diarrhea, nausea, vomiting, and burning of throat, but lasts only hours; if severe, there can be trouble breathing and lowered blood pressure	Toxins are produced by bacteria that feed on unrefrigerated fish from the Scombroideae family —tuna, bonito, mackerel, and skipjack—and some nonscombroid fish, such as Pacific dolphin (mahimahi); the bacteria break down the histidine in fish to form toxic levels of histamine
Shigellosis	*Shigella*	Symptoms appear 1 to 7 days after eating: abdominal pain, cramps, bloody diarrhea, and fever	Found only in the intestines of humans and monkeys, the bacteria is transmitted to food by unsanitary food handlers; typically, affected food is liquid or moist, extensively handled, and not thoroughly cooked, such as tuna, chicken, and potato salads; proper refrigeration prevents illness

(*continued*)

Table 17.2 FOOD-BORNE ILLNESS FACTS (continued)

Illness	Offending Organism	Time of Onset and Symptoms	Method of Transmission and Food Source
Staphylococcal food poisoning	*Staphylococcus aureus*	Symptoms appear rapidly—½ to 4 hr after eating—and are severe: explosive diarrhea, cramps, and vomiting, but do not last longer than a day; often resembles the flu	"Staph"—mistakenly called ptomaine poisoning—only occurs if food is left at the wrong temperature for a length of time; may originate from a food handler's skin infection, boil, acne, or nasal mucus; found in meats, poultry, egg products, meat/fish salads, and cream pastries; common
Trichinosis	*Trichinella spiralis*	Early symptoms (during first week of infection) include diarrhea, nausea, vomiting, fever; later (2–3 weeks) muscle pain, and stiffness develop	Insufficient cooking of affected pork allows larvae to survive and, once eaten, mature into worms in the intestines
Vibrio food poisoning	*Vibrio parahaemolyticus, Vibrio vulnificus*	General symptoms: explosive, watery, or bloody diarrhea and abdominal cramps; in *V. vulnificus*, wound infections and a rapid, fatal blood infection can result	*V. vulnificus* is generally linked to raw oysters (and wounds); *V. parahaemolyticus* can be found in any unrefrigerated, inadequately cooked shellfish, especially shrimp; other types are associated with mollusks
Asiatic cholera	*Vibrio cholerae*	Explosive, watery, or bloody diarrhea and abdominal cramps; can quickly lead to severe dehydration	Contaminated water or food, or other sources tainted by contaminated water

would like the law altered so that additives that cause fewer than one cancer over the lifetimes of 1 million people are deemed legal. Consumer groups, however, argue that additives that even slightly increase an individual's cancer risk should be outlawed.

When making decisions concerning pesticides and what foods are safe for consumption, the consumer may be surprised to learn the following.

• *Pesticide residues in animal products versus produce.* Fruits and vegetables seem to be the focus of

Box 17.4   THE CIRCLE OF POISON

Consumers have a justified concern about pesticides that have not been adequately retested by the EPA since they were approved in the 1950s, 1960s, and early 1970s, even if the potential health risks are low. More troubling are the number of pesticides that have been banned as carcinogens in this country but can still be found in our produce. Pesticides banned in the United States are often sold to other countries—often poorer Third-World countries where environmental standards are not as strict or enforced. If they are then used to grow food crops that are exported to the United States, they wind up on our tables—a dilemma referred to as a "circle of poison." Some members of Congress have tried unsuccessfully to ban this regulatory loophole.

A case in point is heptachlor, an insecticide, and a related compound, chlordane. Both can cause anemia and cancer and affect fertility. (One review, dated 1988, concluded, "There is hardly an animal, a body system or a process that cannot be adversely affected by exposure to chlordane and/or heptachlor.") Since 1988, domestic sales of both chemicals have been halted; forty-eight other countries have either partially or entirely banned their import. However, some Third-World countries still allow and use chlordane and export their food products here. For example, according to an article in *Environmental Action*, a newsletter by the Environmental Action Foundation, a nonprofit environmental organization, in April 1988, a shipment of 42,000 pounds of Honduran beef was imported to the United States containing eight times the allowable U.S. tolerance limit for chlordane. By the time the beef was tested, almost all the meat had been sold.

Such cases have prompted consumer groups to caution against buying imported food. For example, basmati rice from India has been found to have high levels of certain pesticide residues. Coffee is a heavily sprayed crop. Tomatoes from Mexico may contain pesticide residues from products no longer available to farmers in the United States.

Although most imported produce is probably safe, some consumers may choose to select frozen fruits and vegetables over fresh out of season. Most frozen vegetables sold in this country are grown domestically under domestic regulations and picked and frozen within a day, ensuring nutritional quality as well as pesticide use. Fresh off-season produce, by contrast, may have been raised under less strict safety standards and transported for days before purchase. Until legislation or other measures break the circle of poison, the consumer's best approach may be to support local seasonal agriculture and buy frozen foods out of season.

much consumer concern, but pesticide residues may be as great—if not greater—in animal products. The Center for Science in the Public Interest, a consumer watchdog group, notes that residues are more frequently found in meat, poultry, fish, butter, and lard than produce. This makes scientific sense; pesticides are organic chemicals that can become concentrated as they are ingested and moved up the food chain, from food crops to animals. Many of these residues are lipophilic, or attracted to fat. They tend to lodge and remain

Box 17.5　DIFFERENT CLASSES OF PESTICIDES

Currently, the American Chemical Society roster includes some 7 million chemicals; of these, an estimated 15,000 are classified as pesticides (many of which are not registered in the United States).

Pesticides are divided into several classes, the most notable including insecticides, which kill insects; herbicides, which kill weeds; fungicides, which kill fungi; and rodenticides, which kill rodents. The following is a listing of these classes with examples of some common chemicals in each category.

Insecticides

- Organophosphate cholinesterase-inhibiting insecticides: tetraethyl pyrophosphate (Bladan, Tetron), mevinphos (Phosdrin), parathion, chlorpyrifos (Dursban), malathion (Malathion, Cythion).
- Carbamate cholinesterase-inhibiting insecticides: aldicarb (Temik), carbaryl (Sevin), carbofuran (Furan), methomyl, propoxur (Baygon).
- Non-cholinesterase-inhibiting insecticides: pyrethrins and pyrethroids: allethrin, permethrin (Ambush), cypermethrin (Diaminox).
- Miscellaneous insecticides: dicofol (Kelthane), N,N-diethyl toluamide (DEET).

Herbicides

- Dipyridyls: paraquat, diquat.
- Chlorophenoxy compounds: 2,4 dichlorophenoxyacetic acid, 2,4,5 trichlorophenoxyacetic acid.
- Nitrophenolic herbicides: dinoseb, dinocap, dinitrocresol.
- Miscellaneous herbicides: cyanazine (Bladex), molinate (Ordram), alachlor (Lasso).

Rodenticides

- Anticoagulants: warfarin, coumafene, bradifacoum, pindone (Pival).
- Metal phosphides: zinc and aluminum phosphides.
- Miscellaneous rodenticides: sodium fluoroacetate, strychnine.

Fungicides

- Dithiocarbamates: thiuram, ziram, maneb.
- Organochlorine fungicides: hexachlorobenzene, PCNB.
- Dicarboximides: captan, captafol, folpet.
- Miscellaneous fungicides: chlorothalonil, benomyl.

Box 17.6 A PESTICIDE–FOOD INTERACTION

Insecticides containing the chemical carbaryl are aerially sprayed on oak trees to stem infestations of gypsy moths; some 13 million acres of oak trees nationwide have been defoliated by gypsy moth caterpillars. Carbaryl particles hang in the air for some days after spraying.

A person who eats a meal containing bacon, sausage, or any other packaged meat containing nitrites is at particular risk of harm if they then encounter carbaryl-laden air; when carbaryl is swallowed in the presence of nitrites, stomach acids transform it into nitrosocarbaryl, one of the most powerful carcinogens.

Because it is impossible to keep everyone in an area from eating nitrite-containing foods (although this would be a good idea because they pose health risks of their own), residents of an area to be sprayed are evacuated during the danger period.

---

in places such as beef fat (another good reason to trim all visible fat from meat), in organ meats, and in the tissues of fatty predator fish, such as bluefish, and inland freshwater fish, such as carp.

• *Waxing of produce and pesticide residues.* Many consumer activists complain about the practice of spraying wax on fruits and vegetables to enhance the marketability of produce and prevent bacterial contamination. Fruits sprayed with waxes do not shrivel up as quickly as fruits that are left au naturel. The waxes are applied to replace the moisture that is stripped away during post-harvest washing. A wide variety of produce are routinely waxed: apples, avocados, bell peppers, cucumbers, eggplants, grapefruits, lemons, limes, melons, oranges, peaches, pineapples, pumpkins, rutabagas, squashes, sweet potatoes, tomatoes, and turnips.

Waxes are generally considered harmless: The FDA has given the nod of approval to beeswax and shellac. The controversy arises when a wax is mixed with pesticides or fungicides to protect the fruit from spoilage.

Two fungicides allowed for use in produce wax, captan and folpet, are listed by the EPA as probable human carcinogens. Two other chemicals, benomyl and thiophanatemethyl, are possible human carcinogens, approved be-fore current safety data were available. Some states are now considering laws that will require purveyors to label any produce that is waxed. In the meantime, consumers may opt to use unwaxed organic produce or to wash shiny produce with dish detergent and a produce brush or to peel it.

The current data on pesticide risk are too burdened with uncertainty to be able to reliably assess the dangers. The actual risk to an individual's health from pesticide residues in the diet probably is much less than what the public believes. Unfortunately, current scientific information is inadequate to confirm this.

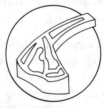

Animal Drugs

Animal foods carry their own unique residue risks. In 1989, the Animal Health Institute, a trade organization for the industry, calculated that U.S. farmers spent an estimated $2.5 billion on feed additives and pharmaceutical and veterinary drugs. Although residues from drugs

Box 17.7   THE PESTICIDE TOLERANCE LEVEL DILEMMA

The following are some of the issues in the debate over the safety of pesticide tolerance levels.

- *Tolerances may be based on old, flawed, or inadequate data.* There are few studies on how pesticides directly affect human health. Instead, to determine a pesticide's safety, EPA toxicologists rely on animal studies conducted by the pesticide manufacturers. In many cases, these toxicity tests are nonexistent or flawed. According to one federal panel, the data to completely assess the health effects of pesticides are publicly available for *only 10 percent* of the active ingredients in pesticide products.

Many of the designated tolerance levels for pesticides were set years before results of thorough testing for chronic health effects, such as cancer, were available. A National Academy of Sciences report in 1987 cited that almost 90 percent of the estimated cancer risk from pesticides in food was linked to older products whose tolerance levels were set before 1972.

In 1982, a congressional committee revealed insufficient carcinogenic data existed for four-fifths (640) of the 800 active ingredients in pesticide products. The committee also concluded that the data supporting a pesticide's tendency to cause a mutation were unacceptable for 90 percent of ingredients.

To remedy the lack of information, a total reexamination process of numerous pesticide ingredients has been ongoing since the mid-1980s, albeit at a snail's pace. The EPA offers reassurance that the tolerance levels err on the side of caution; the amount of a pesticide that remains on food is normally only 1/100th to 1/1,000th the amount known to cause "no effect" in test animals.

- *Programs that monitor pesticide residues in the marketplace are flawed.* The FDA is responsible for determining whether food exceeds recommended tolerance levels for pesticide residues. To do so, the FDA relies on two sampling programs: The first monitors food directly from the fields, testing tens of thousands of shipments of food annually; the second tests for pesticide residues in foods on store shelves.

Critics contend the representative percentage of food tested (approximately 1 percent) is too small. Even if a shipment of food is suspected of exceeding tolerance levels, it is still legal for the goods to be sold while further laboratory tests are performed. What's more, the FDA's routine sampling method cannot determine the presence of approximately one-half of the pesticides used on food.

- *Assumptions about what the "average" American eats are questionable.* Pesticide residues are evaluated in conjunction with information about what the "average" American eats, gleaned from large-scale surveys of food consumption patterns in the United States.

(continued)

Box 17.7   THE PESTICIDE TOLERANCE LEVEL DILEMMA (*continued*)

The last such study, the 1987–1988 National Food Consumption Survey, was severely criticized for its design and implementation. Many experts branded the results unrepresentative, if not statistically invalid. In the face of this, public policy-makers were faced with continuing to use outdated information from a 1977 survey.

and chemicals used to enhance and promote animal growth appear to pose little risk of cancer, many questions about their safety remain unanswered.

Antibiotics. It is still common to add low levels of antibiotics to animal feed to improve the growth rate and curtail the death rate of livestock. Daily ongoing use of antibiotics on livestock eventually can result in an antibiotic-resistant strain of bacteria. When these bacteria are ingested by humans, they can colonize the gastrointestinal tract. Theoretically, if a person develops an infection caused by one of these antibiotic-resistant bacteria, the illness may not respond to treatment.

This scenario is not very likely. Yet it did happen in 1987, when a strain of penicillin- and tetracycline-resistant *Salmonella* infected Californians. The CDC traced the source of the outbreak to consumption of hamburger from cattle given the antibiotic chloramphenicol. A 1989 National Academy of Sciences study of the problem noted that while such direct evidence of human antibiotic resistance caused by use in animal feed is rare, there is a significant theoretical basis for concern.

Milk, the dietary staple of young children, also can contain antibiotics as well as other drugs. In 1990, the FDA reported that eight of seventy samples of milk taken from stores in fourteen cities contained very small levels of drugs, including antibiotics and the suspected carcinogen sulfamethazine (a sulfa drug). The FDA reassured the public that the low levels found caused no public health risk. Yet other government and consumer agencies remain unconvinced; one 1990 General Accounting Office report detailed basic flaws in the FDA surveys of milk safety, concluding that they are not statistically valid and that the FDA is not able to ensure that our milk supply is safe.

Hormones. Although regularly used by beef manufacturers to stimulate growth, hormones are not the threat they once were to our food supply. Today, the cattle industry primarily uses safer, natural sex hormones rather than diethylstilbesterol, a carcinogenic steroid hormone banned in the United States in 1979.

In response to a perceived hormone risk, European countries have outlawed their use in livestock. Although the FDA has suggested banning them in the United States, it currently is legal to feed hormones to livestock. Fortunately, the amounts used are very small.

Natural Toxins

Not all food safety concerns stem from microbial contamination or from chemicals added to the food supply. Equally, if not more insidious, are naturally occurring toxins.

Fish and Shellfish. Both here and abroad, natural toxins in fish and shellfish are a major concern. About one-quarter of the food-borne illnesses reported to the CDC between 1973 and 1987 involved natural food toxins. More than one-half of these cases involve ciguatera poisoning from seafood.

• *Ciguatera poisoning* is the most common fish-borne illness worldwide and the most common

---

Box 17.8   IS THERE A REASON TO GO ORGANIC?

There is no evidence that organically grown foods are more healthful than those produced conventionally, according to a 1990 scientific status summary by the Institute of Food Technologists Expert Panel on Food Safety and Nutrition entitled "Organically Grown Food." The report noted that organic foods have not been well studied. In fact, there are no standards or supervision of products that are labeled organic.

The report also points out, however, that relying on organically produced food may protect our health indirectly by supporting more environmentally benign agricultural practices. Bypassing the use of pesticides and fertilizer nitrates can minimize the pollution of groundwater supplies and protect soil from erosion by reducing dependence on petroleum-based compounds. Such an agricultural system, the report concluded, may offer effective solutions to the environmental damage and nonsustainable aspects of conventional farming practices.

---

nonbacterial food poisoning reported in the United States. The toxin is created by a species of single-celled organisms that attach themselves to coral reef algae and are ingested by small fish feeding off the algae. The toxin is passed along and accumulated in predator fish, especcially fish caught off Caribbean coral reefs, including barracuda, grouper, snapper, and sea bass. People who eat these larger fish can ingest a harmful dose of accumulated toxin.

Ciguatera toxin cannot be detected by odor, color, or taste. It is unrelated to freshness or handling. The toxin is not destroyed by heat, so it survives cooking. Symptoms of exposure, which begin within six hours after eating a contaminated fish, include cramps, gastrointestinal distress, and a characteristic set of neurological symptoms: numbness and tingling of the lips and extremities, a reversal of hot–cold sensation (cold objects can be painful

---

Box 17.9   HOW TO MINIMIZE EXPOSURE TO PESTICIDE RESIDUES

To avoid residues from pesticides, heavy metals, and other pollutants on foods, take the following precautions.

- Eat a well-balanced diet, with less emphasis on animal foods and more on plant foods, such as vegetables, fruits, grains, and beans.
- Trim fat from all red meat, poultry, and fish.
- Avoid, or strictly limit, consumption of organ meats.
- Eat small young fish. Older fish have more time to accumulate organic chemicals in their body. Shop in large commercial markets. Avoid regular consumption of sport fish.
- Remove outer layers of leafy produce.
- Peel skins from waxed fruits.
- Scrub fruits and vegetables with a vegetable scrubber under cold running water.

Box 17.10   MORE PRUDENT FOOD SAFETY SUGGESTIONS

To minimize your risk of illness, consider the following suggestions.

- Check and adhere to "sell by" dates on milk, eggs, and other perishables.
- If hamburger or chicken has an odd or noticeable odor, return it to the store.
- Buy perishables last, including meat, chicken, and eggs, so they don't warm up in your shopping cart, the parking lot, and your car. Refrigerate perishables as soon as you get home.
- Store potatoes in a cool, dry place. Trim away any green eyes.
- Avoid smoked or grilled foods. Baking and roasting are healthier alternatives since they produce very few HAAs; boiling, poaching, and microwaving produce virtually none. (Sautéing has not been studied, but in general, the longer flesh foods are cooked at high temperatures, the more HAAs, so levels may be relatively low.)
- Avoid fried foods; they contain high levels of nitrosamines. Never reuse bacon grease; nitrosamines are concentrated in the leftover fat.
- Use a microwave oven to make bacon; this method forms the least amount of nitrosamines in the bacon. (In some studies, no nitrosamines at all have been detected in microwave-cooked bacon.)
- Insulating meats in aluminum foil, removing the skin from grilled chicken or fish, trimming fat, and avoiding well-done and charred meats all reduce the levels of HAAs. According to some studies, mixing hamburger meat with soy protein before grilling also may reduce the formation of these compounds. (The amino acid tryptophan) in the soy protein interferes with the tendency of creatine in beef to combine with amines to form HAAs.)

---

and burning to the touch), and tooth pain. Medical attention may be required. The acute stage of ciguatera poisoning passes within a day or two, but neurological aftereffects can persist for months or years.

- *Paralytic shellfish poisoning*, although much rarer than ciguatera, also stems from ingesting a naturally occurring toxin. It is often associated with "red tide," the algae bloom of summer. The toxin in this case is produced by a dinoflagellate organism that affects mussels, clams, oysters, and scallops in the United States, usually in the St. Lawrence Seaway Region, and in New England and Pacific coastal states. Like ciguatera, this toxin is not destroyed by heat, and symptoms of paralytic poisoning appear within thirty minutes of eating contaminated shellfish. Characteristics of

the poisoning (which can be fatal) include headache, vertigo, and muscle paralysis. If a person survives the first twelve to eighteen hours of this poisoning, the outlook for recovery is good.

Aggressive monitoring by state authorities in areas where shellfish are collected prevent the sale of those that are contaminated—another reason to buy seafood from a reputable retailer.

- *Scombroid fish poisoning* is not due to a naturally occurring toxin but rather to bacteria acting on fish flesh to produce toxic levels of histamine. Fish such as tuna, mackerel, skipjack, bonito, mahimahi, and bluefish are likely targets. Within an hour of eating affected fish, symptoms occur: flushing, sweating, nausea, gastrointestinal distress, dizziness, headache, and rash. The main danger is possible immediate respiratory distress. This is similar to an allergic reaction. There do not appear to be any long-term effects.

Other natural toxins. A wide array of common foods can harbor other naturally occurring toxins.

- *Polycyclic aromatic hydrocarbons* (PAHs) are carcinogens found in grilled, charred, or smoked foods. During grilling, fat from meat drips down to the hot coals and forms polycyclic aromatic hydrocarbon-laced smoke, which then coats the grilling food.
- *Heterocyclic aromatic amines* (HAAs) are another group of compounds that form when meats are cooked at high temperatures. These potential carcinogens can be formed on the outside of beef, chicken, or fish that is grilled, fried, or broiled (charred meat is a sure sign). HAAs are formed when amines and creatine, both present in muscle tissue, are subjected to temperatures well above the boiling point. Research at the National Cancer Institute suggests that consumption of high levels of these compounds could cause an additional 1,700 cases of cancer for every 1 million Americans.
- *Solanine*, a natural, colorless toxin that may cause severe gastrointestinal effects when eaten in large amounts, is found in the green eyes and sprouts of potatoes, in unripened eggplants, and in green tomatoes.
- *Aflatoxin* is a potent carcinogen produced by a natural mold that can spoil grain, such as corn and peanuts.

Herbs and Nutritional Supplements

Americans spend $3.3 billion each year on vitamin and mineral supplements in their never-ending search for a magic pill to boost health and extend life. Yet, there is much disagreement about whether or not nutritional supplements are necessary insurance for good health or will increase your life span.

Vitamin and mineral supplements are regulatory paradoxes: They are classified as food, not drugs, even though they often act as drugs. This means supplement manufacturers do not have to prove that products are safe or that they have medical benefits; they also need not follow the stringent manufacturing practices for pharmaceuticals, which ensure purity and consistency of drugs. This hole in the regulatory net is a gap the FDA acknowledges needs to be filled.

Vitamins, Minerals, and Unrecognized Nutrients. Two major issues arise when discussing vitamin and mineral supplements. First, because most nutrients can be derived from foods, many experts question the necessity of an individual taking supplements. Also controversial is whether or not supplements of such lesser known nutrients as the bioflavinoids, choline, lecithin, orotic acid, and pancreatin, are necessary or beneficial to health.

The second issue involves supplement safety. Low doses of most supplements are safe. Yet when taken in megadoses, many nutrients have pharmacologic effects and may even be unsafe. For example, excessive quantities of vitamin A—prolonged intake of 15,000 micrograms of retinol—can cause liver damage and birth defects. Vitamin D in amounts only five times over the recommended daily allowance can result in kidney and cardiovascular damage, especially in children. Vitamin B_6 can cause reversible neurological symptoms when taken in doses exceeding 2 grams per day.

Many so-called supplements can be dangerous. Bee pollen extract, touted as an energy booster, has been linked to anaphylaxis, a severe, life-threatening allergic response. Dolomite and bone meal, taken as natural sources of calcium, contain varying levels of lead, which could be particularly dangerous for pregnant and nursing women.

One highly publicized example of self-administered supplementation gone awry occurred in 1989 with L-tryptophan, an amino acid often taken for insomnia. After countless indi-

Box 17.11   HERB ALERT

A wise consumer treads carefully through the unregulated nutritional territory of herbs. Never self-prescribe herbal remedies (that also goes for megadoses of vitamins or minerals). If you are interested in using herbs for medicinal purposes, gather information (including any studies) about the herb, and bring it to your physician for an opinion.

The following is a partial list of many common herbs and their effects.

Herb	Herbalist's Use	Effects/Toxicity
Caraway	Colic	Nausea, vomiting, depression
Castor bean	Laxative, cathartic	Nausea, vomiting, bleeding
Catnip	Euphoriant, stimulant	Hallucinations
Cayenne pepper	Improve circulation, counter irritant	Nausea, vomiting, diarrhea, GI[a] irritation
Chamomile	To relieve flatulence	Decreased intestinal spasms, contact dermatitis
Cinnamon	Stimulant, astringent, to relieve flatulence	Stimulant/irritant to skin or eyes, nausea, vomiting, urinary irritation
Garlic	Hypertension, antiseptic, hyperlipidemia, atherosclerosis	Hypotension, rashes, leukocytosis
Ginseng	Impotence, anemia, depression, diabetes, edema, hypertension	Diarrhea, nervousness, insomnia, anxiety
Grindelia	Expectorant, asthma, bronchitis, mild sedative	Drowsiness, decreased heart rate, increased blood pressure, kidney failure, cardiotoxicity
Jimson weed	Asthma, hallucinogen	Bronchodilation, dry mouth, dilated pupils, hallucinations
Juniper	Gout, diuretic, GI dyspepsia, hallucinogen	Catharsis, kidney failure, seizures, hallucination, renal and GI distress

(*continued*)

Box 17.11   HERB ALERT (continued)

Herb	Herbalist's Use	Effects/Toxicity
Lobelia	Asthma, expectorant	Nausea, vomiting
Morning glory	Hallucinogen, cathartic	Hallucinations, nausea, diarrhea, confusion, coma
Nutmeg and mace	Hallucinogen, GI disorders, rheumatism, abortifacient, to induce menstruation, aphrodisiac	Vomiting, hypothermia, chest pain, dizziness, headaches, nausea, GI disorders
Oleander	Heart stimulant	Vomiting, diarrhea
Olive oil	Laxative	Diarrhea
Pennyroyal oil	Abortifacient, to induce menstruation	Menstrual bleeding, liver failure
Senna	Laxative	Watery diarrhea, abdominal pain
Valerian	Tranquilizer	Tranquilizer, vomiting, drowsiness

[a]Abbreviation used: GI, gastrointestinal.

Source: Goldfrank's Toxicologic Emergencies (Lewis R. Goldfrank, et al, ed.) 4th edition, Appleton & Lange; Norwalk, Ct. 1990, pp. 589–593.

viduals became ill from taking the supplement, the FDA ordered it pulled from the market, but not before twenty-eight people died. Later, a contaminated batch from the main Japanese supplier of L-tryptophan in this country was found to be responsible. This dramatic and deadly example underscores the need for tighter safety regulations.

Herbal Remedies. Growing interest in homeopathy and the "natural" approach has lead some consumers to herbs in the mistaken belief that "natural" is always better. Medicinal herbs, which are unregulated, are like all drugs—toxic at certain doses. For example, comfrey and mistletoe are just two of the hundreds of potentially dangerous drugs (see Box 17.11 and Table 19.1, p. 665).

No government agency regulates the safety and effectiveness of herbal or health food remedies. Yet everything from herbal teas, spices, capsules, and roots can be found in health food stores, various ethnic food markets, and even the local grocery store. Consumers take them for their healing powers but may not realize how unpredictable the benefits can be. Potency and purity are not regulated as with drugs. There is no way to guarantee the same result each time they are taken. For example, buckthorn bark and senna leaves are recommended as laxatives, yet they are so powerful they can cause life-threatening diarrhea (particularly in the very

---

Box 17.12   BIOACCUMULATION AND THE LEGACY OF DDT

Bioaccumulation is an important pathway of exposure, via the food supply, to hazardous chemicals. The term refers to the buildup of dangerously high concentrations of toxins in organisms used for food. Some chemicals that pose bioaccumulation risks are synthetic organic chemicals, such as the pesticide dichlorodiphenyltrichloroethane, or DDT, and polychlorinated biphenyl compounds (PCBs), as well as toxic heavy metals, such as mercury and lead, and radioactive materials. For example, PCBs (which are insoluble in water but soluble in fat) are discharged into a river where they persist for years and can enter the food chain through phytoplankton. (The process of PCB bioaccumulation in the human food chain is depicted in Figure 17.1.)

The pesticide dichlorodiphenyltrichloroethane, or DDT, had a significant role in eradicating the malaria-transmitting mosquito populations. Developed in the 1930s, its use was restricted in 1973 because of environmental concerns. Because DDT is lipophilic, or fat-loving, it is retained in the fatty tissues of birds and animals. It degrades slowly and, thus, is not easily metabolized by animals. Because it is stored for long periods of time in animal tissue, it is easily distributed throughout the food chain.

Such bioaccumulation was shown to have caused a significant decline in certain bird populations, including the peregrine falcon; DDT exposure caused the falcons to produce thinner-shelled eggs. Even though DDT was banned, the resistant compound still persists in the food chain, with most people having a trace of the pesticide in their bodies.

The direct health risk of DDT to humans has never been established; the chemical was banned primarily because of the ecological damage it causes. As no human has ever reportedly died or contracted any health problems from DDT exposure, some public health officials argue that, in certain areas and circumstances, the benefits to humans of eliminating malaria outweigh the ecological concerns regarding DDT.

---

young and old); pennyroyal oil, taken to induce menstruation, has been linked to liver failure and gastrointestinal and vaginal bleeding as well as seizures; excessive amounts of ginseng, the widely available panacea recommended for everything from lethargy to respiratory problems, can cause diarrhea, nervousness, and insomnia.

There are also several not-so-obvious problems with herbal remedies. For instance, an herb may produce no side effects when taken alone, but mixing it with other herbs—as is common to create herbal teas—or with other medications frequently results in adverse reactions. In addition, easily obtainable, unregulated herbal preparations are an invitation for possible contamination. Such was the case when an imported herbal remedy, marketed as an appetite stimulant, contained mercury as one of its ingredients.

Environmental Contaminants

Plants and animals destined to become foods can accumulate environmental contaminants from a host of sources. Pesticides from agricultural runoff, high levels of polychlorinated biphenyls

Box 17.13   LIST OF GRAS SUBSTANCES

Dozens of substances are classified by the FDA as "generally recognized as safe," or GRAS. Translated, that means they can be added to foods in reasonable quantities consistent with "good manufacturing practice" without requiring specific regulatory approval. There are certain regulations for each individual GRAS substance.

Here is a partial list of substances generally recognized as safe:

Acacia (gum arabic)
Acetic acid
Lactic acid
Stearic acid
Sulfuric acid
Agar–Agar
Ammonium bicarbonate
Calcium carbonate
Clove and its derivatives
Cocoa butter substitute, primarily from palm oil
Corn silk and corn silk extract
Ethyl alcohol
Garlic and its derivatives
Gluten, corn
Gluten, wheat
Guar gum
Locust bean (carob) gum
Helium
Hydrogen peroxide
Lecithin
Licorice and its derivatives
Limestone, ground
Magnesium chloride
Maltodextrin
Malt syrup
Nickel
Nitrous oxide
Ox bile extract
Pectins
Propane
Rapeseed oil
Rue
Rue, oil of
Sodium bicarbonate
Sorbitol
Urea

(continued)

Box 17.13   LIST OF GRAS SUBSTANCES (*continued*)

Vitamin A
Wax (Bees)
Wax (Candelilla)
Whey
Yeast, bakers, extract of
Zein

(PCBs), the organic carcinogenic chemicals commonly used as dielectric agents; dioxins; and countless heavy metals are just a few of the toxins capable of making their way from the environment to our dinner tables.

Fish and seafood, which live either part or all of their lives in natural aquatic ecosystems, are particularly susceptible and vulnerable to environmental contaminants. Older, larger inland freshwater bottom-feeding fish, such as carp, spend considerable time in unclean waters and, therefore, are among the most polluted varieties. Predator fish, such as bluefish, accumulate toxins. Bivalves, such as oysters and clams, that live in polluted beds filter the same filthy water over and over. For example, near Monterey, California, the California State Mussel Watch found high levels of twenty-six different pesticides in the shellfish that inhabited nearby waters. As noted earlier, high-fat fish, such as carp, can store toxins and other organic lipophilic compounds in their fat.

One study published in a 1989 issue of the *American Journal of Public Health* estimated that the risk of developing cancer for sportfishermen who ate certain highly contaminated Great Lakes fish once a week for life might be as high as 3.5 additional cancers per 1,000 exposed persons. A more recent small study, which appeared in a 1991 issue of the *New England Journal of Medicine*, reported that Swedish fishermen who ate fish regularly had higher levels of dioxin in their blood than a similar group who did not eat fish regularly.

The most pervasive contaminant in our sea-food supply is mercury. This metal has re-emerged as one of the major contaminants found in fish from lakes across the United States and Canada. Sources of the mercury include volcanoes, mining, metal smelting, and waste dumping. The mercury is dispersed into our air, soil, and water. So serious is the mercury threat that twenty states have issued warnings instructing fishermen to limit and, in some cases, discard the fish they catch from certain lakes that contain seriously high mercury levels. In addition, the EPA has estimated that people who consume more than 30 pounds of fish a year are at higher risk for mercury exposure, particularly pregnant women, and sportfishermen who catch and ingest contaminated fish.

Environmental pollution is not limited to the land and sea. For example, in one study, butter sold in stores next to dry-cleaning establishments had higher levels of perchloroethylene, a carcinogen emitted by the dry-cleaning process, than butter from stores farther away.

Lead, a heavy metal ranked among EPA's most significant environmental pollutants, enters our food supply in a number of ways: leached into tap water delivered from aging pipes or pipes joined with lead solder; leached into food cooked in ceramics glazed using unsafe techniques; leached into wine stored in lead-crystal decanters or poured from bottles with lead-foil caps; leached into food from lead-soldered cans (although 90 percent of the cans in the United States no longer are soldered with lead, many imported cans still are). (See pp. 241–243, 392, and 537–540, for more information on lead.)

Additives

Sugar and salt are two of the most common additives found in everyday foods. Additives are used in a wide variety of processed foods to keep them from spoiling sooner. They also contribute to the flavor and texture of the food.

While most additives used in our foods are safe (see Box 17.13), several warrant closer scrutiny.

- *Acesulfame K* (trade names Sunette and Sweet One) is a sugar substitute. Although the FDA has approved it as safe, arguing that rats develop lung and mammary tumors anyway, the Center for Science in the Public Interest cites a cancer-causing effect in animals and suggests avoiding it.
- Health concerns also have been raised linking *aspartame* (trade name NutraSweet), the artificial sweetener used in over 3,000 products, to a number of symptoms, including headaches, behavioral changes, and dizziness in a small number of sensitive individuals. Persons with the rare disorder phenylketonuria can't metabolize the amino acid phenylalanine (found in aspartame) and should avoid products containing it.
- *Butylated hydroxyanisole* (BHA), a chemical added to oil-containing products to prevent rancidity, has been labeled a possible carcinogen by the World Health Organization; the state of California also lists it as a carcinogen. The FDA is reviewing its status.
- *Monosodium glutamate* (MSG), a natural substance used to enhance flavor in Asian and Latin cuisine, is infamous for its suggested link to Chinese restaurant syndrome, the temporary appearance of symptoms that include numbness, tingling, pressure and tightness, warmth, and flushing, especially in the face, neck, and shoulders. Although bothersome, the symptoms pass within hours and do not cause any lasting harm.

Since it was first described in the late 1960s, there have been hundreds of studies on individuals to determine whether MSG actually causes these symptoms. The results are equivocal: Some evidence indicates that high doses of MSG does cause the syndrome, but the symptoms also can appear after consuming other foods, such as chocolate, alcohol, and coffee.

More serious is the evidence that suggests MSG can provoke an asthmatic attack in a small number of asthma sufferers. Although the FDA recently reiterated its statement that MSG is safe for the vast majority of people, the matter is now being further studied. The World Health Organization recently declared MSG safe as well.

- *Nitrites* are chemicals that combine with naturally occurring substances called amines to produce nitrosamines. Nitrosamines are considered potent carcinogens because high doses can induce cancer in every species of animal tested.

In the 1970s, the USDA banned nitrites from many processed meats. Officials also lowered permissible nitrite levels in a number of products and mandated that bacon manufacturers add ascorbic acid (vitamin C) to their products because ascorbic acid inhibits the formation of nitrosamines.

- *Saccharin*, a weak carcinogen used as an artificial sweetener, was banned in 1977 after laboratory studies linked it to cancer. Public opposition and protest, however, put a moratorium on the ban. Saccharin no longer garners the attention it once did, probably because consumers now have an array of better-tasting artificial sweeteners to choose from.
- *Sulfites*, sulfur-based compounds, are added to food and some over-the-counter medications to preserve freshness and appearance. Sulfites have been linked to triggering life-threatening allergic reactions in a small percentage of people, mostly asthmatics.

Sulfite use has been dramatically curtailed by the federal government. Fresh produce, including that used in salad bars, may no longer contain sulfites. Sulfites may still be found in food and drugs, but manufacturers of these products are required to declare the presence of sulfites on any product that contains more than 10 parts per million. They still are added to some foods, such as dried fruit, and should be well labeled as containing such; they are also sometimes used to treat shrimp to prevent "black spot," and may not be listed on labels. There are six forms of sulfites that may be listed: sulfur dioxide, sodium sulfite, sodium bisulfite, potassium bisulfite, sodium metabisulfite, and potassium metabisulfite. Nearly all wines contain a label saying that it may contain sulfites, because the chemicals can form as a result of the fermentation process, even in wines to which no sulfites have been added.

- *Red dye No. 3* is one of the many synthetic dyes used to give foods color. It was shown to cause thyroid tumors in male rats and has been banned in some foods (see information sheet, "Food, Drug, and Cosmetic Dyes," p. 382).

Irradiation

One approach to protecting foods from bacterial contamination is irradiation. The idea was first proposed more than thirty years ago, and in 1963 the FDA approved the irradiation of wheat. Later, the agency also began permitting the irradiation of spice and teas.

Irradiated food is exposed to high-level ionizing radiation, which controls the growth of harmful microorganisms. The resulting food is radiation-free.

On paper, irradiation appears to be an effective approach for reducing the growing problem of microbial contamination. USDA studies show that treating poultry with irradiation can eliminate most *Salmonella*.

There is no evidence that eating food irradiated at normal low doses causes harm to humans. Yet consumers are not enthusiastic about irradiation. Some mistakenly fear irradiated food is radioactive. Consumer groups are concerned about the formation of unique radiolytic by-products that result from irradiation. Many of these contain potentially toxic free radicals, or unstable molecules that might be capable of damaging cells and causing cancer. The FDA states that the amounts of these unique radiolytic by-products are so small that they are not a public health concern.

Consumer groups argue that the focus should not be on irradiating food to prevent microbial contamination but on cleaning up unsanitary conditions, such as those in the poultry industry, to reduce contamination at its source. Detractors also point out that irradiation may be employed to camouflage spoiled foods, and although the irradiation process may kill *Salmonella*, it doesn't always destroy spore-forming bacteria, such as those that cause botulism.

Consumer opposition has effectively blocked food irradiation in the United States and Great Britain. Although irradiation is approved for use on pork, poultry, and other foods, it is only in use on spices.

WHAT YOU CAN DO NOW

Although the list of potentially dangerous compounds in food is enormous, the actual risk for many of these is quite small. You should keep in mind just how far we've come: According to our national government, our food supply is among the safest a civilized society has ever experienced.

Many of the food risks that plague other countries have been eliminated in the United States. Refrigeration, a virtually universal practice in this country, allows us to keep many nutritious foods fresh, thus bypassing heavily salted or cured foods and preventing spoilage.

When it comes to the safety of our food, prudence is the byword. Assuring an uncontaminated food supply means relying on a complex system of raising or growing, harvesting, processing, and distribution.

Box 17.14   HOW FOOD IS PRESERVED

Without preservation, the shelf life of most foods is very short. Food quickly deteriorates because of microbiologic, physical, chemical, and enzyme-induced decay. The following is a roundup of some of the most common food preservation techniques.

- *Canning* reduces the potential pathogens present to less than 1 in 10 billion organisms. This ratio is based on experience with the most resistant of food pathogens, *Clostridium botulinum*. Canned food that is commercially sterile has a shelf life of about two years. In foods stored for longer periods, deterioration involves changes in texture or flavor rather than to microorganism growth.

- *Pasteurization* is a procedure used for milk and some other foods that utilizes lower heat, generally below the boiling point of water. This destroys only the pathogenic organisms associated with the food. The shelf life of a pasteurized product is generally quite short, as nonpathogenic organisms can still multiply, causing spoilage. Raw milk, which is not pasteurized, is quite dangerous and has been associated with a number of outbreaks of food-borne illness, in some cases leading to death.

- *Irradiation* uses ionizing radiation, primarily in the ultraviolet wavelength range. It produces very little heat—so much so that it is sometimes called cold sterilization—which makes it particularly attractive to foods such as spices, which would change flavor if heated, and animal foods, such as pork and poultry.

- *Drying*, or the process of removing the water from a food, is among the most effective food preservation techniques ever developed. The reason it is so superior is that almost all microbial, enzymatic, and chemical reactions require water. Water is also partially removed when foods are baked, deep-fat fried, extruded, or smoked. Because sugar and salt bind water, they help preserve food as well.

- *Freezing*, like drying, makes the water in food unavailable to microorganisms.

- *Fermentation* is an age-old method of food preservation resulting in such modern-day staples as wine, beer, cheese, bread, vinegar, olives, and pickles. It works by adding friendly organisms to food to produce a more acidic or alcoholic environment. This inhibits pathogenic bacterial growth as well as the bacteria that cause spoilage. These friendly organisms also may occur naturally in a food.

- *Packaging* physically protects food from microbes and pests, such as insects and rodents, and controls the penetration of oxygen, water, and light.

- *Food additives* can also preserve foods. Benzoic acid occurs naturally in cranberries and is often added to carbonated beverages to prevent microbial spoilage. Calcium propionate is added to bread to prevent mold growth. Some additives are not as benign. Sulfites can cause a sometimes fatal allergic reaction in up to 10 percent of asthmatics (see p. 162). Sodium nitrate, added to cured meats such as bacon to prevent botulism, can form nitrites and combine with natural amines in food to form carcinogenic nitrosamines in cooking, and perhaps in the stomach. The FDA also has set limits on the permissible amount of nitrates in cured foods.

The greatest food risk to Americans is food-borne illness caused by pathogens such as *Salmonella*. Pesticides, animal drugs, and environmental contamination pose smaller theoretical risks, and practices such as irradiation may pose little if any risk to consumers.

As demonstrated in this chapter, the complex system of getting food from farm to table is not without flaws. However, the steps outlined in this chapter can help assure the safety of your food supply.

CHAPTER 18

Noise

Noise pollution does not attract as much public attention for research as other environmental problems, but the assault on our ears is just as widespread as the growing mounds of garbage. In a 1990 report to the National Institutes of Health (NIH), a panel of fourteen experts estimated that approximately one in ten Americans suffer from hearing impairment: For at least 10 million of them, the damage is partially attributable to an excessively noisy environment.

Among the disturbing signs that, overall, the aural acuity of our society is eroding is a 1990 report by physicians in Staffordshire, England, who conducted a study on deafness. They were unable to find students who had not been exposed to loud music to serve as control subjects. Settling for a low-exposure group, they found noticeable hearing damage even among these people. For future studies, the researchers say they plan to recruit either Chinese exchange students who grew up without being exposed to amplified music or young people who object to rock music for religious reasons.

Equally troubling are statistics such as those released by the University of Washington Occupational Medicine Clinic in Seattle. Between 1982 and 1987, nearly 10 percent of the 1,424 people evaluated at this clinic showed noise-induced hearing loss. Almost one-half of those studied had been exposed to hazardous levels of noise at their job sites.

The chief environmental culprit behind these reports is the sheer din of modern life. It is not just our hearing that is at risk; exposure to the overabundance of noise can also cause secondary effects such as anxiety, hypertension, and insomnia.

THE EAR: HOW HEARING OCCURS

All of the sounds we hear are produced when sound waves (complex series of air pressure fluctuations) strike our ears and vibrate the tiny inner ear organs that convert sound energy into electrical signals. What we "hear" is the brain's interpretation of these electrical signals. Even when it is functioning perfectly, the human ear does not detect every type of sound wave. For example, we cannot hear dog whistles, which emit sounds that are too high-pitched for human hearing.

What most people think of as the ear is really just the outer ear. It consists of the ear canal and a cartilaginous flap of skin (called the pinna) attached to the side of the head (see Figure 18.1a). The pinna funnels air, compressed by sound waves, into the inch-and-a-half-long ear canal. The compressed air travels down the tube and strikes the tympanic membrane, which vibrates like the surface of a drum, hence, the name eardrum.

The eardrum separates the outer ear from the

middle ear, an air-filled cavity containing three ossicles, tiny bones that transmit vibrations from the eardrum to the inner ear. The first ossicle, the hammer, or malleus, is attached to the eardrum, and it moves when the eardrum vibrates. The hammer taps the second bone, the anvil, or incus, which in turn moves the third bone, the stirrup, or stapes. The footplate of the stirrup then vibrates through a thin membrane, called the oval window, pushing the inner ear fluid. A thin membrane covering a second opening, the round window, expands in one direction whenever the footplate in the oval window is pushed in the opposite direction, allowing the fluid to move.

Displacement of inner ear fluid transmits a wave through a fluid-filled spiral-shaped chamber in the inner ear (see Figure 18.1*b*). This chamber, called the cochlea, contains a long, fibrous membrane (the basilar membrane) covered by the organ of Corti, a structure composed of 5,000 to 30,000 delicate hair cells, each one tuned to a particular sound frequency, like a set of piano keys (see Figure 18.1*c*). When a sound wave stimulates one of these hair cells, it sends a signal to the auditory nerve, which passes the message along to the brain. Scientists still don't understand exactly how the hair cells convert wave motion to electrical impulses.

SOUND VERSUS NOISE

Although there is no quantitative distinction between sound and noise, the term *noise* is sometimes used to refer to sounds that are annoying and potentially harmful to hearing. In nature, there are few sounds that can damage human hearing. In modern life, there are many sounds that can, from jackhammers, jet engines, and motorcycles to power tools, snowmobiles, and lawn mowers. Even sounds that are not perceived as uncomfortable by the listener, such as music heard through headphones, can cause irreversible damage.

Three characteristics of sound determine whether or not it is potentially harmful:

1. *Sound pressure level, or loudness.* When a sound wave travels through air, it produces a small change in atmospheric pressure, which can be measured in decibels. The decibel scale ranges from 0 decibel, the softest sound the average human can hear, on up; most people have a pain threshold of at least 125 decibels, although damage can occur at a much lower level (85 decibels) (see Table 18.1).

2. *Frequency, or pitch.* Each sound wave has its own rate of vibration, which is measured in hertz, the number of cycles per second. The more rapid the vibration, the higher the pitch and the greater the hertz. People respond to frequencies ranging from about 20 to 20,000 hertz but are most sensitive to the sounds in the range of 500 to 3,000 hertz. This is the band that includes human speech.

Whereas the simplest form of noise is a single-frequency sound, such as the pure tone produced by a tuning fork, most environmental noises are spread across a wide band of frequencies. Devices used to evaluate your hearing give more weight to the high frequencies, just as human ears do. In the early stages of hearing impairment, environmental noise typically has the greatest effect on your ability to hear frequencies centered around 4,000 hertz, a bit higher than the pitch of most human speech. That's why it's often more difficult if you have a noise-induced hearing loss to understand a woman's voice than a lower-pitched man's voice. As the noise-induced hearing loss worsens, it spreads to adjacent frequencies (see Box 18.1).

3. *Duration.* The longer you are exposed to a loud noise, the more physical damage to the ear and the more likely it is that hearing loss will occur.

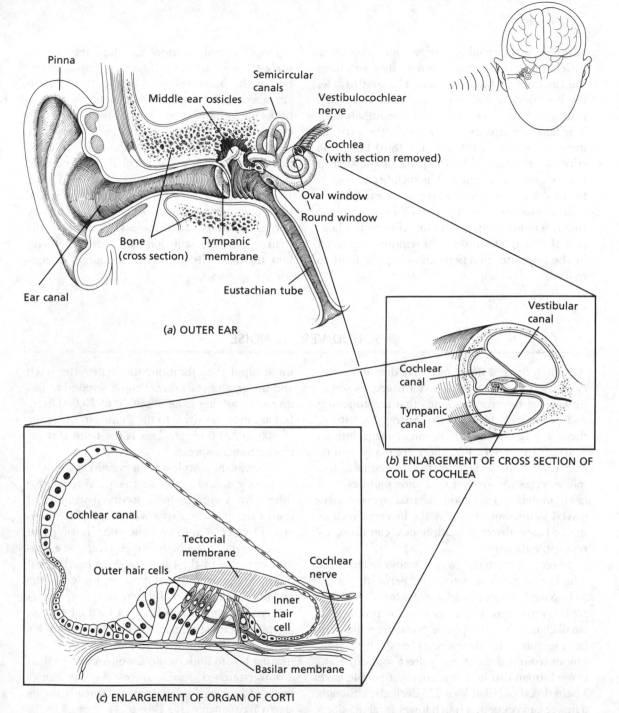

Pinna

Middle ear ossicles

Semicircular canals

Vestibulocochlear nerve

Cochlea (with section removed)

Oval window

Round window

Bone (cross section)

Tympanic membrane

Ear canal

Eustachian tube

(a) OUTER EAR

Vestibular canal

Cochlear canal

Tympanic canal

(b) ENLARGEMENT OF CROSS SECTION OF COIL OF COCHLEA

Cochlear canal

Tectorial membrane

Outer hair cells

Cochlear nerve

Inner hair cell

Basilar membrane

(c) ENLARGEMENT OF ORGAN OF CORTI

Figure 18.1 THE ANATOMY OF THE EAR.

The anatomical parts of the ear that are essential to hearing.

HOW NOISE CAUSES HARM

Intense sounds can cause structural changes in the ear. Noise damage to the ear takes one of two forms: acoustic trauma or noise-induced hearing loss.

Acoustic trauma occurs when a sudden, loud noise, such as an explosion, creates an instant pressure wave. This impulse may rupture the eardrum, dislocate the tiny bones inside the middle ear, and injure the organ of Corti (inner ear). Such impact noises can occur on the job, such as from a machine with a hammering action, or off the job, such as from a rifle or firecrackers.

Noise-induced hearing loss, on the other hand, results from long-term exposure to sounds that are not intense enough to cause acute acoustic trauma. This cumulative type of damage occurs slowly. At first, exposure to noise may cause a temporary threshold shift: For a short time, you cannot hear the weakest sounds that are normally audible. If the noise stops, you usually regain full hearing within a day or so. For some people, however, it may take weeks to recover.

The effects of noise exposure are cumulative. After a series of temporary threshold shifts, a permanent shift occurs. No one can predict how many temporary threshold shifts an individual can tolerate, but this much is clear: When you experience a temporary reduction in hearing, you have injured yourself. The first time this happens, you will probably recover quickly. With repeated injuries, the likelihood of permanent damage increases (see Box 18.2).

How Much Noise Is Too Much?

Scientists have observed that long-term exposure to intense sounds scars and eventually kills some of the sensory hair cells in the cochlea of the ear. They don't understand exactly how this happens, but several theories have been proposed. For example, it's possible that loud noises cause vasoconstriction in the capillaries of the cochlea, reducing the flow of blood to the hair cells. That may deprive the cells of oxygen and nutrients needed to function properly.

Not everyone responds in the same way to noise. Some people appear to be able to tolerate excessive noise without substantial hearing impairment, whereas others exposed to the same noise source suffer a noticeable deterioration. For example, there are cases in which military recruits have suffered permanent hearing damage from one day on the rifle range, whereas their instructors exhibit relatively little hearing loss after years of exposure. Similarly, some individuals exposed to intense sounds on the job, for example, in the mining and steel industries, appear to have no hearing loss after many years of work.

Just as the sun's ultraviolet rays tan some people while burning others, noise affects some individuals more profoundly than others. Scientists know that light-eyed, fair-skinned people are most vulnerable to skin cancer, but determining who is most likely to experience noise-induced hearing loss is much more difficult, which is one reason why people who work in noisy environments should have regular hearing tests to detect early losses.

Although the most obvious physical problem associated with excessive noise is hearing loss, there may also be some secondary effects. When intense sounds strike the ear, they prompt the whole body to mobilize for action. Muscles contract, perspiration appears, and hormones are released into the bloodstream. An adrenalinelike compound called norepinephrine causes vasoconstriction (blood vessels are narrowed). Blood pressure, heart rate, and breathing speed begin to rise, all of which can affect bodily functions.

Although the research is preliminary, some studies have suggested that exposure to loud noise may be associated with a rise in blood pressure, which can lead to hypertension. For example, in 1977, a Dutch study discovered that people living near Amsterdam's Schipol Airport were using more antihypertensive drugs than

Table 18.1 DECIBEL RANGES AND EFFECTS OF COMMON SOUNDS

	Example	Sound Pressure (dBA)	Effect from Exposure
	Jet takeoff (25 meters away)	150	Eardrum rupture
	Aircraft carrier deck	140	
	Armored personnel carrier, jet takeoff (100 meters away), earphones at loud level	130	
	Thunderclap, textile loom, live rock music, jet takeoff (161 meters away), siren (close range), chain saw, boom stereo systems in cars	120	Human pain threshold
	Steel mill, riveting, automobile horn at 1 meter, boom box stereo held close to ear	110	
	Jet takeoff (305 meters away), subway, outboard motor, power lawn mower, motorcycle at 8 meters, farm tractor, printing plant, jackhammer, garbage truck	100	

(continued)

Box 18.1   HOW HEARING IS MEASURED

To measure hearing ability, audiologists use a device called an audiometer, a set of earphones that generates pure tones and words. First, the audiologist puts the earphones over the subject's external ear canal, tunes it to a particular frequency, and presents a series of tones of decreasing loudness. The purpose of this is to determine the hearing threshold level—the softest tone the subject is able to hear—at that particular frequency. The procedure is repeated for a number of frequencies and is used to compile an audiogram, a chart that shows how a subject's hearing compares with the average hearing thresholds for normal healthy ears. Following the pure tone hearing test, words are presented at varying intensities to test understanding.

Table 18.1 DECIBEL RANGES AND EFFECTS OF COMMON SOUNDS (*continued*)

Example	*Sound Pressure (dBA)*	*Effect from Exposure*
Busy urban street, diesel truck, food blender, cotton spinning machine	90	Hearing damage (8 hr exposure), speech interference
Garbage disposal, clothes washer, average factory, freight train at 15 m, dishwasher, food blender	80	Possible hearing damage
Freeway traffic at 15 m, vacuum cleaner, noisy office or party, TV audio	70	Annoying
Conversation in restaurant, average office, background music, chirping bird	60	Intrusive
Quiet suburb (daytime), conversation in living room	50	Quiet
Library, soft background music	40	
Quiet rural area (nighttime)	30	
Whisper, rustling leaves	20	Very quiet
Breathing	10 / 0	Threshold of hearing

Note: Because the human ear is sensitive to such a wide range of sound levels, the decibel scale is designed logarithmically, meaning that acoustic intensity multiplies ten times with every 10-decibel increase. In other words, 10 decibels is 10 times louder than 1 decibel, 20 decibels is 100 times louder, and 30 decibels is 1,000 times louder. Sounds at about 125 decibels or greater, as well as high-frequency tones, are experienced as painful by most people. This table provides examples of the sounds that fall within certain decibel ranges and their effects on human hearing. Abbreviations used: dBA, average-weighted decibels; m, meter.

Source: Chart adapted with permission from *Living in the Environment: An Introduction to Environmental Science* (7th ed.) by G. Tyler Miller, copyright 1992, Wadsworth Publishing Company, p. 235.

Box 18.2　WARNING SIGNS OF DANGEROUS NOISE LEVELS

There are several warning signs that indicate when a noise is loud enough to damage your hearing, but even if you don't notice any of those symptoms, gradual damage may still be occurring. Experts say the best way to protect your hearing is to follow this simple rule: Avoid loud noises whenever possible. When avoidance isn't possible, wear some form of hearing protection.

According to the 1990 NIH consensus panel's report, sound levels below 75 decibels—the approximate level of a vacuum cleaner—are unlikely to cause hearing loss, even over long exposure periods. But daily exposure to sounds above 85 decibels—equivalent to the sound of a power lawn mower—could cause permanent hearing damage.

A noise does not have to be painful to cause hearing loss, but a painful noise should certainly be avoided. People should also avoid any noises that cause the following early signs of hearing loss:

- Tinnitus (ringing in the ear).
- A sensation of "stuffiness" or fullness in the ear.
- A muffling or temporary dullness of hearing.
- Difficulty in understanding speech, including a need to look at people when they're speaking in order to understand them.

---

people in quieter neighborhoods; use of the drugs had doubled in the six years following the construction of a new runway. A 1978 study by Dr. Ernest A. Peterson of the University of Miami School of Medicine reported that high blood pressure was induced in rhesus monkeys and other primates exposed to noise levels of 85 to 90 decibels over extended periods of time; even after the noise stopped, the monkeys' blood pressure remained higher than normal.

Studies like these are necessary for understanding more about hearing loss. Unfortunately, this type of research has not received much financial support, so it is unlikely that we will have definitive answers for some time.

Insomnia may also be a by-product of exposure to excessive noise. The Dutch study found that people living near the Amsterdam airport took more sleeping pills than people living elsewhere, suggesting that the noise may have caused an inability to fall asleep as well as fatigue.

Intense noise can also cause stress, anxiety, and irritability. Noises that are high-pitched and unpredictably intermittent are generally the most annoying.

In one laboratory test, researchers made their subjects angry at one member of the research team. Then they seated each subject in a room equipped with a push-button control and told the person that pushing the button would administer electrical shocks to the unpopular researcher. In these tests, the subjects seated in noisy rooms pushed the button more often and held it down significantly longer than their counterparts in quiet rooms. Although noise seemed to incite hostile behavior in angry subjects, it didn't seem to affect subjects who weren't angry.

In another experiment, someone who had accidentally dropped an armful of books on the sidewalk (actually a researcher faking the incident) asked passing pedestrians for help. In the presence of a noisy lawn mower or jackhammer, passersby were much less likely to stop and lend a hand than when the experiment was conducted on a quiet street.

The effort required to understand speech in a noisy environment may also cause anxiety and fatigue. Loud noises make it difficult to hear approaching vehicles and warning shouts, possibly increasing a person's accident risk both on and off the job. In a noisy factory, workers who have to communicate by shouting may develop vocal-cord problems.

NOISE IN THE WORKPLACE

It is estimated that more than 10 million Americans who work in manufacturing, agriculture, mining, construction, and forestry are exposed to potentially hazardous noise. Noise in the workplace is not only one of the top occupational hazards, it is the most common cause of irreversible hearing loss. Noise can also trigger stress, disrupt or disorient workers, and contribute to industrial accidents by interfering with communication.

Regulating Noise in the Workplace

In the United States, the major agencies regulating noise exposure in the workplace are the Labor Department's Occupational Safety and Health Administration (OSHA), the Environmental Protection Agency (EPA), and the Department of Transportation.

In 1969, OSHA began regulating workplace noise for employers with federal contracts. In 1971 it developed standards for all employers in the manufacturing and maritime industries. In 1972, the Noise Control Act was passed (see Box 18.5); that same year, the Labor Department's National Institute for Occupational Safety and Health (NIOSH), the research arm of OSHA, recommended that noise exposures be limited to 85 decibels, averaged over an eight-hour period, for new businesses. NIOSH also suggested that the secretary of labor study the feasibility of instituting an 85-decibel exposure limit for existing businesses.

The current OSHA noise standard is 90 decibels over eight hours—five decibels higher than the level most experts agree will produce permanent hearing loss after many years. Under OSHA guidelines, workers can be exposed to even higher noise levels for shorter periods of time: A 5-decibel increase is permitted for each halving of exposure time: 95 decibels for four hours, 100 decibels for two hours, and so forth up to 115 decibels for fifteen minutes.

In 1981, however, the agency drafted an amendment requiring employers to institute hearing-conservation programs when noise exposure levels reach 85 decibels. The amendment was postponed but finally implemented in 1983.

OSHA's regulations are now weakly enforced, and employers are required to adhere to noise limits only "to the extent feasible." Over the past decade, this loophole has widened: The number of citations issued to employers lacking noise-reducing controls decreased from 2,292 in 1981 to 191 in 1987. Beginning with a case in 1976, the courts have ruled that OSHA must take economic as well as technical feasibility into account when requiring companies to use engineering controls to reduce noise.

In 1982, OSHA stopped issuing citations to employers who exposed employees to excessive noise levels below 100 decibels, so long as the companies had "effective" hearing-conservation programs. Without changing the law, OSHA effectively raised the noise standard by 10 decibels, allowing workplaces to be ten times noisier than under the 90-decibel standard. Despite the new focus on hearing conservation, fines for violations of the hearing-conservation amendment have steadily declined in recent years. In 1987, U.S. industries paid an average of only $18 per citation.

Noise inspections of factories and other workplaces are infrequent. Anyone who works around heavy equipment or loud noises may be at risk, not just those working in the noisiest occupations (see Box 18.3). However, workers affected by noise-induced hearing loss have some recourse: They can file worker compensation claims or lawsuits. However, the average payment for hearing loss is only about $3,000, and many states require employees to leave the noisy environment before filing a claim, so employees often take no action until they retire.

Box 18.3   THE NOISIEST OCCUPATIONS

According to NIOSH estimates, 14 percent of the American work force are employed in industries where noise levels commonly exceed 90 average-weighted decibels, the level at which hearing impairment can occur if exposure continues over time. (Average-weighted decibels takes into account the more damaging properties of higher frequency tones.)

High to low, in order of the percentage of the work force exposed, the noisiest industries are

Textile mills.
Petroleum and coal products.
Lumber and wood products.
Food and food-related products.
Furniture manufacturers.
Fabricated metal products.
Stone, clay, and glass products.
Primary metal industries.
Rubber and plastics products.
Transportation equipment.
Electrical equipment and supplies.
Chemicals manufacturing.
Clothing.
Paper and allied products.
Munitions and accessories.

Other Environmental Agents

Environmental agents other than noise can contribute to hearing loss. For example, it is well established that aspirin and some antibiotics, such as neomycin and kanamycin, can cause hearing loss. A few studies have also suggested that industrial heavy metals, such as mercury, and solvents, such as carbon disulfide, may affect hearing. People who work with these substances in a noisy environment may experience even greater hearing loss than people who are exposed only to noise.

Protective Action for the Ears

To protect workers' hearing and comply with regulatory standards, employers may try to abate noise at its source. Often this entails something as simple as installing a muffler or sound barrier, tightening a bolt, or mounting a machine on a sheet of rubber. However, some workplace noise can't be controlled at a reasonable cost, even with the best engineering available. In such cases, and in workplaces where employers decide not to adopt noise controls, workers should protect themselves by wearing personal hearing-protection devices—either ear plugs, ear muffs, or canal caps (see Box 18.4).

The current OSHA standard requires employers to set up hearing-conservation programs for workers exposed to 85 decibels or more over an eight-hour shift. Many experts feel that standard protects only up to 94 percent of the population, not everyone.

Companies with hearing-conservation programs conduct regular hearing tests on employees and require employees to wear ear protectors. If you work at a company that does not have a hearing-conservation program and you are experiencing some of the warning signs of hearing loss, you should take measures to protect yourself.

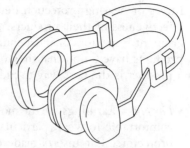

Figure 18.3 EAR MUFFS.

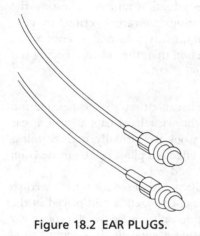

Figure 18.2 EAR PLUGS.

NOISE OUTSIDE THE WORKPLACE

In all cultures, as people grow older, their hearing tends to become less acute. However, in industrialized societies, where many individuals are exposed to noisy environments, pronounced hearing loss is common in old age.

In less technologically advanced societies exposed to less noise, elderly people often have good hearing. For example, the Mabaan tribe in Sudan prizes hearing, and the people of the tribe usually speak very quietly. The loudest noises in the Mabaans' environment, other than the occasional music ceremony, are from livestock. Tests on elderly members of the tribe show their hearing is as good as that of much younger people living in urban areas of developed countries.

Millions of Americans are exposed to loud noise as part of their everyday environment.

Trucks on the road, jackhammers at construction sites, jet engines at the airport, all produce noise above 85 decibels. City streets, blaring stereos, rock concerts, and recreational pursuits, such as working with power tools; riding motorcycles, snowmobiles, and boats; and playing music in a band, may expose the ear to dangerous levels of sound.

It does not matter whether you are exposed to noise from an assembly line, a jackhammer, or stereo headset: If a sound is too loud, it can cause damage, no matter what its source.

Government agencies have made some efforts to curb noise in the workplace, but little has been done to stifle dangerously loud sounds outside of it (see Box 18.5). Some of the worst offenders include the following.

Box 18.4 HEARING-PROTECTION DEVICES

Three basic types of hearing-protection devices are available. The first two are very good at blocking noise, whereas the third should only be used in special cases. All three types can be purchased without a doctor's prescription in a variety of retail stores.

A regulation passed before the EPA's noise office closed requires that manufacturers of hearing-protection devices supply noise-reduction ratings indicating the effectiveness of their products. However, these ratings are rarely verified by government inspectors or independent laboratories, and many scientific reviews of the products have found that they offer far less protection than they claim. Trying out a product is the best way to judge its effectiveness.

- *Ear plugs.* Ear plugs are the most popular devices because they are inexpensive and comfortable to wear, particularly for workers who wear hard hats as well as ear protectors. Ear inserts made of dry cotton or wool are virtually useless unless they're impregnated with a soft wax. However, effective plugs can be made from a variety of materials, including rubber, plastic, and wax.

  Expandable ear plugs are the newest type available. Made of foam or "Swedish wool" (extremely fine mineral fibers), they're pinched together and placed in the ear canal, where they expand to fill the space. It doesn't matter which type of ear plug a worker chooses; what's important is getting a good fit. If a slight tug is required to pull out the plug, it probably fits properly.

  Workers are often tempted to use plugs that are a bit smaller than the size that would be most effective, because the smaller plugs are more comfortable. However, this defeats the purpose of wearing plugs. Also, some activities, such as chewing gum, may loosen the plugs, so workers who wear them should check the fit throughout the day.

- *Ear muffs.* In areas with extremely high noise levels, plugs may not provide sufficient protection, and workers should wear ear muffs, the most effective type of ear protector available. Ear muffs have cups lined with sound-absorbing material that are held against the skull with a spring band or oil-filled ring that provides a tight seal. Workers should not substitute stereo headphones or other muffs that are not designed specifically for hearing protection.

  Ear muffs don't need to be replaced as often as plugs, but they can be uncomfortable in heat. Workers who wear glasses may also find it difficult to keep the muffs tightly sealed to the head, and some workers may be tempted to stretch the muffs to reduce pressure on the head, ruining the muffs' effectiveness. Like ear plugs, ear muffs must be properly fitted. Some employers prefer muffs to plugs because they can tell at a glance whether employees are wearing them.

- *Canal caps.* Canal caps, soft rubber or foam plugs that are held against the ear by a headband, are not a good substitute for ear plugs or ear muffs. However, some

(*continued*)

Box 18.4 HEARING-PROTECTION DEVICES (*continued*)

employees who are exposed only intermittently to noise prefer the caps because they can comfortably be worn around the neck when not in use.

No matter what form of ear protection is used, it should be worn continuously during exposure to loud noise. If the protectors are removed for even a few minutes, their effectiveness will be significantly reduced. For example, earplugs can reduce the amount of noise reaching the middle ear by up to 30 decibels. However, if the plugs are worn only 99 percent of the time, the maximum noise reduction drops to 20 decibels.

Box 18.5 THE NOISE CONTROL ACT

In 1972, Congress passed the Noise Control Act, giving the EPA a mandate to regulate environmental noise. The act placed the EPA in charge of all federal noise activities and ordered other agencies to help develop noise-reduction plans. The EPA's Office of Noise Abatement and Control, which at one time had a staff of 130 and a budget of $10 million, supported scientific research on noise during the 1970s and early 1980s. Most of what we now know about noise is based on fifteen-year-old EPA reports.

In its heyday, the EPA office established noise standards for new trucks and motorcycles and proposed regulations for tractors, buses, lawn mowers, and jackhammers. Some of these regulations remain on the books, but the government in recent years has made no effort to enforce them.

The EPA noise office also started a program to rate the sound levels of consumer products and developed a "buy quiet" program to encourage federal and state agencies to purchase quiet products. A panel of experts attending a 1979 EPA symposium on machinery and construction noise agreed that quieter equipment could be designed "provided that the proper economic incentives were available." The panel drew up a list of one hundred machines that needed to be redesigned to reduce noise.

The EPA's Office of Noise Abatement and Control was closed in 1982, and the noise program now has only one full-time employee. Without federal support, most state and local noise-control programs have also died. According to Dr. Alice H. Suter, who worked in the EPA's noise office and was the principal author of OSHA's hearing-conservation amendment while at OSHA's Office of Health Standards, there were about 1,100 state and local antinoise programs during the peak of activity at the EPA in the 1970s. Suter estimates there are now only 15 such programs.

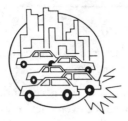

Urban Noise

Vehicles are a major noise source. Some cities have even passed antihonking statutes in a vain attempt to lower the volume; these laws allow police and traffic officers to issue tickets to drivers caught honking when there's no emergency.

In New York City, where the nation's first noise-pollution law was enacted in the 1970s, inspectors issued 749 summonses for noise-law violations in the first six months of 1990. Car alarms create so many problems in Manhattan, the nation's noisiest urban area, that New York Governor Mario M. Cuomo recently signed a bill requiring new alarms to stop after five minutes.

Although automobiles, trucks, buses, trains, and airplanes built in recent years are quieter than their predecessors, land and air traffic has increased, so the total level of noise is higher than it was in the past.

As many as 90 million people are routinely exposed to traffic sounds and other background noises that exceed the EPA's safe day–night level of 55 decibels. The EPA's noise office determined that noise above this level can be detrimental to public health. (The day–night level is the average noise level over a twenty-four-hour period, with sounds occurring between 10 P.M. and 7 A.M. counted as if they were 10 decibels higher.)

The burden of protecting citizens from unsafe levels of noise has fallen on local police and environmental inspectors assigned to enforce community antinoise laws. In San Antonio, Texas, where an ordinance prohibits "vexing, hazardous" sounds of more than 74 decibels, there are two full-time noise cops with a $7,600 noise analyzer. Since 1989, the duo has issued tickets to

a wedding party with a loud band, a church with bell tower chimes that woke neighbors, and a number of nightclubs, including one that now uses its own meter to monitor sound levels.

Most communities aren't as zealous as San Antonio in pursuing noise polluters. Although many cities place limits on car mufflers, radios, and other noise sources, noise problems are usually only investigated when someone complains.

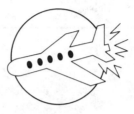

Airport Noise

Although the Federal Aviation Administration (FAA) claims that today's quietest aircraft are one-fourth as loud as those that made up most of the fleet fifteen years ago, consumer advocates complain that the increased traffic at airports and in the air more than makes up for the difference.

• When airplanes fly over Shirley Gazsi's house in Cranford, New Jersey, which is in the flight path of Newark International Airport, she can't hear her stereo or television, and the windows rattle. Gazsi and her neighbors have formed the Coalition Against Aircraft Noise to fight the routing plan that sends planes over their suburbs.
• Mary Williamson lives a few hundred feet from the runway at the Robert Mueller Municipal Airport in Austin, Texas. She has covered her bedroom windows with sheets of soundproofing board, but the roar of jets still wakes her every morning. Williamson says she not only hears the planes, she feels them. She would like the airport to either move or adopt noise restrictions.

The FAA claims that the number of people subjected to "unacceptable" noise has declined from 7 million in the early 1970s to 3.2 million in 1990 and will fall to 1 million by 2010. However, people like Gazsi and Williamson are skeptical of these figures. They also object to the FAA's measurement technique, which averages noise over twenty-four-hour periods and disregards transient noises that are loud enough to disrupt conversations.

Most people working outside the airline industry aren't exposed to loud enough aircraft noises for long enough periods to cause hearing loss. These noises, however, can be extremely annoying to people living near airports and may contribute to a variety of psychological and physical problems (see Box 18.6).

Box 18.6   AIRPORT NOISE

More than 400 U.S. airports are already restricted by local noise laws. John Wayne Airport in Orange County, California, has the strictest laws—only Stage 3 aircraft can land there. (Today's quietest aircraft, called Stage 3, are only 25 percent as loud as the Stage 1 aircraft that made up the majority of the fleet fifteen years ago, according to the FAA.) Other airports have adopted nighttime curfews and noise "budgets." Airport neighbors helped draft a plan for the Seattle–Tacoma International Airport; it's expected to cut noise in half by 2001. The plan allocates noise among various airlines, which can opt for fewer flights using noisy planes or more flights using quieter planes.

Community organizers and politicians have also waged battles against airport construction and objectionable flight routings. In Denver, airport officials had to buy up land for a buffer zone to overcome protests against the construction of a new airport, which will be completed in 1993. In late 1991, the FAA announced that it would investigate the possibility of rerouting flights over New York, New Jersey, and Connecticut in response to requests from members of Congress from the region. At the Dallas–Fort Worth International Airport, officials are considering a plan to pay local residents for the right to fly over their property. Airport planners hope the compensation will eliminate objections to the construction of two new runways.

Battles between airports and their neighbors may create new safety concerns. Airlines have already had to provide special training for pilots who fly into airports that require noise-reducing takeoff maneuvers. Airlines currently refuse to reroute planes over the ocean, but if new runways and flight paths aren't created, congestion may result in more accidents. Scheduling problems will also increase as airlines struggle to comply with a patchwork quilt of local rules.

Some airlines have called for national noise standards. A provision included in a 1990 draft version of a national transportation policy was removed under pressure from government agencies that feared they might be sued for noise violations. The Senate's aviation subcommittee is now considering legislation that calls for a national noise standard to be adopted by 1992.

Meanwhile, the FAA and the National Aeronautics and Space Administration have signed research agreements to jointly study technology for reducing noise, particularly noise from sonic booms. The program's ultimate aim: to make an American supersonic plane acceptable to the public.

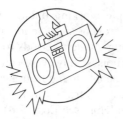

Recreational Noise

Rivaling the proliferation of noise-polluting industrial machinery is the growth of recreational tools and gadgetry that whirr or boom at levels exceeding safe standards.

Rock Music. In industrialized nations, so many young people listen to loud music that it's difficult for researchers to find subjects who haven't been exposed and haven't suffered some noise-induced hearing loss (see p. 630). Although OSHA regulations prohibit employers from subjecting employees to 100-decibel noise levels for more than two hours at a time, rock concerts typically have sound levels above 100 decibels and often last longer than two hours. What's more, the sound systems used at these concerts are powered by tens of thousands of watts of amplification, and there are often 200 or more speakers aimed at the audience. According to some physicians, attendance at as few as ten rock concerts can lead to hearing loss. One expert has stated the ears of young people exposed to rock music are as damaged as those of war veterans exposed to artillery.

Because young people tend to play music at such high volumes, some municipalities prohibit loud use of car radios, some of which are powerful enough to be heard several blocks away, and boom boxes. However, there's no law against the use of personal stereos, which don't disturb the peace but can deliver up to 115 decibels to the ears of the listener.

Sports. People who watch spectator sports, such as auto racing, or who participate in activities such as hunting, motorcycling, boating, and snowmobiling may also be putting their hearing at risk. Protective devices, such as ear plugs and muffs, can help.

FINDING A SOLUTION

"The effect of repeated sound overstimulation is cumulative over a lifetime and is not currently treatable," stated the 1990 NIH Consensus Development Conference on noise and hearing loss. "Hearing impairment has a major impact on one's communication ability, and even mild impairment may adversely affect the quality of life," the panel added. "Unfortunately, although noise-induced hearing loss is preventable, our increasingly noisy environment places more and more people at risk."

There are many ways to counter the growing problem of noise. Sophisticated noise-control technologies could minimize exposure at the source. For example, active noise-cancellation systems could broadcast antinoise sound waves, mirror images of noise sound waves, to cancel out loud sounds. (One such sound processor is under development by car radio manufacturers; it samples wind and engine noises and broadcasts antinoise sound waves to cancel out engine and wind noises.)

However, the best solution to noise-induced hearing loss is prevention. As outlined by the 1990 NIH conference, what is needed are:

- Incentives for manufacturers to design quieter products.
- Regulations governing the maximum noise emission levels of consumer products.
- The reestablishment of a federal agency to plan solutions to noise issues.
- High-visibility media campaigns to develop public awareness of the effects of noise on hearing.
- Health curricula that teach public school stu-

dents how to prevent noise-induced hearing loss.

Noise-induced hearing loss is a problem that can be avoided. If you stay away from loud noises or wear ear protection when you must be exposed to excessive noise, you can spare your hearing. Although everyone's hearing becomes somewhat less acute with age, people who protect their hearing when they are young will be able to hear much better as elders than those who don't take precautions.

CHAPTER 19

Consumer Products

The Consumer Product Safety Commission (CPSC) Notebook on Safety reports that every hour an average of 3 people die and 3,000 others are injured in accidents caused by dangerous product design, consumer carelessness, or poor product labeling. The following cases pulled from government safety reports illustrate a few of the hazards:

- A thirty-four-year-old man received burns on his arm after using a caustic drain cleaner to unclog a bathroom sink. Fifteen minutes after applying the chemical, the water remained backed up in the sink, so he used a plunger to attempt to clear away the clog. The drain cleaner solution splashed on his arm, burning his skin.
- Two children, ages five and six, were electrocuted when a hair dryer fell into the bathtub while they were bathing. The switch was in the off position, but the appliance was plugged in.
- A man was painting his utility room, located off the kitchen and garage. He opened both the garage and kitchen doors to ventilate the room. After painting, he soaked the rag in gasoline to remove the paint he splattered on the floor. When the burner on the hot water heater in the utility room came on, the gasoline vapors in the room exploded, burning his scalp, face, and legs.

In some cases, a product's threat is clear and immediate. Oven and drain cleaners contain caustic chemicals that can cause chemical burns. Hair dryers and other electrical appliances can electrocute or start fires if handled improperly. Countless household cleaners, nail and hair products, and office supplies contain toxic ingredients that can poison if they are swallowed, inhaled, or touched to the skin.

Other times, exposure to a consumer product can cause long-term, chronic health problems. For example, perchloroethylene, a common dry-cleaning chemical, can depress the central nervous system, causing dizziness and nausea, and has been found to cause cancer in animals.

Demonstrating the link between a product's use and such chronic ailments can be problematic (for many of the reasons, discussed earlier in Chapter 2, "Illness and the Environment: Finding the Links," and Chapter 3, "How We Perceive Risks and How Scientists Measure Them," that make it difficult to expressly link specific environmental agents to cancer), although many of the toxic ingredients found in consumer products are known or suspected carcinogens. Other ingredients are known to pose more immediate acute risks to health, such as eye and respiratory tract irritation, headaches, dizziness, visual problems, and memory impairment.

People often take the safety of consumer products for granted, figuring that if the product is on the market, it must be safe to use. The problem with this thinking is threefold.

First, many consumer products are not regulated by the government (although they may be expected to follow certain standards or get approval from a private group, for example, the Underwriters Laboratories, which approves electrical equipment and appliances). These products must be used properly to avoid hazards. Consumers should always read product labels carefully and heed the warnings. (If you have any questions about the safety or use of any consumer products, call the Consumer Product Safety Commission [CPSC] Hot Line at 1-800-638-CPSC or 1-800-492-8104 [in Maryland] or your regional poison control center listed in Appendix B.)

Box 19.1   WARNING: ALWAYS READ LABELS

The CPSC requires warning labels on products that can cause substantial personal injury or illness, such as those containing chemicals that are toxic, corrosive, irritants, flammable, combustible under pressure, or radioactive. Under the Hazardous Substances Act of 1960, hazardous products must carry labels with certain required information:

- A signal word, *danger* or *poison*, with the skull and crossbones on products that are toxic and the word *warning* or *caution* on all other hazardous materials.
- A statement of the type of hazard: "Extremely flammable," "Harmful if swallowed," "Contents under pressure," or a similar statement.
- A list of any precautionary steps or warnings: "Avoid contact with eyes," "Avoid breathing dust," "Do not take internally," or a comparable warning.
- Instructions for first aid in case of swallowing, contact, or other exposure: "Flush with water for fifteen minutes," "Call a physician immediately," or appropriate advice.
- A statement of handling and storage instructions: "Keep away from heat and open flames" or "Keep container closed when not in use."

Second, consumers cannot depend upon currently written labels to obtain full disclosure. There is no requirement that product labels list the exact product ingredients, a provision designed to protect industry trade secrets. Manufacturers do not have to disclose the ingredient list to the government or obtain approval of new formulations before introducing potentially hazardous products. (Because products are frequently reformulated, a system of prior approval is considered to be very cumbersome. The government can pull a product off the shelves when it is proved hazardous.) This problem is not limited to consumers: Poison control centers and government agencies must often guess at product contents when dealing with a consumer complaint because what's in the can is not identified on the label; they provide advice based on the chemicals that are commonly used in similar products. (When personal injury is involved, however, poison centers can get accurate information on the product's contents from the manufacturer.)

Third, children often have easy access to consumer products and are particularly at risk from exposure to both "safe" and dangerous consumer products. A child's growing body is more vulnerable to the long-term effects of exposure to

CONSUMER PRODUCTS

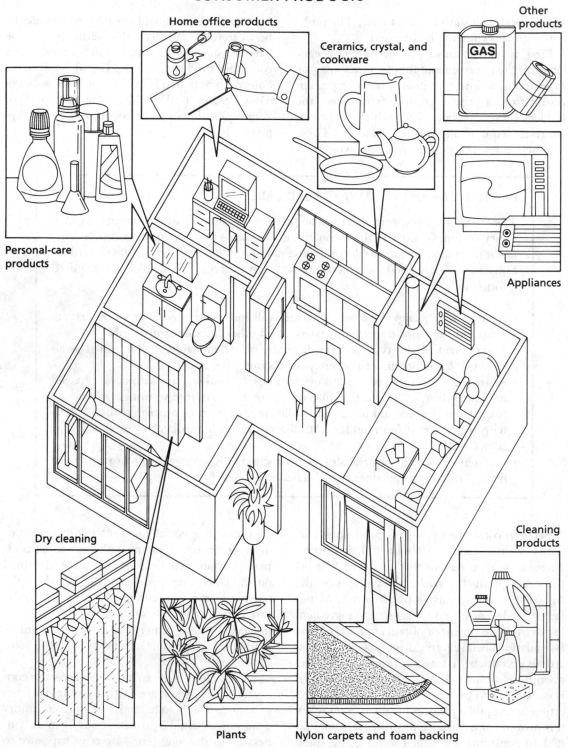

Home office products

Ceramics, crystal, and cookware

Other products

GAS

Personal-care products

Appliances

Dry cleaning

Cleaning products

Plants

Nylon carpets and foam backing

Box 19.2 HOW TO HANDLE EMERGENCY POISONINGS

According to the American Association of Poison Control Centers, follow these emergency procedures in case of an accidental poisoning.

- *Inhaled Poison:* Move the person to fresh air. Open doors and windows as widely as possible. If the victim isn't breathing, begin artificial respiration. (It's necessary to note that there is an extremely minimal risk that the person performing artificial respiration may become exposed to the inhaled poison.)
- *Poison on the skin:* Flood skin with water for ten minutes while seeking medical advice. Wash gently with soap and water and rinse.
- *Poison in the eye:* Flood the eye with lukewarm water poured from a glass two or three inches from the eye. Continue for fifteen minutes while seeking medical advice. Have the victim blink as much as possible during flooding.
- *Swallowed poison:* Unless the victim has an altered level of consciousness, cannot swallow, or is having convulsions, he or she should drink milk or water immediately to dilute the poison. Call a poison control center and ask whether to make the patient vomit. *Do not induce vomiting unless it is recommended.* Vomiting can cause further damage if a caustic substance has been swallowed. Always keep a 1-ounce bottle of syrup of ipecac in the medicine cabinet (to induce vomiting in emergencies when directed by a poison control center or physician) as well as activated charcoal, which can adsorb almost all chemical ingestants, chemically binding them in a way that can prevent them from doing harm. Both syrup of ipecac and activated charcoal are available in most pharmacies. Check the expiration date on the ipecac periodically and replace when expired.

Near every phone in the house, always keep the numbers of the local poison control center, your doctor, police, fire, and ambulance system.

---

toxins and environmental agents (see Chapter 12, "Of Special Concern: Infants and Children"). Small children are notorious for getting into things they shouldn't, such as cleaning supplies, which contain many toxic chemicals. Even products that do not pose a danger when used properly can be hazardous to children who use them improperly, resulting in illness or injury.

This chapter takes a look at a variety of consumer products and outlines hazards associated with products in categories such as electrical appliances, cleaning, personal care, laundry and textiles, home and office equipment, and miscellaneous others, such as houseplants, ceramics, and cookware.

Figure 19.1 CONSUMER PRODUCTS

People often take the safety of consumer products for granted, figuring that if the product is on the market, it must be safe to use. Unfortunately, many categories of products contain items that present health hazards to the consumer, including appliances, cleaning products, personal-care products, laundry products, textiles, home and office products, as well as such natural items as some plants commonly found in homes and offices.

APPLIANCES

Besides the risk of electrocution, electrical appliances pose the specter of two main hazards, one definite—fire—and one a possibility—extremely low-frequency (ELF) electromagnetic fields (EMFs). Annually, 166,000 home fires result in about 900 deaths and 6,200 injuries and another 300 people are electrocuted in home accidents. Many of these deaths and injuries can be prevented. Recently, scientists have noted a potential radiation hazard from electrical appliances and power lines, but the actual risk has not been quantified (see p. 594).

Air Conditioners and Heaters

Poorly maintained air-conditioners and heaters can raise indoor levels of pollen and fungi, resulting in eye, nose, and throat irritation; shortness of breath; dizziness; fever; asthma; and influenza. To reduce risk of contamination, keep the air filter clean by washing or vacuuming it every two weeks or so and by changing it at the suggested intervals.

Electric Blankets

Electric blankets pose a fire hazard if they are not kept in good condition and used properly.

- The wiring should not have any cracks or breaks.
- Blankets should be uncovered when used to prevent overheating.
- Blankets should not be folded or wadded up when in use.
- Pets should be kept off the bed when the blanket is plugged in.

Recent studies have raised concerns about the safety of exposure to ELF EMFs produced by electric blankets (see Chapter 16, "Radiant Energy"). Many household appliances, such as toasters and alarm clocks, generate the same ELF fields as electric blankets, but typically, they are used for only a few minutes a day and at some distance from the body. When sleeping with an electric blanket, the body is literally wrapped in a low-frequency field for seven or eight hours at a time. A 1987 report issued by the Congress's Office of Technology Assessment concluded that the risks presented by EMFs are not yet defined adequately but cannot be categorically denied and that the low-frequency fields "can produce substantial changes at the cellular level."

A number of studies are now underway, but until results are available, people who are at greatest potential risk—pregnant women and children—may choose to avoid electric blankets and mattress pads. (Comforters and blankets will provide the same warmth.)

Although the U.S. Food and Drug Administration (FDA) "sees no reason" to stop using electric blankets, some experts recommend prudent avoidance (i.e., turn off your blanket before you get in bed). Also avoid water-bed heaters and keep bedside clocks at least two feet from your head.

Hair Dryers

Prior to 1979, many hair dryers, both hand-held consumer blow dryers and professional bonnet-style models, contained asbestos in the heat shields, causing the release of asbestos fibers during use. Exposure to asbestos fibers can cause asbestosis and malignancies (see Chapter 6, "Respiratory Ailments"). No hair dryers produced since 1979 contain asbestos, and most asbestos-containing dryers were recalled in the early 1980s as part of an extensive CPSC recall campaign. Because most asbestos dryers have been replaced, the risk to consumers is virtually nil; the risk to professionals is minimal. (For information on brands and models of hair dryers that contained asbestos, call the CPSC at 1-800-638-CPSC.)

Box 19.3   ELECTRICAL SAFETY CHECKLIST

- Are the light bulbs the correct wattage for the size of the light fixtures? A bulb of too high wattage can overheat and start a fire. If unsure about the correct wattage, use a bulb no larger than 60 watts.
- Are the appliance cords in good condition? Frayed, cracked, or damaged cords can cause shocks or start fires.
- Is there a Class C fire extinguisher in the home? This extinguisher is used for electrical fires.
- Are the appliance cords uncoiled? Tightly wrapped cords can overheat.
- Are any extension cords overloaded? (Check the electrical rating on the appliance and the cord.) Overloaded extension cords are fire hazards.
- Do unused wall outlets have safety covers? Children often insert objects in uncovered outlets.
- Do electrical plugs fit snugly into your outlets? Loose plugs can lead to overheating.
- Are the television, stereo, and other appliances placed far enough from the wall to allow air to circulate freely? Blocking air flow can lead to overheating. (Do not stack newspapers or magazines on top of the TV; give your appliances some breathing room.)
- Are all appliances located far enough from water sources, such as kitchen and bathroom sinks? Electrical appliances are hazardous if they come in contact with water.
- Are there ground-fault circuit interrupters (GFCIs) installed in bathrooms and the kitchen? GFCIs are inexpensive devices that prevent electrical shock by limiting the flow of electricity when the electric path is disturbed. Most new homes have GFCIs, but many older homes do not.

  GFCIs are useful in bathrooms, kitchens, garages, and other rooms where risk of electric shock is high. GFCIs can prevent more than two-thirds of all electrocutions that take place in the home each year. Most GFCIs are installed at the outlet, but portable units, for use with electric yard and garden tools, are also available. Test your GFCIs once a month to be sure they're in working order.

  Warning signs of electrical overload or trouble:

Flickering lights.
Warm switch plates.
Blown fuses.
Tripped circuit breakers.

If problems develop, have a licensed electrician do the repairs immediately.

Humidifiers

Particles of mold and bacteria can grow in humidifier reservoirs and spread through the household via the released water vapor to cause eye, nose, and throat irritation, as well as illness. Ultrasonic humidifiers, the most common type, sometimes contain heaters to kill microorganisms before discharging the mist, but even these models can cause irritation by spewing white dust, tiny particles of minerals found in the water. The white dust problem is particularly severe if ordinary tap water rather than distilled water is used. To minimize problems:

- Be fastidious about cleaning the humidifier daily to prevent bacteria and molds from accumulating.
- Use only distilled or demineralized water in humidifiers.
- Do not add bleach or disinfectant to the water, as this can aggravate symptoms.

Ionization-Type Smoke Detectors

Most of the 5,000 Americans who die each year in residential fires die not from burns but from inhaling smoke and toxic gases. A smoke detector will provide an early warning of a fire long before you detect heat, flames, or quantities of smoke.

There are two basic types of smoke detectors: photoelectric detectors, whose alarms are activated when the smoke is dense enough to deflect a beam of light, and ionization detectors, which use a radioactive source to generate an electric field that detects the presence of smoke, setting off the alarm. Because they contain radioactive materials, ionization-type smoke detectors should not be discarded in the trash; they should be carefully wrapped and mailed back to the manufacturer for disposal.

Kerosene and Gas Heaters

If used in a poorly ventilated area, unvented kerosene and gas space heaters produce two risks: They produce dangerous gases, carbon monoxide and nitrogen dioxide, and their fuels are flammable. (See pp. 370 and 552 for the symptoms of exposure and dangers of these gases.)

To reduce exposure and risk:

- Use heaters only in well-ventilated areas.
- Do not use an unvented fuel-burning space heater.
- Always use 1-K fuel in kerosene heaters. Never use gasoline, as even small quantities can cause a fire.
- Only use space heaters with a guard around the flame area or heating coil to prevent burns or fire.
- Keep children, pets, clothing, and draperies away from the heater.
- Never use a space heater overnight in a room where someone is sleeping, as dangerous levels of carbon monoxide can accumulate.

Microwave Ovens

According to the FDA, although almost all microwave ovens emit microwaves, the levels are not enough to threaten human health or cause cancer. (FDA safety standards allow microwave emissions of up to 5 milliwatts per square centimeter at a distance of two inches from the oven; actual emissions are typically under 2 milliwatts, according to FDA tests.) Exposure to microwaves decreases dramatically with distance: Someone twenty inches from an oven would receive only one one-hundredth the radiation of a person two inches away.

To minimize the risk of exposure:

- Keep a reasonable distance from the oven when it is in use.
- Make sure the doors, hinges, latches, and sealing surfaces are in good repair.
- Anyone who wears a heart pacemaker should check with a doctor to make sure the device is shielded against interference from the electromagnetic emissions from microwave ovens; modern pacemakers are shielded, but older models may not be.

Sunlamps

Like the sun, sunlamps give off two types of ultraviolet radiation: UVA and UVB rays. (UVB rays are stronger than UVA rays and thus implicated more strongly with causing skin cancer.) Although some sunlamp manufacturers and tanning salons claim UVA sunlamps are safer than the sun, indoor tanning presents the same risks as outdoor tanning: skin cancer, premature aging of the skin, sunburn, cataracts, damage to the cornea and retina of the eye, and blood vessel damage. (See Chapter 16, "Radiant Energy," for more information on UVA and UVB radiation.)

The radiation from sunlamps can promote photosensitivity and cause a special type of sunburn, particularly in someone taking certain medications, including tetracycline. If you do use a sunlamp, always wear protective goggles.

Televisions

Older television sets may emit low levels of X-ray radiation, but since 1970, the government has limited emissions from television to minimal levels. If you're not sure whether your set meets emission standards, check the back of the set for a label or tag certifying compliance. When viewing a television purchased before 1970, sit at least six feet away from it when watching. These older sets should not be used with home computers or video games because users commonly sit quite close to the television screen.

Wood Stoves

Some homeowners have turned to wood stoves in an attempt to lower their heating bills. However, when not properly installed, maintained, and used, these stoves present significant dangers of fire, carbon monoxide poisoning, and burns to children and adults.

- Install wood stoves with proper clearance, typically three feet from walls, ceiling, furnishings, and other combustible materials.
- Keep clothes, kindling, newspapers, draperies, and other flammable materials away from the flame or hot surface areas.
- Burning wood can produce deadly amounts of carbon monoxide unless the fumes are vented up the flue. Keep the flue clear so that it can draw air properly. Do not burn pressure-treated or chemically preserved wood; they contain toxic ingredients that, when burned, are released into the atmosphere as deadly wastes, fumes, and heavy metals.
- Keep a window open slightly to provide enough air for proper burning and to reduce the risk of carbon monoxide poisoning.
- With both wood stoves and fireplaces, the chimney or chimney pipe should be kept clear of creosote, a black, tarry substance that becomes a fire hazard when it builds up along the chimney wall. Avoid burning resin- or creosote-bearing woods, as well as pine or dry woods. Ideally, check the chimney every few weeks for creosote deposits when the stove or fireplace is in frequent use.

CLEANING PRODUCTS

Many cleaning products carry warning labels but no list of ingredients. Unless consumers write to the manufacturer requesting a list of ingredients, they may find it impossible to know exactly which toxic chemicals a particular product contains. As a result, always heed product warnings, even if a product seems safe.

Ammonia

Common in many household cleaners for its grease-cutting properties, ammonia can irritate the skin, causing rashes, redness, and chemical burns. Ammonia should be used in a well-ventilated area because the fumes can also irritate the eyes and lungs. Ammonia can also cause severe damage if it splashes in your eyes; it can also damage other body parts in industrial-strength concentrations. Never mix ammonia with chlorine bleach because the resulting chloramine fumes are very toxic.

Chlorine and Chlorine Bleach

Chlorine bleach is harmful if swallowed, causes eye irritation if it splashes into the eyes, and should never be mixed with products containing ammonia or acidic toilet bowl cleaners because the resulting chloramine or chlorine fumes can be very toxic.

Some people are sensitive to the fumes from chlorine bleach and may find the residues left on clothing washed with bleach irritating, even if the clothes have been dried. Instead of using bleach in the laundry, you can substitute sodium hexametaphosphate (a crystal that can be ordered from a chemical supply house), which can remove mineral deposits and soap residues from clothing.

Disinfectants

Disinfectants reduce the concentration of germs (just like plain soap and water); they do not kill all germs. Most disinfectants contain toxic substances, such as chlorine, ammonia, phenol, ethanol, and cresol (a chemical that can be absorbed through the skin and can damage the liver, kidney, lungs, pancreas, and spleen or affect the central nervous system, causing depression, irritability, or hyperactivity). Instead of using disinfectants, clean thoroughly with soap and water; hot water alone kills some germs and bacteria. Borax, a safer disinfectant and deodorizer, is available in the laundry section of most supermarkets.

Drain Cleaners

Drain cleaners contain highly corrosive chemicals, typically lye (sodium or potassium hydroxide). Lye is highly caustic; it can burn the skin, eyes, mouth, esophagus, and stomach, and if splashed onto the cornea of the eye, it can cause blindness. Most chemical drain cleaners are too dangerous for use and, actually, do not work very well. Instead of drain cleaners, opt for a safer declogging method, such as a plunger or a plumber's snake, available at most hardware stores. If you still choose to use any type of drain cleaner, wear rubber gloves and protective glasses or wraparound goggles.

Furniture Polish

Many furniture polishes contain toxins, such as phenol and dinitrobenzene, both of which can be absorbed through the skin (see the information sheets on pp. 377 and 405).

One alternative is mineral oil, which is relatively safe (in the past it was used as a laxative). If the mineral oil is aspirated into the lungs when swallowing, it can cause a chronic form of pneumonia.

Glass Cleaners

Most glass cleaners contain ammonia, water, and a colorant. The ammonia can release irritating fumes and cause eye damage if accidentally sprayed in the eye. Aerosol glass cleaners present more problems because the tiny droplets of ammonia in the air can be inhaled or land in your eyes (see Ammonia). A nonammonia alternative is one part vinegar to one part water.

Oven Cleaners

Many oven cleaners contain lye (sodium or potassium hydroxide), which can burn the skin, irritate the lungs if inhaled or aspirated, and burn the esophagus and stomach if swallowed. Aerosol spray containers are especially hazardous because the spray sends tiny droplets of lye into the air where they can be inhaled or land on eyes and skin. If you must use this product, always wear rubber gloves and avoid inhaling the vapors.

Scouring Powders

Most scouring powders contain chlorine bleach, which produces chlorine gas when mixed with water. These fumes can irritate eyes, nose, throat, and lungs. Never mix chlorinated scouring powder with ammonia (see Ammonia) or acidic toilet bowl cleaners, as the resulting fumes can be toxic.

Silver Polish

The active ingredients in most silver and metal polishers are ammonia (see Ammonia) and petroleum distillates. Depending on the chemicals in the product, silver polish vapors may also be harmful.

PERSONAL-CARE PRODUCTS

Many personal-care products and cosmetics don't contain hazardous ingredients but often do contain substances that can be irritating or cause allergic reactions on the delicate areas of the body that many of these products are applied to. The FDA regulates cosmetics, a category that includes any product that is rubbed, poured, sprinkled, or sprayed on the body for cleansing or beautifying without changing the body's structure or functions. Cosmetics must list ingredients, except for fragrances and certain trade secrets, but do not need FDA approval before they can be sold. The FDA can take action against a manufacturer after a sufficient number of consumer complaints have been logged to demonstrate that the product is hazardous.

Regular Shampoo and Conditioner

Shampoos contain cleaning agents or surfactants, which clean the hair and produce lather. Conditioners often clean the hair and produce lather, too; they often contain lanolin derivatives and balsam to keep hair from being stripped of natural oils. Some people may develop an allergic reaction to a particular ingredient(s). Once the offending agent is identified, they should switch to another product.

Dandruff Shampoo

Special dandruff shampoos contain toxic medications to prevent dandruff, such as selenium sulfide (see selenium, p. 411), and resorcinol, which is easily absorbed through the skin. Formaldehyde is commonly used as a preservative; it is a potential human carcinogen and can irritate the skin, eyes, and respiratory passages (see formaldehyde, p. 383).

Powders

Cosmetic powders pose no health risk used under normal conditions. Excessive inhalation of powder can cause coughing or lung irritation. Talc should never be used around a newborn because inhalation may lead to suffocation.

Soaps

Most soaps are alkaline. Some people may develop an allergic reaction to a soap, particularly if it is used on the face. If a reaction develops, it's necessary to pinpoint the offending ingredient in the soap and then switch to a brand that doesn't contain it. For some, switching to a specialty bar that is acidic rather than alkaline will stop the irritation.

Contraceptives

In the United States, contraception choices range from over-the-counter products, such as condoms, spermicides, and sponges, to doctor-prescribed birth-control pills, intrauterine devices, and diaphragms. Each method presents some risk and should be discussed with an individual's doctor.

Condoms are made of latex rubber or lamb

cecum (although commonly referred to as lamb skin, these products are actually made from the first part of the lamb's large intestines). Lamb cecum does not protect you from transmission of sexually transmitted diseases. The latex can cause irritation or an allergic reaction. If that happens, double up when using condoms by using one made from lamb cecum next to the skin and putting one made with latex rubber on top.

Diaphragms and cervical caps are also made of latex rubber, which can cause irritation or allergic reaction. In rare cases, diaphragm use has caused bladder infections, constipation, and in extremely rare instances, toxic shock syndrome (see below)

Most vaginal spermicides (foams, creams, jellies, gels, or suppositories) used with diaphragms, cervical caps, and sponges contain either nonoxynol-9 or octoxynol as the active ingredient. In some cases, a woman or her partner may develop irritation or an allergic reaction to the chemicals; this may be eliminated by switching to another brand. Women who use spermicide for birth control should wait at least six hours after intercourse before douching to ensure the product's full effect.

Intrauterine devices are made of plastic and/or copper. In rare cases, they cause perforation of the uterus.

Sponges are made of polyurethane and used with spermicide and present the same risk of irritation or allergic reaction as the spermicides used alone. Although rare, sponges have been known to break apart inside the vagina and require a doctor's assistance for complete removal; very rarely, sponges have been associated with toxic shock syndrome (one case per 3 million sponges).

Douches

Commercially prepared douche solutions contain strong chemicals, including ammonia, detergents, and artificial fragrance, which can cause vaginal irritation and inflammation or allergic reactions. According to an FDA advisory review panel, there is no need for a woman to douche (the panel blames the practice on "tradition, ignorance, and commercial advertising"). Simply rinse the vaginal area with water when bathing, or use a mild soap externally if desired. To minimize irritation to the genital area, avoid tight, constricting clothes and undergarments, and wear cotton underwear (it absorbs moisture and allows perspiration to evaporate).

Feminine Hygiene Sprays

Despite their names, most feminine hygiene sprays contain only perfume—not antibacterial ingredients—and are not necessary for proper personal hygiene. They can cause irritation and rashes in women and men whose partner uses the product before intercourse. Simply rinse the vagina with water during regular bathing. If an unpleasant odor or discharge is present, do not try to mask the odor; consult a doctor.

Tampons

The major risk of tampon use is toxic shock syndrome, a disease caused by the bacterium *Staphylococcus aureus*. Toxic shock syndrome cases skyrocketed in the early 1980s with the introduction of superabsorbent synthetic fibers, which allowed women to leave tampons in the vagina for extended periods of time. Although changes in the design of tampons has led to a 93 percent drop in the number of toxic shock syndrome cases since 1980, the risk is still present (the federal Centers for Disease Control and Prevention reported 61 cases of toxic shock syndrome in 1989, compared with 890 cases in 1980).

The following are symptoms of TSS; if they occur, call a doctor immediately:

- Fever of 102°F or more.
- Vomiting.
- Diarrhea.
- A sunburn-type rash.
- A precipitous drop in blood pressure, which can cause shock and death.

Box 19.4   GUIDELINES FOR SAFE USE OF TAMPONS

- Women who have had toxic shock syndrome or recently have had a baby should avoid using tampons, especially those with superabsorbent fibers.
- Alternate between the use of sanitary napkins and tampons.
- Use the least absorbent tampon possible. (Tampon boxes must carry uniform absorbency ratings, ranging from junior to regular to super to super plus.)
- Change tampons at least every six to eight hours.
- Avoid using deodorant tampons and sanitary pads. Even people who aren't usually sensitive to perfumes can develop an irritation or allergic reaction to the scents.

Fingernail Polish, Remover, and Fixatives

Although fingernail polish does not always carry a label warning of its toxicity, it should. Most such products contain a number of volatile and very dangerous chemicals, including phenol, toluene, xylene, and formaldehyde resins, which can irritate the lungs or are known or suspected carcinogens (see information sheets for details).

The primary ingredient in nail polish remover is acetone, which can cause nails to become brittle and split. When inhaled, nail polish remover can irritate the lungs and cause dizziness. If swallowed, it can cause restlessness, vomiting, and unconsciousness. If you do use polish and remover, do so in a well-ventilated area, and store both polishes and remover in a locked medicine cabinet if children are present.

Nail products used to remove fake fingernails contain acetonitrile; in the human body, acetonitrile is metabolized to cyanide. If you have children in the house, make sure nail products are well out of reach; fatalities have occurred after children drank these products.

Hair Spray

Many hair sprays contain ethanol, formaldehyde resins, and plastics. People who regularly use such sprays can develop shortness of breath, re-duced lung capacity, or the lung problem thesaurosis if they inhale the toxic mist for extended periods. (Thesaurosis results in enlarged lymph nodes, lung masses, and changes in blood cells. Symptoms subside when the use of hair spray ceases.) When hair spray comes into contact with skin rather than hair, allergic skin reactions and eye and nasal passage irritation can occur.

Avoid breathing hair spray mist. If you must use hair spray, use a pump spray rather than an aerosol; the mist will be less fine and easier to control.

Mouthwash

Do not assume that a product designed to be put in your mouth is safe to swallow; it's not. Most mouthwashes contain ingredients, such as formaldehyde, ammonia, hydrogen peroxide, and alcohol, that can be harmful if swallowed in large amounts. Avoid bad breath by practicing good oral hygiene: Brush and floss daily, and visit your dentist regularly. Keep mouthwash out of the reach of children.

Toilet Paper

Dyes and scents in toilet paper can cause irritation in the genital area. Use unscented white toilet paper.

LAUNDRY PRODUCTS AND TEXTILES

Since World War II, hundreds of synthetic fibers have been developed. The fibers themselves pose no apparent risk, but many have formaldehyde finishes, or resins, to keep them wrinkle free, and agents used to clean them can cause skin or respiratory irritation.

Carpets

Polyurethane foam padding under many rugs and carpets may release toxic gases such as formaldehyde and pentachlorophenol; these can cause tiredness, insomnia, headaches, and respiratory problems. Substitute cotton, cotton/wool, or wool rugs with jute or latex backing for foam backing (see p. 558).

Dry-Cleaning Residues

The chemical most often used in dry cleaning is perchloroethylene, a chemical shown to cause cancer in animals. Perchloroethylene can also cause liver damage, depression of the central nervous system, light-headedness, dizziness, sleepiness, nausea, loss of appetite, and disorientation. According to the Environmental Protection Agency (EPA), recent studies show that people unknowingly breathe low levels of the chemical when wearing dry-cleaned clothes and when breathing air from closets where dry-cleaned goods are stored.

To minimize exposure to perchloroethylene, do not accept dry-cleaned goods that have a noticeable chemical odor or air them out and make certain they are thoroughly dry before wearing.

Flame-Retardant Fabrics

Consumers, especially children, are protected from flammable fabrics by the 1953 Flammable Fabrics Act. All children's sleepwear in sizes 0 to 14 must be flame retardant. From 1972 to 1977, sleepwear manufacturers treated some fabrics with the flame-retardant TRIS (2,3-dibromopropyl phosphate) in order to meet federal flammability standards. TRIS was later identified as a potential carcinogen and banned for use in children's sleepwear in 1977.

Since the late 1970s, many manufacturers have reformulated some polyester and nylon fabrics to make them flame-retardant without being chemically treated. Parents who are concerned about chemicals in fabrics should not necessarily turn to all-cotton sleepwear because cotton is highly flammable. Instead, look for fabrics that meet the flammability standard without chemical treatments, including nylon, polyester, and nylon–polyester blends (see Box 19.5).

Mothballs

In the past, mothballs contained camphor, a highly toxic crystal: As little as 1 or 2 grams could kill a child who might swallow it. Today, mothballs, moth repellents, and moth flakes contain naphthalene or *para*-dichlorobenzene, chemicals that are much less toxic but still carry risks (see Naphthalene information sheet, p. 398). For instance, accidental ingestion of a single *para*-dichlorobenzene mothball is not particularly harmful, but swallowing one that contains naphthalene can cause a breakdown of red blood cells that results in hemoglobinuria (evidenced by a change in urine color), anemia, blue skin discoloration (methemoglobinemia), diarrhea, abdominal pain, lethargy, and convulsions. Naphthalene is also a suspected human carcinogen. People who are deficient in the enzyme glucose-6-phosphate dehydrogenase are especially susceptible to blood toxicity if naphthalene is ingested.

Aromatic cedar can repel moths and is available in many forms, including blocks for drawers and wooden linings for closets.

Permanent Press Clothing and Linens

Formaldehyde, often in combination with other chemicals, is routinely used to add permanent press qualities to clothing, linens, and draperies. Most polyester–cotton blend fabrics have formaldehyde finishes, as do many other fabrics, including some made of pure cotton. Polyester–cotton blend bedsheets have a particularly heavy coating because of their heavy use and frequent laundering. Clothing labeled as permanent press, crease resistant, waterproof, or permanently pleated often has formaldehyde resins combined directly with the fibers, making the formaldehyde permanent.

Washing new clothes before wearing them can lower formaldehyde levels significantly (by about 80 percent), but low levels continue to be released as the resin breaks down during the life of the product. As the product ages, the formaldehyde emissions decrease.

Rug Cleaners

Most rug, carpet, and upholstery cleaners contain perchloroethylene, a known human carcinogen, or naphthalene, a suspected carcinogen. To avoid needing rug cleaners, clean rugs and carpets immediately after a spill to avoid stains. To deodorize, sprinkle baking soda over a dry carpet and vacuum after fifteen minutes.

HOME AND OFFICE PRODUCTS

Almost every home has an office, even if the office is little more than a desk where bills are paid and work is done in the evening and on weekends. A home office may also include a crafts or art studio. (For more information on hazards associated with arts, see Chapter 20, "Art and Hobbyist Materials".) In addition to the typewriter correction fluids, magic markers are found in most such offices.

Asbestos Tile

Asbestos, a mineral fiber found in rocks that is fire-resistant and not easily destroyed or degradable by natural processes, was commonly used in floor tiles and insulation until the 1970s. Asbestos is hazardous only when crumbling and airborne, when microscopic fibers are released into the air and can be breathed deep into the lower portions of the lungs, causing asbestosis (scarring of the lungs that results in limited lung function and death), mesothelioma (cancer of the lining of the lungs and abdomen), lung cancer, and cancers of the digestive tract (see p. 124 and Asbestos information sheet, p. 365).

Asbestos in vinyl floor tiles does not present a health risk unless the tiles are sanded or seriously damaged. If it does need to be removed, asbestos tile or insulation in homes or buildings must be handled by a professional. Contact the state Environmental Protection Agency for a list of licensed asbestos removers, or call the EPA at 1-800-424-9065 for the name of the asbestos coordinator in your region.

Photocopiers

Common fears associated with photocopiers involve three main issues:

Exposure to chemicals. The photoconductive materials in photocopiers (typically selenium and cadmium compounds) do not appear to pose health hazards. Selenium has not been shown to be toxic, and the cadmium compounds, if present, appear at acceptably low levels.

Exposure to light. The fluorescent or halogen lights found in photocopiers emit ultraviolet radiation, which does not pose any risk to the op-

---

Box 19.5 COMBUSTION DANGERS

When fabrics burn, the fumes of the fire can be as deadly as the flames:

- Burning plastics and synthetic fibers found in carpets, draperies, and synthetic fabrics, can generate dense, extremely toxic smoke containing carbon monoxide, aldehydes, hydrogen cyanide, and hydrogen chloride.
- Once ignited, synthetic textiles pose serious fire hazards because they burn fast and their flames spread due to the petroleum content in plastics.
- Synthetic fibers also generate high temperatures quickly when ignited, which can cause fabrics to melt and burn the skin.
- When ignited, some plastics, including polyesters, form a char and resist burning when the flame is removed; other fabrics burn rapidly. (Natural fabrics also react differently to flame: Some fabrics, such as silk and wool, are self-extinguishing, whereas cotton and linen are relatively flammable.)
- The weave of a fabric also contributes to its flammability: The looser the weave, the more flammable the fabric.

  Smoke detectors are your best defense against a potentially devastating fire. Make sure those in your home are in good condition; don't forget to change batteries twice a year (an easy way to remember to do so is when switching to and from daylight saving time.)

---

erator unless the glass plate is removed from the machine; blue light, which can damage the eyes but not at the low levels emitted by copiers; and visible light, which can cause eye discomfort if the operator stares at the moving light. To avoid irritation, look away from the light.

Exposure to ozone. Some high-speed electrostatic photocopiers produce low levels of ozone, a gas that can be very irritating to the eyes and pulmonary system. Ozone irritation typically exists only when the machines are operated in a poorly ventilated area. If ozone frequently builds up in a small, stuffy copy room, consider ventilating the room with a fan that exhausts air outside the building.

Epoxies

Epoxies, rubber cements, super glues, and other adhesives contain a number of potentially dangerous, volatile chemicals, many of which can burn the skin if touched and irritate the eyes and respiratory system if inhaled. Many products contain naphthalene, phenol, ethanol, vinyl chloride, formaldehyde, acrylonitrile, among other chemicals. Most of these release toxic vapors that can cause cancer.

When using epoxies, wear eye protection, rubber gloves, and long sleeves and be sure to work in a well-ventilated space (see Chapter 20, "Art and Hobbyist Materials").

Particle Board Furniture and Cabinets

Many cabinets, desks, and bookshelves built since the early 1980s contain particle board (pressed wood made using adhesives containing urea–formaldehyde resins), which is covered with wood, paper, or vinyl veneer. (Older—and often heavier—cabinets are typically made of covered plywood.) The particle board releases formaldehyde vapors, which can build up inside the cabinets because they are closed and they do not circulate air. To prevent the release of formaldehyde gas, seal particle board with nontoxic wood finish.

Permanent Magic Markers

Solvent-based indelible inks in permanent felt-tipped pens and markers and some ballpoint and fountain pen inks contain acetone, ammonia, benzyl alcohol, toluene, xylene, and other chemicals. Many of these chemicals can cause central nervous system impairment (such as drowsiness, headache, and confusion), nausea and respiratory tract irritation, and some are known or suspected carcinogens.

Switch to water-based markers. If you must use permanent markers, use them in a well-ventilated area.

Video Display Terminals

More than 30 million video display terminals (VDTs) are in use in the United States alone, but not all of them emit electromagnetic radiation. For example, portable computers use liquid crystal display screens that do not give off electromagnetic radiation. However, the monitors used with most desktop personal computers produce electromagnetic fields (EMFs).

Since the widespread introduction of VDTs in the late 1970s, many employees have worried about the possible health risks of spending hours in front of their computer terminals. Much of the fear about radiation abated in the early 1980s, when government researchers found VDTs did not emit significant levels of radiation.

Recent studies, however, focus on the extremely low-frequency (ELF) EMFs surrounding computer monitors. Some studies suggest that radiation from ELFs may be enough to increase the risk of cancer and threaten the fetuses of pregnant women. At least one initial study suggested that women using VDTs are more likely to have miscarriages. However, the increased risk could have been a result of job stress rather than VDT use. Most studies, including a major well-designed and comprehensive study of pregnancies among 730 telephone operators, have not detected any effects (see Chapter 11, "Reproductive Effects and Prenatal Exposures"). The U.S. Department of Labor's Occupational Safety and Health Administration has no standards applying specifically to VDTs and claims the radiation from VDTs falls below the organization's current standards.

As with other types of radiation, ELF radiation drops off dramatically as you move away from the source. Radiation comes from all sides of the monitor, but more from the backs and sides than the front. Some manufacturers have started to market special computers shielded to reduce emissions, but you can protect yourself by staying at arm's length from the monitor.

Liquid Corrective Fluids

Liquid corrective fluids often contain such dangerous substances as trichloroethylene. It is safer to use corrective tape that strikes a white powder over an error or adhesive correction tapes to cover mistakes. If you must use liquid, use a water-based fluid for use with copies rather than originals. A single coat may not cover, but two coats of water-based fluid is safer than a single coat of solvent-based fluid.

OTHER HOUSEHOLD HAZARDS

Some products present risks that can be easily overlooked, either because they are not used very often, such as paint strippers, or because they are used every day, such as ceramic dishes or batteries.

Batteries

Household batteries can cause chemical burns if they leak, overheat, or rupture. For this reason:

- Do not attempt to recharge a battery not intended to be recharged.
- Do not use the wrong size or type of battery in a recharger; for example, an automobile battery charger cannot be used to recharge flashlight batteries.
- Do not use alkaline and carbon–zinc batteries together in the same appliance.
- Do not combine run-down batteries with new or freshly charged ones. Batteries will produce only as much power as the weakest will allow, and the strong batteries will put extra stress on the weaker ones, possibly causing them to overheat or leak.
- Do not reverse batteries in an appliance (placing the positive end where the negative end should be).
- Do not let batteries touch other metallic objects, including keys, tools, and hardware kept in drawers, as they can short out the battery, producing enough heat to cause a burn.

Children have been known to place the small button batteries used in watches, calculators, cameras, and hearing aids in their noses and ears or accidentally swallow them. These batteries are made of salts of various metals, including zinc, cadmium, mercury, silver, nickel, and lithium, usually covered with metal. They range in size from about half the size of a dime to slightly larger than a quarter. In most cases, these small batteries pass through the body uneventfully, but they can cause choking if aspirated and caustic burns, ulcers, and dangerous exposure to heavy metals if they leak. To prevent accidental ingestion, keep batteries away from small children. Do not discard batteries in trash cans when small children have access to them; dispose of them in an environmentally safe way.

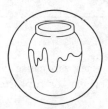

Ceramics and Crystal

Most glazes on ceramic plates, cups, bowls, and pitchers contain lead, but when properly formulated and fired, the metal does not leach into food. Although products made and sold in the United States must meet safety standards, this is not true of all products purchased overseas. Some pottery, especially items made in small cottage industries abroad, may not be properly treated and are one source of lead poisoning. It is impossible to tell whether or not an item leaches lead simply by looking at it. Contact with acidic foods, such as wines, vinegar, and orange, tomato, and other fruit juices, can dissolve the glaze and accelerate the release of lead into the food. When in doubt about any ceramic ware, use plastic or glass containers to store juice and acidic beverages. Unless it has been tested, avoid eating from pottery imported from Mexico, China, Italy, or Spain, as well as U.S. earthenware dishes made before 1971.

A recent report warns that lead can leach out of lead crystal decanters and into the wine, liquor, or water being stored, adding another dose of lead to your body. Pregnant women in particular are warned not to drink from lead crystal goblets.

Cookware

Different materials used in cookware present different health issues:

- *Aluminum* cookware is safe. According to the FDA, the amount of aluminum consumed from the use of aluminum cookware is negligible. Using uncoated aluminum pans for all cooking and food storage every day would release less aluminum than the amount in a single antacid tablet or buffered aspirin (see Chapter 5, "The Brain and Nervous System.")
- *Nonstick* finishes on pots and pans, such as polytetrafluoroethylene (Teflon) or Silverstone, can be cleaned quickly and easily and require less fat for nonstick cooking. Avoid burning the pans; overheating the empty pans

may release polymer fumes. Use only plastic or wooden utensils with this cookware or the finishes may scratch off and contaminate foods with bits of plastic; although not toxic, the substances are indigestible.

- *Copper* cookware typically is lined with tin or stainless steel. Do not use *unlined* copper pots for general cooking because the metal can be dissolved by some foods, such as acids in tomato-based spaghetti sauce.
- *Cast iron* cookware evenly conducts heat and provides a nutritional bonus: Trace amounts of iron leach out into foods cooked in unglazed cast iron pots, providing a hidden source of dietary iron, an advantage to many people, especially women.

Foam Insulation

In the 1970s, many homeowners had plastic foam insulation "blown" or "foamed" into the wall cavities and between the studs and walls in their homes as an energy-saving measure. Many homes then developed high levels of fumes of formaldehyde, an irritating and potentially dangerous substance (see p. 558). The National Academy of Sciences estimates that 10 to 20 percent of the general population may be susceptible to adverse reactions to formaldehyde, even at very low levels. Formaldehyde emissions decline with time, so insulation installed several years ago is not apt to raise formaldehyde levels to dangerous concentrations now.

Gasoline and Other Flammable Liquids

Gasoline, kerosene, lighter fluid, and turpentine are highly flammable and pose a risk of burns. An estimated 60,000 Americans suffer burn injuries each year due to accidents involving these liquids. In many cases, gasoline is used to clean paintbrushes, auto parts, or other greasy products and the vapors are ignited by the pilot light in a nearby natural gas appliance. Even at low temperatures, gasoline and many other flammable fluids continuously give off vapors, which accumulate at floor level (the vapors are heavier than air and will not rise and escape through open windows); however, the vapors do travel with the air current and can ignite at flame sources far from where the substance is being used.

Do not store or use gasoline and other flammable liquids in basements or utility rooms where there are gas appliances such as water heaters, furnaces, or clothes dryers.

Metal and Stone Cleaners

Metal and stone cleaners contain hydrofluoric acid, which can be used in diluted form to clean metals (such as iron, copper, or brass) or brick and stone (particularly fireplaces). During use, the product will be applied to the metal or stone, then diluted with water during the rinsing state. Because most people will use the product outdoors, the diluted acid can be allowed to sink into the ground (pine trees love diluted acid). Yet it must be noted that these cleaners are extremely dangerous if they come in contact with your skin: They can result in life-threatening burns or even loss of fingers.

Paint Removers and Strippers

Many chemical paint removers and strippers contain dangerous chemicals: The suspected carcinogen methylene chloride is found in a number of them. This chemical poses a number of serious health threats: Burns can occur from contact with the skin or eyes; and anyone with a history of heart disease should not use paint strippers or other products containing methylene chloride because once it's metabolized in the liver, it produces carbon monoxide in the blood (see Carbon Monoxide information sheet, p. 370). Many paint strippers also contain methanol, a potentially lethal poison if swallowed, inhaled, or absorbed through the skin (see Methanol information sheet, p. 396).

Many older paint removers and strippers contain benzene, a toxic chemical and known carcinogen (see Benzene information sheet, p. 366), now outlawed for use in commercial products.

Paint dust and the remains after stripping lead-based paint can present a health threat. Lead paint was used in about two-thirds of houses built before the 1940s, one-third of the houses built from 1940 to 1960, and some houses built since then. Assume that all paint applied before 1950 contains significant amounts of lead. Lead poisoning can occur from eating paint chips or by breathing and ingesting lead dust and paint scrapings. For this reason:

- Never eat or smoke near a paint-stripping project.
- Pregnant women, small children, and older people—all particularly vulnerable to lead poisoning and the adverse effects of solvents—should not be in the house when a stripping project is underway.

If you must use paint strippers:

- Always wear protective goggles, gloves, and clothing when handling any product containing methylene chloride, including spray paints, primers, adhesives and glues, wood stains, varnishes, paint thinners, shoe polishes, and water repellents.
- If paint remover splatters on the skin, rinse the area with water, wash with soap and water, then rinse again.
- Use an exhaust fan in a wide open window.

Paint Thinner and Mineral Spirits

Many people wrongly believe paint thinner is harmless and use it to wash paint-covered hands and brushes. If inhaled, thinners can cause upper respiratory irritation upon contact, drowsiness, loss of coordination, headache, nausea, and chapped, dry skin. Use paint thinner in a well-ventilated room and wear rubber gloves. Instead of using paint thinner to clean up after using oil-based paint, coat hands with Vaseline before painting to keep paint from soaking into the skin, and wash with cold cream afterward.

Pesticides

For an extensive discussion of pesticides, see Chapter 17, "Food Safety."

Plants

Each year, about 100,000 accidental plant ingestions are reported to poison control centers. Most plants are nontoxic and pose no significant health risk to anyone who might accidentally swallow them, but some plants are dangerous. A single leaf can block a small child's airway. For this reason:

- Identify all poisonous plants inside and outside the house.
- If small children live in the house or visit often, get rid of all highly toxic plants and select nontoxic alternatives (see Tables 19.1 and 19.2), and move others out of reach of children.
- Never chew on jewelry made from seeds, beans, or grasses of unknown plants.

Indoor plants, such as dumbcane (or *Dieffenbachia*) and philodendron, and outdoor plants and flowers, like jack-in-the-pulpit, lily of the valley, azalea, oleander, and rhododendron are poisonous, causing a variety of symptoms from gastrointestinal to cardiovascular problems, depending on the poison. Rosary pea and castor bean seeds, which are often used as ornaments or in making necklaces and other jewelry in other countries—the seeds are banned in the United States—are quite toxic if chewed.

Rodenticides

A rodenticide is any product commercially marketed to kill rats, rodents, mice, squirrels, gophers, and other small animals. A number of different types of hazardous compounds have been used as rodenticides, including arsenic, thallium, phosphorus, barium carbonate, sodium monofluoroacetate, warfarin, brodifacoum, red squill, and strychnine (see

Table 19.1 TOXIC HOUSE AND GARDEN PLANTS

Common Name	Botanical Name	Toxic Part
Aconite	*Aconite* spp.	Roots, flowers, and leaves
Apple	*Malus* spp.	Seeds
Baneberry	*Actaea* spp.	Red or white (doll's eyes) berries, roots, and foliage
Belladonna	*Atropa belladonna*	All parts, especially black berries
Black locust	*Robinia pseudoacacia*	Bark, foliage, young twigs, and seeds
Bleeding heart	*Dicentra spectabilitis*	Foliage and roots
Buckeye and horse chestnut	*Aesculus* spp.	Sprouts and nuts
Caladium	*Caladium* spp.	All parts
Castor bean	*Ricinus communis*	Seeds
Chinaberry tree	*Melia azerdarach*	Berries
Chokecherry	*Prunus* spp.	Leaves and pits
Common privet	*Ligustrum vulgare*	Black or blue wax-coated berries and leaves
Crocus, autumn	*Colchicum autumnale*	All parts, especially bulbs
Daffodil	*Narcissus pseudonarcissus*	Bulbs
Daphne	*Daphne mezereum*	Berries (commonly red, but other colors in various species) and bark
Death camas	*Zigadenus* spp.	Bulbs
Delphinium	*Delphinium* spp.	Seeds and young plant
Dumbcane	*Dieffenbachia* spp.	All parts
Elderberry	*Sambucus* spp.	Roots, stems, and unripe fruit
Elephant's ear	*Colocasia* spp.	All parts
English ivy	*Hedera helix*	Berries and leaves
Foxglove	*Digitalis purpurea*	All parts, especially leaves, flowers, and seeds
Golden chain (laburnum)	*Laburnum anagyroides*	Seeds, pods, and flowers
Heath family (laurels, rhododendron, and azaleas)	*Rhododendron* spp.	All parts
Holly	*Ilex* spp.	Berries
Hyacinth	*Hyacinthus orientalis*	Bulbs
Iris	*Iris* spp.	Underground rhizome and developed leaves
Jack-in-the-pulpit	*Arisaema* spp.	All parts, especially roots
Purge nut, curcas bean, peregrina, and psychic nut	*Jatropha curcas*	Seeds and oil
Jerusalem cherry	*Solanum pseudocapsicum*	Unripe fruit, leaves, and flowers
Jessamine (yellow and Carolina)	*Gelsemium sempervirens*	Flowers and leaves
Jimsonweed	*Datura stramonium*	All parts, especially seeds and leaves
Lantana	*Lantana camara*	Unripe green-blue or black berries
Larkspur	*Delphinum ajacis*	Seeds and young plant

(continued)

Table 19.1 TOXIC HOUSE AND GARDEN PLANTS (continued)

Common Name	Botanical Name	Toxic Part
Lily of the valley	*Convallaria majalis*	Leaves, flowers, and fruit (red berries)
Mayapple (mandrake)	*Podophyllum peltatum*	Roots, foliage, and unripe fruit
Mistletoe	*Phoradendron flavescens*	Berries
Monkshood	*Aconitum nepellus* and *Aconitum columbianum*	Roots, flowers, and leaves
Narcissus	*Narcissus* spp.	Bulbs
Nicotiana (wild and cultivated)	*Nicotiana* spp.	Leaves
Nightshades (including European bittersweet and horse nettle)	*Solanum* spp.	All parts, especially unripe berries
Oaks		All parts
Oleander	*Nerium oleander*	Leaves, branches, and nectar of flowers
Philodendron	*Philodendron* spp.	All parts
Poison hemlock	*Conium maculatum*	Roots, berries, and foliage
Pokeweed (pigeonberry)	*Phytolacca americana*	Roots, berries, and foliage
Potato	*Solanum tuberosum*	Vines, sprouts (green parts), and spoiled tubers
Rhubarb	*Rheum rhaponticum*	Leaf blade
Rosary pea (jequirty bean, crab's eye, and precatory bean)	*Abrus precatorium*	Seeds
Skunk cabbage	*Symplocarpus foetidus*	All parts, especially roots
Water hemlock (cowbane and snakeroot)	*Cicuta* spp.	Roots and young foliage
Wisteria	*Wisteria* spp.	Seeds and pods
Yellow oleander	*Thevetia peruviana*	All parts, especially kernels of the fruit
Yew	*Taxus* spp.	Needles, bark, and seeds

information sheet on each substance). Many of these, although no longer available to the general public, have been available in commercial products and can be found around the home.

Extreme care should be given to these poisons when handled; some contain toxic ingredients, such as thallium, which can be absorbed through the skin or inhaled, or sodium monofluoroacetate, which can be absorbed through open wounds or inhaled. Other poisons should not be handled because they cause skin burns, such as yellow phosphorus.

Instead of using chemicals, try the old-fashioned mouse trap. Set a number of traps all through the house; rodents sometimes avoid them if they are always in the same place. Keep the bait fresh, and change the location every few days.

Table 19.2 NONTOXIC HOUSEPLANT ALTERNATIVES

Common Name	Botanical Name
African violet	*Saintpaulia ionantha* or *Episcia reptans*
Aluminum plant	*Pilea cadierei*
Aralia (false)	*Dizygotheca elegantissima* or *Fatsia japonica*
Baby's tears	*Helxine soleirolii*
Begonia	*Begonia semperflorens*
Bird's nest fern	*Asplenium nidus*
Boston fern	*Nephrolepis exata*
Bridal veil	*Tradescantia*
Christmas cactus	*Zygocactus truncatus*
Coleus	*Coleus blumei*
Corn plant	*Dracena fragrans*
Creeping Charlie	*Pilea nummularifolia* and *Plectranthus australis*
Creeping Jenny, moneywort, and lysima	*Lysimachia nummularia*
Donkey tail	*Sedum morganianun*
Emerald ripple	*Peperomia caperata*
Fiddleleaf fig	*Ficus lyrata*
Gardenia	*Gardenia radicans*
Grape ivy	*Cissus rhombifolia*
Hawaiian ti	*Cordyline terminalis*
Hens and chicks	*Echeveria* spp. and *Sempervivum tectorus*
Jade tree	*Crassula argentea*
Lipstick plant	*Aeschynanthus lobbianus*
Monkey plant	*Ruellia makoyana*
Mother-in-law tongue	*Sansevieria trifasciata*
Parlor palm	*Chamaedorea elegans*
Peacock plant	*Calathea makoyana*
Piggyback plant	*Tolmiea menziesii*
Pink polka-dot plant	*Hypoestes phyllostachya*
Prayer plant	*Maranta leuconeura*
Rosary vine	*Ceropegia woodii*
Rosary pearls	*Senico rowleyanus* or *S. herreianus*
Rubber plant	*Ficus elastica*
Sensitive plant	*Mimosa pudica*
Snake plant	*Sansevieria trifasciata*
Spider plant	*Chlorophytum comosum*
String of hearts	*Ceropegia woodii*
Swedish ivy	*Plectranthus australis*
Umbrella plant (Schlefflera)	*Brassaia actinophylla*
Wandering Jew	*Tradescantia albiflora* and *Zebrina pendula*
Wax plant	*Hoya carnosa* or *H. exotica*
Weeping fig	*Ficus benjamina*
Zebra plant	*Aphelandra squarrosa*

GETTING RID OF HAZARDOUS PRODUCTS

Americans generate more than 4 million tons of household hazardous waste each year. Much of it ends up in the local landfill, where it may eventually leach into the ground. When dumped into a septic tank, some hazardous products can contaminate underground water supplies.

Although the first step to dealing with the hazardous waste problem is to avoid toxic products when possible, to dispose of a hazardous product consider these options:

• Use it up properly. When possible, finish the product or give the unused portion—left in the original container—to a friend or a community organization. Paint or solvent-based products

more than ten years old should be discarded, because it is highly likely they'll contain hazardous ingredients such as mercury or methylene chloride.

• Take the leftover product to a hazardous waste collection program. Thousands of communities have collection programs; call the local municipal health department, sanitation department, or local environmental protection agency to find out if a program exists in your community. If one does not exist, lobby to have one organized. These programs typically accept pesticides, household cleaners, paints and paint products, automotive products, batteries, solvents, aerosol products, acids, waste oil, and pharmaceuticals (see Box 19.6).

Box 19.6   HOW TO SET UP A HAZARDOUS WASTE COLLECTION PROGRAM

For information on setting up a household hazardous waste collection program, write the League of Women Voters of Massachusetts, 8 Winter Street, Boston, MA 02108, or request a copy of the EPA publication *Household Hazardous Waste: A Bibliography of Useful References and List of State Experts* by calling the EPA's Superfund hot line at 1-800-424-9346.

Disposal for Common Household Hazardous Waste

Auto Batteries. Take used auto batteries to an auto dealer for recycling (required by law in some states).

Floor Polish and Furniture Polish. Use up polishes or give them away. As a last resort, solidify them with kitty litter and toss them in the trash.

Household Cleaning Products. Ammonia, bleach, disinfectants, drain cleaners, oven cleaners, and toilet bowl cleaners can be used up or

given to friends. If your home does not have a septic tank, you can dilute them with water and pour down the drain.

Medical Waste. Carefully place syringes in a used detergent bottle and add a solution of one part bleach and ten parts water. When the bottle is full, tape the lid shut and discard it. Do not discard syringes in containers that will be recycled. Wrap up out-of-date or unneeded drugs—both prescription and over-the-counter products—to prevent children from eating them, then throw them into the trash or flush them down the toilet.

Motor Oil, Transmission Fluid, and Brake Fluid. These can be re-refined and reused. Take them to your service station.

Metal and Stone Cleaners. Any unused hydrofluoric acid should be saved for a household hazardous waste collection program.

Paint. Use it up, give it away, or bring it to a collection site.

Wood-Finishing Products. Do not flush products containing solvents down the drain. Toxic fumes can back up into the house and flammable vapors can collect and explode in the sewer lines or septic tanks. Use it up or give it away.

CHAPTER 20

Art and Hobbyist Materials

Eighteen years ago, sculptor Tony Jones entered his studio and climbed inside a huge polyester and fiberglass outdoor sculpture he was making. He wore a double-nozzle gas mask, which he thought would amply protect him from the resin fumes in the air. Unfortunately, he was wrong; the mask was not the correct type of respirator. After a half hour of silence, two art students working in a neighboring studio checked in on Jones and found him unconscious, overcome by toxic fumes. His head, shirt, and shoes were stuck fast to the sculpture, so the students cut him out and rushed him to the hospital. Jones survived, but he continues to suffer from respiratory problems and an allergy to fiberglass and plastics. His shoes remain glued inside his art work, a reminder of the hidden dangers of many art materials.

More recently, a middle-aged portrait artist saw her physician because of recurrent episodes of dizziness, fuzzy thinking, and tingling in her hands and feet; she was concerned she had pre-senile dementia. Her studio had one window, she kept her door closed to conserve heat, and she cleaned her brushes in a closet using mineral spirits. She noted that she would become "high" every day after cleaning her brushes and that her dizzy spells came on after working intensively in her painting studio for several weeks. In this, and in many cases, a condition brought on by

the use of artists' materials can be resolved after reviewing the artist's practices and work space. A consultation with an occupational health physician traced her symptoms to her use of solvents. She improved the ventilation in her studio by opening the door and putting in a window exhaust fan and cleaned her brushes outdoors, and her symptoms ceased.

Many times, it is difficult to prove that a particular art or hobbyist supply causes an illness, particularly because symptoms of some serious illnesses do not show up until years after the exposure.

The extent of long-term chronic health problems that result from using artist and hobbyist materials is unknown. For years, art historians assumed that Vincent van Gogh painted blurry stars and halos around streetlamps as a matter of artistic style, a ready excuse to use the vibrant yellows and oranges he favored. However, modern physicians now speculate that van Gogh's technique may have had less to do with creative expression than visual distortion brought on by chronic lead poisoning. Such suspicions are well founded: van Gogh was known to eat paint and to have used pigments containing lead as well as cadmium, mercury, and other heavy metals.

One fact remains clear: Materials used in arts, crafts, and hobbies must be handled with respect. Many of these products contain dangerous materials—from carcinogenic methylene chloride in solvents to dangerous heavy metals, such as lead in glazes or silica in clays and casting flour. Used carelessly, they can cause numerous health problems that range in seriousness from mild skin or respiratory irritations to death.

HOW TOXINS FROM ART MATERIALS ENTER THE BODY

Problems from exposure to toxins can be acute—the immediate result of a single encounter—or chronic—the result of repeated exposures to toxic materials over a period of months, years, or even decades. Toxins enter the body in one of three ways: skin contact, inhalation, or ingestion.

Skin contact is the most common entry route for art toxins. Normally, the skin acts as a barrier and prevents injury to the body's systems, but solvent chemicals such as acetone, toluene, methyl alcohol, methanol, and turpentine can be absorbed right through the skin.

Breathing the vapors, spray mists, gases, fumes, smoke, and dusts from art materials is also a common method of entry. Some substances can immediately irritate and eventually burn the throat and lungs. For example, both glacial acetic acid (used as a stop bath in photography) and sulfur dioxide (a gas by-product sometimes released during the firing of certain ceramics) can damage the lung tissues, causing diseases such as asthma or emphysema. Exposure to other materials can cause serious long-term health problems; silicosis can develop after breathing silica dust during stone sculpting, and kidney damage can occur over time from inhaling toluene in solvents.

Although few adult artists intentionally put art materials in their mouths, they often *indirectly* consume toxins through contact with contaminated hands via food, drinks, and cigarettes. For this reason, artists should never eat, drink, chew gum, or smoke in their studios.

Children and other family members may be inadvertently exposed to toxins from art materials through contact with contaminated clothes or objects brought home. Exposure to these chemicals can occur while washing clothes that have been worn in the studio.

WHO IS AT RISK?

Certain groups of people are more prone to developing health problems from exposure to hazardous art and hobby materials, although no one should be considered immune. Children, the elderly, pregnant women, men and women of childbearing age, smokers, people who drink alcohol in excess, people on certain drugs or medications, and people with particular health problems (such as allergies or impaired heart, lungs, liver, and other organs and their functions), are more susceptible to toxic chemicals. Women who are pregnant or nursing need to take particular care, because a developing fetus and infant are susceptible to some toxins found in art materials. Nursing mothers should also beware, because toxins can enter breast milk and linger for some time, posing a potential threat to nursing infants. For example, the carcinogen methylene chloride, which is found in some furniture strippers, can be present in breast milk up to seventeen hours after exposure (see Chapter 11, "Reproductive Effects and Prenatal Exposures").

In comparison with adults, children face greater risks from toxic art materials than adults for a number of reasons. A chemical that might

ART AND HOBBYIST MATERIALS

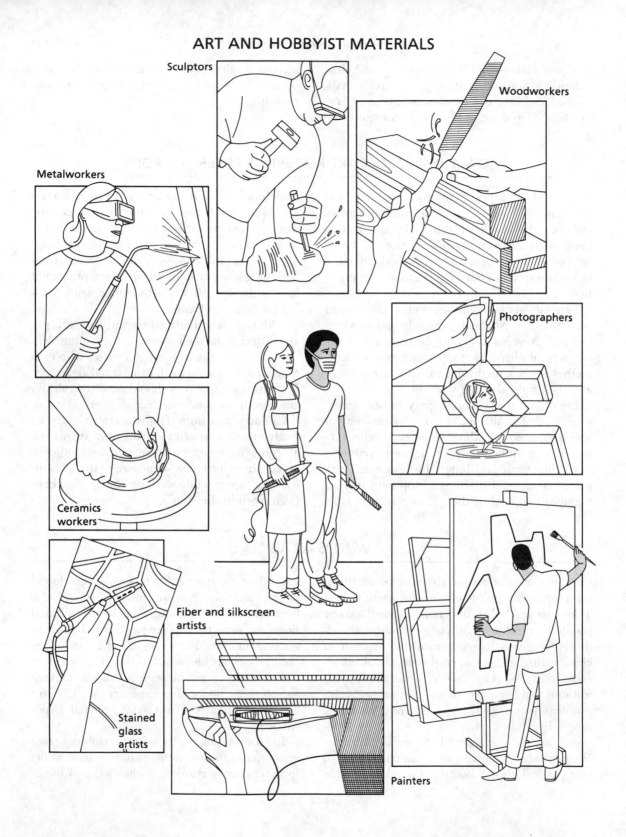

Sculptors

Woodworkers

Metalworkers

Photographers

Ceramics workers

Stained glass artists

Fiber and silkscreen artists

Painters

not be toxic to adults can harm the smaller child. Growing children also have a more rapid metabolism than adults; this means that if a chemical needs to be metabolized to be toxic, children are more at risk. Children also have a greater body surface area relative to their weight than adults and, thus, can absorb greater amounts of toxic substances through their skin. Similarly, children's more rapid rate of breathing, relative to their weight, increases their risk of exposure through inhalation of a toxic agent (see Chapter 12, "Of Special Concern: Infants and Children").

Because of the increased risk factors, children under age twelve should not be exposed to hazardous art materials. Age twelve is the cut-off point, because younger children will not necessarily understand or carry out precautions. Furthermore, many children, especially preschoolers, will put contaminated items in their mouths and may swallow them.

Determining Your Risk of Exposure

An individual's risk of exposure to toxic art and hobbyist materials depends on a host of factors.

How great is the exposure? The body's tolerance for certain chemicals depends on the length and frequency of exposure. Anyone who works long hours with these materials *should not* rely on the safety guideline of exposure limits suggested for workplaces. Most of these exposure limits are intended for industrial workers, who are exposed to chemicals for only at most eight hours at a time and have time before the next shift to detoxify before encountering the chemical again. Many artists, especially when preparing for an exhibit or show, may work day and night, leaving too little time for the chemical to be purged from the body.

Artists who work in home studios must take even greater precautions: Any contamination of the living area can result in twenty-four-hour exposure to dangerous chemicals. At-home artists also risk exposing other family members and visitors, especially children, to the hazards from their materials.

How toxic is the substance? The more toxic the chemical, the smaller the amount it takes to cause problems. Whenever possible, choose the least toxic art material to minimize chances of injury. For example, both toluene and acetone are used as solvents in spray fixatives, but toluene has been shown to damage the central nervous system and kidneys. Acetone is not without risk—it is quite flammable and can cause respiratory irritation—but as long as necessary precautions are taken, acetone solvents can be safer to use than products containing toluene (see Box 20.4).

Is the artist exposed to other environmental toxins? Art materials may represent only one of many sources of exposure to toxins. For example, an artist working with stained glass or ceramic glazes will encounter lead in fumes, dust, and pigments in addition to lead encountered in drinking water, food, and drink, as well as other hidden sources.

Is there interaction between an art-related hazard and other factors? The effects of environmental exposure can be synergistic, not just additive, so that exposure to one substance multiplies the dangerous effects of another toxin. For example, heavy smokers stand at least a ten times greater chance of developing lung cancer

Figure 20.1 ART AND HOBBYIST MATERIALS

Woodworkers, photographers, painters, fiber and silk-screen artists, stained glass artists, potters and ceramic workers, welders and metalworkers, jewelry makers, and sculptors who work in clay, wood, stone, and plastic are all among those who can be affected by toxic materials used in arts, crafts, and hobbies.

Box 20.1   MINIMIZING THE RISK FOR CHILDREN UNDER TWELVE

The following are guidelines from the Center for Safety in the Arts on art material recommendations for children under twelve. The same guidelines apply for people at special risk: pregnant and nursing women, the elderly, and institutionalized adults. Most important, supervise children at all times while using art and hobbyist materials.

Do Not Use	*Substitutes*
Clay in dry form; powdered clay, which is easily inhaled, contains free silica and possibly asbestos. Do not sand dry clay pieces or do other dust-producing activities	Talc-free premixed clay (e.g., Amaco white clay). Wet mop or sponge surface thoroughly after using clay
Ceramic glazes or copper enamels	Water-based paints; artwork may be waterproofed with acrylic-based mediums
Cold water, fiber-reactive dyes, other commercial dyes	Vegetable and/or plant dyes (e.g., onionskins, tea, and flowers) and food dyes
Instant papier-mâchés (inhalable dust is created, and some may contain asbestos fibers, lead from pigments in colored printing inks, etc.)	Make papier-mâché from black-and-white newspaper and library or white paste, or use approved papier-mâchés
Powdered tempera colors (inhalable dust is created and some tempera colors contain toxic pigments, preservatives, etc.)	Liquid paints or paints the teacher premixes
Pastels, chalks, or dry markers that create dust	Crayons, oil pastels, or dustless chalks

---

compared to nonsmokers. Nonsmokers who worked with asbestos in the past have shown a five times greater risk of lung cancer compared to nonsmokers who were not exposed to asbestos. However, people who both smoke *and* worked with asbestos were fifty to ninety times more likely to develop lung cancer than those without either risk factor (see Box 3.2, p. 52).

Box 20.2   HOW TO IDENTIFY SAFE MATERIALS

A nontoxic studio will still offer the full range of materials and will not hamper a child's creativity. In most cases, there are safe alternatives to toxic art materials, yet it is crucial for a consumer to be able to distinguish between products that are safe for children's use and those that are not. Recent laws are making the distinction a bit easier: Art materials that are potentially hazardous if used by children must carry restrictive labeling, such as "Not for Use by Children" or "Keep Out of Reach of Children." Also, those that have been deemed safe for children should be identified by an ASTM D.4236 statement and no hazard labeling on the product.

```
┌─────────────────────────────────────────────────────────────────────────┐
│  Box 20.3  SYMPTOMS OF EXPOSURE TO TOXIC ART MATERIALS                    │
│                                                                           │
│  • See your doctor or an occupational health physician immediately if you │
│    experience health problems, such as headaches, dizziness, fatigue,     │
│    nausea, coughing, or breathing difficulties, during or after work with │
│    art materials.                                                         │
│  • Bring a list of the materials you work with and the ingredients of the │
│    products so that the physician can consider whether the materials      │
│    might be the source of the problem. (Poison control centers can assist │
│    you and/or physicians in assessing the toxicology of the chemicals.    │
│    Please see Appendix B for a center in your region.)                    │
│  • Anyone who works with highly toxic materials such as lead, solvents,   │
│    or silica dust should have regular medical checkups to monitor for any │
│    adverse effects.                                                       │
└─────────────────────────────────────────────────────────────────────────┘
```

HOW TOXIC ART AND HOBBYIST MATERIALS DAMAGE THE BODY

Art and hobbyist materials have been shown to cause skin irritation, lead poisoning, silicosis, liver and kidney damage, nerve damage, reproductive problems, carbon monoxide poisoning, cancer, and asthma, among other ailments.

Some problems resulting from exposure to toxins from art materials are more common than others:

• *Skin* problems, including rashes, burns, and other irritations, are the most frequent problems caused by hazardous chemicals. Although not the most harmful ailments, they can be debilitating and can prevent you from working. Skin irritations may also allow other toxic chemicals to more readily enter the body (see Chapter 4, "Skin Ailments").

• *Acute respiratory diseases* can result from exposure to irritating fumes, such as sulfur dioxide, nitrogen dioxide, or ammonia, which damage the lungs. The chemicals can irritate the upper respiratory system, causing bronchitis (inflammation of the air passages). If the chemicals come in contact with the air sacs in the lungs, chemical pneumonia and/or pulmonary edema can develop.

• *Chronic lung diseases* can be caused by repeated low-level exposures to substances such as ozone, nitrogen oxides, and sulfur dioxide.

Long-term exposure to these chemicals can damage the airways leading to the air sacs. Over the years, certain dusts, including asbestos and silica from clays and many stones, as well as moldy hay, certain wood dusts, and even pet birds, can cause scarring of the lung tissue or pulmonary fibrosis. Some diisocyanates can lead to development of chronic asthma and lung scarring (see Chapter 6, "Respiratory Ailments").

• *Heart damage* (or abnormalities) can result from repeated exposure to a number of chemicals, including halogenated hydrocarbons, such as methylene chloride and methyl chloroform.

• *Other chemicals interfere with the blood*, either by affecting the transport of oxygen through the blood, such as carbon monoxide and methylene chloride, or by inhibiting the formation of red and white blood cells and platelets, such as benzene.

• *Liver damage* results from the potent solvent dimethylformamide. Polychlorinated biphenyls (PCBs) can also damage the liver, as can many solvents (such as toluene, xylene, and especially chlorinated solvents, such as carbon tetrachloride, chloroform, and perchloroethylene), as well as metals such as lead and arsenic (see information sheets for these substances).

• *Kidney damage* can result from exposure to such

substances as lead, arsenic (which has been used in violet color—cobalt arsenate—but which is no longer incorporated in the United States), cadmium, chlorinated hydrocarbons, and turpentine.

- *Nervous system damage* can be caused by heavy metals, such as lead, mercury, and arsenic. Exposure to carbon disulfide can cause brain damage. Many other substances, especially solvents, can depress the central nervous system, resulting in fatigue, dizziness, confusion, sleepiness, lack of coordination, or nausea (see Chapter 5, "The Brain and Nervous System").
- *Reproductive disorders* can result from exposure

to some art materials. For example, solvents containing toluene and xylene may cause menstrual problems in women. Lead can also cause menstrual disorders, loss of sex drive, sperm abnormalities, and atrophy of the testes. Even in small amounts, some chemicals and metals known as teratogens (because they impair fetal growth and development) can damage the fetus. Teratogens include benzene, cadmium, carbon disulfide, carbon monoxide, chlorinated hydrocarbons, ethyl alcohol, glycol ethers, lead, toluene, and xylene (see Chapter 11, "Reproductive Effects and Prenatal Exposures").

HAZARDOUS SUBSTANCES IN ART MATERIALS

Some of the most dangerous ingredients in art products are found in solvents, aerosol sprays, glazes, and acids and alkalis.

Solvents

These chemicals are used in many arts and hobbyist activities to dissolve and remove oil paint, resins, varnishes, rubber cements, and inks. Almost all organic solvents are poisonous if swallowed or inhaled in sufficient quantity; most cause skin irritation after extended contact and some can be absorbed through the skin. Benzene and several other solvents are so toxic they should not be used (see Box 20.4).

There are several types of solvents available. Each presents different hazards.

- *Alcohols* are common solvents. Swallowing even very small amounts of methanol (wood or methyl alcohol) can cause dizziness, intoxication, blurred vision, blindness, liver and kidney damage, or death. Ethanol can irritate the eyes and upper respiratory tract (see information sheets, pp. 379 and 396).
- *Aromatic hydrocarbons* are the most dangerous solvents. Although they can be absorbed through the skin, most problems arise when

they are inhaled. Even low-level exposure to benzene (or benzol) can cause chronic poisoning by destroying the bone marrow, causing aplastic anemia and leukemia. Toluene (or toluol) and xylene (or xylol) may cause liver, kidney, and reproductive system damage. (Crude grades of toluene also may be contaminated with the more toxic benzene.) (See information sheets on these substances.)

- *Chlorinated hydrocarbons* can cause skin irritation and liver and kidney damage, and many are suspected carcinogens. They can be absorbed through the skin. Examples include tetrachloroethane, methylene chloride, ethylene dichloride, perchloroethylene, and trichloroethylene (see information sheets).
- *Esters* and glycol ethers can cause eye, nose, throat, and respiratory irritation. In the workplace, glycol ethers, such as methyl cellosolve, are regulated because of concerns that they may cause birth defects and reproductive damage (see Chapter 11, "Reproductive Effects and Prenatal Exposures").
- *Ketones* can irritate the eyes and upper respiratory tract and depress the central nervous system, causing fatigue, dizziness, confusion, sleepiness, lack of coordination, or nausea. Methyl and butyl ketones cause peripheral neur-

opathy, characterized by numbness and eventual nerve damage with muscle weakness in the limbs (see Chapter 5, "The Brain and Nervous System").

- *Aliphatic hydrocarbons*, such as gasoline, mineral spirits, kerosene, and *n*-hexane, can cause skin irritation. Inhalation can cause a mild narcotic effect and lung irritation. Ingestion can cause pulmonary edema (chemical pneumonia) and possible death. *n*-Hexane can cause peripheral neuropathy.

Box 20.4 TOXICITY RANKINGS OF SELECTED SOLVENTS

When buying art materials containing solvents, always choose the least toxic product. The following is a list of solvent types in descending order, from most to least toxic.

DO NOT USE (KNOWN OR SUSPECTED CARCINOGENS)

Benzene
Carbon tetrachloride
Chloroform
Ethylene dichloride
Trichloroethylene
Perchloroethylene
Dioxane

USE WITH CARE

Toluene
Xylene
Methylene chloride
Styrene
Methyl cellosolve
Phenol
Ketones
Esters
Alcohols
Petroleum distillates

Aerosols

Aerosol mist may contain paint, varnish, adhesive, and other materials, which may be toxic if inhaled. Some aerosols also contain dangerous solvents, such as toluene and chlorinated hydrocarbons.

Acids and Alkalis

These substances are used for cleaning and etching metals and glass, removing paint, and processing photos. Examples include potassium hydroxide (caustic potash), sodium hydroxide (caustic soda), sodium carbonate, potassium carbonate, calcium oxide (quick lime), hydrofluoric acid, and ammonia. These chemicals can burn the skin, eyes, respiratory system, and gastrointestinal system.

Solder

To bond metals in many crafts activities, artists and hobbyists commonly use soft solders (those with melting points below 600°F), which usually contain significant amounts of lead, one of the top environmental toxins. Some exposure to lead occurs during soldering, as lead oxide fumes are released. The greatest danger, though, comes from ingesting lead; typically, an artist will handle solder and, without washing hands, then handle food, gum, or cigarettes—all of which are easily contaminated by this dangerous heavy metal (see Chapter 5, "The Brain and Nervous System," and information sheet, p. 392). "Nonlead" solder may contain a large amount of cadmium, which can also present health hazards if used carelessly (see information sheet, p. 368).

Solvents, aerosols, acids and alkalis, and solders are used in a number of different types of artwork. Each medium and activity presents its own hazards, which are summarized in Box 20.5.

Box 20.5   HAZARDS OF DIFFERENT TYPES OF ART ACTIVITIES

CERAMICS

PROBLEM

- Many clays contain silica. Inhaling silica dust from handling dry clay can lead to silicosis, also known as potter's rot. Symptoms include shortness of breath, susceptibility to infections, and severe scarring of the lungs. Some clays also contain talc and asbestos (see Chapter 6, "Respiratory Ailments").
- Ceramic glazes often contain toxic metals, such as lead, barium, and lithium, which should not be ingested or inhaled.
- During firing, toxic fumes may be released. For example, carbon monoxide, sulfur dioxide, and formaldehyde can be released from clays; and lead, cadmium, fluorine, chlorine, and sulfur dioxide can be released from the breakdown of some raw glazes.

WHAT TO DO

- Use talc-free clays, and use wet clay whenever possible.
- Be certain the work area is thoroughly ventilated. Wear an appropriate, fitted dust respirator and keep it uncontaminated (see Box 20.7). Wet mop daily to remove dry clay dust.
- Wear toxic dust respirators when mixing glazes from powders. Use spray glazes in a ventilated spray booth.
- Make sure the kiln and the area around it are properly ventilated.

FIBER ARTS

PROBLEM

- Knitters, weavers, and others involved in fiber arts face a hazard of fiber dust, which can cause respiratory irritation and allergies when inhaled. Years of exposure to cotton, flax, and hemp dust can cause byssinosis, or brown lung, which

(continued)

Box 20.5   HAZARDS OF DIFFERENT TYPES OF ART ACTIVITIES (*continued*)

resembles chronic bronchitis or emphysema (see Chapter 6, "Respiratory Ailments").

WHAT TO DO

- Use yarns that have been cleaned and processed before sale.
- Make certain the studio is properly ventilated. If this is impractical, use a respirator (see Box 20.7).

JEWELRY

PROBLEM

- Silver soldering can be hazardous. The lowest-melting silver solders can contain up to 30 percent cadmium. Cadmium fumes can cause chemical pneumonia. Chronic exposure can cause kidney damage, lung damage, and lung cancer (see information sheets, pp. 368 and 412).
- Silver solders often contain fluoride fluxes to help the metals fuse together. Fluoride can cause respiratory irritation and nosebleeds.
- Asbestos exposures in jewelry makers' studios have resulted in mesothelioma (see p. 125).

WHAT TO DO

- Use cadmium-free solders.
- Use borax fluxes instead of fluoride.
- Be certain the area is well ventilated and/or use an appropriate respirator (see Box 20.7).

METALWORK

PROBLEM

- In the casting process, the metal is melted and poured into a mold. Metal fume fever, with symptoms that include headache, fever, dizziness, nausea, and chest, muscle, and joint pains lasting twenty-four to thirty-six hours can develop if metal and alloy fumes are inhaled, especially from oxides of zinc, copper, iron, magnesium, and nickel.
- Inhalation of lead fumes (present in bronze or lead casting) can cause lead poisoning. Some crude ores contain significant amounts of mercury, which may be inhaled during smelting; this may cause a chemical pneumonitis or damage the nervous system. Similarly, nickel fumes can cause lung or nasal cancer, manganese can cause chemical pneumonia and Parkinson's disease, and chromium can cause lung cancer and kidney damage (see information sheets for these substances). Do not use beryllium alloys; they can cause scarring of the lungs.
- Exposing the eyes to infrared radiation can cause cataracts.

(continued)

Box 20.5   HAZARDS OF DIFFERENT TYPES OF ART ACTIVITIES (*continued*)

WHAT TO DO

- Cast metals only in well-ventilated areas. A melting furnace should have a canopy hood exhausting to the outdoors. Use a respirator (see Box 20.7).
- Wear protective goggles when casting metals.

PAINTING

PROBLEM

- Many pigments contain toxic compounds. For example, chromium and cadmium pigments are suspected carcinogens. The cobalt arsenate form of cobalt violet is extremely toxic (it is no longer in use in the United States). Mercury in some latex paint may be a concern (see information sheets for chromium, cadmium, cobalt, and mercury).
- Mineral spirits and turpentine, which are often used as thinners and are in some oil and acrylic paints, are hazardous through skin contact, inhalation, and ingestion.

WHAT TO DO

- Whenever possible, substitute a nontoxic or less toxic pigment for a more toxic one.
- Use solvents and solvent-based products only in well-ventilated areas. Where this is impractical, use an appropriate, fitted respirator (see Box 20.7).

PHOTOGRAPHY

PROBLEM

- The greatest hazards occur during the preparation and handling of concentrated solutions of photo-processing chemicals. Each solution presents a different hazard. The developer contains hydroquinone and Metol (monomethyl *p*-aminophenol sulfate), which can cause skin irritation, loss of skin pigment, and allergic reactions. Concentrated glacial acetic acid, used in the stop bath, can burn the skin on contact, and inhaling it can irritate the throat and lungs. The fixer often emits sulfur dioxide, which can irritate the lungs, cause chronic lung damage, and is of special concern to people with asthma. Many photo bleaches, reducers, toners, hardeners, and stabilizers can burn or cause other irritations.

WHAT TO DO

- Wear protective gloves and goggles when preparing solutions.
- Mix chemicals in a well-ventilated area. Kodak recommends at least ten air changes per hour for black-and-white processing. If this is impractical, be certain to use a respirator (see Box 20.7).

(*continued*)

Box 20.5   HAZARDS OF DIFFERENT TYPES OF ART ACTIVITIES (*continued*)

PLASTICS SCULPTURE

PROBLEM

- A number of types of plastic resins, such as amino, phenolic, or formaldehyde resins, are toxic if inhaled, swallowed, or touched. Polyester resins often contain styrene, which is toxic through inhalation and skin contact. Acrylic resins often contain methyl methacrylate, which can cause headaches and irritability when inhaled, and benzoyl peroxide, a flammable skin and eye irritant (see information sheets on these substances).

WHAT TO DO

- Wear gloves when handling resins.
- Use local exhaust ventilation or a window exhaust fan (see Box 20.7).
- It may be necessary to wear a chemical respirator.

STONE SCULPTURE

PROBLEM

- Inhaling silica dust can result in silicosis, also known as grinder's consumption, which limits breathing capacity and results in scar tissue in the lungs, or silico-proteinosis, which resembles pulmonary edema. Stones containing large amounts of free silica include quartz, granite, sandstone, brownstone, slate, opal, amethyst, onyx, and soapstone. Soapstone, serpentine, and greenstone may also contain asbestos, which can cause lung cancer and asbestosis if inhaled (see Chapter 6, "Respiratory Ailments").

WHAT TO DO

- Avoid working with silica- or asbestos-containing materials. If you must use them, use a fitted appropriate respirator and make sure it is uncontaminated. Keep the area properly ventilated (see Box 20.7).
- Take steps to avoid tracking silica dust outside the studio (e.g., to your home) to avoid contaminating others.

SILK SCREEN

PROBLEM

- The biggest problems involve solvents, which are used in virtually every step of the printing process. Most solvents are skin and respiratory irritants and can cause long-term health problems, particularly central nervous system impairment.

(continued)

Box 20.5   HAZARDS OF DIFFERENT TYPES OF ART ACTIVITIES (*continued*)

WHAT TO DO

- Make sure the studio is properly ventilated. Local ventilation over the working area is best. If this is impractical, use a chemical respirator (see Box 20.7).
- Wear gloves and avoid contact with all solvents.
- Switch to water-based inks if possible.

STAINED GLASS

PROBLEM

- Making stained glass involves the use of solders, many of which contain significant amounts of lead. Lead poisoning can occur from inhalation of the lead dust or fumes, especially if the solder is overheated, and from inadvertent ingestion of lead from handling the solder and then, without washing hands, handling food, gum, or cigarettes. The risk exists with both lead came (a slender, grooved bar used to hold together panes in stained glass or latticework windows) and copper-foil techniques. With lead came, there is the additional risk of inhaling or accidentally ingesting lead dust from cutting or sanding the came (see information sheet, p. 392).
- Many of the patinas used on the leading can be toxic. For example, copper sulfate is toxic through ingestion and inhalation.

WHAT TO DO

- Make certain the studio is adequately vented. If this is impractical, use an appropriate respirator. Clean up carefully after cutting lead came.
- Avoid inhalation, ingestion, and skin contact with substances used to color the leading.

WOODWORK

PROBLEM

- Skin irritation is caused by some woods, such as South American boxwood, ebony, American and African mahogany, rosewood, walnut, satinwoods, and western red cedar (see information sheet, p. 401).
- Chronic inhalation of sawdust can cause respiratory disease. Dust from South American boxwood, cork oak, and redwoods can cause an acute illness resembling pneumonia. Beech, iroko, and teak dusts can cause asthma, and western red cedar dusts can cause asthma and fibrosis of the lung.

(continued)

Box 20.5 HAZARDS OF DIFFERENT TYPES OF ART ACTIVITIES (*continued*)

WHAT TO DO

- Avoid direct skin contact with woods causing skin irritation.
- Keep work areas well ventilated. Wear appropriate respirators if working with irritating wood (see Box 20.7).

PREVENTING TOXIC EXPOSURE

Knowing that there are a good number of toxins used in art and hobbyist materials, it seems surprising that some of the extremely toxic ones, for example, benzene, have not been banned outright from these uses. These products are still on the market because they have desirable properties that some artists want in their work, such as the specific quality of flake white paint versus a titanium white. For the hobbyist, white is often white, and these differences may not be as important, so the hobbyist can opt for a safer product.

Reading the Labels

For years, artists had no way of knowing what chronic health problems they might develop from using certain art materials. But the federal Labeling of Hazardous Art Materials Act, which became effective November 1990, should ensure that manufacturers disclose all acute and chronic problems that could be caused by the use of their art products. The law uses broad strokes to define art materials as any substance or product marketed or represented as suitable for use in any phase of the creation of any work of visual or graphic art of any medium.

By law, art materials that potentially cause acute or chronic health problems must carry warning labels stating the potential hazard, naming the hazardous ingredients, and listing guidelines for safe use. Products that do not pose any hazards bear the label ASTM D.4236, which means they are in accordance with the voluntary chronic hazard labeling standard of the American Society for Testing and Materials. Manufacturers must have their products evaluated by a toxicologist at least once every five years. The law also prohibits the purchase of art materials that may pose chronic health hazards by schools for use in preschool classes to grade 6.

Art materials may also carry a voluntary label indicating that the product meets voluntary standards for quality and performance established by an independent trade association. Products meeting the standard, which was developed in 1985 by toxicologists and representatives from industry and artists organizations, bear one of the three labels certified by the Art and Crafts Materials Institute:

- "AP" (approved product) for nontoxic products.
- "CP" (certified product) for nontoxic products proved to be of high-quality materials.
- A health label that lists all toxic ingredients and describes the safety precautions.

These standards and regulations are helpful to all those who use hobbyists' materials. However, artists who travel and study abroad should note that supplies available overseas are not reviewed or regulated for safety.

In addition, these days most artists are quite aware of the dangers in artists' materials. They have made an effort to educate themselves about how to properly and safely use materials that contain toxic substances in an effort to keep these materials on the market.

In many cases, the simplest solution for the artists and hobbyists concerned about toxins in their materials is to switch to a less toxic alternative product. For example, painters can replace flake white paint, which contains lead carbonate, with zinc white or titanium white paints. Artists using ceramic glazes containing lead can switch to lead-free products. Even if substitute products are not available, careful artists can safely use some products as long as they conscientiously protect themselves.

The Safe Studio

When working with potentially dangerous art materials, you can minimize your risk by following basic preventive measures.

Know Your Materials. In addition to the information now required on product labels, detailed information on product hazards and precautions are available on Material Safety Data Sheets, which are prepared by the manufacturer. By law, manufacturers must provide this information on chemicals listed as toxic by the Environmental Protection Agency. If a manufacturer refuses to give you a data sheet, switch products. The regional poison control center in your area can also provide information on the materials you use (see Appendix B for a listing).

Keep All Materials Labeled. Do not transfer anything to unlabeled containers.

Prepare for Emergencies. Keep a stocked first-aid kit in your studio. Post a list of emergency telephone numbers beside the phone. Keep the appropriate type of fire extinguisher handy, and be sure there is a functional smoke detector in the work space (see Box 20.6).

Box 20.6 THE WELL-STOCKED FIRST-AID KIT

Every artist's studio should have a complete first-aid kit, and everyone using the studio should know where it is kept. Although the specific first-aid supplies an artist might need depends on the work done in the studio, every kit should include these basics:

- One-half pint of syrup of ipecac (up to 2 tablespoons are given to induce vomiting).
- One tube of burn ointment.
- Paper cups.
- A variety of sizes of adhesive bandages.
- A variety of sizes of bandage compresses.
- Telfa pads.
- Sterile eye pads.
- Adhesive tape.
- Scissors.
- Tweezers.
- One bottle of aspirin.
- An eyewash cup for washing the eye.

Most importantly, the kit should contain a list of emergency telephone numbers, including numbers for the regional poison control center, area hospitals, and doctors. When an emergency occurs, call your regional poison control center for instructions on how to administer first aid.

Choose and Use Safe Supplies. First, try to substitute nontoxic materials for more toxic ones. However, if an art material contains a toxic ingredient, use it sparingly and try to choose a form of the material that is less likely to enter the body. For example, use a product in liquid form instead of an aerosol or a solid form instead of a powder. Do not use such proven or suspected carcinogens, such as benzene.

Follow Special Precautions When Working at Home. Never work in kitchens or bedrooms. Keep children out of the studio. Keep pets out of your work area as well. Some animals are very susceptible to even small amounts of toxic materials, and pets often track powders and dusts throughout the house.

Provide Adequate Ventilation. In most cases, an open window is not enough ventilation. If exposure to toxins is intense or prolonged, an exhaust fan will be necessary to remove the toxin at the source. Cross-ventilation is *not* necessarily adequate ventilation. Don't count on an air-conditioner for ventilation; most recirculate almost all the air and, even when set on vent, they do not get rid of all the contaminants. Using a fan to move the air in an unventilated area can reduce concentrations of some toxic fumes, but may spread them to other areas and possibly expose others to the substance. When it is impractical to provide adequate ventilation, use a fitted and appropriate respirator (see Box 20.7).

Clean Up Carefully. Wet mop frequently. Don't sweep; it stirs up dust. When storing left-over supplies, never use milk containers or soft drink bottles; children or careless adults may accidentally drink from them. Store powders in airtight jars or tins to prevent dust from escaping.

Never Eat, Drink, Chew Gum, Apply Makeup, or Smoke in the Studio. Wash your face and hands before eating since even small amounts of toxins on your lips or fingers can cause problems. Carefully clean under your fingernails and do not bite your nails. Use soap and water—not solvents—to clean your skin. For cleaning up after using oil-based paints, use baby

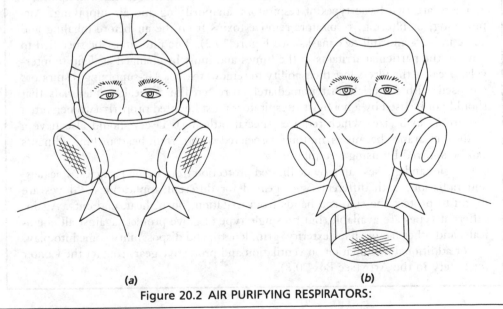

(a)   (b)

Figure 20.2 AIR PURIFYING RESPIRATORS:

(*a*) with a face mask and (*b*) without a face mask.

Box 20.7   WHEN ADEQUATE VENTILATION IS IMPRACTICAL

When the materials used in an art or craft produce fumes, the work space or studio should have good ventilation, ideally two windows for cross-ventilation. It is critical to prevent fire and explosions and to remove toxic vapors, gases, and dusts from the air. Recommendations on many art materials indicate that they should be used with "adequate ventilation," without defining what that means.

Often, the artist or hobbyist sets up wherever he or she can find the space, with or without windows. Even if there is ventilation, it may be too cold out to open the windows while working in the room.

There are two basic types of ventilation—dilution ventilation and local exhaust ventilation. Dilution, or general, ventilation involves mixing toxic fumes with uncontaminated air by using an open window or a fan. In dilution systems, fresh air should pass through breathing zones before being contaminated and exhausted. Air-conditioning cannot be used as general ventilation, because the systems often recirculate toxic vapors or spread it to other parts of the house or building.

Local exhaust ventilation captures toxic fumes or dusts before they mix with room air. Local exhaust ventilation is necessary when the materials are highly toxic or when large amounts of toxins are produced, such as when using aerosol sprays or when doing plastic sculpture or kiln firing. Local exhaust systems include a hood, ducting, and an exhaust fan and are considered safer, because they prevent the artist from being exposed to the toxic material.

One solution for a worst-case scenario—a closed work space with poor ventilation—is protective gear such as a respirator; this is often used as a last resort (after substituting less toxic materials), because it can be uncomfortable and limit mobility.

There are two basic types of respirators: air purifying and air supplying. Air-purifying, or filtering, respirators remove toxins from the air before inhaling and come in half- and full-face masks (see Figure 20.2). The filter must be specified to remove the particular irritants in the fumes and must be changed at definite intervals, because the filters lose their ability to remove toxins. Air-supplying respirators are used with materials that immediately threaten life or health—materials that should not be used by a hobbyist. Respirators must be fitted properly (women often require a small size, which requires special ordering). Users should also have a medical clearance because symptoms associated with certain heart or lung ailments can be spurred by using a respirator.

Goggles and glasses can provide limited protection from flying particles, splashes, and radiation, with different types geared for different applications. Gloves are useful to protect the skin and hands from irritation, burn, heat, and cuts. Again, different types are available, but no single type of glove protects against all chemicals, and other factors like dexterity, grip, length, and disposability come into play.

For additional information on ventilation and protective gear, contact the Center for Safety in the Arts (see Box 20.8).

oil, then soap and water. Don't drink in the studio because dust and fumes can settle and dissolve in your beverage. Never smoke in your studio; it creates a fire hazard, stresses the lungs, and can transfer toxins from your hands to your mouth.

Wear Protective Clothing. Remove your work clothes when you leave the studio. Wash them separately from other clothes, and wash them often. Wear protective gear: appropriate safety goggles when grinding, sanding, welding, or working with chemicals that could splatter; appropriate protective gloves when working with dangerous chemicals; earplugs or earmuffs when working under noisy conditions; and a properly fitted respirator over the nose and mouth when working with powders, dusts, and fumes, although a respirator is not a substitute for adequate ventilation.

Box 20.8 RESOURCES

The Art and Craft Materials Institute, Inc., 100 Boylston Street, Boston, MA 02116; 617-266-6800. The group sponsors a certification program for children's art materials and a voluntary labeling program for all art supplies.

Center for Safety in the Arts, 5 Beekman Street, New York, NY 10038; 212-227-6220. The group is a national clearinghouse for research and education on hazards in the arts. The group sponsors the Art Hazards Information Center, which answers questions on art hazards.

Adhering to this list of safety precautions and procedures may force you to rethink and alter your work schedule, habits, and maybe even the manner in which you create your art. Yet the payoff—protecting and preserving your health—makes following these instructions well worth the effort.

CHAPTER 21

The Workplace

When a doctor visits a working class home," wrote Bernardino Ramazzini, the renowned seventeenth-century Italian physician, "he should take time for his examination, and to the questions recommended by Hippocrates, he should add one more: 'What is your occupation?' "

Ramazzini knew what he was talking about. The keenly observant doctor, today considered the father of occupational medicine, spent much of his life documenting a litany of health hazards specifically associated with particular trades such as metal digging, gilding, and glassmaking.

Ramazzini's concerns that occupational hazards were transforming the workplace into a spawning ground for misery and disease proved prescient. Dr. Alice Hamilton, America's first physician specializing in occupational medicine, documented a remarkable variety of ailments in the U. S. workplace during the late nineteenth and early twentieth century. She witnessed irrational behavior among hat workers routinely exposed to mercury, nerve-damaging lead poisoning in bathtub enamelers, "dead fingers" in workers who used jackhammers, and bizarre psychoses exhibited by rayon industry workers exposed to carbon disulfide.

Although the annual number of fatal occupational injuries in the United States has declined in recent years, the problem of workplace safety and health is far from resolved. Trauma—accidents—still take a hefty toll in the workplace, accounting for more than 10,000 deaths in 1988, according to the National Safety Council. An-other 72,000 American lives were lost to occupational diseases in 1989, reported the National Safe Workplace Institute. (In terms of relative risks, a person is 1.9 times more likely to die from an occupational disease than from diabetes and twice as likely to die from a work-related accident than in a fire or by drowning.)

Nonfatal work-related illnesses and injuries are high: More than 6.3 million cases of occupation injuries and illnesses were reported to the U.S. Department of Labor's Bureau of Labor Statistics in a 1991 survey. Almost one-half of the injuries sustained on the job were so serious that the afflicted workers had to restrict or lose work time, a consequence that contributed to an astounding 60 million workdays lost or restricted in 1991.

The sources of workplace danger are as varied as the symptoms and the injuries they elicit (see "The Twenty Common Symptoms and Exposures in the Workplace," p. 422). For instance, many chemicals carry their own peculiar risks of skin allergies; heightened levels of mental stress and excessive noise on the job contribute to a broad array of complaints and disabilities; and rapid, repetitive performance of the same tasks day in and day out can result in any number of musculoskeletal disorders.

In addition, because there is a long period of time between exposure and symptoms, and because those symptoms often mimic those seen in other illnesses, many workers and health care professionals do not realize that work is the source of the malady.

WORK-RELATED HAZARDS

Environmental hazards in the workplace fall into four general categories:

1. Chemical agents.
2. Physical agents, such as noise or vibration.
3. Biological agents, such as bacteria or viruses.
4. Muscle or connective tissue strains and injuries precipitated by using poorly designed tools, maintaining awkward positions, and performing repetitive motions.

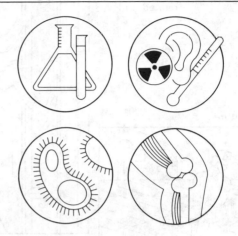

Yet none of these categories are unique to an on-the-job environment. For example, homeowners who paint their houses every few years subject themselves to a number of risks, including exposure to hazardous fumes, injuries from back-wrenching positions, and falls from precariously placed ladders. However, workers who paint houses for a living face these dangers every day and risk the ill effects from the cumulative toxicity of the materials they work with.

Indeed, so rich is the workplace as a spawning ground for illness and injury that much of what we today know about hazards in the environment emerged initially from studies of workplace hazards.

Box 21.1 THE MOST RISKY OCCUPATIONS

The following table is an analysis of occupational injury and illness incidence rates per 100 full-time workers in an industry. These numbers also include work-related fatalities, although the Bureau of Labor Statistics itself acknowledges that these figures are probably significantly understated.

Industry	*Approximately total cases per 100 workers*
Construction	13.0
Manufacturing	12.7
Agriculture (includes forestry and fishing)	10.8
Transportation and public utilities	9.3
Mining	7.4
Wholesale and retail trades	7.6
Services	6.2
Finance, insurance, and real estate services	2.4

Specific risks vary greatly among occupations. Printers frequently encounter hazardous fumes and noise levels, and office workers often suffer from back pain and other ergonomic problems caused by seating positions. Health care workers face many of the same hazards associated with chemical and construction industries, such as exposure to chemicals like ethylene oxide, the de-

WORKPLACE HAZARDS

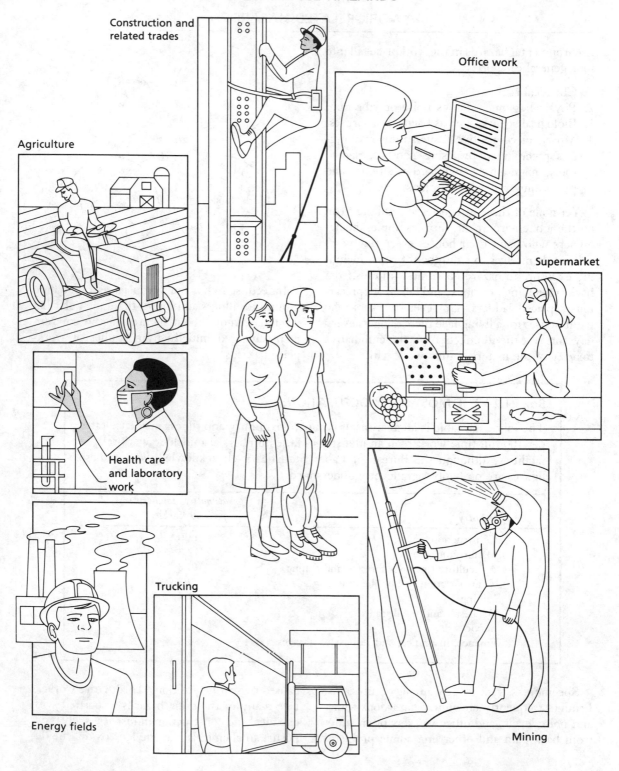

Construction and related trades

Office work

Agriculture

Supermarket

Health care and laboratory work

Energy fields

Trucking

Mining

Table 21.1 THE TEN LEADING WORK-RELATED DISEASES AND INJURIES IN THE UNITED STATES[a]

1. Occupational lung diseases: asbestosis, byssinosis, silicosis, coal workers' pneumoconiosis, lung cancer, occupational asthma

2. Musculoskeletal injuries: disorders of the back, trunk, upper extremity, neck, lower extremity; traumatically induced Raynaud's phenomenon

3. Occupational cancers (others than lung): leukemia; mesothelioma; cancers of the bladder, nose, and liver

4. Severe occupational traumatic injuries: amputations, fractures, eye loss, lacerations, traumatic deaths

5. Cardiovascular diseases: hypertension, coronary artery disease, acute myocardial infarction

6. Disorders of reproduction: infertility, spontaneous abortion, teratogenesis

7. Neurotoxic disorders: peripheral neuropathy, toxic encephalitis, psychoses, extreme personality changes (exposure-related)

8. Noise-induced loss of hearing

9. Dermatologic conditions: dermatoses, burns (scaldings), chemical burns, contusions (abrasions)

10. Psychologic disorders: neuroses, personality disorders, alcoholism, drug dependency

[a] The conditions listed under each category are to be viewed as *selected examples*, not comprehensive definitions of the category. *Source:* NIOSH.

velopment of back problems (from moving patients), and the effects of stress, and are additionally imperiled by harmful viruses and other disease-causing organisms.

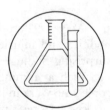

Chemical Hazards in the Workplace

Of the known chemicals, some 100,000 may be harmful to health, and at least 10,000 of these can be found in the workplace. Hazardous chemicals can be inhaled (via airborne dust, droplets, or gas), absorbed through the skin, or (more rarely) ingested as dust or in liquid form.

Chemicals can harm the body in a variety of ways. Certain kinds of dust, such as asbestos and silica, can permanently scar the lungs and decrease respiratory efficiency, or, as is the case with asbestos, result in cancer. Some gases, such as carbon monoxide, do not directly harm the lungs but interfere with the ability of red blood cells to carry life-sustaining oxygen from the lungs to body tissues, causing chemically-induced asphyxiation.

Many jobs bring chemical substances in direct contact with the skin, causing troublesome irritation or inflammation. Repeated skin contact with some chemicals over a period of time (a few days to a few months) can induce the allergic condition contact dermatitis (see Chapter 4,

Figure 21.1 WORKPLACE HAZARDS

Although the sources of workplace danger are as varied as the symptoms and the injuries they cause, occupationally related hazards fall into one of four general categories: chemical, physical, and biological agents and ergonomic (mechanical) stresses resulting from muscle or connective tissue strains and injuries. Almost every occupation presents some type of environmental health hazard, although some are considerably more risky than others. Chemicals in the workplace is rated by the EPA as one of the top environmental health risks faced today.

Box 21.2 SURPRISINGLY RISKY OCCUPATIONS

High-Tech Electronics

So rapid has been the expansion of the electronics industry that the full spectrum of its threats to workers remains unknown. Microchip plants often have poor ventilation. Particularly in developing countries, there is a concern that cost-saving measures may be exposing employees to dangerous levels of lead, methylene chloride (a possible carcinogen), and other solvents. Workers in this industry are often subject to painful burns caused by contact with hydrofluoric acid.

Firing Range Work/Police Target Instruction

Bullets are made of lead, and every time a pistol is fired, lead dust and fumes are released into the air. Many workers in indoor firing ranges are continually exposed as there is no efficient way to rid the air of lead. In factories using lead, high-powered exhaust fans are placed right on top of equipment, which is difficult in firing ranges.

Janitorial and Maintenance Work

Janitorial workers generally handle numerous dangerous solvents used in cleaners. In hospitals they may come in contact with used syringes and other potentially harmful wastes.

A Peculiar Workplace Hazard for Women

Many working women face a peculiar hazard. According to a May 1992 study by NIOSH, homicide is the leading cause of occupational fatalities and injuries for women in the workplace. Two factors contribute to this surprising finding: Relatively few women work in the most hazardous occupations, such as mining and construction, but they make up the greatest percentage of people who work in places that are likely targets for robbery, such as all-night grocery stores, photo-development booths, and other small retail establishments.

"Skin Ailments"). Chemicals, particularly some solvents and pesticides, also can be absorbed directly through the skin, seeping into the tiny blood vessels just beneath the skin's surface and circulating through the body, causing damage to internal organs such as the nervous system, kidneys, and liver.

The National Institute of Occupational Safety and Health (NIOSH) conducts research and makes recommendations to the Occupational Safety and Health Administration (OSHA) based on scientific evidence as to what levels of chemicals pose acceptable health risks. OSHA sets standards based on the lowest levels that seem possible for industry to achieve. (See the information sheets for current standards and recommendations.)

There are a number of more toxic chemicals that are common in the workplace, notably carbon monoxide, heavy metals such as lead and mercury, and certain solvents, all prevalent in large quantities in certain industries.

Box 21.3 MENTAL STRESS ON THE JOB

According to a report by the Bureau of National Affairs, on the average, 1 million employees each day are absent from work because of stress-related disorders, and 40 percent of job turnover is due to stress. Manifestations of job-related stress include headaches, backaches, fatigue, insomnia, allergies, gastrointestinal problems, and hypertension (high blood pressure). Stress can also aggravate the effects of other occupational health hazards.

According to the National Safe Workplace Institute, these factors contribute most to stress on the job:

- Repetitive and boring work.
- Excessive monitoring by supervisors.
- Fear of death or injury on the job.
- Sexual harassment.
- Insufficient control over work situation (the combination of having little latitude in making job decisions and high psychological demands).
- Lack of recognition.
- Heavy workload.
- Fear of job loss or of being demoted.
- Underutilization of skills.
- Lack of support from supervisors and co-workers.

- *Carbon monoxide*, a colorless, odorless, and tasteless gas, binds to hemoglobin in red blood cells 240 times more strongly than oxygen, displacing the life-sustaining gas from those cells and depriving the brain and other organs of oxygen. Cigarette smoke contains 700 to 800 parts per million of carbon monoxide, and cigarette smokers may have as much as 7 percent of their blood's hemoglobin bound by carbon monoxide.

  Some of the earliest human exposures to carbon monoxide probably resulted from cooking fires, with subsequent sources including coal-fired home furnaces, internal combustion engines, and various manufacturing operations. Today, the effects of carbon monoxide are numerous and widespread. It is produced in large amounts during certain industrial processes, such as petroleum refining and steel manufacturing. Carbon monoxide also is a problem for internal combustion engine workers, including welders, garage workers, small-engine and forklift truck operations, motor vehicle drivers, and indoor ice rink workers. Even spectators of such events as tractor pulls, which involve heavy machinery, may be exposed to carbon monoxide. (See information sheet, p. 370 for more information on the symptoms of exposure.)

- *Solvents*, or organic (carbon-containing) liquids that dissolve organic solids, are used in nearly every industry (see Table 21.2). These chemicals may enter the body directly through the skin or through the lungs by inhalation. Solvents can damage the skin and, once in the body, can cause skin, bone marrow, kidney, and neurologic damage and, in some cases, cancer. Many solvents are potent nervous system poisons and can cause a number of neuropsychological symptoms including unexplained fatigue, irritation, depression, memory loss, and disruptions in coordination and

Table 21.2 COMMON SOLVENT-CONTAINING PRODUCTS

Product[a]	Solvent
Aerosols	Dichlorodifluoromethane (propellant 12), trichlorofluoromethane, isobutane, toluene, chlorinated hydrocarbons
Fingernail polish	Acetone, aliphatic acetates, benzene, alcohol, phenol, toluene, xylene, formaldehyde
Gasoline	Petroleum hydrocarbons, paraffins, olefins, naphthenes, benzene, toluene, xylene
Cements, glue	Toluene, acetone, isopropanol, methanol, propanol, ethanol, n-hexane
Lacquer thinners	Toluene, aliphatic acetates, alcohols, ketones, hydrocarbons
Cleaning fluid	Ammonia, naphtha, perchloroethylene, trichloromethane, potassium hydroxide (lye)
Paint strippers	Benzene, methylene chloride, methanol
Plastic cement	Toluene, acetone, aliphatic acetates, n-hexane
Typewriter correction fluid	Trichloroethane, trichloroethylene

[a]Other common solvent sources include dry-cleaning fluids, transmission fluids, windshield washer fluids, brake fluids, degreasers, refrigerants, disinfectants, aerosol deodorants, insect sprays, paints, varnishes, and room deodorizers.

sex drive (see Chapter 5, "The Brain and Nervous System").

Industries that use solvents may be required to have exhaust ventilation to keep inside air levels safe. In some cases, workers can reduce the risk of exposure by substituting a nonsolvent substance (see Chapter 20, "Art and Hobbyist Materials").

• *Lead* is a well-known public health risk for children who are exposed to or inhale the metal in the environment from old paint, soil near roadways, or drinking water. It also represents a significant occupational hazard for adults, given its extensive production in smelting operations, radiator repair, battery manufacturing, and construction. Lead is a particularly sinister substance because it is not easily cleared from or detoxified within the body; thus, its toxicity is cumulative. Exposure is generally from inhalation of either airborne particles of lead or lead oxide fumes, which are released when the metal is heated. Symptoms arise when toxic levels are reached in the body, either within days, in cases of acute high-dose poisoning, or after years of chronic low-dose exposure (see Lead information sheet, p. 392, and Chapter 12, "Of Special Concern: Infants and Children"). The effects of lead on the male reproductive system are not well understood, but the metal is toxic to sperm, and men who

---

Box 21.4 USING SOLVENTS SAFELY

Follow these precautions when using solvents:

• Wear an appropriate, fit-tested respirator when using solvents.
• Do not smoke while using solvents or use them near an open flame.
• Do not use solvents to clean your skin (i.e., paint remover).
• Do not allow children in newly painted rooms.

Box 21.5   MINIMIZING EXPOSURE TO LEAD AND MERCURY

When lead and mercury are used regularly, OSHA standards for these toxins should be enforced. If mercury or lead levels exceed the OSHA standards, employers should provide workers with respirators in accordance with the provisions of the OSHA Respirator Standard.

In areas where lead or mercury are used, also follow these precautions to minimize risk of exposure:

- To avoid accidental ingestion of lead, do not smoke, eat, or chew tobacco in the workplace.
- Wear protective clothing whenever working with lead or mercury.
- Change work clothing daily before going home. To avoid contaminating street clothes, leave all lead- or mercury-contaminated clothes at work, and have them washed at work, separate from street clothes. Also, vacuum lead-impregnated garments with a High Efficiency Particulate Air filter (HEPA) vacuum. This is a special type of vacuum that filters out very small particles so that toxic dust contaminants, such as lead, are not released into the air.
- Do not store work clothes and street clothes in the same locker.

Additional precautions for working with lead:

- Do not open windows or use fans, as breezes can stir up lead dust.
- Do not dry sweep lead-dust-covered floors.

Additional precautions for working with mercury:

- Have available and know how to use a standard mercury clean-up kit, consisting of a mercury binding resin.
- Do not use materials such as carpet in areas where mercury is used (such as dental treatment areas), as carpeting retains mercury and mercury binding resins work well only on smooth surfaces.
- Store mercury-containing materials, such as dental amalgams, in air-tight containers.

have been exposed to minimal amounts have lowered reproductive capacity (see Chapter 11, "Reproductive Effects and Prenatal Exposures").

The Occupational Safety and Health Administration (OSHA) has a standard for airborne lead that factories should not exceed; when the standard is surpassed, employers are required to check their employees' blood levels for lead at least every six months. The OSHA maximum allowable blood concentration for lead is 50 micrograms per 100 milliliters of blood. When a worker's blood levels exceed that standard or if the worker is clinically ill, he or she must avoid exposure to lead at the work site until the lead level declines. Lower levels (30 to 40 micrograms per 100 milliliters of blood) should be of concern to those planning on having children (see Box 21.5).

- *Mercury* was recognized by the ancient Egyp-

Box 21.6 HOW TO TELL IF YOUR JOB IS TOO NOISY

The National Institute of Occupational Safety and Health (NIOSH) recommends that noise levels on the job not exceed 85 decibels over an eight-hour work day to prevent hearing loss. Companies should institute appropriately designed hearing-conservation programs at sites where noise levels consistently exceed 85 decibels. The noise level is too high if:

• You must raise your voice to be heard by your co-workers.
• Your ears ring after leaving work.
• You suffer temporary hearing loss after leaving work.

---

tians as so toxic that they allowed only slaves and convicts in mercury mines. Tragic tales of mercury poisonings pepper medical history, including the 1810 disaster aboard a British ship in which broken vials of mercury caused the death of every bird and animal on board while poisoning 200 sailors and killing three.

Although the Environmental Protection Agency (EPA) banned the use of mercury in indoor paint in 1990, it is still encountered in various chemical forms in pesticide manufacturing, paper mills, electrical component manufacturing, medical instruments, the felt industry, and dentistry (for use in amalgam fillings). Today, the most serious exposures occur in a variety of occupations: gold miners in the Amazon region who use mercury to purify gold-containing material taken from river sediments and persons involved in thermometer repair and manufacturing are at greatest risk (see Box 21.5).

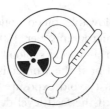

Physical Hazards in the Workplace

There are many work-related physical hazards to health. The most common include the following:

• *Excessive noise* is so prevalent on the job that hearing loss is a major cause of work-related disabilities and significant preventable illness (see Box 21.6). Job-related exposure to *vibration* (often produced at the same time as noise) is responsible for a signficant number of cases of the circulatory ailment called Raynaud's phenomenon, or white finger syndrome (see p. 192).

• *Radiation* encountered on the job can damage health in a number of ways. The highly penetrating rays of ionizing radiation from X rays and radioactive materials are encountered in the health care, construction, and mining industries, as well as in manufacturing and defense industries.

One potential, physical hazard that may be encountered in a number of workplace situations are *electric* and *magnetic fields* (nonionizing radiation). Power lines, residential electrical wiring, and electrical devices generate extra-low-frequency (ELF) fields, the health effects of which are under investigation (see p. 596). Radar, communication equipment, and cooking devices generate microwaves. Furnaces and other industrial sources of heat emit infrared radiation, which is particularly dangerous to the eyes and is the cause of glass-blowers cataract, a clouding of the rear surface of the ocular lens following chronic exposure to high-temperature furnaces. Arc-welding equipment and the sun emit high doses of ultraviolet radiation, which poses a risk of skin cancer or

Table 21.3 ESTIMATED IDEAL TEMPERATURES FOR VARIOUS JOBS

Job	*Temperature (°F)*
Office work	65–72
Light but active industrial work	60–67
Heavy industrial work	55–65

cataracts for welders or workers whose jobs include much outdoor work. (For a complete discussion of radiation, see Chapter 16, "Radiant Energy.")

• *Extremes of heat, convection, and humidity* are aspects of the workplace over which workers usually have little control, but these environmental factors can significantly affect worker safety. Both temperature and humidity affect the rate at which the body can cool itself, and studies indicate a strong correlation between accident rates and workplace temperatures above or below optimum. The optimal conditions for peak performance and comfort depend, in part, on acclimatization to the physical activity level of the job (see Table 21.3).

Higher temperatures prevail in many occupations. Farmers, miners, foundry workers, construction workers, and many factory workers often must work under extremely hot conditions. Most people in good health can

---

Box 21.7   AVOIDING HEAT-RELATED DISORDERS ON THE JOB

There are two heat ailments that workers should be on guard against. The first is *heat exhaustion*, which leaves its victims feeling tired and nauseated. Other symptoms include rapid, shallow breathing; a weak, slow pulse; and moist, clammy, cold skin. In this condition, the blood vessels become very dilated (enlarged), lowering blood pressure to dangerous levels. Victims recover rapidly when brought to a cooler environment and undressed, given fluids to restore water and lost electrolytes, and allowed to rest with head lowered.

The second condition, *heatstroke*, is a medical emergency characterized by a sharp rise in body temperature, confusion, bizarre behavior, and even convulsions. Victims usually do not sweat, and the skin is warm and dry. *Left untreated, this condition can be fatal.* It can be helpful to lower the victim's body temperature with cold water, ice, wet sponges, or cloths. Victims should be taken to a hospital as soon as possible.

To protect yourself from heat ailments on the job:

• Drink a glass of water, fruit juice, or a beverage containing electrolytes (such as sports drinks) every half hour in hot conditions.
• Take rest breaks in the shade or cool area at least every hour or two, as needed.
• If you are new to a job or have been away for more than a few days, ask to be allowed to work half days for the first week in hot conditions. This will allow sufficient time for acclimatization.
• In very hot conditions (like the gold mines in South Africa), employers are required to provide dry-ice vests or similar devices for cooling.

acclimate to a hot workplace within a week to a month.

People who might be prone to health risks in hotter temperatures include those who are new to the environment, are returning from a vacation or a convalescence, have heart disease, are overweight, and are dehydrated (perhaps from drinking alcohol). Anyone working in a hot environment should heed the symptoms that indicate a heat-related disorder is present, including muscle cramps, dizziness, pallor, and cool, moist skin (see Box 21.7).

Cold temperatures present a different set of problems. Since the body's physiological means of acclimating to lower temperatures are limited to constricting blood vessels to conserve heat at the core, proper clothing is essential. (Happily, we do habituate to cold; we become a little less uncomfortable to lower temperatures in time.) Athletes, commercial fishermen, farmers, miners, and meat packers are among the workers who must cope with cold environments. The major health risks from cold are hypothermia, frostnip, frostbite, and trench foot; higher accident and error rates are also common, perhaps from stiffness, a reduction in finger flexibility, and shivering at cold temperatures. Cold sensitivity varies among individuals, but the factors that may predispose to

---

Box 21.8 AVOIDING COLD-RELATED DISORDERS ON THE JOB

There are three ailments of most concern. *Hypothermia*, or low body temperature, is a drop in the body's core temperature. It can occur after exposure to cold air for long periods of time (particularly when the body is damp) or after direct exposure to cold water for as little as a few minutes. Victims of hypothermia may shiver uncontrollably for a while and then become more relaxed. They lose judgment and coordination and eventually become unconscious and die if not taken to safety.

Frostbite and the less serious *frostnip* result when skin and sometimes muscles, usually in the nose and hands and feet, undergo irreversible damage from freezing temperatures. The skin turns gray and hardens. Victims of severe frostbite should be hospitalized for gradual rewarming, a very painful process. If the freezing is not too severe, the tissues will recover, but affected areas can remain painful for years, especially when exposed to cold temperatures. Serious cases of frostbite may result in blistering and, ultimately, amputation of the affected extremities.

To protect yourself from cold-related injuries on the job:

- Wear several layers of clean clothes to provide multiple insulating layers of air. These trap heat more effectively than a single thicker layer does. The internal layer should be cotton, silk, propylene, or other fabric that draws perspiration away from the skin. The external layer of clothing should be windproof.
- Wear insulated boots and layered socks.
- Wear specially designed boots and gloves in arctic conditions.
- In case of frostbite, do not attempt to rewarm until any risk of further cold injury is past. Do not massage or rub affected areas with snow.
- Dry off and replace wet clothing with dry clothes. If available, get into a warm sleeping bag until help arrives.

Box 21.9   SYMPTOMS OF ALTITUDE DISORDERS

Even the most physically fit individual can be affected by altitude sickness, also known as acute mountain sickness. This condition occurs because air at higher altitudes, for example, 6,000 feet, is less pressurized than air at sea level. In other words, while the same amount of oxygen is present for breathing, it isn't as readily available to the lungs and blood, resulting in an accumulation of fluid between the cells in the body. Overall symptoms of altitude sickness include headache, nausea, fatigue, the inability to sleep, and restlessness.

Individuals who ascend above 10,000 feet may be felled by high-altitude pulmonary edema (HAPE) or high-altitude cerebral edema (HACE), two serious, medical emergencies that can be remedied by descending to altitudes below 8,000 feet. HAPE, which results from an accumulation of fluid in the lungs, is characterized by symptoms of initial rapid breathing, which can escalate to breathlessness, and a dry cough, which eventually develops into a pink, frothy sputum. HACE, which results from a fluid accumulation in the brain, can include symptoms of headache, loss of appetite, nausea, lethargy, and vomiting.

Box 21.10   LYME DISEASE

Lyme disease gets its name from a cluster of cases reported in the town of Old Lyme, Connecticut, in 1976. Since the first U.S. cases were reported in the 1970s, the disease has spread to forty-three states. The condition was first called Lyme arthritis, after its most distinctive symptom, but the name was changed to Lyme disease as doctors became aware of the many other problems the infection can cause.

Lyme disease is spread by the deer tick, which is roughly the size and color of a poppy seed. Fortunately, most ticks do not carry the organism that causes Lyme disease (*Borrelia burdorferi*). At least half of all tick bites aren't noticed at all. The bite is often painless, and the tick falls off the body after feeding for twenty-four to forty-eight hours.

Most infections are marked by a rapidly expanding red rash three to four inches across. Common symptoms are aches, pain, fever, chills, swollen glands, headache, lethargy, and general malaise typical of viral diseases such as the flu. In days to weeks after infection, most patients develop muscle and joint pain with redness and swelling affecting the knees and other large joints. Without treatment, 50 percent of Lyme disease patients will develop acute arthritis, which usually affects the knee or other large joints. The arthritis becomes chronic in 10 percent of cases. Fifteen percent of untreated patients develop meningitis or painful nerve conditions within three months of infection.

Antibiotic treatment almost invariably cures the infection. Curing the infection, however, won't reverse any permanent damage that's been done by Lyme disease.

greater sensitivity remain obscure (see Box 21.8).

- *Atmospheric pressure changes* are most likely to affect commercial and recreational divers, caisson workers, airline pilots, and mountain guides and trekkers, who work at or move between atmospheric pressures higher or lower than those found at sea level.

Divers and caisson workers can face serious decompression problems, known as the bends, when they ascend from high-pressure aquatic depths to the normal atmospheric pressure at the water's surface. (Divers can avoid this ailment by rising slowly, in stages, and by breathing a mixture of helium and oxygen rather than nitrogen and oxygen.) Decompression problems in these workers can lead to joint pain and injury, limb weakness, confusion, coma, and even death.

- Airline personnel, although not subject to as extreme pressure changes as divers, are subject to barotrauma and decompression sickness and may experience pain from body cavities such as the sinuses, ears, or dental caries. (You may have experienced minor ear discomfort during an airplane ascent or landing.) The headache caused by barotrauma may be severe and is sometimes a harbinger of neurologic injury (see Box 5.1, p. 89).

Mountain guides and others who work at high altitudes (thus under low atmospheric pressure) may be subject to light-headedness and shortness of breath because the air at those altitudes contains relatively little oxygen. Over time, the body can adjust to these conditions by increasing its production of red blood cells. Particularly rapid ascent above 8,000 feet can lead to acute mountain sickness, characterized by severe headaches and a loss of judgment, or a life-threatening episode of pulmonary or cerebral edema. In these cases, the only treatments are to descend or breathe oxygen. To avoid these consequences, high-altitude workers must acclimatize slowly to higher altitudes before taking on any strenuous tasks (see Box 21.9).

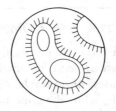

Biological Hazards in the Workplace

Disease-causing biological agents, such as molds, fungi, bacteria, and viruses, share many work environments. There may be higher concentrations of molds and fungi in indoor air, and some studies indicate that these organisms may be responsible for allergic reactions or ailments often attributed to sick-building syndrome (see Chapter 14, "Air"). Harmful organisms may also be present in drinking water or in the water droplets condensed and diffused by air-conditioners. Most notably, air-conditioners with water reservoirs (fungi or bacteria can grow more readily in water) have been linked to outbreaks of Legionnaires' disease, a form of pneumonia (see Box 1.3, p. 27).

Workers who must spend large amounts of time outdoors, including farmers, foresters, contractors, and gardeners, are at greater risk of acquiring diseases spread by biting (i.e., ticks) or stinging insects (i.e., bees), animals, and snakes. Ticks and mosquitoes can spread such debilitating ailments as Lyme disease, Rocky Mountain spotted fever, and viral encephalitis (see Box 21.10). Allergic reactions to a wide variety of plants, particularly poison ivy, the most widespread skin irritant, also are hazards.

Farmers and others who come in direct contact with soil or farm animals also risk infection with a countless array of zoonotic diseases, illnesses resulting from infectious agents that attack humans and animals (rabies is a common example). Zoonotic diseases are linked to a wide variety of bacteria, parasites, and viruses that can infect the body in a myriad of ways: Breathing the air where turkeys are raised, for exam-

Box 21.11   QUESTIONS TO ASK ABOUT HEALTH HAZARDS ON THE JOB

The Hazard Communication Standard requires your employer to designate some-one to answer your questions about potentially dangerous chemicals and other health hazards. Here are some questions you might ask:

- Will/Do I come into contact with harmful or excessive dusts, fumes, gases, vapors, or mists?
- Will/Do I work with radioactive materials, microwaves, or lasers?
- Will I be/Am I exposed to drugs, hormones, molds, parasites, bacteria, animals, or animal products?
- Are some materials apt to cause skin irritation? If so, will/do I need special pro-tective clothing, cleansers, or lotions to clean and protect my skin?
- Are all components of machines in good condition and maintained regularly? Can the equipment being used pass a safety inspection?
- What sort of job and safety instruction do employees receive? How soon after starting work does a new employee receive training?
- Will I be exposed to excessive noise?
- Are there exhaust systems to carry off dangerous dusts and fumes?
- What monitoring systems are available to detect leakage of dangerous chemicals?
- Are there showers and changing rooms, if needed?
- Should I wear gloves, aprons, or other personal protective clothing? What about earplugs or muffs, goggles, a hard hat, or respirator? (If yes to the last, request instructions in proper usage.)
- Can I safely clean my work area of routine dust and spills? How do I do this?
- Are fire precautions in place, including smoke detectors, regular fire drills, and fire extinguishers?
- Is first aid equipment available?
- Where do I find Material Safety Data Sheets on each chemical I work with? (Is someone available to explain technical terms and answer questions?)

If you work in an office, ask these questions:

- Does the air seem stuffy, especially in the midafternoon?
- What office machines are used and what chemicals are used in them?
- Are photocopiers located in separate rooms with additional exhaust ventilation?
- Is smoking permitted? If so, do the smoking areas have dedicated separate venti-lation?
- Is my office located close to other work areas that produce pollutants, such as printing departments, loading docks, or laboratories?
- Are the vents unobstructed by furniture or partitions? Are they operating con-tinuously?
- Are work stations comfortable and adequately lighted?

If your employer cannot or refuses to answer your questions, contact your local health department or OSHA (see Appendix B).

ple, may lead to psittacosis, a pulmonary disease linked to bacteria present in the stools of these birds; or farmers who drink raw milk from cows they raise run the risk of ingesting *Campylobacter* bacteria. Other microorganisms these workers may be exposed to can cause diseases such as toxoplasmosis (which, if contracted by a pregnant woman, can cause miscarriage or brain damage to her developing fetus), tetanus, anthrax, histoplasmosis, tularemia, and tuberculosis.

What is most ironic is that health care workers—those whose jobs are devoted to helping and healing the ill—are often at greatest risk for a myriad of health problems, most notably infection with tuberculosis bacterium, human immune deficiency virus (HIV), and the hepatitis B virus. Laboratory workers and animal handlers also come in contact with a vast array of biological hazards and potential ailments on a daily basis.

Similarly, several studies also have documented an increased risk of infection with cytomegalovirus among child-care workers, many of whom are young women of childbearing age. Infected women can pass the virus to their newborns during delivery. About 10 percent of newborns who demonstrate serious congenital cytomegalovirus infections develop symptoms affecting vision, hearing, and intellectual development.

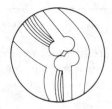

Ergonomic Hazards in the Workplace

The human body can perform awkward, seemingly unnatural movements and endure considerable discomfort, but only for a limited period of time. Almost *one-half* of reported occupational disorders stem from bone, muscle, and connective tissue hazards that strain the body's physical limits and result in inflamed tendons, back pain, displaced vertebrae, nerve damage, and disabling pain in the joints or back.

In recent years, ergonomic specialists focused more attention on injures that result from the repetition of relatively simple motions rather than immense strains. Typical victims of these cumulative trauma disorders include key-punch operators who sit hunched while typing hundreds of characters per minute; slaughterhouse workers, who carve the same cut of beef hour after hour, day after day; checkout clerks, who repeatedly guide groceries over laser scanners; and electronics workers, who spend whole days handling thousands of tiny microchips with various kinds of tweezers (see Chapter 10, "Musculoskeletal Ailments").

MINIMIZING OCCUPATIONAL RISKS

Although references dating back hundreds of years have documented health hazards common to certain professions, occupational safety and medicine emerged as distinct disciplines only in the late nineteenth century. Not until the early twentieth century were the first workers' compensation laws passed in the United States. Since then, many of the advances in workplace safety and health have stemmed from the efforts of unions to protect workers' health and have been buttressed by various state and federal agencies and regulations (see Table 21.4). Recently, industry has become more noticeably active in creating safer, healthier workplaces in the United States, perhaps motivated by workers' compensation liability and costs.

Table 21.4 AGENCIES THAT REGULATE WORKERS' HEALTH

Agency (Department)[a]	Responsibilities
Federal	
National Institute for Occupational Safety and Health (NIOSH) (Centers for Disease Control and Prevention, Department of Health & Human Services)	• Performs occupational safety and health research • Recommends standards to OSHA • Educates and trains occupational safety and health specialists • Provides worker safety and health training and education • Provides grants to research centers • Consults with employers
Mine Safety and Health Administration (Department of Labor)	• Establishes safety standards • Develops programs to ensure compliance • Inspects and enforces safety standards • Provides worker education and training
Occupational Safety and Health Administration (OSHA) (Department of Labor)	• Develops standards for workplace safety and health • Develops programs to ensure compliance • Inspects and enforces standards • Provides worker education and training • Consults with employers • Monitors state programs
Bureau of Labor Statistics (BLS)	• Provides data on work-related illnesses and injuries • Collects data for OSHA logs
Environmental Protection Agency (EPA)	• Provides worker protection for agricultural pesticide workers • Provides worker protection regulations for significant new uses of chemicals
National Institute of Environmental Health Sciences (NIEHS)	• Provides information to regulatory agencies • Conducts the national toxicology program, which tests chemicals for toxicity and carcinogenicity
Department of Transportation	• Establishes safety standards for trucking and shipping industries • Develops programs to ensure compliance • Inspects transportation workplaces and enforces guidelines for health and safety
Private Sector	
National Safe Workplace Institute (NSWI)	• Investigates workplace-related injuries and accidents • Publishes reports and newsletters on workplace safety and health
Bureau of National Affairs	• Publishes and provides subscription services on such topics as the environment, safety, labor laws, and employee relations • Publishes daily reports on business and labor news

[a]See Appendix B for addresses and phone numbers.

Box 21.12   WHAT TO DO WHEN YOU SUSPECT UNSAFE CONDITIONS

If you suspect that environmental agents in your workplace are damaging your health, you have a number of options.

- You can report unsafe and unhealthy working conditions to OSHA by filing a complaint under Section 8f1 of the 1970 Job Safety Act. Federal law protects workers from being fired or discriminated against for being a whistleblower. Contact the Occupational Safety and Health Administration, U.S. Department of Labor, 200 Constitution Avenue, NW, Washington, DC 20216.
- NIOSH publishes many pamphlets with safety information on a wide range of occupations and may also conduct health hazard evaluations or provide technical assistance. Contact the National Institute for Occupational Safety and Health, 4676 Columbia Parkway, Cincinnati, OH 45226, or call the toll-free number 1-800-356-4674.
- The National Safe Workplace Institute, a privately funded watchdog group, publishes a number of reports and a monthly newsletter on workplace safety and health. Contact the National Safe Workplace Institute, 122 S. Michigan Avenue, Suite 1450, Chicago, IL 60603; 312-939-0690.
- You may be able to find a specialized occupational health clinic to consult. New York is one of the first states in the country to have set up a network of such clinics, which are available to all workers in the state and staffed by specialists in occupational medicine. The clinics conduct medical screenings for groups of workers who have worked with dangerous materials, provide diagnoses of people's work-related medical problems, arrange for industrial hygiene evaluations of workplaces, make appropriate referrals to other medical specialists, and help workers make worker's compensation claims. Contact the Occupational Health Clinic Network Office, New York State Department of Health, 2 University Place, Albany, NY 12203; 518-458-6228.

    New Jersey and Massachusetts plan to start similar programs. In all states, you may contact the state department of health for help in locating a specialist in occupational health.
- The Committees on Occupational Safety and Health (COSH) are a group of twenty-five regional organizations dedicated to providing education and training to workers about safety and health on the job. Call them to ask about planning a survey of your workplace. Contact NYCOSH, 275 Seventh Avenue, New York, NY 10001; 212-627-3900. This office will refer you to the COSH location nearest you.

One especially significant regulation, the Hazard Communication Standard (HAZCOM, or the "right to know" law), adopted in 1985, requires all employers except federal and local government agents, which have their own regulations, to do the following:

- Have a written hazard communication program available to employees.
- Label all chemical containers and have a complete inventory of chemicals in the workplace.
- Make Material Safety Data Sheets (MSDS) readily available, with detailed information

about individual chemicals in use in the workplace.

- Train employees to read an MSDS before they work with hazardous chemicals. The general intent of OSHA and the EPA (with respect to hazardous waste workers) is to ensure that people are trained before they work with dangerous chemicals.

By law, if you do not get the information requested about hazardous chemicals within three workdays, you have the right to refuse to work with that substance until the information is provided. (The employer may assign you to different duties but may not, by law, discriminate against you.) (See Box 21.11.)

Protecting Yourself

Despite such laws, it's important for you to take responsibility for protecting yourself and your family from occupational hazards. To do so you should:

- Find out which hazards are present in your occupation. Your employer or union representatives should have written material on the subject. See Box 21.11 for questions to ask your employer.
- Wherever required, wear appropriate and properly fitted personal protective clothing, including ear, eye, and respiratory devices recommended for your job.

- Be attuned to early symptoms related to hazards associated with occupations. Should any arise, see a physician with occupational health training, as well as your personal doctor. See Box 21.12 for information on what to do when you suspect unsafe conditions.
- Keep a historic record of your work experiences and exposures to different chemicals and to the physical and other hazards discussed in this chapter. Many occupation-related diseases do not occur for years after exposure, making such a log invaluable for an accurate diagnosis and determination of their causes.

Protecting Your Family

Hazards at the workplace can take a toll on a worker's family as well. Toxic industrial dusts tainted with lead, asbestos, silica, mercury, and pesticides, for example, can be unknowingly carried home on clothing and hair.

To avoid inadvertently exposing your family to the hazards of your job, if you work with hazardous substances:

- Try to shower at the job site after your shift. Do not wear work clothes home.
- Have your work clothes laundered at the workplace, not at home. (In some industries, disposable clothing is the most practical and safe alternative.)

PROFILES OF HIGH-RISK OCCUPATIONS

Mining

Mining is one of the most dangerous occupations in the world. While the image of miners working in cramped, hot, poorly ventilated underground mines lingers, it has changed to some degree: Today, most miners in the United States extract coal from cramped, ventilated, underground mines or in surface mines that are less dangerous.

In 1990, there were approximately 170,000 miners in the United States. To ensure these workers' health, mines must meet specific requirements, including proper ventilation to prevent explosions and minimize health hazards; the Mine Safety and Health Administration inspects underground mines four times a year and surface mines twice a year. Yet in 1990, over 1,000 citations were issued for mines exceeding dust standards; also, in 1991 more than 500 coal-mining firms were given citations for tampering with the results of dust samples taken to protect coal miners from black lung disease.

Both trauma from accidents or explosions and chemical hazards are common causes of death and disability in this line of work. Although the families of miners most fear the wail of sirens indicating a cave-in or explosion, miners are much more at risk of suffering a slow death from lung disease. Also implicated in a number of mining-related injuries and deaths are the massive machines used in surface mining.

Miners make up the majority of people who die from pneumoconioses, which is a group of occupational diseases. These ailments include coal worker's pneumoconiosis, also known as black lung disease, which accounts for nearly half of the annual deaths due to pneumoconioses caused by exposure to coal dust (in 1988, coal worker's pneumoconiosis claimed over 2,000 lives); silicosis, a potential threat to the more than 1.1 million workers in the United States who are exposed to silica dust, including gold and silver miners, tunnelers, and foundry, granite, and ceramics workers; and asbestosis, one of the most prevalent diseases treated in occupational health clinics that is attributed to exposure to asbestos fibers. (For more information on these diseases, see Chapter 6, "Respiratory Ailments.")

Protecting Miners' Health. In 1969 Congress passed the Federal Coal Mine Health and Safety Act, which established a coal dust standard (since revised downward to the current 2 milligrams per cubic meter) and provided for surveillance of worker health. Under this law, the coal industry is required to use ventilation and other measures, such as spraying water, to control airborne dust levels. The law also established a fund, financed by the coal industry, to support miners disabled by black lung disease and provide a right of entry for the Public Health Service to conduct further research on the health risks of coal mining.

Construction, Renovation, and Related Fields

The construction trades rival mining and agriculture in terms of workplace hazards. Ironworkers, painters, plumbers, welders, laborers, electrical workers, carpenters, heavy-equipment operators, and others face a myriad of chemical and physical health hazards daily, from mechanical trauma to inhalation of asbestos, toxic gases, and dangerous particles.

Trauma from accidents is a common cause of death and disability. Many workers also suffer other trauma-related injuries, from falling objects, tumbles from unsecured ladders and scaffolding, debilitating strains due to lifting heavy objects, and unsafely operating or maintaining machinery. The most common traumas are eye injuries caused by flying particles or by chemical or radiation burns.

Construction workers are often subject to extreme weather and ultraviolet radiation from the sun.

Noise and vibration from the use of power equipment, such as jackhammers and power saws can lead to such health problems as hearing loss and back pain (see Chapter 18, "Noise," and Chapter 10, "Musculoskeletal Ailments").

Ultraviolet radiation emitted by arc-welding equipment can cause skin and eye damage when proper precautions are ignored. (In a Swedish shipyard, 2,000 eye injuries due to such radiation were recorded in one year among 3,000 welders.)

Construction workers must often sit or stand in awkward positions for long periods of time and are prone to ergonomic stresses. For example, welders frequently develop shoulder pain from the static positions they assume. Hand tools, if not properly selected or designed for the job, are another source of potential ergonomic injury. (Ergonomically designed tools are available and best to use whenever possible.)

Workers in these trades routinely are exposed to potent and damaging chemicals, notably the following:

- *Asbestos* is commonly encountered by construction workers when renovating buildings with asbestos insulation; applying and removing asbestos from steam pipes and furnaces; and working with asbestos-insulated shingles, tiles, paint fillers, and wiring. While the EPA banned many uses of asbestos in 1974, it was commonly used in buildings between 1930 and the late 1960s (see Chapter 6, "Respiratory Ailments," and the Asbestos information sheet, p. 365).
- *Lead* is a significant problem for many in the construction trades, especially ironworkers. A blood test for lead every six months is recommended for workers who may be exposed to lead (in selected instances, more often) (see the Lead information sheet, p. 392).
- *Toxic gases* are a particular hazard for workers who join metals through welding, soldering, and brazing, processes that create nitrogen dioxide, ozone, carbon monoxide, and lead oxide. Inhalation of welding gases can cause chronic bronchitis, emphysema, pneumonia, and asthma. (If inhaled in large amounts, as may accumulate in confined spaces, nitrogen dioxide and ozone can cause pulmonary edema, a serious ailment in which the lungs fill with fluid.) Welding also disperses iron oxide dust and toxic fumes that can cause welder's lung, an acute inflammatory response. Similarly, inhalation of zinc oxide fumes released from zinc-containing welding flux can cause the flulike metal fume fever, or the "zinc shakes," characterized by fever cycles followed by severe chills; the condition resolves once exposure to the gases is eliminated.

Protecting Construction Workers' Health

To prevent injuries:

- Wear a hard hat on any construction site.
- Wear hearing protection in high-noise areas.
- Wear protective eye covering when welding or performing any task that may create metal, wood, dust, or sand particles.
- Wear protective footwear (steel-tipped shoes).

- Know the safe operation of machinery and tools.
- Make sure ladders and scaffolding are secure.

When working with chemicals:

- Know what chemicals may be encountered in your job (see Box 21.11).
- Wear whatever protective clothing is recommended.
- Use respirators when painting in enclosed, unventilated spaces or when performing tasks that yield large amounts of dust.
- Handle any amount of asbestos with extreme caution. Even efforts to contain a limited amount of asbestos require use of approved fitted respirators and disposable protective overalls. In all other cases, follow the detailed and extensive guidelines for handling asbestos to avoid contamination. Have a physical examination every year, which includes a spirogram to measure lung capacity. A chest X ray may also be recommended.

When dealing with physical hazards:

- Dress appropriately for the weather. To prevent sun exposure, wear a hat, long sleeves, and sunscreen.
- Use specially designed shields when welding to prevent eye damage from high-intensity light.
- Use ear protection devices when working in a noisy environment, and have an audiometric hearing examination every year.
- Take a ten-minute break every hour when using equipment that generates vibration, such as a jackhammer.
- Wear antivibration gloves when using hand tools that produce vibration.

Erogonomic considerations:

- Use the proper tool for the job and learn its correct operation. Hands are stronger and less vulnerable to injury when wrists are kept straight.

Box 21.13   CHILDREN: A HIGH-RISK GROUP IN AGRICULTURE

One of the most dangerous environments for children is the family farm. Between 1.5 million and 2 million children work in American agriculture, many of them operating dangerous equipment. Each year, many of these children are crushed by combines, suffocated in bins of flowing grain, and exposed to dangerous levels of pesticides. A recent Purdue University study found that 300 children die from farm-related injuries each year. Another 23,500 children are injured on the farm, some of them losing limbs. One in every five agriculture deaths is a child under sixteen.

A safety movement aimed at preventing childhood farm accidents, called Farm Safety Just for Kids, was started in 1987 by an Illinois mother whose child died after falling into a bin of corn as he was helping his stepfather. As a result of the group's efforts, one grain wagon manufacturer is testing a safety grate to keep children from falling into corn loads. Other companies are painting warnings on their equipment. The New York State legislature is considering a bill that would forbid children less than sixteen years old from operating corn pickers.

- Take a ten-minute break every hour when working in cramped, awkward positions.
- Minimize working in awkward positions that require excessive bending, stooping, or working with hands overhead.

Agriculture

The romantic pastoral images of life on the farm quickly fade with the sobering statistics on the physical, biological, and chemical health hazards encountered there. According to the National Safety Council, farming is one of the most dangerous lines of work.

The primary cause of death and disability in agriculture is trauma. Each year, accidents cause approximately 2,000 deaths and 200,000 disabling injuries and, all too often, these deaths involve a child under sixteen (see Box 21.13). Most fatal accidents involve farm machinery; other accidents occur from encounters with kicking and biting farm animals.

Farming accidents often prove more dangerous because farmers usually work alone and in sites not easily accessible to emergency vehicles. Exposure to bacteria in soil and feces can complicate infections.

Recovery from farm injuries is often complicated by the injured farmer's desire to return to work quickly. Most states' workers' compensation laws either exempt agricultural workers or small operations with less than five employees. In addition, many rural communities offer few other employment options, and rehabilitation services are often far away.

There also are numerous chemical hazards on most American farms, including pesticides and toxic gases.

Pesticides (fungicides, insecticides, and pesticides) pose a particular risk. When inhaled, the phenolic compounds in many weed and brush control products can raise body temperatures and cause liver, kidney, and brain damage. Herbicides, such as paraquat, can be absorbed through skin contact, inhalation, and ingestion and can result in lung damage. Defoliants containing chlorophenoxy compounds, such as Agent Orange, are skin irritants and have been known to cause neurological damage. Cotton defoliants and crabgrass killers may contain arsenic, which can cause liver, kidney, and nervous system damage when ingested or absorbed through the skin. Most pesticides are skin irritants as well, and insecticides containing nicotine can damage the nervous system once absorbed through the skin.

Hazardous exposures most often take place when workers return to a sprayed site too soon. Each pesticide has a defined waiting period during which everyone should stay out of the treated area; the period varies, depending on the decomposition of the pesticide and weather conditions. Children, who are even more sensitive to the adverse effects of these chemicals, should stay away even longer (see information sheets on the specific substances).

Toxic gases can overwhelm and kill unsuspecting farm workers. Manure-holding tanks or pits inside livestock containment buildings can accumulate fatal concentrations of gases such as methane or hydrogen sulfide. Freshly filled silos can fill with nitrogen oxide, which, when inhaled, can cause the severe disorder silo filler's disease, characterized by a difficulty in breathing several hours after entering a silo. If not treated, the condition can prove fatal.

Pig farmers are at particular peril because of the practice of confining pigs indoors to keep production prices down and to raise uniformly lean pigs throughout the winter. Strong gases such as ammonia, carbon dioxide, carbon monoxide, methane, and hydrogen sulfide can collect in these pig nurseries. In the 1980s, nineteen American farmers died from inhaling hydrogen sulfide from decomposing pig waste; hydrogen sulfide is as lethal as the hydrogen cyanide used in executions. Along with the gases, the dust of pig dander and particles of feed and dry manure cause an abnormally high incidence of respiratory ailments, ranging from coughs to lung scarring and pneumonia (see Box 6.1, p. 111).

Pig farmers dislike wearing the cumbersome respirators that filter out dust and toxic gases. Effective ventilation in the buildings are too costly for most farmers. (In addition to ear, nose, throat, and lung problems, pig farmers are at risk for broken bones, bites, and other injuries.)

Farmers are the occupational group most dis-abled by respiratory disease, according to NIOSH. For example, farmer's lung, a serious hypersensitivity pneumonitis that affects breathing, is the result of an immunological overreaction to mold spores from hay or grain.

Agriculture workers often are exposed to extremes of temperature and humidity, harmful ultraviolet radiation from sunlight, and excessive noise and vibration from farm tools and machinery. Skin conditions due to exposure to heat and sunlight are particularly prevalent. Farmers have a high rate of hearing loss due to noise exposure and are subject to whole-body vibration while riding on tractors or other farm equipment.

Biological hazards are common, too, including mold spores, grain dust, dried fecal matter, and bacteria, which cause infection and a number of respiratory disorders.

Chronic bronchitis, a generalized inflammation of the lungs, is diagnosed in up to 58 percent of workers in livestock confinement facilities. Smokers are at added risk for bronchitis because grain dust and tobacco act synergistically to damage lung airways.

Farmers are also subject to zoonotic diseases caused by infectious agents that attack humans and animals, such as rabies.

Protecting Agricultural Workers' Health

Preventing injuries:

- Know the correct use and maintenance of equipment.
- Only use newer model tractors that offer roll-over protection (designed not to crush during an accident) and power takeoff shields, which protect against getting caught in a rotating shaft (or install these devices on existing tractors).

When using chemicals and pesticides:

- Follow package directions for mixing and loading pesticides, and do so in well-ventilated areas.

- Wear gloves when using pesticides to avoid skin exposure.
- After pesticide use, take a shower and wash clothing.
- Clean up spills according to package directions.
- Wait the prescribed time period before going into an orchard or field that has been sprayed with pesticides.
- To avoid ingestion of pesticides, do not smoke, eat, or drink when pesticides are being applied.
- When emptying manure pits in poorly ventilated buildings, wear a respirator with an external air supply to prevent breathing deadly gases.
- To prevent silo filler's disease, stay out of and away from silos for at least three days after filling. If you must enter a silo within ten days after filling, run the blower at least a half hour in advance and wear the proper respirator, safety harness, and safety lines with someone standing by on the outside in case of an emergency.

For protection from physical hazards:

- Wear clothing appropriate to the weather. (*Warning:* Loose clothing may be a safety hazard.) Wear hats, long-sleeved shirts, and sunscreens to prevent sun exposure.
- Use a well-padded seat to improve comfort and lessen vibration. Have the seat's condition (shock absorbers and stabilizers) checked annually.
- Adjust seating so that joints are for the most part in neutral positions, neither heavily flexed nor extended.
- Buy the quietest possible farm equipment with sound-tight cabs and improved mufflers. If this is not possible, wear protective hearing devices when operating noisy equipment.
- Take breaks every hour during mower or tractor use to reduce chances of vibration injury.

For protection against biological hazards:

- Wear a NIOSH-approved disposable half-face dust mask inside confined buildings. If you experience symptoms, wear a plastic mask with replaceable filters or a powered respirator.
- Provide appropriate sanitization and health care for animals.
- Get appropriate vaccinations.

Health Care and Laboratory Workers

You may think of hospitals as safe havens, but workers in the health care field are exposed to a wide array of environmental hazards.

The most serious health threat to physicians, nurses, medical technicians, and other health care workers are biological hazards: Physicians and nurses are two to five times more likely than the average person to have been infected with the virus that causes hepatitis B; they are more likely than the average person to be exposed to tuberculosis via respiratory droplets in the air; and they are routinely exposed to chicken pox, measles, and Rubella (German measles). Acquired immune deficiency syndrome (AIDS) is also high on the list of health care workers' concerns, a legitimate anxiety because of the current lack of a cure, although only a few health care professionals have contracted the disease from occupational exposure. AIDS and hepatitis B can only be transmitted through contact with an infected patient's blood or other body fluids.

Needle-stick precautions, infection control procedures, and vaccinations are particularly important for health care workers. The Centers for Disease Control and Prevention have published regulations for the use of barrier devices, such as disposable gowns, gloves, and masks, to protect health care workers from pathogens in blood or other body fluids. They also suggest that health care employers look to new medical technology that can eliminate the presence of needles wherever possible. Proper use of these devices along with periodic tuberculosis skin (cutaneous sensitivity) testing, vaccination against hepatitis B, and immunization against measles, mumps, and rubella are important for health care workers.

Other types of biological agents can present a

health hazard to this group of professionals. Animal fur, dander, saliva, urine, and other body products can cause laboratory animal allergy in some workers. To minimize this danger, the animal care environment should include cages with filters and rooms with exhaust ventilation and no recirculation of air. When such facilities are unavailable, face masks, gowns, and gloves will provide some protection for animal workers.

Health care environments commonly expose workers to chemical hazards, ranging from anesthetic gases to ethylene oxide, anticancer drugs, and formaldehyde.

Anesthetic gases, such as nitrous oxide, are used in dentistry, outpatient surgery, and to a lesser extent in major surgery. Long-term exposure has been shown to impair work performance and cause liver, kidney, and neurological disease and is associated with increased rates of miscarriage among female workers and wives of male workers. Although no longer used, there is some indication from animal studies that the historical anesthetics chloroform and trichloroethylene may be carcinogenic. (Anesthetic gases should be used only in areas with proper ventilation and no recirculation of air. When using these gases, make sure that face masks are well fitted on patients.)

Ethylene oxide, a highly reactive gas used to sterilize medical supplies and equipment that would be damaged by heat sterilization, has been associated with miscarriage, leukemia, and stomach cancer (see Ethylene oxide information sheet, p. 380, and Chapter 11, "Reproductive Effects and Prenatal Exposures"). When using instruments, cloth, or textile material sterilized with ethylene oxide, specialized rooms and equipment are necessary to allow the gas to escape. Government regulations require that air samples be taken every three months in areas where ethylene oxide is in use.

Anticancer drugs used in chemotherapy can harm health care workers if they inhale the drugs (some are in aerosol form) or spill them on their skin. Exposure to anticancer drugs can produce headaches, light-headedness, dizziness, nausea, and skin irritation. Unchecked exposure may result in liver damage, and some studies suggest that pregnant workers who are exposed to the drugs have a higher rate of reproductive problems (see Chapter 11, "Reproductive Effects and Prenatal Exposures"). There is also concern that these drugs may cause cancer at some future date in the workers.

People who work with these drugs should follow the specific precautions and use the equipment specified for them. All such medications should be prepared inside a specifically designed air-flow cabinet that is ventilated to the outside (see Figure 21.2), and gowns, gloves, and masks should be worn when administering them.

Formaldehyde, a highly irritating liquid used in sterilization and embalming and as a means to preserve animal and human tissues in laboratories, can cause eye and skin irritation, chest tightness, headache, and irritability. Mercury,

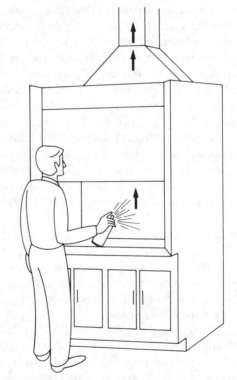

Figure 21.2 A VENTILATED LABORATORY HOOD.

the primary ingredient in amalgam fillings, presents a hazard to dentists and dental workers (see the information sheets for the specific chemicals and their effects).

Musculoskeletal stressors, including the lifting of patients and accidental falls, often lead to back and other musculoskeletal injuries in health care workers; a recent study found nurses and nurses' aides to suffer more back injuries than workers in construction and other occupations thought of as more strenuous. (See Box 10.5, p. 207, and Figure 10.7, pp. 209–211, for information on avoiding back injury.)

Mental stress is a health risk in the health care environment. According to a NIOSH study, seven of the top forty occupations with the highest rates of stress-related disease (high blood pressure, heart disease, and ulcers) were in health care fields (clinical lab technician, health technology technician, licensed practical nurse, nurses' aide, dental assistant, health aide, and registered nurse). In addition, five of the twelve occupations with the highest mental health admissions were in health care (health technology technician, licensed practical nurse, clinical laboratory technician, nurses' aide, and dental assistant).

Shift work, engaged in by 37 percent of health care workers, can require people to change their sleeping and working patterns in a manner contrary to normal biological rhythms, particularly in the case of night shifts. Because shift workers who rotate can adjust about one hour each day, it is best to keep people at each rotation for several weeks rather than constantly switching their schedules.

Nurses experience stress from their typically heavy workload, close contact with dying patients, and the overwhelming emotional needs of patients and their families. Partially in response to stress, physicians suffer substantial problems with drug abuse and suicide.

The biotechnology industry has undergone a remarkable expansion since the early 1970s, when biologists first gained the ability to alter genetic sequences. Work with genetically engineered organisms carries unique genetic and chemical risks, in addition to the standard biological risks faced by traditional health care and medical laboratory workers. Among the chemical risks are:

- *Methotrexate*, a common ingredient in cell-culture media that support the growth of engineered strains of bacteria, is toxic to certain human cells. So routine is its use that many workers tend to ignore its dangers.
- *Trichloroacetic acid, perchloric acid, and hydrazine*, used routinely to extract nucleic acids from cells or tissues, are highly toxic chemicals. For example, exposure to hydrazine fumes can result in a number of symptoms including temporary blindness. Proper ventilation of these chemicals' fumes is important in any biotechnology lab.
- *Acetonitrile*, used in the high-pressure liquid chromatography process, represents the most common cause of acute overexposure in the biotechnology industry. Overexposure by any route can cause central nervous system damage, blood disorders, and cyanide poisoning.
- *Ethidium bromide*, a key reagent for performing DNA sequencing, is a potent carcinogen, eye irritant, and skin sensitizer. Gloves and eye protection are called for whenever this compound is employed.

Protecting Health Care Workers' Health

The following rules will help prevent infection in health care settings:

- Obtain all available preventive vaccinations such as rubella, mumps, tetanus, polio, and hepatitis B.
- Always wear gloves when handling blood or body fluids. If there is a chance of splashing, wear eye and face protection.
- If a patient is diagnosed with tuberculosis, isolation precautions are necessary. Patients must be in private rooms and should be encouraged to wear masks to prevent the spread of the tuberculosis bacilli. Workers also

should wear masks whenever visiting in their rooms.

- Wash your hands before and after contact with each patient.
- Discard needles and sharp instruments in containers specifically designed for their disposal. Never try to recap a syringe.
- If you have a needle-stick injury involving any patient, tell your supervisor, or visit the employee health service immediately. It may be possible to minimize the chance of hepatitis or HIV infection by taking appropriate immunizations and medications.

Truck Driving

Truck drivers, particularly drivers of long-haul tractor trailers, are at risk of accidents (trauma); physical hazards, such as noise and vibration; chemicals, such as fuel emissions; and stress-related factors, including sleep deprivation.

Accidents are a primary cause of occupational death and disability among truck drivers. According to the latest figures from the national Traffic Safety Council, trucks were involved in one-fifth of all vehicle accidents with approximately 10,700 truck drivers and truck occupants fatalities.

Key among the factors that lead to truck driving accidents is a lack of proper vehicle maintenance or training for the drivers, unsafe driving practices (including speeding, tailgating, and erratic lane changes), substance abuse, and driver fatigue. In a telling study of interstate trucking, investigators found that one in four trucks stopped for inspection by the Federal Bureau of Motor Carrier Safety had defective brakes, and one in five drivers had been driving for more nonstop hours than permitted by law. Unfortunately, the monitoring of such unsafe practices by the government is not likely to improve in the near future: The bureau is so understaffed that if trucking companies' equipment and records were checked in sequence, an interstate trucker would probably only be examined once every forty-two years.

Truck drivers are subject to whole-body vibration, excessive noise, and heat stress. For instance, truck cabs vibrate at up to 20 cycles per second (hertz), well above the 5-hertz level that studies indicate can lead to experiencing chest pain, balance problems, and fatigue, and above the 10-hertz level, which can impair visual acuity and general coordination.

Drivers of older trucks often endure noise levels above 85 decibels, the level at which a person is at risk of hearing loss, and are subject to noise intensities above 100 decibels for brief periods of time. High noise levels contribute not only to hearing loss but may also contribute to accident rates from a loss of control on the road or an inability to communicate.

Heat can become a problem for drivers in cabs without air conditioning or who frequently work in a hot environment. Heat stress usually manifests as sweating and increased heart rate. Heat stress can lead to a number of physical disorders, including weakness, fatigue, dizziness, and muscle cramps, and can affect mental skills, leading to accidents (see Box 21.7).

Chemicals, notably carbon monoxide and diesel fumes, endanger the health of truck drivers who are caught in heavy traffic in poorly maintained vehicles with leaks in the ventilation and exhaust systems. These gases cause light-headedness, fatigue, headache, nausea, poor mental performance, and reduced visual acuity.

Mental stress and other psychosocial factors, such as irregular work–rest cycles, sleep deprivation, heavy work loads, delays and schedule shifting, poor family and social relationships, and economic pressures, can lead to substance abuse and contribute to accidents directly and indirectly.

Protecting Truckers' Health

- Make sure the truck is well maintained.
- Follow highway safety rules. Observe speed limits.
- Use a well-padded seat to improve comfort and

lessen vibration. Have the seat's condition (shock absorbers and stabilizers) checked annually.

- Get enough sleep.
- If at all possible, install air-conditioning.
- Adjust seating so that joints are for the most part in neutral positions, neither heavily flexed nor extended.
- Do not use alcohol, amphetamines, and stimulants. Do not abuse caffeine.
- Take ten-minute stretch and rest breaks at least every three hours.

Textile Manufacturing

The mechanics of producing fabric create many health hazards for textile workers. All the fibrous plants from which cloth is made—cotton, flax, hemp—release bits of fibrous dust that linger in the air, thus creating a serious health threat to the millions of textile workers in the United States.

Creating fabric entails a series of complex processes, many of which put the worker in direct contact with numerous chemicals: First, fibers must have their impurities removed. Next, they must be straightened, spun, woven, dyed, finished, and then put through the process of burling, which involves the removal of knots, loose threads, and other particles. Scouring and bleaching are additional procedures used to make fabric.

Exposure to chemicals is common for some workers in this industry. Sulfur dioxide or hydrogen peroxide may be used during the scouring and bleaching processes. Mercerization, a technique used to prevent fabric from shrinking during normal washing, utilizes a sodium hydroxide solution, and creating a durable permanent-press fabric requires formaldehyde-containing resins. Additional chemicals implemented in textile processes include antistatic compounds, antibacterial and antifungal agents, moisture repellents, and chemicals that make a fabric water- and flameproof.

Dyes are also a problem for textile workers. Unusually high rates of bladder cancer occur in textile workers who have been exposed to benzidine-related dyes (benzidine is the chief ingredient in three colors: direct black 38, direct brown 95, and direct blue 6). Liquid benzidine can enter the body directly through the skin; in vapor form, it enters through the lungs. Even low concentrations of benzidine seem capable of causing bladder cancer, leading NIOSH to recommend that use of all benzidine-based dyes be discontinued.

Nearly a million textile workers are exposed to cotton dust, particularly those who operate cotton gins, bale cotton, and card and spin. These workers are most at risk of contracting the respiratory disorder byssinosis, (brown lung) and chronic bronchitis (see Chapter 6, "Respiratory Ailments").

Textile manufacturing is one of the noisiest of all industries. Noise levels commonly exceed the 85-decibel level that NIOSH recommends to limit hearing loss. Hearing loss is common, and excessive noise contributes to accidents and stress.

Protecting Textile Workers' Health

- Industry is required to equip machinery with exhaust systems. Local exhaust systems consist of a hood with a duct directly over the source of the dust.
- Steaming cotton before processing may reduce dust. The cotton industry is researching whether this is feasible.
- Wear a NIOSH-approved respirator when cleaning dye spills and appropriate protective clothing. Always use an appropriate vacuum or wet cloth—no sweeping.
- If you work with potentially hazardous dyes, your company should have a medical surveillance program developed and implemented by a board-certified occupational health physician. In the case of certain dyes, this may include monitoring the urine for early signs of bladder cancer.

Leather Tanning

The process of turning animal skins into leather is a complex alchemy, and many of the chemicals used to perform this task cause health problems. According to 1989 figures from the Bureau of Labor Statistics, leather workers report a high incidence of skin diseases. Also problematic are respiratory ailments, certain types of cancer, injuries, and infectious diseases.

Some of the more common and toxic chemicals encountered in leather tanning are sulfuric acid, chromium sulfate, calcium oxide, ammonia gas, benzidine, and solvents, including dimethylformamide (see information sheets for further information on these chemicals).

- *Sulfuric acid* is often used to treat a hide in its initial preparation stage. Sulfuric acid fumes are extremely irritating to the respiratory tract. People usually cannot stand to be in an area with high concentrations and if they remain, pulmonary edema (fluid in the lungs) can result.
- *Chromium compounds,* in which some hides are soaked during the chrome tanning process, can injure the skin, nasal membranes, and lungs. The lining of the nose can be so damaged that it leads to perforation of the nasal septum. The most serious result of chronic chromium exposure is lung cancer, which often develops more than twenty years after exposure.
- *Ammonia* will burn wet skin and may burn the lungs, leading to pulmonary edema. Most often it is simply irritating, triggering symptoms such as watery eyes. Over time, the cornea may be damaged. Chronic exposure to low levels of ammonia gas can lead to bronchitis and emphysema.
- Dimethylformamide is associated with chemical hepatitis and testicular cancer.

Protecting Leather Workers' Health

- There are OSHA standards that specify the amount of chemicals, such as dimethylformamide, in the air in tanneries that should not be exceeded; if exceeded, the employer must provide respirators in accordance with the provisions of the OSHA Respiratory Protection Standard. Concerning the use of chromium compounds, which are considered to be carcinogenic by NIOSH at any detectable level, wear a respirator.
- When trimming and buffing hides, wear a dust mask.
- Wear gloves, aprons, and boots made from an impermeable material appropriate for the chemicals used.
- Wear goggles when working in areas with lime, ammonia, or sulfuric acid.

Wood and Paper Industries

Wood dust, a ubiquitous component in the wood and paper industries, poses the greatest health hazard to laborers in these lines of work. The most immediate danger of the easily ignited dust is the possibility of fire or explosion from the buildup of large amounts of dust.

Yet this fine powder also can cause other health problems: Skin rashes and irritation of mucous membranes lining the nose and throat are the most common adverse effects of exposure to dusts from pine, oak, and mahogany. Western red cedar dust is a potent allergen for many people, causing asthma, skin rashes, and conjunctivitis (pink eye). The dusts of a few tropical woods, such as satin wood, cause toxic neurological responses: headaches, nausea, vomiting, fatigue, and loss of appetite. Furniture workers and others exposed to wood dust may be prone to nasal and sinus cancer forty years after their first exposure to the dust.

Chemicals are another problem for workers in this industry.

- *Sulfur dioxide,* a colorless gas that is a severe eye, mucous membrane, and skin irritant, was once a ubiquitous hazard in paper mills. The gas principally damages the upper respiratory passages (it causes spasms that prevent the gas from going deeper into the lungs). Many workers may adapt to low levels of the gas, and after a few days do not even notice its odor, but some 10–20 percent of healthy adults are still affected by the chemical and are unable to work in the paper industry.

The long-term effects of working with low concentrations of sulfur dioxide remain unknown, although chronic irritation of the nose and throat and diminished capacity to smell and taste have been documented. Chronic bronchitis and emphysema may result from long-term exposure.

- *Acrylamide*, used in the paper industry as a strengthener, is absorbed through the skin and causes peeling and redness of the hands, numbness of the lower limbs, and excessive sweating of the hands and feet. It can also cause nerve damage, characterized by tingling of the fingers; further exposure may lead to loss of balance and coordination. Symptoms may be reversible if exposure is halted early. NIOSH considers acrylamide a suspected human carcinogen.

Protecting Wood and Paper Industry Workers

- Sand only in areas with ventilation and exhaust controls. Sanding machines should be equipped with hoods, dust collecting bags, or exhaust ducts.
- Clean up wood dusts by wet sweeping. Do not vacuum unless using a machine that does not emit dust in the exhaust.
- Wear safety goggles to prevent eye injury.
- Wear approved respiratory protection gear in dusty areas.
- Wear the appropriate gloves. They can help prevent contact with potentially irritating substances that can lead to skin rashes or allergics.
- Keep dry (wet skin increases allergic reactions). If your clothes get wet, change into dry ones.
- Change clothes regularly. Wear coveralls.

Office Work

The office environment carries a number of inherent risks. Office workers suffer from a wide variety of disorders including eye and neck strain, repetitive motion disorders, stress-related cardiovascular disease, ulcers, back problems, and respiratory ailments.

Office workers inside factories often overlook the fact that they may be exposed to the pollutants common to the plants in question. For example, when OSHA inspected a small Cleveland-based lead smelter in May 1990, office workers *as well as* plant workers had blood lead concentrations above OSHA standards.

Ergonomic factors are significant in office-related ailments. Sedentary work often creates problems of poor physical fitness and flexibility. Everyday aches and pains can usually be blamed on the stationary sitting position office work requires. Serious problems often occur as a result of twisting, flexing, or hunching in ways that put your bones and muscles under additional stress (see Chapter 10, "Musculoskeletal Ailments").

According to a recent NIOSH study, operators of video display terminals have the highest rate of stress-related disorders. In addition, eyestrain can afflict anyone who does a lot of close work, particularly at a video display terminal. Keeping the eyes fixed on one focal point is tiring and can lead to headaches (see Box 10.6, p. 212).

Repetitive motion disorders, such as carpal tunnel syndrome, affect people whose jobs require them to make the same motion repeatedly. Data entry clerks, typically required to make a minimum of 8,000 keystrokes per hour, are particularly vulnerable to carpal tunnel syndrome (see p. 214).

Indoor air pollution, exacerbated by ventilation systems not adding enough fresh air from outside, or overly low humidity in office buildings can also affect workers' health (see Chapter 14, "Air," for a complete discussion).

Plastics, Chemicals, and Rubber Manufacturing

About fifty chemicals produced in the United States are produced in excess of 1 billion pounds annually, and a majority of these substances are used in the plastics and rubber industry. Thousands of workers risk unhealthy chemical exposures during the production of these compounds and from their application in industrial and consumer products.

A few of the more commonly produced chemicals are polyvinyl chloride, benzene, and diisocyanate polymers (polyurethane).

Polyvinyl chloride (PVC) is a widely used plastic, employed in the manufacture of such varied products as tape cassettes, upholstery, toys, and medical equipment. Vinyl chloride monomer is used in the production of PVC and has been linked to a wide variety of health ailments, the mostr significant being liver cancer but also including central nervous system disorders and pulmonary abnormalities. PVC also is compounded with other chemicals, such as talc, to produce a final product. If this additive is inhaled, it can cause numerous health problems: Talc has been linked to many respiratory ills (bronchitis is common among workers exposed to talc).

Workers exposed to vinyl chloride during the manufacturing of PVC may develop acroosteolysis, a syndrome affecting peripheral nerves in the hands and fingers, characterized by numbness, tingling, excessive sensitivity to cold and pain, and dissolution of the bones. Supermarket meat wrappers, who may be exposed to decomposing PVC fumes when PVC meat wrapping is heat-sealed without proper exhaust ventilation, can suffer a syndrome of respiratory irritation. The fumes may also exacerbate workers' asthma.

Benzene, a coal-tar naphtha first produced in the nineteenth century, is one of the most essential and most dangerous chemicals used in the pharmaceutical and petrochemical industries. Chronic exposure to benzene suppresses the body's production of red blood cells, can cause irreversible aplastic anemia, and is linked to two cancers, leukemia and lymphoma.

Benzene is also common in detergent and petroleum product manufacturing. Gasoline in the United States contains up to 2 percent benzene; in Europe, concentrations range from 5 to 16 percent. Although small amounts can be absorbed through the skin, inhalation of vapors is the usual route of exposure. Because benzene is rather sweet smelling, workers may not be aware of unhealthy exposures. Symptoms of high exposures include headache, dizziness, fatigue, loss of appetite, irritability, nervousness, and nosebleed (see Benzene information sheet, p. 366).

Isocyanates, such as those used to make polyurethane, are ingredients in adhesives, tires, boats, car bumpers, insulation, upholstery, wire coating, and various plastic foams. Chronic exposure can cause occupational asthma, which often leads to permanent respiratory impairment. Symptoms of exposure include eye, skin, and throat irritation and shortness of breath. Diisocyanates can also cause neurological symptoms including headache, dizziness, loss of balance, fatigue, and tension. The metabolic breakdown products of certain diisocyanates are carcinogenic in animals (see information sheet, p. 376).

Protecting Plastics and Rubber Workers' Health

- Design engineering processes so that they are totally enclosed to eliminate unnecessary exposures.
- Follow all components of a respiratory protection program and wear specifically designed respirators in areas where you may be exposed to chemicals.
- Wash skin immediately after exposure to chemicals.
- If clothing becomes contaminated with chem-

icals, change immediately and shower to prevent skin exposure and fire hazards.
- When working in confined spaces, follow confined space regulations, including, being appropriately trained, using a buddy system, and using an appropriate air-supplied respirator.
- If you experience shortness of breath or dizziness during work, see your physician. You may need to see a physician board trained in occupational medicine.

Prevention and Environmental Action

CHAPTER 22

The ABCs of Staying Healthy

S taying healthy in a risky environment means more than just sidestepping encounters with noxious agents. It is also a matter of utilizing the home, work, and outdoor environments in ways that *promote* health. This chapter integrates what we know about environmentally based health risks into an overall personal preventive health program.

The first step in prevention is taking stock of personal health risks. This means identifying the factors of "nature and nurture" that may increase our susceptibility to disease and making an educated guess of how large or small a role they are likely to play in our health over the years. Ultimately, we want to develop a rational plan for healthy living, a program that supports wellness rather than disease.

There are many practical measures to take around the home or workplace to minimize environmental hazards. Many of these are highlighted to give you an idea of what preventive steps you can take.

ASSESSING YOUR HEALTH RISKS

How do you go about assessing risks to your health? The question has as many answers as there are individuals. After all, each of us brings "nature"—a genetic heritage—as well as "nurture"—a blend of life-style, biological, and occupational factors. Each of these elements contributes to promoting either well-being or illness.

A Risk Assessment Exercise

Read the following profiles of two different people and try to identify and prioritize their health risks and needs.

Profile 1. A forty-nine-year-old man lives in a major East Coast city. He works long hours as a securities analyst, a job he finds often stressful but satisfying, in a tightly sealed modern high-rise office building. While at work, he suffers from stinging eyes, a runny nose, and headaches and finds that he frequently gets upper respiratory infections.

Mealtimes are irregular; he often eats fast-food lunches and take-out dinners from neighborhood restaurants. He's fifteen pounds overweight, smokes a pack of cigarettes a day, and drinks two or three glasses of wine every night to unwind. He'd like to begin an exercise program but feels he doesn't have enough time in his schedule. Divorced for two years, he lives alone and has been slow to develop new friendships and relationships.

This man lives in an apartment in an older building that contains intact, sealed asbestos insulation. He also owns a small country home in

Bucks County, Pennsylvania, and spends much of his free time there.

His father died of a heart attack at age fifty-three.

Profile 2. A twenty-seven-year-old woman lives with her husband and three-year-old son in a small midwestern town. She started work on the production line in a meat packing house seven months earlier, where she makes the same cut on an animal carcass thousands of times a day. Lately, she has been waking up in pain in the middle of the night with her fist clenched so tight that it takes several minutes for her fingers to open and close normally. Some of her co-workers have had surgery for similar hand disorders and have not yet been able to return to work. She also feels tense much of the time and finds it difficult to relax.

She and her husband, a teacher who is twenty pounds overweight, recently finished renovating the old farmhouse where they live. They did the remodeling work themselves, using a heat gun to remove the paint and restore the natural woodwork. They swept up thoroughly each day after their work.

Recently, a company that represents interstate waste haulers applied to the county commissioner for a permit to open a transfer depot for solid household waste ten miles from her house. She worries that having the depot so close to home might expose her family to hazardous waste.

While this woman and her husband work, her mother, who recently underwent surgery for breast cancer, takes care of their son. Although the child appears to be healthy, he has been complaining lately of stomachaches. The grandmother said that recently the boy has been acting fussy and does not seem interested in any of his usual play activities. Both parents have noticed that he seems slower to express himself than his three-year-old cousins; they have wondered aloud whether his development is normal for a child his age.

The couple enjoys bicycling and preparing meals together to entertain family and friends. They often serve chips and dips as appetizers and barbecue hamburgers and hot dogs outdoors. Winter meals feature meat and potatoes, sometimes with a vegetable, followed by ice cream or cake for dessert.

As a hobby, this woman makes stained glass ornaments and decorative windows, using the kitchen as a studio—a craft she would like to pursue full-time. Not only would working out of the home be professionally satisfying, it would give her more time with her son. For this reason, they have just built a workshop for her in the basement of their home.

Identifying their health risks. These two people have different lives, jobs, health concerns, and priorities. Each have risks based on their family history, life-style, and occupations.

PROFILE 1. You might think that the asbestos in this man's basement is his major risk, but the asbestos is well encapsulated and would only present a threat if airborne. On the other hand, should the encapsulation begin to deteriorate, asbestos would move to the top of his health priority list and demand immediate professional attention.

Because his father died of heart disease, this man's inherited predisposition to developing cardiovascular disease is his most significant health risk. Viewed in this light, his smoking, high-fat diet, weight, and lack of exercise pose the most serious threats to his health, and all of these factors are within his power to modify. Of these threats, smoking stands out as the most damaging behavior, putting him at high risk for developing lung cancer, heart disease, or a chronic respiratory ailment.

His consumption of alcohol not only contributes extra calories to his diet, but if consumed in more than moderate amounts, it can raise his blood pressure, further increasing his risk of heart disease. If he drives after drinking even as few as two beers, he is also endangering both his life and the lives of others.

Although the asbestos at home does not pose a serious health hazard at present, conditions at his place of work may. His office building, with its minimal ventilation and air-tight windows, encourages the buildup of indoor air pollutants. Spending ten to twelve hours a day in this environment could be exposing him to accumulated concentrations of noxious substances, such as tobacco smoke and formaldehyde fumes (see Box 14.7, p. 557). Of course, his frequent smoking in this office only worsens the already marginal air quality.

A less obvious but possibly more significant risk for this man may be found in his weekend house; the cottage is located in an area known to have high concentrations of the radioactive gas radon. If present, radon may pose little risk since this man only spends a few days a month there. However, it bears investigation since this man is also a smoker; exposure to radon combined with smoking tobacco greatly increases the odds for developing lung cancer (see p. 558).

This man's sedentary life-style compounds the problems caused by smoking and being overweight. By lacking a network of social supports, he may be subject to more stress-related disorders. (Researchers have ranked separation and divorce as the second most stressful kind of life event experience after death of a spouse.)

To sum up, his health priorities are the following:

- Stop smoking. This is the single most important change that this man can make toward preventing disease and premature death and maintaining health.
- Eat a balanced, low-fat diet.
- Begin an exercise program under the supervision of his doctor.
- Reduce alcohol consumption to no more than two small glasses of wine a night.
- Ask co-workers if they also suffer the symptoms of sick-building syndrome. Make inquiries about the frequency of maintenance on the building's ventilation system. Install some potted plants in his office to help remove noxious

gases from the air (the spider plant, golden pathos, and philodendron are the most effective air cleaners).
- Take a brisk walk at lunchtime to get fresh air and some exercise.
- Test his country house for radon (see Box 14.8, 559). If testing reveals an unacceptable level of radon gas, he should contact his regional Environmental Protection Agency (EPA) office and request a list of approved remediation contractors.
- Socialize by joining a company athletic team or volunteering his time and expertise to a community group.
- Continue to monitor the asbestos in the basement. If it shows signs of disintegration, then he needs to act. Otherwise, he need not worry about it.

PROFILE 2. This woman and her family have two pressing medical priorities that stem from the environment and demand immediate attention.

First, her son's behavior could be due to lead poisoning and must be investigated right away. There are two likely ways in which the boy has been exposed: Much of the paint on the walls of the family's old farmhouse probably contained lead. When it was removed during renovation using the heat gun, lead fumes were present in the air, and lead-containing dust most likely then settled to coat the floors, windowsills, and the soil just outside the house—places the boy was crawling about as an infant and playing in as a toddler. Cleaning up thoroughly by sweeping did not remove the danger; the lead dust was then dispersed into the air. Since this woman has been making stained glass, using the kitchen as a workshop, lead from the solder used in this craft may have settled on the kitchen surfaces, and the child may have inadvertently ingested it as well. Children are much more vulnerable to the effects of lead, so immediate action is needed (see Lead information sheet, p. 392).

Second, although this woman had worked on the packing line for just a few months, she already has the symptoms of carpal tunnel syndrome, a musculoskeletal disorder that can be caused by repetitive motions, such as the repeated cuts that she makes at work (see Chapter 10, "Musculoskeletal Ailments"). Unless she is able to adjust the way in which she works and treats the condition, it could get progressively worse, ultimately interfering with her ability to continue working at this job.

Although she is only in her late twenties, the fact that her mother has had breast cancer means that she is at increased risk for developing breast cancer. She will need to follow guidelines for early detection of this cancer (see Box 7.4, p. 151).

What about the waste transfer station? Although it bears attention, this potential environmental hazard may be of less serious or immediate concern. She can work through her department of health to ensure that the waste being hauled is monitored to ensure that it is only nonhazardous litter and trash from people's households, not industrial waste.

To summarize her health priorities:

- The family members should be tested for lead poisoning. There are effective treatments to remove the lead from the blood, when it is detected early, before it becomes stored in the body. Because the danger of lead dust exposure remains, remove the boy from the premises during renovations and have the soil around the farmhouse checked for lead as well (see Chapter 12, "Of Special Interest: Infants and Children").
- Request that her production line job be rotated every few hours. If she and co-workers are trained to rotate to other jobs, they may be able to prevent permanent damage to their wrists and hands.
- Devise a long-range plan to launch her handicrafts business full-time. It's unlikely that she'll be able to adapt her job, even with rotations to different positions, to her body. By taking concrete steps toward changing her avocation into a vocation, she can better cope with the physical and mental stress of her as-

sembly line work by knowing that she has a target date for starting a new career.
- Install an exhaust fan that is vented to the outside in her workshop. Some of the crafts materials she works with emit toxic fumes. Keep her son away from her work area, especially since she works with lead solder (See Chapter 20, "Art and Hobbyist Materials").
- Reduce stress. Exercise is an excellent way to cut down on stress. Because she and her husband enjoy similar outdoor activities, such as bicycling, it allows them to spend more time together.
- Reduce the amount of fat and increase the amount of fruits and vegetables in her diet. This family's diet is well above the recommended limit of 30 percent of total daily calories from fat and is seriously deficient in fruits and vegetables (see p. 736).
- Have a physical breast exam each year, self-examine her breasts once a month (see Box 7.4, p. 151), and have a baseline mammogram by age thirty-five if not earlier. After age forty, annual mammograms are recommended. Her risk of breast cancer is also an additional reason for her to avoid a diet high in fats.
- Attend public hearings on the waste transfer depot, and form and voice an opinion. If she feels strongly that the waste depot poses a health hazard to the community, take action (e.g., sign petitions that urge the county not to allow the transfer station.)

Components of Self-Assessment

The types of factors used to assess our major health risks fall into three major categories. First are the factors that are beyond our abilities to control, such elements of nature as gender, age, and inherited susceptibility to disease. Second are factors that are at least partially under individual control, such as where we live, our work, and our recreational activities. Third are the factors entirely within our power to control, including whether we smoke cigarettes, what we eat, whether we drink alcohol, abuse substances, build a network of friends and social supports, and find ways to mitigate the stresses of everyday life.

When the various components within these three broad areas are seen independently, it's apparent that there is much that an individual can do to take preventive action.

Nonmodifiable Risk Factors. Each person's unique genetic makeup—the contribution of nature—is a given. Family history of disease, age, and gender—although these are factors that cannot be altered per se, they can be affected by many of the other modifiable behaviors.

HEREDITY. Many of us know certain families whose members tend to develop cardiovascular disease, become obese, or have a long life or a short one. A single gene, passed on from one generation to another, can lead to disorders such as hypercholesterolemia, an excessive amount of cholesterol in the blood that leads to premature death from heart disease. The role of heredity is not limited to such major illnesses as heart attacks but is also involved in many other disorders as well.

The relative role of genetics and environment has been tested by observations of twins and adoptees. A key study was carried out in Denmark a few years ago with adults whose birth parents were known but who had been adopted early in childhood. Adoptees whose biologic parents had died of cardiovascular disease at a comparatively young age (less than age fifty) were more than four times as likely to die of this cause themselves than would normally be expected. Going one step further, it was found that premature death of biologic parents from *any* natural cause doubled the risk of death in their children, even though the children were raised by other parents. This indicates that genetic influences play a major part in the development of serious illnesses.

Although it may be tempting to point to he-

redity alone as a cause of disease, the situation is not that clear-cut. Geneticists acknowledge that an interaction between genetic and environmental factors can lead to an even greater susceptibility—or resistance—to disease than the influence of genes alone or environment alone.

GENDER. Another determinant of health is gender: There is no question that women live longer than men for reasons that are not fully understood. However, there is much to learn about how and why differences in gender express themselves in different health profiles.

For example, until menopause, women have a very low risk of heart attack, but after the cessation of the menstrual cycle, the risk of heart attack soars. Women over age sixty-five have a higher incidence of high blood pressure and stroke than men. Is this an unmodifiable trait or partly influenced by cultural and environmental factors?

Women may have longevity, but ironically, studies have shown that women with heart disease have been found to receive less aggressive treatment than men with the same condition, perhaps part of the reason women are more likely to die from their heart attacks than men in later years (see Chapter 9, "Heart and Circulatory Ailments").

AGE. Age does not *cause* disease, but for many ailments, the passage of time contributes to the likelihood of their arising. More than one-half of all heart attacks occur in people over age sixty-five, and the progressive accumulation of debris and cholesterol inside the walls of arteries over years can contribute to atherosclerosis, the main cause of coronary heart disease.

The risk of developing cancer also increases with age, both because of longer-term exposures to potential carcinogens, from tobacco smoke, chemicals, and radiation, as well as the cumulative effects of other behaviors that affect the evolution of cancer, such as diet. Some theorists also propose that changes in the immune system that occur with aging may make it harder for the body to eliminate carcinogens or to police and repair damaged cells that can go on to become malignant (see Chapter 7, "Cancer").

Partially Modifiable Risk Factors. Some risk factors can be modified partially but not entirely. These include occupational risks and hazards present in the house or community environment. Although sometimes we are able to act in ways that reduce or eliminate these risks, for instance, moving from a house situated near a leaking waste dump or finding another job, such changes are not always practical or possible.

OCCUPATIONAL ENVIRONMENT. Most of us do our jobs without considering the risks inherent in the workplace. Even when we work at a trade in which physical health hazards are an ever-present danger, such as farming, logging, mining, construction trades, and certain types of manufacturing, it is easy to be lulled into minimizing work-related hazards since we derive such high economic, social, and psychological benefits from work.

In fact, the workplace is one of the most significant sources of exposure to all varieties of health hazards. For example, the EPA cites work-related exposures to chemicals as one of the top environmental risks we confront.

Accidents; biological agents (including viruses, bacteria, molds, and parasites); chemical agents; tasks that strain or injure bones, muscle, or connective tissue; and mental stress are all occupationally related risk factors. Anyone planning a preventive health program must take them into account (See Chapter 21, "The Workplace").

Ironically, we owe a debt to the frequency of toxic exposures on the job. Because people who work with toxins often are exposed every day and for a protracted amount of time, the workplace has served inadvertently as an environmental "laboratory": Many hazardous substances regulated today were first identified because of their effects on workers.

Although risks inherent in the workplace are often begrudgingly accepted as a trade-off for the economic and social benefits of working, it is possible—and often legally required—to minimize many of them. There are state and federal regulations to prevent and make workers aware of occupational hazards.

Unfortunately, employers may have little incentive to implement these regulations, and their enforcement is not guaranteed. It behooves the individual, working in concert with co-workers, unions, and government regulatory agencies, to identify and understand the hazards particular to his or her own worksite and be ready to act vociferously in his or her own behalf to safeguard health. Also, it is always important to follow safety guidelines and to take the appropriate protective measures for a particular task.

For help in assessing occupational health risks, please see Box 21.11 (p. 701). If you believe that your employer is violating safety regulations, you may have recourse to government regulatory agencies such as the Occupational Safety and Health Agency. See Table 21.4, p. 703, and Appendix B for a discussion of these agencies.

COMMUNITIES AND HOUSES. Our houses, backyards, and communities, the places where we spend our leisure time and nonwork activities, are so familiar that it is all too easy to overlook them as potential sources of threats to health. Many of the potential environmental hazards we face are present in these sites.

For example, the integrity and safety of drinking water depends in large measure upon where we live. It directly affects each of us individually if the local water supplies are polluted by chemical wastes from industry or the runoff of pesticides applied to gardens and croplands (see Chapter 13, "Water").

The materials used to build houses, schools, and community buildings can expose us to various environmental hazards: Lead exposure is often due to the type of plumbing in a building (see p. 538). Asbestos was ubiquitously used in insulation materials and is embedded in our walls and around pipes (see p. 125). Indoor air pollutants—carbon monoxide, nitrogen dioxide, formaldehyde, and volatile organic chemicals—can emanate from materials commonly found within the house (see Figure 14.2, pp. 554–555).

Just outside our front door, the air we breathe may contain high levels of ozone or other outdoor air pollutants, particularly if we live in an urban area (see Chapter 14, "Air").

The very soil upon which our houses are built may be a source of trouble. In every state, EPA monitors have found houses with elevated levels of radon, not just in areas thought to be radon "hot spots" (see p. 558). Or, in extreme cases, we may have inadvertently built our communities on soil tainted by highly toxic materials. (See Chapter 15, "Soil," for a discussion of the Love Canal incident).

Whether or not we are subjected to excessive noise from airplanes, burglar alarms in cars, boom box radios, gasoline-powered leaf blowers, jackhammers, modern garbage trucks, or traffic often depends upon the location of our houses (see Chapter 18, "Noise").

Even leisure time activities pursued at home, from gardening to crafts activities, may involve toxic substances that can invite trouble (see Chapter 20, "Art and Hobbyist Materials").

The home and the automobiles that enable us to navigate our communities are a significant site of accidents and a leading cause of death or injury each year in the United States. Vehicle accidents are a much greater hazard to us than most other environmental threats, and their risk rises greatly when people do not wear seat belts or when they ignore the simple rule of never driving after drinking.

Young children are at particularly high risk of home-based accidents (see Chapter 12, "Of Special Concern: Infants and Children") as are the elderly (see Box 10.3, p. 204).

Modifiable Risk Factors. There are a number of important risk factors entirely within our power to modify. These include smoking, diet, abuse of alcohol and other substances, social interactions and networks for support, and how we cope with stress. Increasingly, scientists are finding that these factors exert a great deal of influence on our state of wellness or disease. These modifiable behaviors can play a major role in eliminating or reducing other health risks that are not under our control.

SMOKING. The single most important preventable cause of death in our society is within our control: tobacco smoking.

According to a 1989 report from the surgeon

Box 22.1 FIRE HAZARDS

Fire may be more of a hazard in the home than in the workplace. The main causes of home fires include heating equipment—both furnace and radiator units as well as portable heaters, cooking fires, overheated electrical wires, and smoking. Municipal laws usually require businesses and institutions to have regular fire drills so that occupants of a building are prepared to exit quickly and calmly if necessary. Every household would do well to follow the same practice and to install and regularly test and maintain fire detectors in the home.

Whether a family consist of one person or ten, it is important that everyone knows how to leave the building safely in the event of a fire. Safety experts advise people to plan escape routes including two different exits from each room in the house or apartment. Just as schools and institutions practice regular fire drills, families are advised to have their own regular fire drills and a method for meeting and accounting for each person after they exit the building.

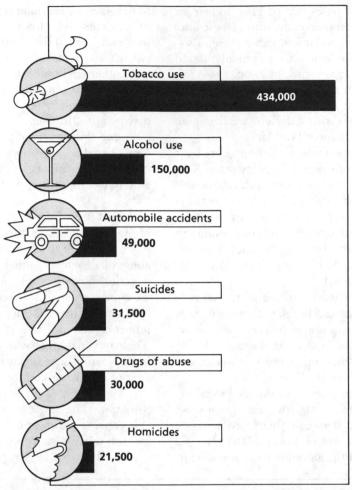

Tobacco use
434,000

Alcohol use
150,000

Automobile accidents
49,000

Suicides
31,500

Drugs of abuse
30,000

Homicides
21,500

Figure 22.1 ANNUAL DEATHS DUE TO TOBACCO SMOKE.

The mortality statistics connected with tobacco use are staggering, however they are expressed. For example, from 1992 through 1996, the American death toll from smoking is expected to exceed the combined death toll of every war in the country's history. As this figure shows, the five next greatest causes of death added together total barely more than one-half the fatalities caused by smoking.

Source: Based on figures from the National Center for Health Statistics.

general's office, one of every six deaths in the United States can be attributed to smoking (see Figure 22.1). All forms of tobacco smoke contain a mixture of thousands of chemical substances, among them nicotine, tar, carbon monoxide, benzene, arsenic, nitrosamines, and polonium-210, a radioactive isotope. This combination is so harmful that tobacco use is linked to an estimated one-third of all cancer deaths, more than all other carcinogens added together.

Everyone around a smoker—spouses, business associates, children—is affected by the smoker's habit. Tobacco smoke released into the environment is the most significant indoor air pollutant (see p. 556). Nearly 85 percent of the smoke that fills a room is secondhand, or passive, smoke, given off by the burning end of a cigarette. Such smoke contains more highly concentrated amounts of tar, nicotine, ammonia, and carbon monoxide than mainstream smoke, as well as greater concentrations of several known carcinogens, including benzo[*a*]pyrene, benzene, and nitrosamine (see Figure 22.2).

Infants and children exposed to cigarette smoke are more likely to develop a host of respiratory ailments, such as bronchitis, ear infections, and colds, and may be at increased risk of cancer (see Chapter 12, "Of Special Concern: Infants and Children").

Birth of the Habit. The typical smoker starts during childhood or adolescence—the marketing studies of at least one cigarette manufacturer refer to teens as "12- to 17-year-old adults." Teenagers who see smoking portrayed as a glamorous activity by peers, elders, films, and cigarette ads are easy prey for the lure of the habit.

Once they start smoking, it is difficult to quit.

Box 22.2   SMOKING FACTS AND FIGURES

- Smoking plays a significant role in the top five leading causes of death in the United States, namely, heart disease, stroke, cancer (particularly of the lung, head, and neck), respiratory disease, and accidents (especially accidental fires).
- According to the 1989 report of the U.S. surgeon general, an estimated 390,000 Americans die each year from diseases caused by smoking.
- The good news is that the prevalence of smoking among adults decreased from 40 percent in 1965 to 28 percent in 1988, according to the U.S. Office of Smoking and Health.
- The bad news is that, at this rate, 22 percent of Americans will still be smokers in the year 2000, and the incidence of smoking among teenage girls in the United States is alarmingly high and on the rise.
- According to federal reports, smoking is more prevalent among minorities, blue-collar workers, and less educated Americans than among the overall population.
- According to the U.S. Office of Smoking and Health, an estimated 52 percent of smokers begin smoking by age eighteen, and 90 percent begin smoking by the time they reach twenty-one.
- As many men have dropped the smoking habit, more women have picked it up. Women tend to be slower to quit smoking than men. As a result, the rate of lung cancer deaths in women is rising to the point that it is surpassing breast cancer as a major cause of death among females.
- Cigarette smoking has also been linked to an increased incidence of heart disease and stroke among women.
- A woman who smokes during pregnancy risks delivering a baby with developmental problems and a low birth weight.
- A person who smokes and is also exposed to such agents as asbestos or radon has a vastly higher risk of developing lung cancer than a smoker who isn't in contact with these substances.
- An estimated 46,000 to 54,500 deaths occur yearly from the effects of secondhand, or passive, smoking, that is, inhaling the smoke of other people.

> ## Box 22.3　HOW TOBACCO HURTS
>
> Tobacco affects organs throughout the body, especially the circulatory and respiratory systems. Although medical scientists have not yet identified the exact components of cigarette smoke that exacerbate cardiovascular disease, studies have implicated nicotine and carbon monoxide as major factors.
>
> With each puff of a cigarette, the lungs take in large amounts of carbon monoxide (a gas that also comes out of the exhaust pipe of an automobile). Carbon monoxide combines with the hemoglobin of red blood cells more readily than does oxygen, reducing the supply of oxygen delivered to the heart, brain, and other organs.
>
> The powerful and addictive substance in cigarette smoke, nicotine, makes the heart beat faster and constricts tiny blood vessels (arterioles) in the body, putting an added strain on the heart. Nicotine appears to increase the chance that platelets will stick to the walls of blood vessels, thus promoting the buildup of cholesterol deposits. When enough material accumulates in a blood vessel leading to the heart, it can totally block the flow of blood and result in a heart attack.
>
> Nicotine causes physical dependency by producing changes in the body's chemistry. It stimulates nerve cells, causing the release of chemicals called neurotransmitters; the cells signal the body to step up the heart rate, to release hormones that affect the central nervous system, and to alter the body's metabolism. This results in the physical "rush" that smokers come to crave.
>
> Cigarette smoke damages the hairlike structures called cilia, which line the respiratory system and help it to ward off infection. Cigarette smoke also can damage the tiny air sacs in the lungs and lead to emphysema as well as other respiratory diseases. Some cigarette tars stick inside the lungs, depositing chemicals that may promote cancer.
>
> Smokeless tobacco is also a health hazard that leads to nicotine addiction and increases the risk of disease or death from mouth and throat cancer.

Teenage and older smokers often don't appreciate the addictive nature of nicotine until they are already hooked (see Box 22.3).

Nicotine, a psychoactive drug, rivals heroin in its ability to addict. Smokers actually must inhale a certain amount of nicotine a day—the level varies from smoker to smoker—in order to stave off the physiological and psychological distress of withdrawal.

The discomfort of withdrawal may be surprisingly inconsequential for some smokers who quit, but others experience anxiety, difficulty concentrating, drowsiness, headaches, or mood swings. These symptoms tend to persist for about a week after quitting, then disappear.

However, the craving for nicotine lingers and may even last for years.

The Benefits of Quitting: Health benefits begin to accrue as soon as a smoker stops smoking. Within five years, the risk of heart disease for an ex-smoker matches that of a nonsmoker. The risk of stroke and peripheral arterial disease of the arms and legs also is reduced. The lungs begin to clear out poisons from the chemicals in cigarette smoke, and the mucus that clogged breathing passages is cleared.

Smokers who give up the habit, even after several years of smoking, reduce their risk of lung cancer to near that of nonsmokers within a decade. According to the 1990 surgeon general's report on the health benefits of smoking cessation, the risk of malignancies of the mouth, larynx, esophagus, pancreas, and bladder also plummets.

Of course, smoker's spouses, children, friends, co-workers, and family members—all of whom were exposed to environmental tobacco smoke—benefit as well.

Stopping Smoking: Most smokers determined to break the habit quit once, fail, and try to quit again. Typically, this quit–fail cycle may repeat itself as many a six or seven times before a smoker succeeds.

Smoking is a behavior that practically takes on a life of its own for smokers. Quitting—and staying off cigarettes—is an ongoing process.

Regardless of the method a smoker chooses to quit, the support of others is key in achieving success. When analyzing controlled studies that looked at the various interventions used to stop smoking, researchers found that success had less to do with method and more to do with consistent reinforcement: The support of family members, personal physicians, co-workers, and acquaintances. A strong nonsmoking message in the home, the workplace, school, and recreational setting provides greater incentive to quit smoking for good.

Box 22.4 WHY SMOKERS SMOKE

People cite many reasons for smoking: relaxation, stimulation, even the feeling of holding a cigarette or a lighter. Generally, however, smokers smoke out of habit. Specific activities or situations usually serve as cues for wanting to have a cigarette. Among these are:

- Waking up.
- Driving to work.
- Finishing a meal.
- Feeling tired.
- Having a drink.
- Watching TV.
- Having sex.
- Reading.
- Drinking coffee.
- Doing a presentation at work.
- Dealing with a job crisis.
- Taking a break.
- Working against a deadline.
- Going to a social gathering.
- Meeting new people.
- Hearing good or bad news.

The first step in quitting smoking is to become aware of the reasons why you smoke. Review the list of triggers listed above and see which ones are applicable to you.

The American Lung Association suggest that smokers find alternatives to smoking as they prepare to quit, such as exercise or a new hobby. Smoking often is a years-long habit, but with patience and determination, it can be broken.

Box 22.5   TIPS TO HELP STOP SMOKING AND STAY A NONSMOKER

- Make the decision to quit and focus on how good it will be to be free of the habit. There are smoking-cessation systems that fit all types of personalities.
- Get in shape physically. Get sufficient rest. Work on eliminating sources of stress in your life.
- Enlist a friend or a co-worker who is an ex-smoker to be on call to offer support when you feel that your resolve to stay off cigarettes is weakening.
- Convince a fellow smoker to quit along with you.
- Set a specific date to quit. Many have kicked the habit during the American Cancer Society's Great American Smokeout held every November.
- Take note of the times you routinely smoke a cigarette. Do something different or change your schedule to avoid taking a cigarette break.
- Remove all reminders of cigarettes—ashtrays, matches, lighters—so that you won't have any visible cues.
- Remind yourself of the negative effects that cigarette smoke has on your body. These include bad breath, discolored teeth, smelly hair, stained fingers, excess phlegm in the lungs and breathing passages, burning eyes, irritation of the throat, a decreased ability to smell and taste, premature facial wrinkles, shortness of breath, greater susceptibility to upper respiratory illnesses such as colds and the flu, and an increased risk of heart disease and cancer.
- Seek out new activities, especially ones that you can "get your hands into," such as cooking, pottery, woodworking, gardening, or knitting.
- Find places where smoking is prohibited, such as theaters, libraries, museums, or stores, and spend some of your free time there.
- Stock up on low-calorie substitutes for cigarettes. Raw vegetables, fruit, and sugarless gum and candies are good choices. When smokers quit, they usually experience an increased appetite for snacks and munching during the first few weeks of living without cigarettes.
- Brush your teeth often and compare the fresh taste in your mouth with your old cigarette breath.
- Avoid activities and people that you associate with smoking, especially during the first few months of quitting.
- Think about your health. Go for a brisk walk and savor the fresh air. Schedule a daily walk or some other exercise into your routine.
- If the craving for a cigarette strikes, do something to distract your attention. Do some deep breathing or stretching exercises or, if possible, take a walk.
- Plan to reward yourself for your accomplishment. Beware of rewarding yourself with food, though, because smokers who quit have a tendency to gain weight.
- Don't cave in to the belief that you can become a part-time smoker after you've quit. Quitters who think that they can smoke just one cigarette soon go back to being full-time smokers.
- Relapse occurs more often than not. If you slip and have a cigarette or start smoking all over again, be reassured that you're not alone. Set a new quit date and better luck next time!

Box 22.6   WEIGHT GAIN AFTER QUITTING

On the average, a person who gives up cigarettes gains from six to eight pounds within five years of quitting. About one in ten will gain up to thirty pounds.

Although researchers aren't certain why weight gain occurs after quitting, it is thought to be partly due to the fact that nicotine speeds up the metabolism, the rate at which the body burns calories. When nicotine is no longer available, the metabolism slows down and more food is converted to fat, resulting in a temporary weight gain.

In addition, smokers who have just quit often eat as a substitute for smoking. Attention to diet and exercise, essential to everyone's health, is especially important for smokers who quit to maintain weight within the desired range.

Despite the modest weight gain that occurs after smokers quit, experts view it as much less of a health problem than smoking.

How Smokers Stop: In 1986, the Office of Smoking and Health conducted the Adult Use of Tobacco Survey to find out how smokers who quit permanently manage to achieve their goal. Researchers from the University of Wisconsin, the Office on Smoking and Health, and the Office of Technology Assessment then analyzed the data in an attempt to determine which methods were successful. The results showed that most smokers who quit on their own used a "cold turkey" approach.

• *Going cold turkey.* Those who have successfully given up smoking often say they simply made the decision to stop smoking and were determined to stick to it. Up to 90 percent of smokers who quit end up doing so on their own, without the help of a formal program. According to the analysis conducted by the Wisconsin and federal researchers, smokers who went cold turkey had twice the success rate of smokers who relied on a formal program.

Of course, this is not the entire story: The success of cold turkey quitters is self-reported, which means there are no reliable figures to back up the reports. Moreover, going cold turkey is often the last resort of a very determined person who may already have attempted to quit several times. Trying, failing, and trying again may be simply part of the process of successfully quitting for many people.

• Smoking-cessation programs: Formal smoking-cessation programs seek to help smokers replace behaviors linked to smoking with nonsmoking activities. A major element of these programs is building group support to help participants assist one another in successfully kicking the habit. All of them rely on similar basic strategies: Set a date to quit; keep a log of every cigarette smoked accompanied by a note that records the smoker's feelings at the time of making the log entry; change routines that are centered around smoking; and, eventually, quit for good. These programs seem to be especially helpful for highly addicted smokers who have had no success in quitting on their own (see Box 22.4).

A number of nonprofit organizations offer smoking-cessation programs including the American Cancer Society, American Lung Association, and the American Heart Association. Community centers, church groups, and commercial services also operate programs. Employees of companies that sponsor wellness programs may be able to sign up for a free series of smoking-cessation sessions. The cost of these programs varies as does their success rate.

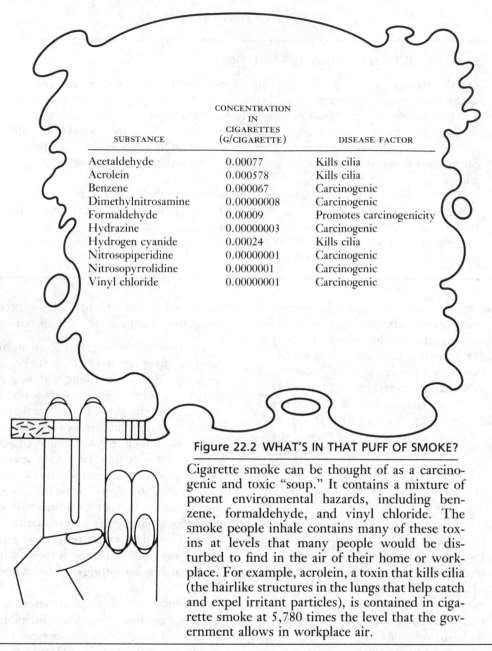

SUBSTANCE	CONCENTRATION IN CIGARETTES (G/CIGARETTE)	DISEASE FACTOR
Acetaldehyde	0.00077	Kills cilia
Acrolein	0.000578	Kills cilia
Benzene	0.000067	Carcinogenic
Dimethylnitrosamine	0.00000008	Carcinogenic
Formaldehyde	0.00009	Promotes carcinogenicity
Hydrazine	0.00000003	Carcinogenic
Hydrogen cyanide	0.00024	Kills cilia
Nitrosopiperidine	0.00000001	Carcinogenic
Nitrosopyrrolidine	0.0000001	Carcinogenic
Vinyl chloride	0.00000001	Carcinogenic

Figure 22.2 WHAT'S IN THAT PUFF OF SMOKE?

Cigarette smoke can be thought of as a carcinogenic and toxic "soup." It contains a mixture of potent environmental hazards, including benzene, formaldehyde, and vinyl chloride. The smoke people inhale contains many of these toxins at levels that many people would be disturbed to find in the air of their home or workplace. For example, acrolein, a toxin that kills cilia (the hairlike structures in the lungs that help catch and expel irritant particles), is contained in cigarette smoke at 5,780 times the level that the government allows in workplace air.

Source: Adapted with permission from *The Well Adult* by Mike Samuels and Nancy Samuels, copyright 1988 by Summit Books (Simon & Schuster), p. 143.

Note: When inquiring about success rates be sure to ask: Is the one-year quit rate based on actual follow-up of the smokers who completed the program or does it represent only the comments of selected participants?

Box 22.5 contains a number of tips that may help a smoker quit.

· *Medications:* Nicotine gum and transdermal nicotine patches can help a smoker quit by providing the addictive nicotine without the other

---

Box 22.7 SUMMARY OF NRC GUIDELINES FOR A HEALTHY DIET

- *Limit fat intake to 30 percent or less of daily calories.* Saturated fats, which include butter, cheese, and meat drippings, should account for 10 percent or less of this amount. Some health experts now suggest aiming for an even lower fat intake and advise that a more prudent dietary goal should be 20 to 25 percent of calories from fat.
- *Limit cholesterol to not more than 300 milligrams a day.* Animal products such as meat, dairy products, egg yolks, and fatty foods are major sources of cholesterol.
- *Eat six or more servings of breads, cereals, and legumes daily.* Preferably, the breads and cereals should be whole grains.
- *Consume five servings a day of fruits and vegetables.* Emphasize green and yellow vegetables and citrus fruits.
- *Limit protein intake to moderate levels.* Eat no more than two three-ounce servings a day of lean red meat, poultry, or fish. Seek out alternative protein sources that are comparatively low in fat, such as yogurt, cottage cheese, tofu, and legumes. (The body can extract additional protein from legumes when eaten in combination with grains, such as rice.)
- *Maintain an appropriate body weight.* Balance food intake and physical activity.
- *Limit or eliminate alcohol consumption.* If you do choose to drink, limit consumption to the equivalent of one ounce of pure alcohol a day. In practical terms, that translates into no more than two twelve-ounce bottles of beer, two small glasses of wine, or two average-size cocktails.
- *Dietary supplements are not recommended.* Eat a variety of foods to obtain the vitamins and minerals your body needs. Avoid taking any supplements that exceed the recommended daily allowances.
- *Limit salt intake.* Consume no more than 2,400 milligrams a day (an amount that roughly corresponds to about a teaspoonful of salt). Cut down on salt in food preparation and do not add it to foods at the table. Because many processed foods (lunch meats, canned and commercially prepared soups, fast foods, frozen meals, and cheese) contain large amounts of sodium, consume these sparingly.
- *Maintain an adequate calcium intake.* This measure is crucial to preventing osteoporosis later in life (see p. 200). When using dairy products (a good source of calcium), choose low-fat or nonfat products. Incorporate nondairy sources (see Table 10.1, p. 200) in the diet as well.

---

toxic chemicals contained in cigarettes. These prescription medications help smokers avoid withdrawal symptoms, but the dependency on nicotine is simply transferred to the gum or the patch; the user must still be weaned from the device. Some smokers report that, despite wearing the patch, another behavior associated with smoking remains: the desire to have something in their mouths (see Box 22.6).

Clonidine, an antihypertensive medication, is sometimes prescribed to smokers trying to quit. Clonidine has been used in the treatment of mild alcohol and drug withdrawal symptoms, but its effectiveness in combating nicotine withdrawal symptoms remains unclear.

DIET. For decades, the major national voluntary health organizations and expert committees have stressed the role of diet as a controllable risk factor in preventing disease. Diet plays a significant role in the risk of developing such chronic health problems as heart disease, cancer, stroke, and diabetes.

The first group to focus on a specific disease with respect to diet was the American Heart Association. In the early 1960s, they proposed a set of dietary guidelines to reduce the risk of cardiovascular disease. Since then, the American Heart Association has periodically revised its recommendations to reflect new scientific findings (see Chapter 9, "Heart and Circulatory Ailments"). Similarly, in the late 1970s, the National Cancer Institute issued dietary guidelines to reduce the risk of cancer, and they regularly revise these recommendations as well. Other bodies of experts have issued dietary recommendations as well. All told, the recommendations are remarkably consistent, and in 1989, they were summarized in the recommendations set forth by the National Research Council (NRC) in its major report on diet and health (see Box 22.7).

We recommend adopting the following guidelines issued by the council: lower the amount of fat in the diet, maintain an appropriate body weight, consume a sufficient amount of complex carbohydrates and fiber, exercise regularly, avoid or consume only a moderate amount of alcohol, and eat a variety of foods.

The two most crucial elements of a simple and safe diet are balance and variety. Most of us have a limited culinary repertoire; we cook perhaps just eight to ten basic meals on a regular basis, week after week. To implement the dietary recommendations suggested by the council, changing our diets becomes a matter of making certain those ten routinely prepared menus are healthy ones and then expanding their number. In this case, variety is not just the spice of life: It increases the odds that we will ingest proper nutrients and helps limit our exposure to toxic substances that might be present in one particular foodstuff.

Nutritionists have used a number of visual guides to represent the components of a healthy diet. Many of us grew up with the "basic four," created in the 1950s, which represented the diet as a pie chart made up of four food groups. Each group—grains, dairy products, proteins, and fruits and vegetables—was allotted an equal share of the pie; a person ate a "good diet" if they ate at least one food from each group at every meal.

Thinking on diet and nutrition has changed significantly. As the dangers of eating a diet too high in fat and cholesterol were discovered and benefits of eating more grains, fruits, and vegetables came to light, the emphasis placed on each food group shifted. A healthful diet is now described as containing proportionately greater amounts of breads, grains, and cereals, as well as fruits and vegetables, than meats and dairy products. Fats and sugars should be greatly reduced to a minimal amount.

To help illustrate the new thinking, in 1992 the U.S. Department of Agriculture released the "eating right pyramid," a diagram that depicts the various food groups in terms of their recommended proportion in the diet rather than assigning them equal shares of a pie chart (see Figure 22.3 and Box 22.8).

To help you determine what constitutes a healthful diet, we have coordinated the NRC guidelines with the eating right pyramid.

Fats and Sugar. The eating right pyramid places fats, oils, and sweets in a category all their own accompanied by the admonition "use sparingly." A high intake of fat of *any* kind is a major cause of obesity and has been associated with colon and breast cancer, and there is a substantial and growing body of evidence that saturated fat and cholesterol in the diet contribute to heart and blood vessel disease as well as stroke.

The typical American diet still derives about 37 percent of its calories from fat, substantially higher than the upper limit of 30 percent suggested by the NRC. (Some health experts be-

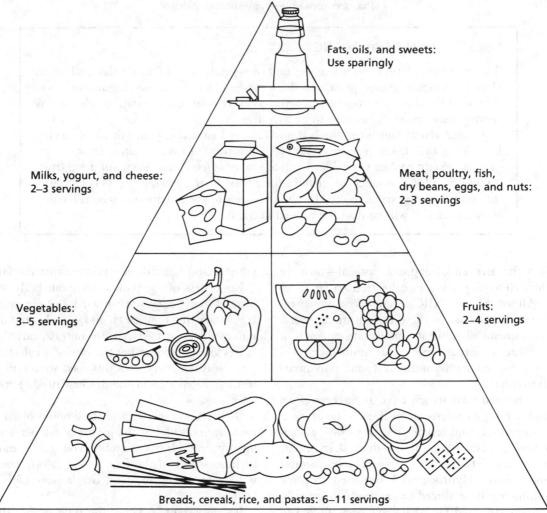

Fats, oils, and sweets:
Use sparingly

Milks, yogurt, and cheese:
2–3 servings

Meat, poultry, fish,
dry beans, eggs, and nuts:
2–3 servings

Vegetables:
3–5 servings

Fruits:
2–4 servings

Breads, cereals, rice, and pastas: 6–11 servings

Figure 22.3 THE EATING RIGHT PYRAMID.

Unlike the "basic four" model of nutrition, which assigned equal value to meats, dairy products, fruits and vegetables, and grains, the eating right pyramid emphasizes the proportions in which we should eat from these groups. The proportions are intended to plan a diet that provides enough nutrients, without too much of the fat that is contained in the foods near the top of the pyramid. (It's worth noting, however, that beans, included with meats, eggs, and nuts because they are high in protein, are generally very *low* in fat.) It is essential that your meals not only fit the numeric ranges but also stay true to the *proportions* suggested by the pyramid: The lower a food group's position, the greater the role it should play in your diet overall. In other words, you could, while staying in the ranges given, eat more meat and dairy servings than fruit and vegetable servings on a given day (three plus three as opposed to three plus two); however, *in the long run*, you should eat more servings of vegetables and fruits than of meats and dairy products. (The size of what constitutes a serving may be smaller than you think. For example, a three-ounce serving of meat is about the size of a deck of playing cards. For a further explanation, see Box 22.8.)

Source: U.S. Department of Agriculture.

Box 22.8   WHAT'S A SERVING?

The recommendation to eat five servings of vegetables and fruits a day and six to eleven servings of grains, pasta, and rice may seem like a lot of food to eat every day. Although the dietary recommendations constantly refer to a serving, the size of this serving may remain a mystery to many eaters.

To help clarify this issue, the National Cancer Institute explains that one serving is 1 slice of bread, 1 cup cereal or ½ cup cooked pasta or rice, ½ cup of fruit, ¾ cup of juice, ½ cup cooked vegetable, 1 cup of a leafy vegetable, or ¼ cup of dried fruit. Typically, a food producer or manufacturer may see the serving size as being quite different from the size expected by the consumer or the nutritionist who is looking to assure that it will contain the needed nutrients.

---

lieve that an even lower goal is optimal—no more than 20 to 25 percent of calories from fat.)

Although the NRC recommendations referred to total fat in the diet, nutrition experts recommend dividing it equally among each of the three different types of fat in the diet: saturated fat, monounsaturated fat, and polyunsaturated fat.

Saturated fats, which have an adverse effect on the body's cholesterol level, are solid at room temperature and come mostly from animal sources, including meat, poultry, dairy products, chocolate, lard, and tropical oils (coconut and palm). (Hydrogenated fats used in some commercially produced baked goods are actually hidden saturated fats that have been altered to make the product last longer.)

Monounsaturated fats, those contained in avocados; almonds; olives; and peanut, canola, and cottonseed oils, are believed to help protect the blood vessels by lowering low-density-lipoprotein cholesterol (see Chapter 9, "Heart and Circulatory Ailments").

Polyunsaturated fats, such as corn, soybean, sunflower, and safflower oils; mayonnaise; and fish oils, work to lower cholesterol in the bloodstream. Fish oils that contain eicosapentaenoic acid (EPA) and docosahexaenoic acid (DHA), better known as omega-3 fatty acids, which are found in such fish as mackerel,

salmon, and bluefish, are polyunsaturated fats.

Regardless of the type of fat, your body still metabolizes it at the rate of 9 calories per gram. If you take in too much fat and don't burn it up, it immediately gets stored. In contrast, carbohydrates are metabolized at the rate of 4 calories a gram and the body uses this food source more readily. Keep this in mind when making food selections.

(Note: You can estimate the amount of fat in food by multiplying the grams of fat per serving by nine. If the number you get is more than one-third of the food's total calorie count per serving, then the food is relatively high in fat.)

It's important to know the type of fats that occur in food and be able to determine how much fat you're actually getting in a serving. It helps to carefully read food labels. Labels are now increasingly informative as the U.S. Food and Drug Administration has revised its standards regarding what information manufacturers are required to place on labels and what wording they are allowed to use.

Because it's difficult to tally the amount of fat in each meal, an alternate way of beating the dietary fat trap is to identify the main sources of fat in your diet and then consciously cut back by substituting low-fat versions of foods for those laden with fat. Table 22.1 provides some low-

Table 22.1 TRIMMING DIETARY FAT

	High-Fat Foods	*Low-Fat Alternatives*
Fruits and vegetables	• Vegetables cooked with fat (including french fries) or in cream • Avocados and olives • Coconuts and coconut milk • Cream of vegetable soups	• Any fruits and vegetables (except for avocados, coconuts, and olives) eaten raw or cooked without fats, cream, or heavy sauces • Fruit and vegetable juice • Soups without cream
Breads, grains, and cereals	• French toast, pancakes, and waffles • Granola • Fried rice • Stuffed pasta • Snack chips, snack crackers, and popcorn popped in oil and topped with butter or margarine	• Breads, rolls, bagels, and English muffins • Cereals except granola • Plain rice • Plain pasta or noodles • Saltines, soda crackers, pretzels, and popcorn (preferably air-popped) without butter or margarine
Dairy products	• Cream • Hard and whole-milk cheeses • Whole milk and buttermilk • Sour cream and creamed cottage cheese • Ice cream • Cream cheese • Whipped cream	• Non-dairy creamer • Low-fat or imitation cheeses • 2% milk, skim milk, and buttermilk • Low- or nonfat yogurt and cottage cheese • Ice milk and frozen yogurt • Neufchatel cheese and "light" cream cheese (use sparingly) • Nondairy whipped topping
Meats and protein foods	• Hamburger • Untrimmed meat and meats with skin • Sausages, hot dogs, and high-fat lunch meats, such as salami and bologna • Bacon • Fried meats, including fish and poultry • Fish packed in oil • Egg yolks or whole eggs • Peanut butter, nuts, and seeds	• Legumes • Skinless light poultry meat • Well-trimmed red meats • Soybean products (tofu, soy protein, and tempeh) • Low-fat and pressed lunch meats and chicken or turkey lunch meats • Water-packed tuna • Fish prepared without fat • Egg whites • Chestnuts
Sweets and beverages	• Baked sweets, including cakes and pastries	• Angel food cake • Low-fat cookies and cakes

(continued)

Table 22.1 TRIMMING DIETARY FAT (continued)

	High-Fat Foods	Low-Fat Alternatives
	• Chocolate, caramel, and fudge • Creamy beverages, including cappuccino and mixed drinks made with cream or ice cream	• Carob • Hard candy • Coffee, tea, and soft drinks • Alcoholic drinks made without cream • Sorbet
Oils and sauces	• Cooking oils and fats • Cream sauces • Regular salad dressing • Gravy • Butter • Mayonnaise (substitute yogurt)	• Low-calorie salad dressing • Vegetable-based or low-fat sauces or purees • Margarine or reduced-fat spreads (use sparingly)

and moderate-fat alternatives to higher-fat food items.

Sugar is a simple carbohydrate that provides calories but no nutrients. The complex carbohydrates, which include cereal grains and potatoes, are excellent sources of nutrients. Both the simple and the complex carbohydrates contain the same amount of calories—4 per gram. Although sugar is not associated directly with heart disease or cancer, sugary foods often contain substantial amounts of fat. Using large amounts of sugar does promote tooth decay and may encourage excess weight gain, which can have other adverse health effects.

Protein: Protein in the diet comes from such sources as eggs, milk, legumes (including beans and peas), nuts, meat, fish, poultry, and cheese. These items are depicted in the pyramid as foods that should be limited to two to three servings a day.

Although regular consumption of protein is essential to good nutrition, too much protein may increase the risk of certain diseases. People commonly believe that consuming extra protein will make them stronger, but excess protein that is not used as an energy source by the body is converted to fat. Excess amounts of protein also force the kidneys to work harder to rid the body of additional metabolic waste products.

Protein derived from meat often delivers excess saturated fat, which is believed to be a major contributor to heart disease, cancer, and stroke. Small amounts of meat—not more than 3 ounces daily—are sufficient to meet the nutritional needs of most people.

There are numerous excellent alternative sources of protein, many of which are relatively low in fat, such as legumes, egg whites, yogurt, cottage cheese, tofu, low-fat and nonfat dairy products, and food combinations, such as rice and beans.

Vegetables and Fruits: The eating right pyramid guidelines recommend an intake of five servings of fruits and vegetables, approximately twice that of meats or dairy products. Essential to a healthful eating plan, vegetables and fruits are sources of soluble and insoluble fiber and provide substances that appear to prevent the development of cancer. Most Americans' diets are notoriously deficient in vegetables and fruits: a National Cancer Institute study found that only about 9 percent of American adults eat the recommended five servings a day, and 11 percent admitted to skipping this food group entirely.

The National Cancer Institute scientists concluded that about 25 percent of the U.S. population increase their risk of developing cancer as a result of eating *too little* produce. (The weight of scientific evidence says that not including a substantial amount of vegetables and fruits in the diet poses a far greater risk to health than the relative theoretical risk of developing cancer from exposure to pesticide residues in produce. See p. 150.)

Soluble fiber in vegetables apparently helps to lower blood levels of cholesterol and glucose, which, if elevated, can exacerbate the symptoms of diabetes.

Insoluble fiber, which is often compared to a sponge because it absorbs many times its weight in water in the intestine, helps digested food to pass through the intestines more quickly. Although there is no conclusive evidence that fiber protects against colon cancer, it is thought that the quicker waste passes through the bowels, the less time the intestinal wall is exposed to carcinogens. A high-fiber diet also reduces the risk of constipation.

Retinoids, found in fruits and vegetables, are substances that have been shown in laboratory studies to lower the incidence of some cancers, including cancers of the esophagus, pancreas, colon, skin, breast, and bladder. Beta-carotene, a form of vitamin A present in the yellow, orange, and red fruits and vegetables, seems to be an important retinoid that helps protect against cancer. Retinoids are thought to be cancer-protective compounds because they can neutralize the effect of unstable free-radical molecules, which are produced by chemical activity in the body and appear to set the stage for damage to the cell. Sources of these retinoids include carrots, spinach, tomatoes, apricots, cantaloupes, and peaches.

Scientific evidence points to cruciferous vegetables (so named because their flowers are cross shaped), including broccoli, brussels sprouts, cabbage, cauliflower, and kohlrabi, as a source of cancer-protective substances. Broccoli has been shown to be rich in sulforaphane, a chemical that has been associated with improving cancer resistance in laboratory animals.

Carbohydrates. The lion's share of the eating right pyramid is claimed by the carbohydrates, the food group that provides the most basic form of nutrition to people around the world. Six to eleven servings daily of cereals, breads, rice, and pasta are recommended.

The body derives most of its energy from the complex carbohydrates, a collective term for cereal grains, potatoes, pasta, rice, barley, beans, and corn. The carbohydrate family also includes the simple carbohydrates, such as the sugars, a source of quick energy. Complex whole-grain carbohydrates (as opposed to refined carbohydrate products), such as whole-grain cereals, breads and pastas, provide fiber as well as an economical and healthful source of energy.

ALCOHOL. The dietary role that alcohol plays in health is a scientific question that remains unanswered. Moderate alcohol consumption in the form of red wine has been much studied for its possible protective effect on the heart. Some studies have suggested that a moderate amount of alcohol may increase the level of high-density-lipoprotein, or "good," cholesterol in the blood (see Chapter 9, "Heart and Circulatory Ailments," for a discussion of cholesterol types).

Moderate alcohol consumption has been associated with an increased risk of breast cancer, although the results of studies have been mixed. The risk of cancer of the esophagus seems to multiply when alcohol is used in combination with cigarettes.

There is no recommended standard for a safe level of alcohol consumption. For those who drink alcohol, the Committee on Diet and Health of the NRC recommends that intake be limited to 1 ounce of pure alcohol per day. The allowable amount of a given drink thus depends on its alcohol percentage (the proof number of a liquor is equivalent to twice its percentage of alcohol). One ounce of 80-proof whiskey, for example, contains 40 percent alcohol, or 0.4

ounces of pure alcohol; thus, not more than 2.5 ounces of the 80-proof whiskey should be consumed per day. Likewise, a typical brand of beer will contain 10 to 12 percent alcohol, and therefore not more than two 12-oz. cans should be consumed daily to limit intake to 1 ounce of pure alcohol. (See Chapter 11, "Reproductive Effects and Prenatal Exposures," for information on alcohol consumption during pregnancy.)

According to government studies, one in ten Americans has a problem involving alcohol abuse. Alcohol is responsible for an estimated 100,000 deaths each year. Heavy alcohol consumption can produce physical dependency and toxic effects in the liver and other organs. It also is a major contributing factor to accidents in the car, home, and workplace, as well as in boating accidents that result in drownings.

Alcoholism is a complex illness, and an individual may need extensive help to control it. One factor that has been explored in the development of alcoholism is heredity, as many alcohol abusers have a parent who similarly abused the substance. A study of the children of alcohol abusers who were adopted and reared in nonalcoholic households found that these children have a higher incidence of alcoholism than those of nonalcoholic parents. However, the extent of genetic influence is still unclear, as there also are people who are genetically predisposed and yet have not had problems with alcoholism. (See Box 22.9 to help determine if you or a loved one has an alcohol abuse problem.)

A study funded by the Department of Veterans Affairs of male alcoholics who quit drinking found that those who achieved sobriety were able to reduce their death rate to a level as low as that of nonalcoholics over the ensuing one to eleven years. However, alcoholics often themselves present an obstacle to treatment; typically an alcoholic will deny that he or she has a drinking problem. Many businesses refer their employees to employee assistance programs (EAPs) when managers begin to notice a pattern of reduced productivity, absenteeism, or drinking on the job. Treatment for alcoholism can range from psychiatric therapy to participation in Alcoholics Anonymous programs to hospitalization for the problem.

PHYSICAL FITNESS: The more scientists and exercise physiologists study fitness, the more benefits appear to result from it. People who are fit have stronger and more flexible muscles, a stronger heart, and stronger lungs and bones.

Regular physical activity reduces the risk of coronary disease, lowers blood pressure and cholesterol levels, and helps to attain and maintain optimal weight. Exercise can ward off or reverse some of the loss of muscle mass and strength that inevitably comes with aging and is a potent protector against the thinning of bones that leads to osteoporosis. Exercise, which has long been a part of the prescription for controlling adult-onset diabetes, may actually help prevent this form of diabetes that affects people over forty.

Regular exercise (at least three times a week for a minimum of twenty minutes per session, depending on the type of activity) may confer mental health benefits as well. People who exercise regularly often report greater feelings of self-esteem and fewer feelings of mild to moderate depression and anxiety. However, actual studies of the relationship between exercise and mood have not been able to prove that workouts are psychologically beneficial.

According to recent studies, regular physical activity may also help ward off cancer. A 1991 study of 17,148 male Harvard alumni who were followed as a part of long-time survey indicated that those who engaged in moderate physical activity (burning 1,000 calories per week) were up to 50 percent less likely to develop colon cancer. The protective effect was apparent in alumni who regularly and consistently exercised over an eleven- to fifteen-year period.

Scientists cannot not explain why physical activity seems to help combat cancer. One theory suggests that exercise helps food to pass through the intestines more quickly, thus reducing the amount of contact between any toxic materials or carcinogens and the wall of the colon.

Box 22.9   ARE YOU OR A LOVED ONE ABUSING ALCOHOL?

If you answer yes to several of the following questions, you may have a serious problem with alcohol.

- Do you try to get someone to buy liquor for you because you are ashamed to buy it yourself?
- Do you buy liquor at different places so no one will know how much you purchase?
- Do you hide empties and dispose of them secretly?
- Do you reward yourself with a little drinking bout after working hard?
- Do you have blackouts (loss of memory) after drinking?
- Do you ever telephone the host of a party the next day and ask if you hurt anyone's feelings or made a fool out of yourself?
- Do you take an extra drink or two before leaving for a party even if you know liquor will be served?
- Do you often wonder if anyone knows how much you drink?
- Do you feel wittier or more charming when you are drinking?
- Do you feel panicky when faced with nondrinking days?
- Do you invent social occasions for drinking?
- Do you ever carry liquor around with you?
- Do you become defensive when someone mentions your drinking?
- Do you become irritated if unexpected guests reduce your liquor supply?
- Do you drink when under pressure or after an argument?
- Do you drive even though you've been drinking but feel certain you are in complete control?

Source: Alcoholics Anonymous.

Components of Physical Fitness: There are four basic elements of physical fitness and, ideally, you should develop a physical fitness program that builds on all four of them:

- *Cardiorespiratory endurance.* The most basic element of the four, cardiorespiratory endurance is the ability of the heart and lungs to sustain moderately strenuous activity over an extended period of time. Activities that fit the criteria for this category are usually referred to as aerobic, which means that the body uses oxygen to produce the energy required to do the activity. Brisk walking, running, bicycling, rowing, and cross-country skiing are forms of aerobic exercise.

- *Muscular strength.* Strength is defined as the force exerted by a muscle or a group of muscles in the effort of a single contraction. Although strength training, or resistance training, has long been associated with muscular bodybuilders, fitness experts now recommend that people work out with weight machines or free weights, such as dumbbells, in addition to doing aerobic exercise. Ninety-year-olds who took part in an eight-week weight-training program were found to build muscle mass, a physical benefit that gave them greater mobility.

- *Muscular endurance.* If you have poor endurance, the ability of a muscle to repeat an activity several times without feeling sore or

PREVENTION AND ENVIRONMENTAL ACTION

tired, it can effectively reduce your muscle strength. For instance, it may not be difficult to lift one heavy grocery bag, but to lift twelve heavy bags and then be asked to hold one for several minutes may be extremely taxing for someone who has not built any muscle endurance. Workouts with weight machines or free weights or doing calisthenics such as sit-ups or push-ups can increase endurance. The key to achieving endurance is to gradually increase the number of repetitions with each series of exercises.

• *Muscular flexibility*. Flexible muscles, those that can move a joint through its full normal span of motion, are essential for protection against joint and muscle injuries.

How Much Exercise Is Enough? You needn't become a track star or triathlete to become fit or enjoy the health benefits of exercise. The basic requirement for people of all ages is to burn 1,000 calories a week doing moderate exercise and physical activity. (Burning just 150 calories a day during leisure time activity will decrease

cardiovascular risk, whereas expending up to 400 calories a day will reduce heart disease risks even further.)

Moderate activity covers a considerable range. You can burn body fat washing windows, gardening, or walking a dog, as well as by doing aerobics or mountain biking. Some examples of calorie-burning exercises are listed in Table 22.2

Another benefit of moderate activity: You are more likely to stick with it in the long run. The vigorous calisthenics and strenuous workouts that characterized the fitness boom was more of a fitness bust. Less than 10 percent of American adults actually stuck to this grueling regimen. The key is to make activity a natural part of your life-style.

The American College of Sports Medicine, the body of experts that sets standards for exercise recommendations, revised its exercise guidelines in 1990 to include strength training in addition to aerobic exercise (see Box 22.10). Cardiovascular endurance remains the most basic element of physical fitness, but muscle endurance, flexibility, and strength are important as well.

Table 22.2 GOING FOR THE CALORIE BURN

	Calories expended per half hour	
Activity	Man (175 lb.)	Woman (140 lb.)
Sitting	50	40
Standing	60	48
Light activity	150	120
Cleaning house		
Typing/filing		
Playing golf		
Strolling		
Moderate activity	230	185
Brisk walking (3.5 mph)		
Gardening		
Bicycling (5.5 mph)		
Dancing		
Strenuous exercise	365	290
Jogging (a 9-min. mile)		
Swimming		
Very strenuous exercise	460	370
Running (a 7-min. mile)		
Racquetball		
Skiing		

Box 22.10   GUIDELINES FOR PHYSICAL ACTIVITY

The American College of Sports Medicine recommends the following:

- Engage in physical activity three to five days a week.
- Exercise at an intensity that either raises the heart rate to 60 to 90 percent of its maximum or raises the body's oxygen intake to 50 to 85 percent of its maximum.
- Perform aerobic activity continuously for twenty to sixty minutes. If the activity is of low or moderate intensity, it is recommended that the nonathletic adult continue it for a longer period of time.
- Perform activities that use the large muscle groups as part of a continuous rhythmic motion. Walking, hiking, running, and stair climbing are among these.
- Add resistance training of a moderate intensity at least twice a week to exercise the major muscle groups of the body. Perform a minimum of eight to ten exercises and repeat each one eight to twelve times.
- Be sure to warm up before and cool down just after exercise.

Newcomers to weight training are advised to take some kind of instruction before jumping into this activity. An experienced teacher can show beginners how to warm up, breathe properly, plan balanced workouts, and properly use weights of an appropriate size without injury.

Although individuals are urged not to overexert themselves, the American College of Sports Medicine reminds exercisers that participation at lower levels of aerobic activity than those recommended may not produce enough oxygen utilization for cardiovascular fitness. On the other hand, some researchers have found that people whose energy expenditure is slightly below the aerobic threshold, as low as 40 to 50 percent of maximal heart rate, have shown a reduced risk of heart disease and death. These lower levels of activity still may be sufficient to help reduce the risk of various chronic degenerative diseases, such as osteoporosis and diabetes.

Caveat: Anyone who has been physically inactive or is over forty-five years of age and wants to begin an exercise program is advised to get a doctor's approval first.

Exercise and Pollution: It has not yet been determined whether exercising in polluted air causes permanent lung damage, but it definitely can produce a variety of irritating symptoms. Symptoms such as difficulty in breathing, pain or tightness in the chest and windpipe, coughing, and throat irritation occur in aerobic exercisers, particularly when ozone levels are high or if the exerciser already suffers from a respiratory condition. Headaches are not uncommon, probably as a result of breathing in excess carbon monoxide, which interferes with the blood's ability to transport and deliver oxygen.

Respiratory specialists advise people who exercise outdoors to be mindful of the time of day, time of year, and prevailing weather conditions. It is best to plan exercise early in the morning, especially in urban areas: Air quality worsens during heavy traffic times, such as the morning or late afternoon rush hours, and ozone levels tend to be lower in the morning and peak by midafternoon (ozone levels are highest on hot, sunny days). The American Lung Association recommends that people who have asthma or other chronic lung diseases limit strenuous outdoor exercise on days when air quality is poor. Check with local radio or television stations for announcements of days when the air

Box 22.11   SYMPTOMS OF STRESS

The symptoms of stress include a variety of physical and mental symptoms, including:

• Loss of appetite.	• Difficulty sleeping.
• Fatigue.	• Frequent illness.
• Irritability.	• Digestive upset.
• Inability to concentrate.	• Headaches
• Muscle spasms.	• Craving for sweets.
• Teeth grinding.	• Jaw clenching.
• Increased drinking.	• Decrease in self-esteem.

It's important to keep in mind that many of these symptoms also may signal the presence of an organic illness, so seek medical attention if any of them persist.

quality index exceeds 100, the level deemed "unhealthy" (see Chapter 14, "Air").

STRESS. Scientists have long debated the complex manner in which the mind affects the body and vice versa, and the controversies are reflected in the area of stress research. There is still no consensus of a definition for stress, although there is some agreement on the stress reaction.

A typical stress reaction is the body's physical, chemical, and mental response to frightening, threatening, or even exciting circumstances, all of which are called *stressors*. The immediate physiological reaction is a series of biochemical responses termed the *fight-or-flight response*, in which the brain and nervous system stimulate the production of hormones; these trigger or step up the action of some body

Box 22.12   STRESS AND WORK

Researchers who have studied work and stress have organized all occupations into four basic categories. *Active jobs* are highly demanding but call for high-level and challenging problem solving. *Low-strain jobs* are those that allow workers to set their own pace in regard to hours and schedules. *Passive jobs* make little demand on a worker's skills or abilities. *High-strain jobs* demand that a worker perform but offer no latitude for decision making. Here are some examples of these jobs:

Active jobs	*Low-strain jobs*
Executive	Carpenter
Engineer	Repairperson
Bank officer	Naturalist

Passive jobs	*High-strain jobs*
Janitor	Waiter/waitress
Sales clerk	Nurse's aide
Security guard	Gas-station attendant

Box 22.13 MODIFYING STRESS

Equally important to stress modification is the ability to modify anger.

- Learn to recognize your own hostile thoughts and the anger of those you may be confronting.
- Notice how you instinctively react to situations, both your mental and physical reactions.
- Empathize with the person who is angry or who provoked your anger.
- Listen with care to what an angry person says to you.
- When you respond, don't yell and perpetuate your anger.
- Focus on the issue at hand without bringing up incidental or unrelated problems.

Among the things you can do to modify stress in your life are the following:

- *Seek a sense of control in your work.* Strive to achieve your personal goals. Going back to school to finish a college degree or learning a new skill or sport can offer a high degree of satisfaction.
- *Begin a fitness program.* Exercise counteracts stress by relaxing muscles and sending more oxygen to body tissues, including the brain.
- *Establish friendships.* Researchers who study social support have found that people who have someone they can turn to are more likely to survive heart attacks and less likely to become sick than people who are socially isolated.
- *Learn a relaxation technique and use it regularly.* Meditation, progressive deep-muscle relaxation, biofeedback, and guided imagery techniques are among the most popular. There are many self-help books and cassettes available on relaxation.

---

systems while decreasing the activity of others.

Stressors need not be negative situations. Although the death of a loved one, being physically injured, or losing one's job will almost universally be experienced as negative and stressful, many situations that challenge a person to grow personally are also stressors. Taking a new job, facing a deadline, or beginning a marriage can all lead to symptoms typical of stress.

When stress is short-term, the body apparently can return to its harmonious state fairly quickly, but prolonged exposure to stress is thought to increase the risk of illness or disease. Many diseases, from asthma and migraine headaches to eczema and ulcers, have been linked with stress.

Stress and control: How we cope with situations varies greatly between individuals, and a key factor appears to be the element of control. People who have some say over their circumstances appear to be less negatively affected by them.

Some researchers believe that having a high degree of personal control over your work can provide positive stressors: "High-control" jobs have not been associated with a higher risk of illness, such as heart attack. Jobs that are highly demanding but offer workers little latitude for making decisions—and therefore no control over their work—may carry a higher risk of heart attack (see Box 22.12).

Stress and hostility: The type A personality theory emerged in the 1960s as the possible answer to why people who are aggressive, competitive, ambitious, driven, and hostile seemed to have an increased risk of heart attack. After decades of acceptance, new research has shown that the only one of these personality traits that appears to have an effect on health is hostility.

Studies suggest that hostility, or chronic anger, can induce the condition ischemia, in which an insufficient amount of blood (and hence oxygen) reaches the heart muscle. Other studies have associated people with high hostility levels with a higher rate of heart attacks and premature death.

Some experts question whether people who are chronically angry have a cynical attitude about adopting good health habits. Whatever the case, managing hostility as well as stress seems to be crucial for people who are chronically angry to promote a healthful environment (see Box 22.13).

A PROGRAM FOR STAYING HEALTHY

The basic recommendations for creating an individual overall program for staying healthy stress two concepts intrinsic to good health: balance and moderation. Of course, before launching into your personal program, it helps to first define your goals. Then, using the basic concepts of healthful dietary and exercise programs in conjunction with the numerous self-help and preventive guidelines discussed throughout this book, you can design your own program for meeting your goals.

It is important to remember, though, that the details of a preventive health program and whether or not you follow healthful habits are in your hands. You decide what you eat, whether and how much you exercise, and how you manage anger and cope with stress.

In putting together your program, you will be faced with a wealth of information on health, fitness, and wellness. It is important to evaluate it carefully before selecting it as part of your daily activities (see Box 22.14). Look at the reliability of the source; a health program that sounds too good to be true probably is just that. Finally, remember to be patient with yourself. Change doesn't occur overnight.

Health Checkups

Adopting a healthier life-style certainly does not mean you will never need to see a doctor again, but it may shift the motivation for your meetings from disease to health promotion. Although the annual physical was the stanchion of previous generations of preventive health care, this is no longer the case. Instead of giving the same battery of tests to everyone, the U.S. Preventive Services Task Force, an independent group of

---

Box 22.14   SOURCES OF RELIABLE INFORMATION

It is essential to critically evaluate health information. Always question the source of health information. Reliable sources include major national health organizations, such as the American Heart Association, American Cancer Society, and American Lung Association; government agencies, such as the Consumer Affairs Office of the Food and Drug Administration, regional offices of the Environmental Protection Agency, and cooperative extension services of the U.S. Department of Agriculture; and respected consumer groups, such as Consumers Union and the Center for Science in the Public Interest. Other such groups are listed in Appendices A and B.

Box 22.15   TESTS EVERYONE NEEDS

The American College of Physicians and the Blue Cross and Blue Shield Association have adopted preventive screening guidelines that are consistent with those published by the U.S. Preventive Services Task Force. They recommend that healthy adults should be tested as follows:

- *Hypertension.* Adults with blood pressure below 140/85 should be screened every one or two years. Yearly testing is advised for people with a diastolic pressure (the lower second number) between 85 and 89 (people with a diastolic reading 90 or above should consult their physician); black people, and people with other risk factors for hypertension.
- *Coronary artery disease.* Cholesterol tests are recommended at least once in early adulthood and then at five-year-intervals until the age of seventy. Electrocardiograms and exercise stress tests are not recommended as routine tests.
- *Breast cancer.* An annual clinical breast exam is recommended in women without symptoms beginning at age forty. Annual mammography screening is recommended in women fifty and older who have no symptoms of breast disease. Women with a family history of breast cancer are advised to receive annual mammograms when they reach the age of forty.
- *Cervical cancer.* A Pap smear is recommended every three years beginning at the age of twenty. Women with an increased risk of cervical cancer should receive this test every two years.
- *Colorectal cancer.* People age fifty and over should receive an annual fecal occult blood test. They should be screened with sigmoidoscopy every three to five years.
- *Lung cancer.* Screening is not recommended in adults without symptoms.
- *Diabetes mellitus.* All pregnant women should receive screening for gestational diabetes. It is not recommended that healthy adults without symptoms receive screening tests.
- *Osteoporosis.* Routine screening of women who are perimenopausal (about to enter menopause) for osteoporosis is not recommended, except for women at particular risk, including those who have had early menopause, have a low calcium intake, or have had their ovaries removed.

---

physicians convened by the government, recommends that preventive service and tests be tailored to each individual, taking into consideration a person's age, heredity, personal risk factors, and symptoms.

In addition, some screening tests are deemed essential and should be routinely given, even in the absence of symptoms, because they can detect the presence of disease in its earliest stages,

a time most amenable to treatment or cure. These tests include blood pressure tests, blood cholesterol measurements, and mammography (see Box 22.15).

There is no one screening program that suits everyone. How often and how early these tests are given to you may be influenced by your genetic makeup, including whether or not you have a family history of a certain disease; occu-

---

Box 22.16   HOW TO CHANGE A BEHAVIOR

Before beginning a program designed to change any health behavior, it's important to first have a clear definition of what you consider to be a successful result. One way to do this is to write out a statement that says: "I will be successful if I do _____ ."

Your idea of success could be to stop smoking, exercise for half an hour three times a week, lose a certain amount of excess weight, cut down on alcohol intake, or socialize more.

In some cases, your goals of behavioral change may conflict, so a wise course is to concentrate on one thing at a time and achieve success gradually. There are six basic points to follow in working toward changing a health habit on your own:

1. Assess the risks you face from continuing this habit.
2. Identify the problem areas and set priorities.
3. Pick only one or a few goals to work with at one time.
4. Set reasonable, attainable short-term goals and more far-reaching goals for the long haul.
5. Plan to reward yourself when you meet your goals.
6. Be prepared for relapses. They are a part of the process.
7. Incorporate your new healthy behavior into your life-style. Use your success in one area as a model for making other positive life-style changes.

Keep these points in mind as you assemble your list of habits that call for change. The principles apply to all areas of life-style choices.

---

pation; and activities. Much of this information is conveyed by you to your physician during the initial medical exam when he or she discusses your medical history. You can greatly assist this process if you bring to your physician's attention the unique circumstances that exist in your life—your home, your hobbies, leisure time activities, your occupation, including potential worksite exposures of which you are aware—and giving the most complete medical history possible for yourself and your family.

Achieving Personal Change

Effecting change in the external environment, whether by lobbying for reductions in pollution or deciding to recycle more of one's household waste, *is* helpful and often crucial to personal and community health. However, when we think in terms of the impact of the environment on our health, it is important not to neglect an essential factor in the equation—our own bodies. Effecting personal change is more immediately within our ability and can often dramatically affect our susceptibility and vulnerability to agents that exist beyond our control. Box 22.16 outlines some of the basic points for working toward changing a health habit.

Changing habits is not easy and rarely happens overnight, although a crisis sometimes jolts a person into awareness of the need for change and precipitates the process. Most often, such a realization comes more slowly, building to a crescendo that is experienced as "just" deciding to change and doing it. It remains true, however, that it is easier to achieve change by setting specific, attainable goals that give you a feeling of accomplishment when you reach them; in short, it helps to have a plan.

CHAPTER 23

Taking Action in the Face of Uncertainties

T hree weeks before the 1992 spring semester at the State University of New York at New Paltz was scheduled to begin, a car struck a utility pole and caused a power surge. The resulting explosion in electrical transformers spewed forth a toxic cloud of polychlorinated biphenyls (PCBs), a probable carcinogen banned by the U.S. Environmental Protection Agency (EPA) in 1977. (PCBs were used as insulating fluids and are still present in older equipment, particularly electrical equipment.)

The toxic gas affected five buildings on campus. In the transformer room of one building, levels of PCBs as much as 3,200 times the level considered safe under state guidelines were measured (although samples from other areas of the other buildings showed no contamination). Twenty-two people directly exposed to PCB-contaminated smoke were treated at nearby hospitals and released. The 990 students who had remained on campus between semesters were immediately evacuated from their dormitories, abandoning potentially contaminated clothes, books, and other possessions. The start of classes

was postponed while the cleanup operation got underway.

Neither the officials who ordered the evacuation nor the students who were evacuated knew precisely what risks the students faced nor how great those risks were; our knowledge of PCBs' health effects is riddled with uncertainties. The chemical is known to cause chloracne, a skin disease; weakness; and fever (see Chapter 8, "Immunological Alterations"). In animals, PCBs have been shown to induce tumors of the liver, pituitary gland, gastrointestinal tract, and blood (lymphomas), but in humans, studies to date have not shown the same definitive link. Therefore, the EPA classifies them as a "probable" human carcinogen. (See Table 23.1 for a description of the EPA classification of carcinogens.)

However, once the accident had occurred, the people involved were not in a position to debate academic or clinical nuances. They had a clear and immediate choice to make—to evacuate or not to evacuate. To ensure the greatest safety, they chose the former.

SAFEGUARDING HEALTH IN SPITE OF UNCERTAINTIES

Many of us may never be directly involved in a toxic accident, as the students at New Paltz were. Nonetheless, all of us have to take certain

actions—whether choosing a home site, selecting foods to eat, or writing laws and regulations—armed with only incomplete knowledge

Table 23.1 EPA CLASSIFICATION OF CARCINOGENS

Group	Category	Scientific Evidence
A	Human carcinogen	Sufficient human epidemiologic studies
B1	Probable human carcinogen (high probability)	Limited human epidemiologic studies; sufficient evidence in animals
B2	Probable human carcinogen (low probability)	Inadequate human epidemiologic studies; sufficient evidence in animals
C	Possible human carcinogen	Absence of human data; limited evidence in animals
D	Not classified	Inadequate evidence in animals
E	No evidence of carcinogenicity for humans	At least two negative animal studies *or* one negative animal and one negative human study

Note: Over 400 chemicals have been shown to cause cancer in animals; only 30 have been *proven* as causing cancer in humans.

about environmental risks. When it comes to protecting human life or our natural resources—air, food, water, the diversity of species on the planet, or the ozone layer above it—we do not have the option of waiting until the gray areas of scientific uncertainty resolve into black and white.

Governmental Action: The History

The need to act on incomplete information applies not only to reactive situations, such as evacuating from a possibly dangerous area, but also to the proactive steps, such as government regulations, which endeavor to prevent such crises from arising in the first place. The L-tryptophan incident recounted earlier (see p. 32) is a telling reminder of what can happen when such safeguards are not in place. Because L-tryptophan is sold as a nutritional supplement rather than as a drug or a foodstuff, it still does not fall under the province of any regulatory agency.

In the past, public health scandals or disasters have prompted expansions in health regulations. For example, the Food, Drug and Cosmetic Act, which regulates food purity today, is an outgrowth of the Pure Food and Drug and the Meat Inspection acts, passed in 1906 after Americans were outraged by such published exposés as Upton Sinclair's novel *The Jungle*, a slashing indictment of the appalling conditions in Chicago's stockyards. (see Chapter 17, "Food Safety"). Since then, the Food and Drug Administration, which enforces the act, has based many of its regulatory decisions on proving the *safety* of products before approving them (rather than only proving them unsafe before banning them), so as to err on the side of caution.

In fact, the history of environmental legislation is a record of our efforts to act despite the unknowns. For example, when the landmark Walsh–Healy Act of 1936 was passed (see p. 32), the government called upon major industrial and health care providers to establish exposure guidelines for many toxic chemicals despite the lack of conclusive proof of what level of exposure to the substances was dangerous. The consensus levels established with this act have provided the basis for subsequent laws protecting worker health, such as the 1970 Occupational Safety and Health Act, which now also covers a broader range of hazards, such as noise.

The EPA, formed in 1970 to oversee the safety and quality of our environment, enforces the fourteen major environmental laws that have been passed by Congress, administers Superfund legislation to clean up toxic and abandoned waste sites, and awards grants for local sewage treatment plants.

Box 23.1   MAJOR ENVIRONMENTAL LAWS

The Federal Insecticide, Fungicide, and Rodenticide Act, 1947 (FIFRA)
(amended 1972, 1975, 1978, and 1980)

The Insecticide, Fungicide, and Rodenticide Act requires all pesticides to be labeled and registered and requires the EPA to determine whether a given pesticide causes unreasonable adverse effects on the environment or health. The act provides for inspections of pesticides and requires manufacturers to inform the EPA of the contents and environmental and health effects of each pesticide.

The Federal Clean Air Act, 1955
(Amended 1960, 1970, 1977, and 1990)

Originally passed to mandate federal assistance to the states in reducing pollution, this law has been strengthened to require the federal government, states, and cities to meet a wide range of ambient air-pollution standards. Among its current requirements: reducing 1988-level chlorofluorocarbon emissions 20 percent by 1993 and 50 percent by 1999; industry efforts to reduce emissions of 189 toxic chemicals by 90 percent between 1995 and 2003, using the best available technology; the sale of at least 150,000 electric vehicles in California by 1996; the introduction of cleaner-burning gasoline in American cities with the dirtiest air; and emissions reductions for diesel truck, automobiles, and coal-burning power plants.

The National Environmental Policy Act, 1970.

The Environmental Policy Act established the federal policy of implementing all programs in a manner as environmentally sound as feasible. It required all federal agencies proposing activities with possible environmental consequences to complete an environmental impact statement, detailing the likely environmental effects of the action.

The Clean Water Act, 1972
(Amended 1977 and 1987)

The Clean Water Act seeks to regulate, in cooperation with the states, the quality of all American surface waters. The act provides for technical and financial assis-

(continued)

Box 23.1   MAJOR ENVIRONMENTAL LAWS (*continued*)

tance to the states in developing water-treatment facilities and emissions-control technologies. Its requirements include designation of all bodies of water by states as to their uses (e.g., drinking water, fishing, and recreation) and restricting pollution to levels appropriate to those uses; secondary treatment of waste water by all municipal sewage systems; restrictions on landfill and dredging in wetlands; and limits on industrial discharges into water.

The Safe Drinking Water Act, 1974
(Amended 1977 and 1986)

The Safe Drinking Water Act requires the EPA to regulate levels of pollutants in public drinking-water systems and provides for protection of underground water sources. The act also prohibits the use of lead pipes, solder, or flux in the installation or repair of public water systems.

The Resource Conservation and Recovery Act, 1976
(Amended 1980 and 1984)

The Resource Conservation and Recovery Act provides for the Hazardous Waste Management Program, a system responsible for tracking hazardous wastes and overseeing their disposal. It regulates the disposal and treatment of hazardous waste and prohibits open dumps.

The Toxic Substance Control Act, 1976

The Toxic Substance Control Act authorizes the EPA to compile an inventory of existing toxic chemicals and requires manufacturers of new chemicals to notify the EPA of their possible environmental or health effects. The EPA then has the right to prohibit their manufacture if the risks are considered too great. The act also empowers the EPA to test chemicals already in use.

The Comprehensive Environmental Response, Compensation, and Liability Act, 1980
(Amended 1988 and 1990)

This act establishes the Superfund, a fund empowering the EPA to administer the cleanup of hazardous wastes. Thus far, the EPA has placed over 1,200 sites on a Superfund priority list for cleanup.

Environmental Policy: How Much Risk Is Tolerable?

The various environmental laws specify goals for safety but vary greatly in terms of specifying timetables, standards, and methods to be used in reaching them.

For example, the Food, Drug and Cosmetic Act uses an approach that approves substances at levels that pose "no unreasonable risk," a loosely defined term. Embedded within it, however, is the Delaney Clause, which specifies that *no* additive in *any* amount may be permitted in food if it has been found to induce cancers in humans or animals. (A similar "no-risk" approach underlies the discharge goals of the Safe Drinking Water Act and the Clean Water Act.)

Although these standards may seem similar, they are actually significantly different in concept and practice. The latter no-risk standard is potentially far more restrictive than a negligible-risk standard, such as the former. The difference between these approaches is at the crux of many contemporary controversies of environmental and health regulation.

The spirit of the no-risk Delaney Clause is to protect us from unnecessary risks from exposure to carcinogens added to food, the idea being that no amount of a carcinogen large enough to be detected should be trusted. However, scientists today have access to tools that can detect amounts of substances far smaller than those imagined when the legislation was passed in 1951. The implications of these advances has fueled a heated debate among scientists, food manufacturers, legislators, and regulators: Does such a zero-risk standard make sense, particularly because we now know that some natural substances in food, not covered by the Delaney Clause, not only cause cancer but may be more dangerous than tiny amounts of additives?

The adoption of a negligible-risk standard over a zero-risk standard was involved in the EPA's 1992 rescinding of a ban on a group of pesticides, the EBDCs (named for the active chemical ingredient, ethylene bisdithiocarbamate). New experimental work by four leading chemical manufacturers and the government's National Toxicology Program showed the fungicides to be less potent carcinogens in animals than did the earlier studies on which the ban had been based. In addition, direct studies showed that residues deemed as negligible remained in treated foods found in grocery stores. (For more complete discussions of pesticides and pesticide regulation, see Chapter 17, "Food Safety," and Chapter 12, "Of Special Concern: Infants and Children".) This action and others of its type indicate that the EPA is moving away from a zero-risk standard toward a negligible-risk standard.

The choice of either a zero-risk or a negligible-risk philosophy has repercussions in expenditures, regulations, timetables, and the standards the public allows policymakers to set, and setting a philosophical precedent has been the subject of intense debate. Zero-risk advocates often argue that no cost is too high to pay for protecting the environment and that every possible hazard reduction must be carried out; negligible-risk advocates often maintain that many environmental regulations are too costly to follow and must be loosened or abandoned.

However, the reality of such decisions is not as clear-cut as these arguments make it out to be. It could be either impractical or dangerous to ignore the concerns of one side in favor of the other. Without denying the logic of utilizing improved scientific knowledge, it remains possible that the elimination of zero-risk standards could be used as a pretext to weaken environmental regulation solely for economic gain. Furthermore, some toxic substances are turning out to be dangerous in *lower* concentrations than was initially believed, and setting a negligible-risk standard for hazards, such as low-level ionizing radiation, is proving to be more difficult than was expected.

On the other hand, the EPA has reported that the cost of controlling environmental pollution now runs to more than $100 billion a year and is rising. With federal, state, and local governments hard-pressed financially, we may simply be unable to afford to be as stringent as possible in all areas of regulation.

Today's Priorities for Action

Although much remains to be done in terms of regulation, many sources of environmental pollution have been substantially reduced by government mandate. Previous laws and EPA programs have focused most on controlling "end-of-pipe" pollution, cleaning up or minimizing the damage of effluents and emissions. A shift toward preventing pollutants from being generated in the first place may be beginning. The Scientific Advisory Board to the EPA, a group of independent scientists who evaluate the available scientific evidence and acquaint EPA regulators with the latest findings, has recommended that, among other priorities, the EPA take stock of the wide range of environmental hazards and more formally rank the risks as well as concentrate monies on pollution reduction and preventive programs.

Setting limits and determining priorities for environmental hazards are complicated by many factors, some of which reflect the assessment of the risks that are posed and some of which reflect concerns beyond the analysis of the hazards themselves.

The requirements for economic growth are often presented as being at odds with environmental goals. Preventing global warming by reducing industrial emissions of carbon dioxide may cut into the profits of an industry forced to buy new equipment, for example. Politicians may be slow to order changes even when the science indicates it necessary, fearing the anger of influential business leaders or laid-off workers. Automobile manufacturers may fight alterations in design that reduce noxious emissions but add to the price of production.

The Physician's Role

The following case was reported in the *Wall Street Journal* in 1991: A healthy, vital engineer who happened to be taking a commonly prescribed antiulcer drug mowed the grass around his house, edged the shrubs, and worked in the garden, all of which had been treated with a common organophosphate pesticide in levels that are well within the acceptable range for most people. Within a few hours, he felt dizzy and nauseous and had a runny nose, tightness in his chest, and a pounding headache. His wife, who had also worked in the garden, was fine.

Ten days later, he was still sick. The symptoms then progressed: the head pain worsened,

he developed tics in his eyes and difficulty walking, and he now apparently suffers neurological impairment. After six years, twenty doctors consulted, and numerous tests, a toxicologist, three neurologists, and two neuroophthalmologists who examined the man all concluded independently on the diagnosis: poisoning by the organophosphate pesticide used to treat his lawn.

How was this man poisoned when his wife, working outdoors with him, was unhurt? The poison that he inhaled and absorbed through his skin was not eliminated from his body. The doctors suggest that taking the antiulcer medication suppressed the normal role of the liver in metabolizing the poison and eliminating it, allowing it to build to toxic levels and cause severe harm.

The doctors continue to treat this man based on this diagnosis, but his case is considered too weak to win in a court of law.

Whereas courts can debate the legal aspects of a case like this one indefinitely, a doctor treating the physical effects of the poisoning must act with little hesitation, with or without definitive proof. Acting under time constraints in the face of uncertainty is a large part of a physician's job. To create a truly complete medical background for you, a doctor would need to consider genetic predispositions, occupational exposures, the possible effect of exposure to air, water, or soil pollution in the neighborhood where you live, cultural hazards such as your diet, sexual habits, whether or not you smoke (or someone else in the home smokes)—the list and the research could continue indefinitely. When it is unlikely that a single one of the factors caused the problem, it remains difficult to know if three or four or ten of them together might have been responsible or, as in the case of the engineer, if just two independently harmless factors taken together caused a mighty harm.

As a result, physicians are often caught in the crossfire of environmental debates: The advice that they give using limited information does not always mirror the research conclusions of other scientists, the rulings of a court, or the prevailing policies of the moment. With fewer outside interests' concerns to balance, a doctor is more likely to err on the side of caution. For example, doctors may recommend well in advance of official warnings that a woman who is pregnant or thinking of becoming pregnant not drink any alcohol, not because light drinking of alcohol is proven dangerous to a developing fetus but because it simply is not known at what point a developing fetus is most at risk of being harmed by such exposure.

Individual and Community Action

Like doctors, individuals are caught in the position of needing to make decisions and plan strategies with incomplete information. We may not know which foods are the safest or which additives can cause cancer without a doubt, but in the end, we have to eat *something*. We may not know every possible effect of every possible substance used in our local industries or whether a certain building material is absolutely, positively free from substances that can hurt us, but in the end, we have to live *somewhere*. We must work at jobs, raise our children, and buy and use products without having absolute proof as to which choices are harmful or harmless.

No one can avoid risk; it is inherent in the process of life. But individuals can still act to minimize many risks, based on what we do know. This applies not only to personal actions but also to collective action on the part of communities or groups. Alone, we can decide whether or not to use a pesticide, eat a type of food, perform a hobby or job, or reduce our household waste and consumption, but we cannot pass laws, change regulations, or set societal priorities single-handedly. However, by working through advocacy groups, volunteer organizations, and unions, individuals can and have effected change. The increased public attention to the environment in the late 1960s, which culminated in the April 1970 Earth Day observation, ushered in the creation of the EPA in 1970 and the passage that same year of the Occupational Safety and Health Act. On a smaller scale, protests, complaints, and boycotts have motivated fast-food companies to reduce wasteful packaging and to stop purchasing livestock that graze on deforested land. As we have seen, public opinion sways government and business officials more than the assessments of scientists. By speaking together, like-minded individuals can force the world to listen.

Although we may not know all there is to know about the world around and within us, there is much that we do know, and we can use this information to our benefit. By becoming familiar with the information presented in this book, it is hoped that you will come to think about environmental risks not with paranoia but with purpose.

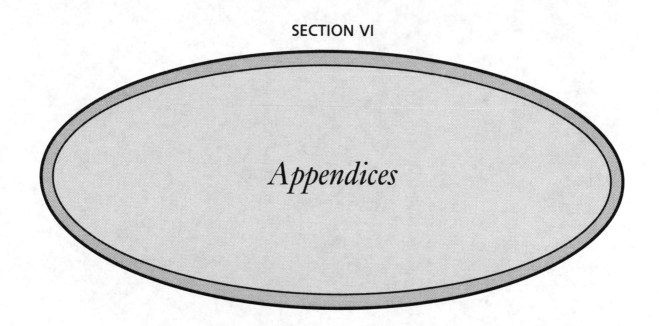

Appendices

Resources for Further Environmental Information

T he following listing is intended to help you find a source for questions about environmental problems in the home, school, or workplace for issues relating to product safety or the safety of food or drugs or if you wish to become involved in community action on environmental issues.

Many of the government agencies provide published information and answer telephone queries, particularly about the regulation of toxins and products and the safety of air, water, and food.

GOVERNMENT ORGANIZATIONS

The Food and Drug Administration (FDA)

In addition to overseeing the body of government regulation on the safety of food and drugs, the FDA also provides public education services, publishing a wide array of pamphlets on the issues of consumer safety that fall under its jurisdiction. Up to ten publications can be ordered for free. To order, call the FDA Consumer Affairs and Information Staff at 301-443-3170; a representative can guide you to FDA publications covering your topic of interest. Or write Consumer Affairs and Information Staff, Department of Health and Human Services, 5600 Fishers Lane, Room 16–85, Rockville, MD 20857.

The Consumer Product Safety Commission (CPSC)

The CPSC, charged with overseeing the safety of consumer goods and implementing federal laws in that area, maintains an automated Product Safety Hot Line, which contains recorded information on consumer recalls, CPSC actions, and general product safety. You can also call the hot line to register a complaint about an unsafe product. The hot line toll-free number is 1-800-638-CPSC; in Maryland, the number is 1-800-492-8104. To ask for publication information on a consumer safety topic, write Publication Request, Consumer Product Safety Commission, Washington, DC 20207.

The Environmental Protection Agency (EPA)

The EPA was created by executive order in 1970 to administer the body of environmental and conservation laws that had previously been the responsibility of various departments. Today, in addition to its regulatory duties, the agency administers a number of public information programs. These include:

The EPA Public Information Center, 202-260-2080. The center handles most general public requests for environmental or environmental law information and publications.

Toxic Substances Control Act (TOSCA) Hot Line, 202-554-1404. This EPA-administered hot line provides information over the phone and through publications on questions dealing with environmental toxins. In some cases, the hot line refers callers to EPA departments specializing in their area of concern.

National Pesticides Telecommunications Network, 800-858-PEST. The network provides information on pesticide products, recognizing and managing pesticide poisonings, toxicology, symptoms of pesticide poisoning, safety information, health and environmental effects of specific pesticides, pesticide cleanup and disposal procedures, and the proper use of pesticides. The network also provides referrals for pesticide analysis and the treatment of illness.

Safe Drinking Water Hot Line, 800-426-4791. Hot line operators respond to calls regarding the safety of drinking water, including bottled water and home water treatment. The service explains federal regulations and EPA policies, gives updates on the status of regulations and laws, provides information on ordering pertinent EPA publications, and offers referrals to federal, state, and local contacts on local water conditions, bottled water, and home water treatments. Hot line consultants cannot discuss specific manufacturers or recommend brand names.

Regional EPA Offices If you have an environmental question or concern specific to the state, geographic region, or locality where you live, you may wish to contact one of the EPA's ten regional offices, which cover the fifty states and the U. S. territories.

Region 1: Connecticut, Maine, Massachusetts, New Hampshire, Rhode Island, Vermont
John F. Kennedy Federal Building, Room 2203
Boston, MA 02203
617-565-3420
Hours: 8:00 A.M.–5:00 P.M. EST/EDT
Regional administrator: Julie D. Belaga

Region 2: New Jersey, New York, Puerto Rico, U.S. Virgin Islands
Jacob K. Javits Federal Building
26 Federal Plaza
New York, NY 10278
212-264-2657
Hours: 8:00 A.M.–5:30 P.M. EST/EDT
Acting regional administrator: William Muszynski

Region 3: Delaware, District of Columbia, Maryland, Pennsylvania, Virginia, West Virginia
841 Chestnut Building
Philadelphia, PA 19107
215-597-9800
Hours: 8:00 A.M.–4:30 P.M. EST/EDT
Regional administrator: Edwin B. Erickson

Region 4: Alabama, Florida, Georgia, Kentucky, Mississippi, North Carolina, South Carolina, Tennessee
345 Courtland Street, NE
Atlanta, GA 30365
404-347-4727
Hours: 7:00 A.M.–5:45 P.M. EST/EDT
Regional administrator: Greer C. Tidwell

Region 5: Illinois, Indiana, Michigan, Minnesota, Ohio, Wisconsin
77 West Jackson Boulevard
Chicago, IL 60604
312-353-2000
Hours: 8:00 A.M.–4:30 P.M. CST/CDT
Regional administrator: Valdas V. Adamkus

Region 6: Arkansas, Louisiana, New Mexico, Oklahoma, Texas
First Interstate Bank Tower at Fountain Place
1445 Ross Avenue, 12th Floor, Suite 1200
Dallas, TX 75202
214-655-6444
Hours: 8:00 A.M.–4:30 P.M. CST/CDT
Regional administrator: B. J. Wynne

Region 7: Kansas, Missouri, Iowa, Nebraska
726 Minnesota Avenue
Kansas City, KS 66101
913-551-7000
Hours: 7:30 A.M.–5:00 P.M. CST/CDT
Regional administrator: Morris Kay

Region 8: Colorado, Montana, North Dakota, South Dakota, Utah, Wyoming
999 18th Street, Suite 500
Denver, CO 80202-2405
303-293-1603
Hours: 8:00 A.M.–4:30P.M. MST/MDT
Regional administrator: Jack W. McGraw

Region 9: American Samoa, Arizona, California, Guam, Hawaii, Nevada, U.S. Trust Territories of the Pacific
75 Hawthorne Street
San Francisco, CA 94105
415-744-1305
Hours: 8:00 A.M.–4:30 P.M. PST/PDT
Regional administrator: Daniel W. McGovern

Region 10: Alaska, Idaho, Oregon, Washington
1200 Sixth Avenue
Seattle, WA 98101
206-553-4973
Hours: 8:00 A.M.–4:30 P.M. PST/PDT
Regional administrator: Dana Rasmussen

INDEPENDENT ORGANIZATIONS

The Children's Defense Fund

The Children's Defense Fund lobbies on the behalf of children on children's issues including health, education, and social issues. For information, write to them at 25 E Street, NW, Washington, DC 20001.

The Environmental Defense Fund (EDF)

EDF is a national nonprofit organization with a staff of full-time scientists, lawyers, engineers, and economists that conducts research, lobbies, and works with business to address environmental and conservation problems. Among the issues on which it has focused are ozone depletion, deforestation, recycling, and protection of Antarctica's natural resources. For more information, contact the group at 257 Park Avenue South, New York, New York 10010, or call EDF Public Information at 212-505-2100.

The Natural Resources Defense Council (NRDC)

NRDC is a private nonprofit environmental advocacy group that supports scientific research, legal actions, and community education on environmental issues. The group produces publications on environmental issues that it makes available to the general public as well as to schools and teachers. For literature or other inquiries, write to Membership and Public Education Department, NRDC, 40 West 20th Street, New York, NY 10011.

The Sierra Club

The Sierra Club is a nationwide organization that sponsors outings and activities relating to environmental issues and education. The group also works for political change on environmental issues. For information, write to the Sierra Club headquarters at 730 Polk Street, San Francisco, CA 94109, or call 415-776-2211.

The Worldwatch Institute

This independent nonprofit organization produces publications and scientific research on world problems including global pollution, overpopulation, and conservation of resources.

To purchase publications or receive a listing of available materials, write to the Worldwatch Institute at 1776 Massachusetts Avenue, NW, Washington, DC 20036, or call 202-452-1999.

Whom to Contact About Environment-Related Health Problems

There are numerous resources available for investigating health problems potentially related to environmental factors. The following guidelines may help overcome the first hurdle: determining the appropriate agency to contact or finding an appropriate medical expert.

The regional poison control center for your area is an excellent place to start a search. These centers, listed later in this appendix, are staffed by medical practitioners who can help during a poisoning emergency and who are well connected to the other medical resources in your region, such as local or state public health offices or specific medical specialists.

Other resources include the local health department, the department of occupational and/or environmental medicine in a nearby university medical center, a health clinic specializing in occupational medicine (some are listed in this appendix), or the Environmental Protection Agency office for your region (listed in Appendix A).

When selecting a medical specialist, be aware that those physicians who are board certified in toxicology, preventive medicine, or occupational medicine have received special training in areas related to environmental factors and disease.

They are probably your best first consult and should be able to refer you to other specialists to handle a specific problem, such as a neurologist, obstetrician, or pulmonary specialist.

The directory of members of the American College of Occupational and Environmental Medicine (ACOEM), one of the twenty American Board of Medical Specialties–recognized medical specialties, is another resource. Do not confuse ACOEM with the American Board of Environmental Medicine, a group that largely represents the clinical ecology perspective and which is not a specialty recognized by the American Board of Medical Specialties. ACOEM's address is: American College of Occupational and Environmental Medicine, 55 W. Seegers Road, Arlington Heights, IL 60005, 708-228-6850.

The Association of Occupational and Environmental Clinics also can provide a list of clinics nationwide specializing in occupational health. This association is a professional organization of clinicians specializing in occupational health issues; be aware, though, that excellently trained medical experts to handle your environmental or occupationally related health problem can be found in many clinical settings not included in this directory. It can be contacted at: Association of Occupational and Environmental Clinics, 1010 Vermont Avenue, NW, #513, Washington, DC 20005, 202-347-4976.

For information specifically on cancer and carcinogens, there is a toll-free number within the contiguous forty-eight states: 1-800-4-CANCER; in Hawaii, call 1-800-524-1234; and in Alaska, call 1-800-636-6070. The number will connect you with one of the twenty-five regional cancer care facilities serving thirty-three states. In states where there is no coverage, you will be connected with the National Cancer Institute Cancer Information Service.

For information on workplace-related ailments, check the listing in this appendix of the major agencies of the numerous public and private organizations that regulate the health and safety of the workplace.

For concerns about potential reproductive health effects from environmental agents, check with your nearest regional Poison Control Center or specialists at nearby university medical centers. Refer to the recommendations in Chapter 11, "Reproductive Effects and Prenatal Exposures." Specialized teratogen information programs also exist; a list of these can be found in *Maternal-Fetal Toxicology: A Clinician's Guide*, edited by Gideon Koren (Marcel Dekker, pp. 332–333).

AMERICAN ASSOCIATION OF POISON CONTROL CENTERS

The centers listed are certified by the American Association of Poison Control Centers. Each serves a large geographic area, is open twenty-four hours a day, provides direct dialing or toll-free access, is supervised by a medical director, and has registered pharmacists or nurses available to answer questions. Staff members are trained to resolve toxicity situations in the home of the caller; in some cases, they may refer callers to a local hospital. The centers draw on toxicology resources including a computer data base that covers some 350,000 substances and is updated quarterly. They also offer educational services to the public and health care professionals. In some states, these large centers coexist with smaller poison control centers that provide more limited information.

ALABAMA

Regional Poison Control Center
Children's Hospital of Alabama
1600 Seventh Avenue South
Birmingham, AL 35233-1711
Emergency numbers: 205-939-9201; 800-292-6678 (AL only); 205-933-4050

ARIZONA

Arizona Poison and Drug Information Center
Arizona Health Sciences Center
Room 3204-K
1501 North Campbell Avenue
Tucson, AZ 85724
Emergency numbers: 602-626-6016; 800-362-0101 (AZ only)

Samaritan Regional Poison Center
Good Samaritan Regional Medical Center
1130 East McDowell Road
Suite A-5
Phoenix, AZ 85006
Emergency number: 602-253-3334

CALIFORNIA

Fresno Regional Poison Control Center
Fresno Community Hospital and Medical Center
P.O. Box 1232
2823 Fresno Street
Fresno, CA 93715
Emergency numbers: 209-445-1222; 800-346-5922

San Diego Regional Poison Center
  UCSD Medical Center
  225 Dickinson Street
  San Diego, CA 92103-8926
  Emergency numbers: 619-543-6000; 800-876-
    4766 (619 area code only)

*San Francisco Bay Area Regional Poison
Control Center*
  San Francisco General Hospital
  1001 Potrero Avenue, Building 80, Room 230
  San Francisco, CA 94122
  Emergency number: 415-476-6600

*Santa Clara Valley Medical Center Regional Poison
Center*
  751 South Bascom Avenue
  San Jose, CA 95128
  Emergency numbers: 408-299-5112; 800-662-
    9886 (CA only)

*University of California, Davis, Medical Center
Regional Poison Control Center*
  2315 Stockton Boulevard
  Sacramento, CA 95817
  Emergency numbers: 916-453-3414; 800-342-
    9293 (North CA only)

UCI Regional Poison Center
  UCI Medical Center
  101 The City Drive, Route 78
  Orange, CA 92668-3298
  Emergency numbers: 714-934-5988; 800-544-
    4404 (South CA only)

COLORADO

Rocky Mountain Poison and Drug Center
  645 Bannock Street
  Denver, CO 80204-4507
  Emergency number: 303-629-1123

DISTRICT OF COLUMBIA

National Capital Poison Center
  Georgetown University Hospital

3800 Reservoir Road, NW
Washington, DC 20007
Emergency numbers: 202-625-3333; 202-784-
  4660

FLORIDA

*Florida Poison Information Center at Tampa General
Hospital*
  P.O. Box 1289
  Tampa, FL 33601
  Emergency numbers: 813-253-4444; 800-282-
    3171 (FL only)

GEORGIA

Georgia Poison Control Center
  Grady Memorial Hospital
  80 Butler Street, SE
  P.O. Box 26066
  Atlanta, GA 30335-3801
  Emergency numbers: 404-589-4400; 800-282-
    5846 (GA only)

INDIANA

Indiana Poison Control Center
  Methodist Hospital of Indiana
  1701 North Senate Boulevard
  P.O. Box 1367
  Indianapolis, IN 46206-1367
  Emergency phone: 317-929-2323; 800-382-
    9097 (IN only)

KENTUCKY

*Kentucky Regional Poison Control Center of Kosair
Children's Hospital*
  P.O. Box 35070
  Louisville, KY 40232-5070
  Emergency numbers: 502-629-7275; 800-722-
    5725 (KY only)

MARYLAND

Maryland Poison Center
  20 North Pine Street
  Baltimore, MD 21202

Emergency numbers: 410-528-7701; 800-492-2414 (MD only)

National Capital Poison Center
(DC suburbs only)
Georgetown University Hospital
3800 Reservoir Rd., NW
Washington, DC 20007
Emergency numbers: 202-625-3333; 202-784-4660 (TTY)

MASSACHUSETTS

Massachusetts Poison Control System
3000 Longwood Avenue
Boston, MA 02115
Emergency numbers: 617-232-2120; 800-682-9211 (MA only)

MICHIGAN

Blodgett Regional Poison Center
1840 Wealthy, SE
Grand Rapids, MI 49506
Emergency numbers: 800-632-2727 (MI only); 800-356-3232 (TTY)

Poison Control Center
Children's Hospital of Michigan
3901 Beaubien Boulevard
Detroit, MI 48201
Emergency number: 313-745-5711

MINNESOTA

Hennepin Regional Poison Center
Hennepin County Medical Center
701 Park Avenue
Minneapolis, MN 55415
Emergency numbers: 612-347-3141; Petline: 612-337-7387; TDD 612-337-7474; 612-337-7474

Minnesota Regional Poison Center
St. Paul-Ramsey Medical Center
640 Jackson Street

St. Paul, MN 55101
Emergency number: 612-221-2113

MISSOURI

Cardinal Glennon Children's Hospital Regional Poison Center
1465 South Grand Boulevard
St. Louis, MO 63194
Emergency numbers: 314-772-5200; 800-366-8888

MONTANA

Rocky Mountain Poison and Drug Center
645 Bannock Street
Denver, CO 80204
Emergency number: 303-629-1123

NEBRASKA

The Poison Center
8301 Dodge Street
Omaha, NE 68114
Emergency numbers: 420-390-5555 (Omaha); 800-955-9119 (NE only)

NEW JERSEY

New Jersey Poison Information and Education System
201 Lyons Avenue
Newark, NJ 07112
Emergency number: 800-962-1253

NEW MEXICO

New Mexico Poison and Drug Information Center
University of New Mexico
Albuquerque, NM 87131
Emergency numbers: 505-843-2551; 800-432-6866 (NM only)

NEW YORK

Long Island Regional Poison Control Center
Nassau County Medical Center

2201 Hempstead Turnpike
East Meadow, NY 11554
Emergency number: 516-542-2323

New York City Regional Poison Control Center
N.Y.C. Department of Health
455 First Avenue, Room 123
New York, NY 10016
Emergency numbers: 212-340-4494; 212-POISONS; TDD 212-689-9014

OHIO

Central Ohio Poison Center
Columbus Children's Hospital
700 Children's Drive
Columbus, OH 43295
Emergency numbers: 614-228-1323; 800-682-7625 (OH only); 614-228-2272 (TTY)

Cincinnati Drug and Poison Information Center and Regional Poison Control System
231 Bethesda Avenue, ML #144
Cincinnati, OH 45267-0144
Emergency numbers: 513-558-5111; 800-872-5111 (OH only)

OREGON

Oregon Poison Center
Oregon Health Sciences University
3181 SW Sam Jackson Park Road
Portland, OR 97201
Emergency numbers: 503-494-8968; 800-452-7165 (OR only)

PENNSYLVANIA

Central Pennsylvania Poison Center
University Hospital
Milton S. Hershey Medical Center
Hershey, PA 17033
Emergency number: 800-521-6110

The Poison Control Center serving the greater Philadelphia metropolitan area

One Children's Center
34th and Civic Center Boulevard
Philadelphia, PA 19104
Emergency number: 215-386-2100

Pittsburgh Poison Center
3074 Fifth Avenue at DeSoto Street
Pittsburgh, PA 15213
Emergency number: 412-681-6669

RHODE ISLAND

Rhode Island Poison Center
593 Eddy Street
Providence, RI 02902
Emergency number: 401-277-5727

TEXAS

North Texas Poison Center
P.O. Box 35926
Dallas, TX 75235
Emergency numbers: 214-590-5000; 800-441-0040 (TX only)

UTAH

Intermountain Regional Poison Control Center
50 North Medical Drive, Building 428
Salt Lake City, UT 84132
Emergency numbers: 801-581-2151; 800-456-7707 (UT only)

VIRGINIA

Blue Ridge Poison Center
Box 67
Blue Ridge Hospital
Charlottesville, VA 22901
Emergency numbers: 804-924-5543; 800-451-1428

National Capital Poison Center (North VA only)
Georgetown University Hospital
3800 Reservoir Road, NW
Washington, DC 20007

Emergency numbers: 202-625-3333; 202-784-4660 (TTY)

Emergency numbers: 304-348-4211; 800-642-3625 (WV only)

WEST VIRGINIA

West Virginia Poison Center
West Virginia University Health Sciences
Center/Charleston Division
3110 MacCorkle Avenue, SE
Charleston, WV 25304

WYOMING

The Poison Center
8301 Dodge Street
Omaha, NE 68114
Emergency numbers: 402-390-5555 (Omaha); 800-955-9119 (NE)

OCCUPATIONAL HEALTH CONCERNS

Note: For a description of the responsibilities of each agency, please see Table 21.4 (p. 703).

Government Agencies

Bureau of Labor Statistics (BLS)
U.S. Department of Labor
2 Massachusetts Avenue, NE
Washington, DC 20212
phone: 202-606-6180

Centers for Disease Control and Prevention (CDC)
1600 Clinton Road NE
Atlanta, GA 30333
phone: 404-639-3311

Department of Health and Human Services (HHS)
Hubert H. Humphrey Building
200 Independence Avenue SW
Washington, DC 20201
phone: 202-619-0257

Department of Transportation
Federal Aviation Administration (FAA)
Office of Aviation Medicine
800 Independence Avenue SW
Washington, DC 20591
phone: 202-366-4000

Mine Safety and Health Administration
(Division of Department of Labor)
Balston Center Tower 3
4015 Wilson Boulevard
Arlington, VA 22203
phone: 703-235-1385

National Institute of Environmental Health Sciences (NIEHS)
National Institutes of Health
P.O. Box 12233
Research Triangle Park, NC 27709
phone: 919-541-3345

National Institute for Occupational Safety and Health (NIOSH)
(Division of Centers for Disease Control and Prevention)
1600 Clinton Road NE
Atlanta, GA 30333
phone: 404-639-3771

Occupational Safety and Health Administration (OSHA)
(Division of Department of Labor)
200 Constitution Avenue NW
Washington, DC 20216
phone: 202-219-6091

Private Sector Agencies

Bureau of National Affairs
1231 25th Street, NW
Washington, DC
phone: 202-452-4200

National Safe Workplace Institute
122 South Michigan Avenue
Chicago, IL 60603
phone: 312-661-0690
FAX: 312-661-0777

Further Reading

N umerous scientific and medical books and journals; consumer publications, newspapers, and magazines; and taped interviews provided sources for this book—far too many to include in this list. We offer the following list as a rudimentary guide or a starting point for readers who wish to read further. It includes only *some* of the major medical and scientific texts in the field of occupational/environmental medicine, only *some* of the major medical and scientific journals, and a handful of consumer-oriented books.

Be aware that the U.S. Government Printing Office has many books and pamphlets available on subjects pertaining to health and the environment. To purchase a publication or to request a listing of materials in a particular area, call 202-783-3238, or write Superintendent of Documents, U.S. Government Printing Office, Washington, DC 20402-9325.

For readers interested in reading more about the subject of risk and risk communication, there is a large and varied scientific literature. We suggest looking at the work of Vincent T. Covello and of Peter Sandman and publications available through the Environmental Communication Research Program at Cook College, Rutgers University, P.O. Box 231, New Brunswick, NJ 08903-0231 (write them for a bibliography).

MEDICAL TEXTS

Dreisbach, Robert H., and Robertson, William O. *Handbook of Poisoning*, 12th ed. Norwalk CT: Appleton & Lange, 1987.

Goldfrank, Lewis, Flomenbaum, N., Lewin, N., Weisman, R., and Howland, M. A. *Goldfrank's Toxicologic Emergencies*, 4th ed. Norwalk, CT: Appleton & Lange, 1990.

Hartman, David. *Neuropsychological Toxicology, Identification and Assessment*. New York: Pergamon Press, 1988.

Koren, Gideon. *Maternal-Fetal Toxicology: A Clinician's Guide*. New York: Marcel Dekker, 1990.

Lave, Lester, B., and Upton, Arthur C. (eds.). *Toxic Chemicals, Health, and the Environment*. Baltimore: Johns Hopkins University Press, 1987.

Lippmann, Morton. *Environmental Toxicants: Human Exposures and Their Health Effects*. New York: Van Nostrand Reinhold, 1992.

Moeller, Dade W. *Environmental Health*. Cambridge, MA: Harvard University Press, 1992.

National Research Council. *Health Effects of Exposure to Ionizing Radiation*. Washington, DC: National Academy Press, 1990.

Occupational Medicine: State of the Art Reviews series. Philadelphia: Hanley & Belfus, Inc.

Alcoholism and Chemical Dependency in the Workplace. Curtis Wright (ed.), Vol. 4, No. 2 (April–June 1989).

Back Pain in Workers, Richard A. Deyo (ed.), Vol. 3, No. 1 (January–March 1988).

Health Problems of Health Care Workers. Edward A. Emmett (ed.), Vol. 2, No. 3 (July–September 1987).

Health Hazards of Farming. D. H. Cordes and Dorothy Foster Rea (eds.), Vol. 6, No. 3 (July–September 1991).

Occupational Cancer and Carcinogenesis. Paul W. Brandt-Rauf (ed.), Vol. 2, No. 1 (January–March 1987).

Occupational Hand Injuries. Morton L. Kasdan (ed.), Vol. 4, No. 3 (July–September 1989).

Occupational Pulmonary Disease. Linda Rosenstock (ed.), Vol. 2, No. 2 (April–June 1987).

Occupational Skin Disease. Robert M. Adams (ed.), Vol. 1, No. 2 (April–June 1986).

Prevention of Pulmonary Disease. Philip Harber and John R. Balmes (eds.), Vol. 6, No. 1 (January–March 1991).

Problem Buildings: Building-Associated Illness and the Sick Building Syndrome. James E. Cone and Michael J. Hodgson (eds.), Vol. 4, No. 4 (October–December 1989).

Worker Fitness and Risk Evaluations. Jay S. Himmelstein and Glenn S. Pransky (eds.), Vol. 3, No. 2 (April–June 1988).

Paul, Maureen, and Kurtz, Sabrina. *Reproductive Hazards in the Workplace: Syllabus for Clinicians.* Occupational and Environmental Reproductive Hazards Center, University of Massachusetts Medical Center, 1990.

Rom, William (ed.). *Environmental and Occupational Medicine*, 2d ed. Boston: Little, Brown, 1992.

Schardein, James L. (ed.), *Chemically Induced Birth Defects.* New York: Marcel Dekker, 1985.

Singer, Raymond M. *Neurotoxicity Guidebook.* New York: Van Nostrand Reinhold, 1990.

Sullivan, John B., and Krieger, Gary R. (eds.). *Hazardous Materials Toxicology.* Baltimore: Williams & Wilkins, 1992.

Zenz, Carl. *Occupational Medicine: Principles and Practical Applications*, 2d ed. Chicago: Year Book Medical Publishers, 1988.

MEDICAL JOURNALS

American Journal of Epidemiology
American Journal of Industrial Medicine
American Journal of Public Health
Annual Review of Public Health
British Journal of Industrial Medicine
Cancer Research
Environmental Health Perspectives

Journal of the American Medical Association
Journal of National Cancer Institute
Journal of Occupational Medicine
Journal of Toxicology
Lancet
New England Journal of Medicine

U.S. GOVERNMENT PUBLICATIONS

National Cancer Institute. *Asbestos Exposure: What It Means, What to Do.* NIH Publication No. 89–1594, November 1988.

U.S. Department of Agriculture. *Food Safety and Quality: FDA Surveys Not Adequate to Demonstrate Safety of Milk Supply.* Washington, DC: 1990.

U.S. Department of Health and Human Services. *The Surgeon General's Report on Nutrition and Health.* Washington, DC: U.S. Government Printing Office, 1988.

U.S. Department of Health and Human Services, Agency for Toxic Substances and Disease Regis-

try. *ATSDR Case Studies in Environmental Medicine* (series).

U.S. Environmental Protection Agency. *Citizen's Guide to Ground-Water Protection.* Washington, DC: 1990.

U.S. Environmental Protection Agency and Sandman, Peter. *Explaining Environmental Risk.* Washington, DC: Office of Toxic Substances, 1986.

U.S. Environmental Protection Agency. *Lead and Your Drinking Water.* Washington, DC: 1987.

U.S. Environmental Protection Agency. *Unfinished*

Business: A Comparative Assessment of Environmental Problems, Vol. 1 (February 1987), p. 100.

U.S. Food and Drug Administration. *Food Risk: Perception vs. Reality*, FDA Consumer Special Report. Washington, DC: 1990.

U.S. Preventive Service Task Force. *Guide to Clinical Preventive Services*. Baltimore, MD: Williams & Wilkins, 1989.

U.S. Public Health Service. *Nicotine Addiction: The Health Consequences of Smoking: A Report of the Surgeon General*. Rockville, MD: 1988.

U.S. Public Health Service. *Reducing the Health Consequences of Smoking: 25 Years of Progress: A Report of the Surgeon General*. Rockville, MD: 1989.

U.S. Public Health Service. *The Health Consequences of Involuntary Smoking: A Report of the Surgeon General*. Rockville, MD: 1986.

GENERAL BOOKS

Ahmed, F. E. (ed.). *Seafood Safety*. Washington, DC: National Academy Press, 1991.

Barnett, Robert. *The American Health Food Book*. New York: Dutton 1991.

Brookins, Douglas G. *The Indoor Radon Problem*. Irvington, NY: Columbia University Press, 1990.

Cohen, Bernie. *Radon: A Homeowner's Guide to Detection and Control*. Mount Vernon, NY: Consumer Reports Books, 1988.

Brown, Lester R., et al., ed. *State of the World*. New York: W. W. Norton, annual.

Cohn, Victor. *News and Numbers*. Ames, IA: Iowa University Press, 1989.

Covello, V. T., et al. (eds.). *Effective Risk Communication*. New York: Plenum, 1989.

Evans, Mark I., Dixler, A. O., Fletcher, J. C., and Schulman, J. D. *Fetal Diagnosis and Therapy: Science, Ethics, and the Law*. Philadelphia: J. B. Lippincott, 1989.

Gabler, Raymond, and the editors of *Consumer Reports Books*. *Is Your Water Safe to Drink?* Mount Vernon, NY: Consumers Union, 1988.

Graham, J. D., et al. *In Search of Safety: Chemicals and Cancer Risk*. Cambridge, MA: Harvard University Press, 1988.

Gross, P. A., et al. *Managing Your Health*. Mount Vernon, NY: Consumer Reports Books, 1991.

Haas, François, and Haas, Sheila Sperber. *The Chronic Bronchitis and Emphysema Handbook*. New York: Wiley, 1990.

Haas, François, and Haas, Sheila Sperber. *The Essential Asthma Book*. New York: Scribners, 1987.

Hall, Eric J. *Radiation and Life*, 2d ed. New York: Pergamon Press, 1984.

Huff, Darrell. *How to Lie with Statistics*. New York: W. W. Norton, 1954.

Jacobson, Michael F., Lefferts, Lisa Y., and Garland, Anne Witte. *Safe Food: Eating Wisely in a Risky World*. Los Angeles: Living Planet Press, 1991.

Kavaler, Lucy. *Noise, the New Menace*. New York: The John Day Co. (HarperCollins), 1975.

Legato, Marianne, and Colman, Carol. *The Female Heart: The Truth about Women and Coronary Artery Disease*. New York: Simon & Schuster, 1991.

Legato, M. S., Harper, B. L., and Scott, M. J. (eds.). *The Health Detective's Handbook: A Guide to the Investigation of Environmental Health Hazards by Nonprofessionals*. Baltimore, MD: Johns Hopkins University Press, 1985.

McCann, Michael. *Health Hazards Manuals for Artists*. New York: Nick Lyons, 1985.

Miller, G. Tyler, Jr. *Living in the Environment*, 7th ed. Belmont, CA: Wadsworth Publishing, 1992. Designed for introductory courses in environmental science and used as part of the Annenberg/CPB Project PBS television series "Race to Save the Planet."

Moses, Lincoln. *Think and Explain with Statistics*. Reading, MA: Addison-Wesley, 1986.

National Academy of Sciences. *Diet and Health: Implications for Reducing Chronic Disease Risk*. Washington, DC: National Academy Press, 1989.

Robins, P. *Sun Sense*. New York: The Skin Cancer Foundation, 1990.

Rouche, Berton. *The Medical Detectives*. New York: Truman Valley Books/Plume, 1947/1991.

Index